Innovative Techniques in Ophthalmology

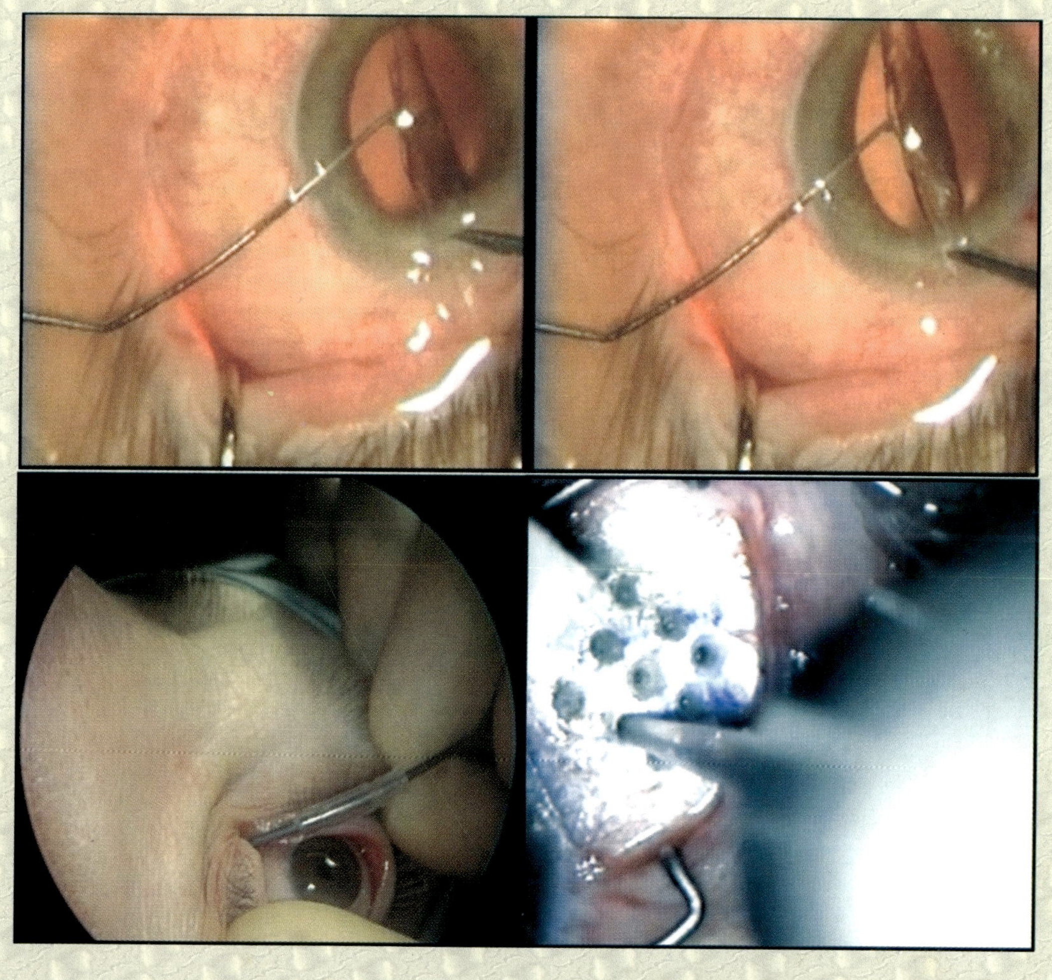

INNOVATIVE TECHNIQUES IN OPHTHALMOLOGY

Editors

Ashok Garg
MS PhD FIAO (Bel) FRSM ADM FAIMS FICA
International and National Gold Medalist
Medical Director
Garg Eye Institute and Research Centre
235-Model Town, Dabra Chowk
Hisar 125 005, India

I Howard Fine
MD
Clinical Professor of Ophthalmology
Oregon Health and Science University
Chief Consultant
Drs Fine, Hoffman and Packer, LLC
1550-Oak St, Ste 5, Eugene
OR 97401, USA

Ioannis G Pallikaris
MD
Professor and Head
Deptt. of Ophthalmology
University of Crete, VEIC, PO Box 2208
Heraklion 71003, Crete, Greece

David F Chang
MD
Clinical Professor of Ophthalmology
University of California, San Francisco
Private Practice, 762, Altos Oaks Drive
Los Altos, CA-94024, USA

Hiroshi Tsuneoka
MD
Associate Professor
Department of Ophthalmology
Jikei University School of Medicine
4-11-1 Izumihonchou, Komae-shi
Tokyo, 201-8601, Japan

Jerome Jean-Phillippe Bovet
MD
Consultant Ophthalmic Surgeon FMH
Clinique de L'oeil
15, Avenyue Du Bois-de-law Chapelle
CH-1213, Onex
Switzerland

Foreword: Jorge L Alio

JAYPEE BROTHERS
MEDICAL PUBLISHERS (P) LTD
New Delhi

Published by

Jitendar P Vij

Jaypee Brothers Medical Publishers (P) Ltd

EMCA House, 23/23B Ansari Road, Daryaganj

New Delhi 110 002, India

Phones: +91-11-23272143, +91-11-23272703, +91-11-23282021, +91-11-23245672

Fax: +91-11-23276490, +91-11-23245683

e-mail: jaypee@jaypeebrothers.com

Visit our website: www.jaypeebrothers.com

Branches

- 2/B, Akruti Society
  Jodhpur Gam Road Satellite
  Ahmedabad 380 015
  Phone: +91-079-30988717 e-mail: jpamdvd@rediffmail.com
- 202 Batavia Chambers, 8 Kumara Krupa Road
  Kumara Park East, **Bangalore** 560 001
  Phones: +91-80-22285971, +91-80-22382956, +91-80-30614073
  Tele Fax : +91-80-22281761 e-mail: jaypeemedpubbgl@eth.net
- 282 IIIrd Floor, Khaleel Shirazi Estate, Fountain Plaza
  Pantheon Road, **Chennai** 600 008
  Phones: +91-44-28262665, +91-44-28269897 Fax: +91-44-28262331
  e-mail: jpchen@eth.net
- 4-2-1067/1-3, 1st Floor, Balaji Building, Ramkote Cross Road
  Hyderabad 500 095, Phones: +91-40-55610020, +91-40-24758498
  Fax: +91-40-24758499 e-mail: jpmedpub@rediffmail.com
- 1A Indian Mirror Street, Wellington Square
  Kolkata 700 013, Phones: +91-33-22456075, +91-33-22451926 Fax: +91-33-22456075
  e-mail: jpbcal@cal.vsnl.net.in
- 106 Amit Industrial Estate, 61 Dr SS Rao Road
  Near MGM Hospital, Parel, **Mumbai** 400 012
  Phones: +91-22-24124863, +91-22-24104532, +91-22-30926896
  Fax: +91-22-24160828 e-mail: jpmedpub@bom7.vsnl.net.in
- "KAMALPUSHPA" 38, Reshimbag
  Opp. Mohota Science College, Umred Road
  Nagpur 440 009 (MS)
  Phones: +91-712-3945220, +91-712-2704275 e-mail: jpmednagpur@rediffmail.com

Innovative Techniques in Ophthalmology

First Edition : **2006**

ISBN 81-8061-754-8

Typeset at JPBMP typesetting unit

Printed at Sanat Printers, Kundli.

Dedicated to

- My Respected Param Pujya Guru Sant Gurmeet Ram Rahim Singh Ji for his blessings and motivation.
- My Respected Parents, teachers, my wife Dr Aruna Garg, son Abhishek and daughter Anshul for their constant support and patience during all these days of hard work.
- My dear friend Dr Amar Agarwal who invented the technique of Phakonit (Bimanual Phaco) for the first time in the world in 1998 for his advice and guidance.

— Ashok Garg

- Our patients who entrust their vision to our surgical intervention and who stimulate us to continually seek improved technology and techniques.

— I Howard Fine

- All my colleagues at Vardinoyannion Eye Instutute of Crete (Greece).

— Ioannis G Pallikaris

- My wife, Victoria and my children Courtney and Alex.

— David F Chang

- My wife, Aiko Tsuneoka, who gave me constant support for long time and to Dr Kunihiro Nagahara who taughe me to master the modern phaco surgery.

— Hisoshi Tsuneoka

- Yveric, Luc and Fanny Laure.
- Silvio Korol, who was not only a teacher but also an intellectual guide and a friend.

— Jerome Bovet

Contributors

Ahmed Galal MD PhD
Vissum/Instituto Oftalmologico
De Alicante, Alicante, Spain

Alok K Ravi PhD
Deptt of Pharmacology
Dr RP Centre for Ophthalmic Sciences
AIIMS, New Delhi 110 029, India

Amar Agarwal MS FRCS FRC Ophth
Consultant
Dr Agarwal's Eye Hospital
19, Cathedral Road
Chennai 600 086, India

Andre Mermoud MD
Professor in Ophthalmology
Hospital Ophtalmique Gules Gonin and
University of Lausanne
Avenue de France 15
1004, Lausanne, Switzerland

AnnMarie Hipsley PT PFS PhD
Director of Research
Global Vision Research Group Ltd
ACE Vision Group, PO Box 328
Blacklick, OH, 43004-0328, USA

Anthony J Maloof MD FRANZCO FRACS
Director of Ophthalmic Surgery
Western Sydney Eye Hospital
Westmead Hospital
Howkesbury Road
Westmead, New South Wales (NSW)
2145, Australia

Arif Adenwala MS
Consultant
Aditya Jyot Eye Hospital Pvt Ltd
Plot No 153, Road No 9
Major Parmeshwaran Road
Wadala, Mumbai 400 031

Ashok Garg MS PhD FRSM
Medical Director
Garg Eye Institute and Research Centre,
235, Model Town, Dabra Chowk
Hisar 125 005 (India)

Ashok Grover MD FRCS
Chairman, Deptt of Ophthalmology
Sir Ganga Ram Hospital
Director, Vision Eye Clinic
12/27, West Patel Nagar
Near Arya Samaj Mandir
New Delhi 110 008, India

Athiya Agarwal MD DO FRSH
Consultant, Dr Agarwal's Eye Hospital
19, Cathedral Road
Chennai 600 086, India

Barbara Kusa MD
Centre Microchirurgia
Ambulatoriale, Via Donizetti, 24
20052, Monza, Italy

Bojan Pajic MD
Director Glaucoma Services
Chief Cornea and Refractive Surgery
Deptt Vision Care, Klinik Pallas
LouisGiroud Str 20, 4600 Olten
Switzerland

Charalambos Siganos MD PhD
Department of Ophthalmology
University of Crete, Heraklion
Crete, Greece

Daljit Singh MS DSC
57, Joshi Colony
Amritsar, India 143 001

David F Chang MD
762, Altos Oaks Drive, Suite-1
Los Altos, CA 94024, USA

Dimitrii Dementiev MD
Chief and Medical Director
Blue Eye Centro di
Microchirurgia Oculare Eye
Clinic Arese 20020 (MI)
Via Campo Gallo 21/10
Milan, Italy

Fabrizio I Camesasca MD
Deptt of Ophthalmology
Istituto Clinico Humanitas
Rozzano, Milano, Italy

Francisco J Gutierrez-Carmona
MD PhD
Associated Professor
Ophthalmological Research Institute
Ramon Caftroviejo Complutense
University of Madrid
Spain 28034

Franco Bartoli MD
Refractive Laser Centre
Corso Vittorio Emanuele 87
10100, Torino, Italy

Frederic Hehn MD
Centre de La Vision
Nations-Vision
23, Boulevard de l'europe
54500, Vandoeuvre, France

George Baikoff MD
Clinique Monticelli
88, Rue du Commandant Rolland
13008, Marsielle, France

George D Kymionis MD PhD
Department of Ophthalmology
University of Crete
Heraklion, Crete, Greece

GV Narendra MS
Retina Foundation
Aso Palov Eye Hospital
Shahibaug, Near Under Bridge
Raj Bhavan Road
Ahmedabad 380 004, India

Hany S Elsaftawy MD
Professor of Ophthalmology
Research Institute of Ophthalmology
Cairo, Egypt

Hiroshi Tsuneoka MD
Associate Professor
Deptt of Ophthalmology
Jikei University Daisan Hospital
4-11-1, Izumihoncho, Komae
Tokyo 201-8601, Japan

Hitendra Mehta MS
Aditya Jyoti Eye Hospital Pvt Ltd
Wadala
Mumbai 400 031, India

I Howard Fine MD FACS
Oregon Eye Surgery Centre
1550, Oak Street
5, Eugene
OR 97401, USA

Ioannis G Pallikaris MD PhD
Professor and Head
Department of Ophthalmology
University of Crete
Heraklion
Crete, Greece

Jairo E Hoyos MD PhD
Instituto Oftalmologico Hoyos
Rambla de Sabadell 62 1°
08201 Sabadell
Barcelona, Spain

Jairo Hoyos-Chacon MD
Instituto Oftalmologico Hoyos
Rambla de Sabadell 62 1°
08201 Sabadell
Barcelona, Spain

Jens Funk MD
Professor of Ophthalmology
Augenklinik-Universitats Klinikum
Killian Str 5, 79106 Freiburg, Germany

Jerome Jean-Philippe Bovet MD
Consultant Ophthalmic Surgeon
FMH, Clinique de l'oeil
15, Avenue du Bois-de-la-Chapelle
CH-1213 Onex, Switzerland

Jorge L Alio MD PhD
Instituto Oftalmologico de Alicante
Avda Denia 111, 03015
Alicante, Spain

Jose-Luis Rodriguez Prats MD PhD
Instituto Oftalmologico De Alicante
Alicante, Spain

JT Lin PhD
4532, Old Carriage Trail
OVIEDO, Florida 32765, USA

Kamal Nagpal MS
Retina Foundation
Aso Palov Eye Hospital
Shahibaug, Near Under Bridge
Raj Bhavan Road
Ahmedabad 380 004, India

Kukrenkov Vetchiaslav MD
Arese 20020 (MI)
Via Champo Gallo, 21/10, Italy

Madhurjya Gogoi MD
Deptt of Pharmacology
Dr RP Centre for Ophthalmic
Sciences, AIIMS
New Delhi 110 029, India

Manish Nagpal MS FRCS
Consultant, Retina Foundation
Aso Palov Eye Hospital
Shahibaug, Near Under Bridge
Raj Bhavan Road
Ahmedabad 380 004, India

Marguerite B McDonald MD
Medical Director
Southern Vision Institute
New Orleans, Louisiana, USA

Maria I Kalyvianaki MD
Department of Ophthalmology
University of Crete
Heraklion, Crete, Greece

Mark Packer MD
Oregan Eye Surgery Centre
1550, Oak Street
5, Eugene, OR 97401, USA

Mark S Humayun MD PhD
Professor of Ophthalmology
Doheny Retina Institute
Doheny Eye Institute
Kech School of Medicine
Univ of South California
1450, San Pablo St, DEI-3600
Los Angeles, CA 90033, USA

Matteo Piovella MD
Centro Microchirurgia Ambulatoriale
Via Donizetti 24, 20052, Monza, Italy

Melania Cigales MD
Instituto Oftalmologico Hoyos
Sabadell (Barcelona), Spain

Mona Pache MD
Augenklinik-Universitats Klinikum
Killian Str 5, 79106 Freiburg, Germany

Mordechai Goldenfeld MD
The Sam Rothberg Glaucoma Centre,
Goldschleger Eye Institute
Sheba Medical Centre
Tel-Hashomer, Israel

Nilesh Kanjani MS
Consultant
Dr Amar Agarwal's Eye Hospital
19, Cathedral Road
Chennai 600 086, India

Nishant Patel MS
Aditya Jyot Eye Hospital Pvt Ltd
Plot No 153, Road No 9
Major Parmeshwaran Road
Opp SIWS College, Gate No 3,
Wadala, Mumbai 400 031, India

NR Biswas MD DM
Deptt of Pharmacology
Dr RP Centre for Ophthalmic
Sciences, AIIMS
New Delhi 110 029, India

PN Nagpal MS
Director
Retina Foundation
Aso Palov Eye Hospital
Shahibaug, Near Under Bridge
Raj Bhavan Road
Ahmedabad 380 004, India

Richard J Fugo MD PhD
100, West Fornance Street
The Fugo Building
Norristown, PA 19401, USA

Richard S Hoffman
Oregon Eye Surgery Centre
1550, Oak Street, # 5 Eugene
OR- 97401, USA

Roberto G Carassa MD
Director, Glaucoma Service
Deptt. of Ophthalmology and Visual
Sciences, University Hospital
S Raffaele Via Olgettina 60
20132 Milano, Italy

Roberto Pinelli MD
Director
Istituto Laser Microchirurgia Oculare
Crystal Palace, Via Cefalonia
70, 25124, Brescia, Italy

Rohit R Lakhanpal MD
Doheny Retina Institute
Doheny Eye Institute
Kech School of Medicine
Univ of South California
1450, San Pablo St, DEI-3600
Los Angeles
CA 90033, USA

Sarmi Malik MS
Ganga Ram Eye Hospital
Rajender Nagar
New Delhi, India

Shlomo Melamed MD
Professor of Ophthalmology
Sackler Med'cal School
Tel Aviv University
Head and Chairman
Sam Rothberg Glaucoma Centre
Goldschleger Eye Institute
Sheba Medical Centre
Tel-Hashomer, Israel

S Natarajan MS
Chairman and Medical Director
Aditya Jyot Eye Hospital Pvt Ltd
Plot No 153, Road No 9
Major Parmeshwaran Road
Opp SIWS College
Gate No 3, Wadala
Mumbai 400 031, India

Soosan Jacob MD DNB FERC
Dr Agarwal's Eye Hospital
19, Cathedral Road
Chennai 600 086 (India)

Stefano Cavazza MS
Ospedale Maggiore
Largo B, Nigrisoli 2, 40100
Bologna, Italy

Suhas Dongargaokar MS
Retina Foundation
Aso Palov Eye Hospital
Shahibaug
Near Under Bridge
Raj Bhavan Road
Ahmedabad 380 004, India

Sunita Agarwal MS DO PSVH
Dr Agarwal's Eye Hospital
19, Cathedral Road
Chennai 600 086, India
15, Eagle Street, Langford Town
Bangalore, India

Sylvian Roy MD
Hospital Ophtalmique Gules Gonin
and University of Lausanne
Avenue de France 15
1004, Lausanne
Switzerland

T Agarwal FORCE DO FICS
Director, Dr Agarwal's Eye Hospital
19, Cathedral Road
Chennai 600 086, India

Vikentia J Katsanevaki MD PhD
Vardinoyannion Eye Institute
University of Crete, Greece

Vivek Kadambi MD DOMS
Director, Kadambi Laser Vision Clinic
and Research Foundation Pvt Ltd
157, Defence Colony
4th Main Road, Indiranagar
Bangalore 560 038, India

Zia Chaudhuri MS MNAMS FRCS
Consultant, Deptt of Ophthalmology
Sir Ganga Ram Hospital
Rajinder Nagar
New Delhi 110 060

Foreword

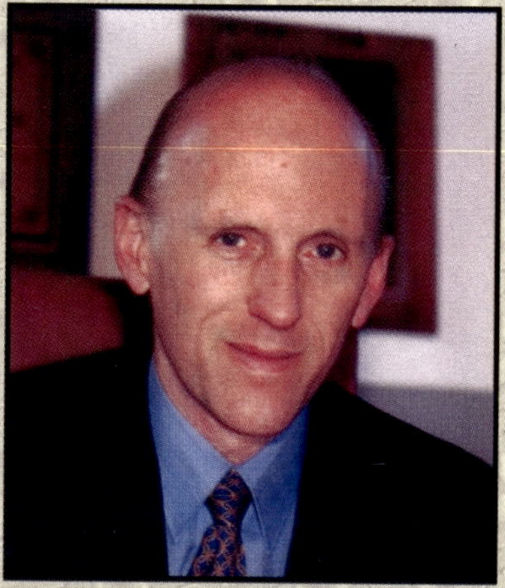

Among the many progresses that surgical medicine has made in the last decades, one of the most relevant and acknowledged ones in the human surgical science is indeed ocular surgery. Progresses in cataract surgery were considered by the US Academy of Sciences as the most important progress in a single surgical procedure in human surgery that took place during the 20th century. Now, in the 21st century, we are facing major changes in our practice as ocular surgeons and indeed innovative techniques like the ones that are gathered in this book are to be not only important, but fostering others in the future that will lead us to a complete transformation in our surgical practice.

Cross-hybridisation between science and technology has been the driving force in the progress of ocular surgery. Ophthalmology has brought a tremendous attraction for scientists of all kinds that has introduced us in concepts such as neurophysiology, neurosciences, regenerative medicine, applied optics to human vision, lasers and other pieces of high technology that are, at this moment, creating a progressive change in our everyday approach to eye disease.

The most recent progress has been made in cataract surgery among others, but indeed not the only one. Microincisional surgical techniques (all of them gathered with the acronym, MICS), new intraocular lenses that are capable to suppress or decrease eye aberrations after surgery, new knowledge in applied optics that is creating a new environment for cataract surgery are addressed in this book. Refractive surgery indeed is part of the progress as well, as today the practice of refractive surgery has to be considered not only related to relieve from spectacle use our patients, but rather to improve their vision by using different innovative techniques and devices that are creating not only a new perspective of visual quality, but also a new hope to many patients with eye disease such as keratoconus. Glaucoma is another area of interest of this book. Glaucoma, one of the most frequent blinding conditions of the human being, is now being approached not only with new pharmacology, but also with new surgery. New approaches made glaucoma surgery to be able to face these cases with an armamentarium that improves their performance and speeds up the surgical process. New examination techniques are indeed of major relevance for our practice, as they bring us the information that is needed to make a correct diagnosis and to define the best approach to solve an ocular problem. Among these examination techniques, those that are based on diagnostic imaging are the most relevant at this moment in the decision making process of anterior segment and posterior segment surgery. New lasers are approaching lacrimal surgery, one of the least developed in the last 40 years of our practice, with a new perspective of conservative procedures that can solve the problems of chronic tearing without creating any external scar in the patient with reliable outcomes. The book ends with the perspectives of something that might be considered today utopia: artificial vision. Nobody can really predict what will be in the next 20 years our perspective for visually impaired people, but indeed the progress in this area, coming from serious research in neuroprocessing and neuroscience, is bringing hope to those who have none.

Dr Ashok Garg has made with this book a commitment with ocular surgery. He is aware of the fact that the progress in ocular surgery is based on these innovative techniques that at this moment

are leading the most important surgeons in the world to face old problems with new tools, hopeless conditions with new positive perspectives and leading a generation of ocular surgeons who are going to transform the practice of ocular surgery in the coming years.

We welcome this important book of Dr. Ashok Garg that will open the minds of many of us to many new technologies that at this moments are emerging in different parts of the world. The important and most relevant social issue that are witnessing in this century is globalisation. Ocular surgery is global and Dr Ashok Garg has been approaching this book on innovations in ocular surgery under the most modern global approach, in which science and knowledge may be created and developed elsewhere around the world. I would like to thank Dr. Ashok Garg and Co-editors for this great effort and all the contributors of the different chapters for their creativity, work and understanding of the philosophy of excellence in their approach to ocular surgery.

Dr Jorge L Alio
MD PhD
Professor and Chairman of Ophthalmology
Medical Director
VISSUM, Instituto Oftalmologico de Alicante
Alicante, Spain
Tel. 34-965-150-025
E-mail : jlalio@vissum.com

Preface

Ophthalmology has come of age specially in the last decade with the evolution of various innovative high-tech procedures and medical management. Today ophthalmic surgery is state-of-art surgery for the management of various anterior and posterior segment diseases. Minimally invasive cataract surgery, glaucoma surgery, refractive and retinal surgery, etc have improved the visual outcome dramatically to the patient satisfaction.

In this book a number of leading international ophthalmologists have shared their experiences in form of chapters for the benefit of ophthalmologists covering all aspects of ophthalmology. A wide array of Modern Surgical Techniques are covered in this book. An interesting Interactive DVD ROM provided with this book depicts various latest surgical procedures performed by International Masters.

Our special gratitude extends to Shri JP Vij, Chairman and Managing Director, Mr Tarun Duneja (GM Publishing) and all staff of M/s Jaypee Brothers Medical Publishers Pvt. Ltd. who gave prompt attention and active support in the publication of this usefu book.

We hope this book on New Innovative Techniques will be a useful companion to ophthalmologists worldwide in their day-to-day practice.

Editors

Contents

SECTION 2: REFRACTIVE SURGERY TECHNOLOGIES (PRESBYOPIA, LENTICULAR AND CORNEAL-BASED REFRACTIVE TECHNIQUES)

SECTION 3: GLAUCOMA TECHNOLOGIES (LASER and MINIMALLY-INVASIVE GLAUCOMA SURGICAL TECHNIQUES)

DVD Contents

Section 1

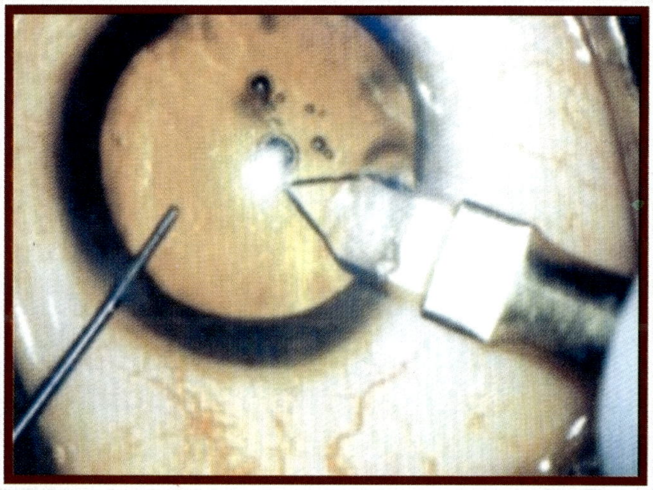

Cataract Surgery and Related Technologies (MSICS, Microphaconit, Minimally Invasive Cataract Surgery)

1

Ocular Anesthesia in MICS

Ashok Garg (India), Franciso J Gutiérrez-Carmona (Spain)

INTRODUCTION

Anesthesia for Cataract Surgery has undergone tremendous changes and advancements in last century (Table 1.1). In 1846 general anesthesia techniques were developed which were not found suitable and satisfactory for ophthalmic surgery. In 1884 Karl Köller discovered surface anesthesia techniques using topical cocaine for cataract surgeries which found favor with the ophthalmologists. However due to significant complications and side effects of cocaine this technique was abandoned.

Also in 1884 Herman Knapp described retrobulbar injection as local anesthetic technique for ocular surgery. He used 4 percent cocaine solution injected into the orbital tissue close to posterior part of the globe to achieve adequate anesthesia but in the subsequent injections patients experienced pain. In 1914 van Lint introduced orbicularis akinesia by local injection to supplement subconjunctival and topical anesthesia. However this technique found favor only after 1930 when procaine (Novocaine) a safer injectable agent made it feasible.

Table 1.1: Evolution of anesthetic techniques for cataract surgery

Techniques	*Years*	*Authors*
General anesthesia	1846	Morton
Topical cocaine	1884	Köller
Injectable cocaine	1884	Knapp
Retrobulbar (4% cocaine)	1884	Knapp
Orbicularis akinesia	1914	Van Lint, O'Brien, Atkinson
Hyaluronidase	1948	Atkinson
Posterior peribulbar	1985	Davis Y Mandel
Limbal	1990	Furata and coworkers
Sub-tenon anesthesia	1990	Hansen
Anterior peribulbar	1991	Bloomberg
Subconjunctival	1991	Petersen
Topical anesthesia	1992	Fichman
Pinpoint anesthesia	1994	Fukasaku
Topical plus intracameral	1995	Gills
No anesthesia	1998	Agarwal
Cryoanalgesia	1999	Gutiérrez-Carmona
Xylocaine jelly	1999	Koch, Assia
Hypothesis, no anesthesia	2001	Pandey and Agarwal
Viscoanesthesia	2002	Werner, Pandey, Apple

With the development of hyaluronidase as an additive to the local anaesthetic solution Atkinson in 1948 reported that large volumes could be injected with less orbital pressure and improved safety injections into the cone (retrobulbar) were recommended and gained rapid favor becoming anesthetic route of choice among ophthalmologists.

In Mid 1970s, Kelman introduced an alternative technique of local anesthesia for ocular surgery known as peribulbar injection. However till 1985 this new technique was not published in ophthalmic literature. In 1985 Davis and Mandel reported local anesthetic injection outside the cone into the posterior peribulbar space (periocular).

Further modifications of both retrobulbar and periocular injection techniques were made by Bloomberg, Weiss and Deichaman, Hamilton and colleagues, whitsett, Murdoch Shriver and coworkers. These modifications consisted of more anterior deposition of anesthetic solution with shorter needles and smaller dosages.

With the introduction of small incision cataract surgery, phacoemulsification and other microsurgical procedures in ophthalmology, use of shorter needles with smaller dosages became more common. Fukasaku and Furata et al reintroduced subconjunctival anesthetic techniques. Fichman in 1992 first reported the use of topical tetracaine anesthesia for phacoemulsification and intraocular lens implantation starting an era of topical anesthesia in ocular surgery.

With the advent of many ocular anesthetic techniques in past two decades indicates the need for the development of an ideal anesthetic and technique for ocular surgery. Every existing technique has its own advantages and disadvantages. General anesthesia for cataract surgery is virtually out of favor with ophthalmologists. Retrobulbar anesthesia, periocular (peribulbar, sub-conjunctival, sub-Tenon or parabulbar, orbital and epidural) and topical Anesthesia or a combination of peribulbar and topical are being used in present day ocular surgery.

Now with the advent of under 1.0 mm incision technique, foldable and rollable intraocular lenses, no anesthesia cataract surgery is becoming increasingly popular, this technique was designed by Agarwal (India) in 1998.

In 1999, Gutiérrez-Carmona (Spain) designed the cryoanalgesia technique for cataract surgery modifying Agarwal's method.

ANESTHESIA FOR MICROPHACO

Microincision cataract extraction may be performed under general anesthesia, local anesthesia or topical anesthesia, depending upon condition of patient cataract status and surgeon choice.

Usually for microphaco general anesthesia is not given. It is advisable only in highly anxious/nervous patient or when cataract surgery requires a long time for completion. Patients who are extremely apprehensive, deaf, mentally retarded, unstable or cannot communicate well with the surgeon are more suitable for general anesthesia. General anesthetic facilities with expert anesthetist are mandatory.

Local anesthesia in microphaco have superseded general anesthesia due to their indisputable advantages, such as the potential for ambulatory surgery, rapid recovery and lack of complications. However local anaesthetic surgery using the retrobulbar or peribulbar technique is not without possible complications, such as perforation of the eyeball accompanied by retinal detachment and severe intraocular hemorrhage, retrobulbar hematoma, diplopia, direct optic nerve trauma caused by the retrobulbar needle, increased intraocular pressure, postoperative ptosis, or systemic complications such as accidental administration of anesthetic to the bloodstream or nervous system.

Moreover, in the last decade, topical anesthesia in microphaco has gained more interest on the part of surgeons as it eliminates the risks involved in using general and local anesthesias. However, this method should be performed by an expert surgeon who has mastered the technique and who can perform it rapidly. No anesthesia microphaco surgery is also becoming popular among ophthalmologists worldwide.

LOCAL ANESTHESIA

Local ocular anesthesia is the mainstay of microphaco. Local anesthesia minimizes the risk of wound rupture a complication frequently associated with coughing during extubation and postoperative nausea and vomiting (in general anesthesia) (Figure 1.1). Generally the use of 1:1 mixture of 2 percent xylocaine and 0.50 percent bupivacaine alongwith adrenaline and hyaluronidase in facial, retrobulbar and peribulbar blocks achieve rapid Anesthesia, akinesia and postoperative analgesia for several hours.

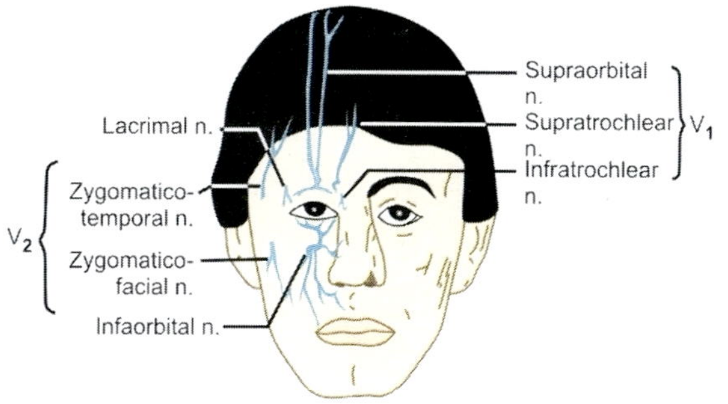

Figure 1.1: Diagrammatic surface distribution of sensory nerves. Note branches derived from ophthalmic nerve (V_1) and maxillary nerve (V_2) a division of the trigeminal nerve

On the other hand, we have sub-Tenon or parabulbar anesthesia performed with a blunt cannula which avoids the complications arising from the use of needles. Intraoperative analgesia and akinesia are similar to the peribulbar technique.

Care should be taken to avoid intravascular injections of anesthetic agents because refractory cardiopulmonary arrest may result from an inadvertent intravenous or intra-arterial injections.

Many patients express pain of facial and retrobulbar injections and other complications so these techniques are now out of favor.

Out of various local anesthesia techniques available today, only following techniques are commonly used for microphaco surgery.

Peribulbar (Periocular) Technique

Since the exit of retrobulbar akinesia, peribulbar akinesia is considered a safe and effective technique of local anesthesia for microphaco. It is method of choice with eye surgeons for giving local anesthesia to cataract. As the name indicates, peribulbar anesthesia is a technique in which a local anesthetic is injected into peribulbar space and is not aimed at blocking a particular nerve.

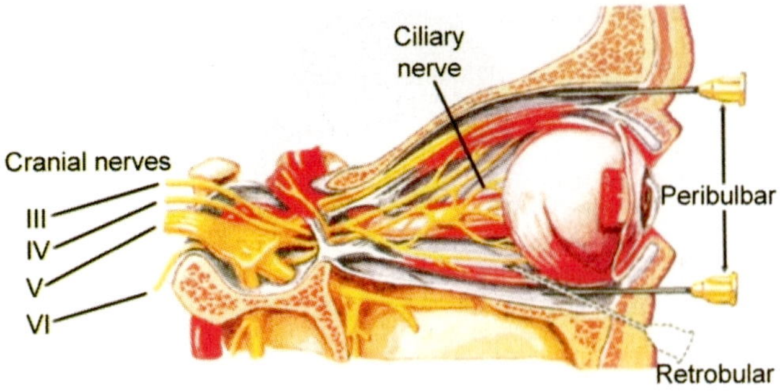

Figure 1.2: Needle positions for peribulbar and retrobulbar akinesia (*Courtesy:* Ciba Geigy clinical symposia)

Technique

Periocular anesthesia is administered at two sites: lower temporal quadrant and nasal to caruncle (Figure 1.2).

The required local anaesthetics are lidocaine 1 percent and bupivacaine 0.75 percent with hyaluronidase. Bupivacaine is preferred as it is a longer acting anesthetic agent which can provide prolonged anesthesia and analgesia.

In the first stage, injection of 0.5 cc of 1 percent lidocaine with a 26 gauge needle is done under the skin at about 1 cm away from the lateral canthus in the lower lid, along the orbital rim. The same needle is passed deeper to inject 0.5 cc of lidocaine into the orbicularis muscle and 1.0 cc into the muscle sheath. A second injection is done in the similar fashion in the upper eye lid just below the supraorbital notch. Pressure is applied at both for a minute using gauze pieces.

In the second stage, combination of 6.0 ml of 0.75 percent bupivacaine, 3 ml of 1 percent lidocaine and 0.25 cc of hyaluronidase is filled into a 10 ml disposable syringe fitted with a, 1-1/4 inch 23 gauge, hypodermic needle. The needle is first introduced deep into the orbit through the anesthetized site in the lower eyelid. One ml is injected just beneath the orbicularis muscle and then the needle is advanced up to the equator of the globe to inject 2 to 3 ml of the solution. The same procedure is followed in the upper nasal quadrant through the preanaesthetized site to inject 1 ml and another 1 ml may be injected around superior orbital fissure, by deeper penetration.

At the end of the procedure, fullness of the lids is noted due to the volume of the injected. Firm pressure with the flat of the hand is applied over the globe and is maintained for a minute. Then, before surgery, any pressure device as per the surgeon's choice like Honan's balloon, super pinky ball, balance weight or simple pad-bandage is applied for 20 to 30 minutes, to achieve the desired response of hypotony.

The efficacy of the anesthesia is evaluated after about 10 minutes of injection and if inadequate, 2 to 4 ml more can be injected. In case of persistent inferior or lateral movement injection lower temporal quadrant and in case of persistent movements upwards of nasally, the upper quadrant could be infiltrated in the same fashion.

Hyaluronidase is essential as it helps in the spread of the drug. Otherwise, there are chances of the eye being proptosed due to high orbital pressure induced by the large quantity of the fluid injected.

Single injection of 5 to 6 ml of anesthetic mixture injected from any site posterior to equator of the globe also achieves same results. For convenience, however, it may be done through lower lid the junction of lateral and middle one-third, along the floor of the orbit.

Adequacy of akinesia is determined by the absence of ocular movements in all directions.

This technique is certainly better than retro-ocular technique and has least complications.

Advantages

The advantages reported are:

1. The injection is done outside the muscle cone and so, the inherent complications of passing the needle into the muscle cone is completely eliminated.
2. It does not enter the retrobulbar space and thereby avoids retrobulbar hemorrhage, injury to optic nerve and entry of anesthetic agents into subarachnoid space and other complications like respiratory arrest.
3. Since the needle is constantly kept parallel to the bony orbit, it avoids injury to globe and entry of anesthetic agents into the eyeball.
4. It causes less pain on injection.
5. The procedure is easier and can be performed without causing damage to vital structures.
6. It does not reduce vision on table.
7. No facial block is required.

Drawbacks

The possible drawbacks of this procedure are:

1. Chemosis of conjunctiva.
2. Delayed onset of anesthetic effect and
3. Potential risk of orbital hemorrhage. Though it occurs rarely, the magnitude of the problem is comparable to retrobulbar hemorrhage and necessitates postponement of surgery.

Mechanism

The exact mechanism is not known but this procedure may best be described as 'Infiltration Anesthesia' where nerve endings in all tissues in the area of injection get anesthetized.

Peribulbar anesthesia is a safe and reliable technique for achieving akinesia and anesthesia of the globe.[6] In case of inadequate anesthesia, repeat injections in the similar manner can be safely used to achieve the purpose.

Superior rectus injection The induction of temporary paralysis of the superior rectus muscle is essential for any intraocular operation where the surgical field is upper half of the eye. This injection also affects the action of levator palpebrae superioris.

In this injection patient is asked to look down. The upper lid is retracted and 2.5 cm long needle is passed into Tenon's capsule at the temporal edge of the superior rectus muscle. The needle is directed posteromedially and about 1 ml of anesthetic mixture of 2 percent xylocaine is injected around the muscle belly behind the equator. This injection can also be made through the skin of the upper orbital sulcus.

Tenon's capsule injection The Injection of anesthetic mixture can be given into Tenon's capsule around the upper half of the eyeball and into the belly of superior rectus muscle. It is considered safer than the retro-ocular injection across the post-ganglionic fibers of the cillary body and may be effective in inducing extraocular muscle akinesia.

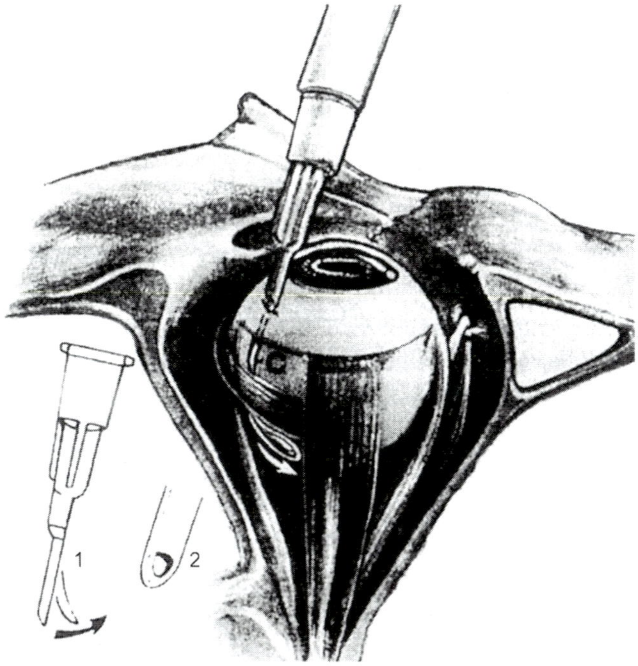

Figure 1.3: Parabulbar (flush) local anesthesia (cross-section view)

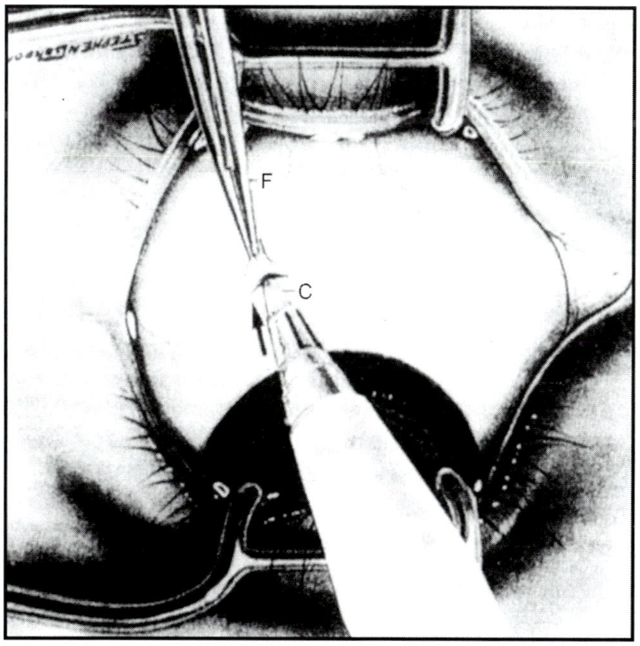

Figure 1.4: Parabulbar (flush) local anesthesia (surgeon view)

Parabulbar (Flush) or Sub-Tenon Akinesia

This is a very valuable alternative technique to the retro and peribulbar methods. In this technique, we attempt to place the anesthetic in the intraconical space, near the ciliary ganglion. This method consists of a limbal sub-Tenon administration of retrobulbar anesthesia using a blunt irrigating cannula (Figures 1.3 and 1.4). This technique can be used for anterior and posterior segment surgery.

Technique

We use a blunt or Greenbaum cannula with the anesthetic or mixture chosen. The patient needs to look up and in the direction of the eye to be operated on so that we can see the inferior nasal quadrant. We place topical anesthesia and next we perform an conjunctival and Tenon incision with Wescott scissors creating a deep tunnel. We introduce the blunt cannula through the tunnel, injecting the anesthetic. After, we place a Honan's balloon or super pinky decompressor for 10 minutes at 30 mm Hg.

Complications

Retrobulbar hemorrhage This can be produced when we perform the mucous-Tenon dissection, or when we introduce the cannula through the tunnel or when we vary this technique by using a continuous infusion with catheter.

Conjunctival edema This is produced when we inject the anesthetic in the subconjunctival space and not in the sub-Tenon space, diminishing the possibility of achieving complete denervation of the eyeball.

Hyposphagma This is frequently produced postoperatively, leading to undesired aesthetic results.

Topical Anesthesia

Since the advent of retrobulbar and peribulbar techniques in the early part of this century, both procedures are mainstay of local anesthesia for intraocular surgery till today. They do carry the risk of perforation of globe, optic nerve and the inadvertent injection of anesthetic at wrong places.

These accidents are mainly due to:

- Carelessness on the part of ophthalmologist who considers the procedures lightly and occurs more often with senior eye surgeons
- Using long needles for these techniques endangers the perforation of globe, piercing the optic nerve and entering crowded retrobular space and even touching the intracranial space on forceful injection of copious amounts
- Anesthetics given through local injection with little knowledge of anatomy of this area
- Retrobulbar hemorrhage with its adverse effects on nerve and globe is very common complication of this technique
- Injury caused by perforation of globe can lead to hole formation, retinal detachment, vitreous hemorrhage and central and branch vein occlusions.

To overcome all these practical difficulties use of topical anesthesia in intraocular surgery has been widely suggested and used at an international opthalmic level.[3] Topical anesthesia meaning topical application of 4 percent xylocaine or 0.5 to 0.75 percent proparacaine one drop 3 to 4 times at regular intervals in the eye has become increasingly popular and accepted.[7] In present day high tech intraocular surgery specially phacosurgery topical anesthesia is the anesthesia of choice with the eye surgeons world wide.

Indications to use Topical Anesthesia

- Its indications in intraocular surgery are mainly when performing phacoemulsification and IOL implantation through a clear corneal tunnel and corneoscleral incisions
- Topical anesthesia is ideally suited for small incision and stitchless cataract surgery. However, it is not a advocated to perform standard/manual extracapsular cataract extraction and IOL implantation
- Proper selection of patient is of great importance in this technique. It is important to have a patient who will comply with the instructions given during surgery.
- Patients who are non-cooperative, hard of hearing, with language problem and anxious patients are poor candidates for surgery under topical anesthesia. Capsulorhexis requires the maximum cooperation of the patient
- Intraocular surgery likely to be problematic in patients with rigid small pupils responding poorly to dilating drops and eyes with lenticular subluxation and high

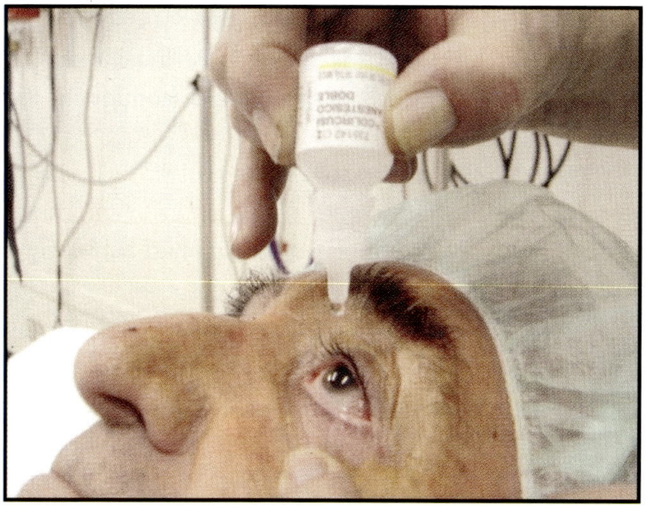

Figure 1.5: The assisting nurse places anesthetic drops in order to achieve topical anesthesia

grade nuclear sclerosis are relative contraindications for topical anesthesia

- Eye surgeon operating with topical anesthesia should be proficient and experienced at phacoemusification
- This procedure requires the use of foldable IOL either as a silicone lens or an acrylic lens. This is essential because corneal tunnel suture lens incision cannot be larger then 3.5 mm. Otherwise corneal complications may arise and the incision would not be self-sealing.

How to achieve surface anesthesia for intraocular surgery
Generally 3 applications of 4 percent xylocaine or 0.4 percent benoxinate HCl or 0.5 to 0.75 percent proparacaine 10 minutes apart starting 30 minutes before surgery are recommended (Figure 1.5). A drop is thereafter instilled prior to the incision. 1 cc of 4 percent xylocaine or 0.4 percent benoxinate HCI or 0.5 to 0.75 proparacaine (from fresh vail) is drawn into sterile disposable syringe and OT staff person is asked to instil a few drops of the same prior to cauterization of bleeders and if required during surgery conjunctival anesthesia is used (pinpoint and mini pinpoint surface anesthesia).[9]

Apart from giving topical anesthesia one has to give systemic analgesia. Besides it, surgeon should have a commanding hypnotic voice (vocal local anesthesia).

- Most surgeons doing corneal tunnel incision under topical anesthesia prefer to do it from temporal side.

Can one convert half way through surgery under topical anesthesia?
Intraoperative conversion from topical to peribulbar anesthesia can definitely be achieved if surgical situation warrants it. Since corneal tunnel incision is sutureless and self-healing a peribulbar injection can safely be given during the surgery.

Advantages of Topical Anesthesia

1. Phacoemulsification experts feel that use of topical anesthesia with a clear corneal tunnel self-healing incision is a significant advancement in intraocular surgery. With topical anesthesia visual recovery is immediate.
2. It prevents the well known complications of retrobulbar and peribulbar injections as mentioned in the early part of this chapter.
3. It lessens the time of operating room use thereby lowering costs.
4. There is no immediate postoperative ptosis as seen in retrobulbar or peribulbar and van Lint, O'Brien infiltrations lasts for 6 to 8 hours due to temporary akinesia of the lids.
5. With topical anesthesia photon laser intraocular surgery can be OPD procedure.
6. Faster visual recovery and ability for patients to remain on anticoagulation therapy.
7. In practice we have seen the anxiety of patients to peribulbar and retrobulbar injections prior to surgery. With topical anesthesia this problem is over and patient compliance will be better during intraoperative period.
8. There is no need for a qualified anesthesiologist in the operating theater during the operation, although a number of ophthalmologists prefer an anesthesiologist by their side for local anesthesia (retrobulbar and peribulbar anesthesia).
9. No risk of postponement of intraocular surgery as seen in cases of retrobulbar hemorrhage.

Again its main advantages is that it provides for immediate postoperative visual recovery.

Disadvantages of Topical Anesthesia

1. Only a highly experienced surgeon can operate with topical anesthesia. The eye can move which makes

the operation more difficult. If the eye movement occurs when capsulorhexis is being done, an undesirable capsular tear may take place leading to failure of this important step of the operation.

2. The chances of intraoperative complications with topical anesthesia can be high if the surgeon is not highly skilled. If such complications arise surgeon should be ready to convert to other methods of local anesthesia during the intraoperative stage, because topical anesthesia along may not be adequate to handle intraoperative complications. Surgeon should be of cool temperament who can handle such a situation without anxiety.
3. Topical anesthesia is not indicated in all patients specially in anxious stressed patients, people with hearing difficulties, children and very young patients.
4. As in our country a large number of patients come from rural areas who are illiterate and poor. Their compliance remains very poor and they do not respond adequately to the command during surgery with topical anesthesia.
5. The presence of very opaque cataract is a contra indication to the use of topical anesthesia. This is because surgeon depends on the patient ability to visually concentrate on the operating microscope light in order to avoid eye movement during the operation. Patients, who are not able to fix the eyes, may lead to complications.
6. Some patients may feel pain during surgery with topical anesthesia. One patient observed a lot more pain and felt as if a sword was being used to cut him up. The pain continued postoperatively for quite some time.
7. In principle, adequate selection of patients is fundamental when considering the use of topical anesthesia.

In spite of these hurdles topical anesthesia will be a safe and common technique for local anesthesia during intraocular surgery in the near future.

Intracameral Anesthesia

This an adjunct method with topical anesthesia designed by Gills in 1995. This results in the blocking of the sensitivity in the long ciliary nerve branches, so that the zonular stretching and the scraping of the iris during phacoemulsification do not produce discomfort in the patient.

This technique consists of injecting 0.1 ml of 1 percent preservative-free lidocaine in the anterior chamber, avoiding the risk of intraocular toxicity and achieving a good analgesia of the iris.

Topical and intracameral anesthesia can be used in patients treated with anticoagulants.

Studies by some authors comparing topical and topical plus intracameral anesthesia have demonstrated that neither topical nor topical plus intracameral anesthesia result in important differences in patient complaints or in complications.[11] However, the use of intraoperative lidocaine is safe and effective in controlling intraoperative discomfort.[10]

No Anesthesia Cataract Surgery

This non-pharmacological technique was first carried out by Amar Agarwal (India) in 1998.[1] Neither topical nor intracameral anesthetics agents are used.

Technique

- Before performing the surgery, we must inform the patient that he will feel contact and that he can move his eyes
- Use a speculum such as Castroviejo, Clarke or Liebermann
- Viscoelastic HealonÒ is injected into the anterior chamber using a needle through the area where the second (paracentesis) site is made
- A straight rod is used to stabilize the eye with the left hand
- With the right hand, a 3.2 mm groove is made in clear-temporal cornea using a diamond knife (Figure 1.6)
- A 5.0 to 5.5 mm wide capsulorhexis is performed using a 26 gauge bent needle cystotome
- Hydrodissection is performed with BSSÒ
- Phacoemulsification is performed using the karate chop technique using less ultrasound power to avoid

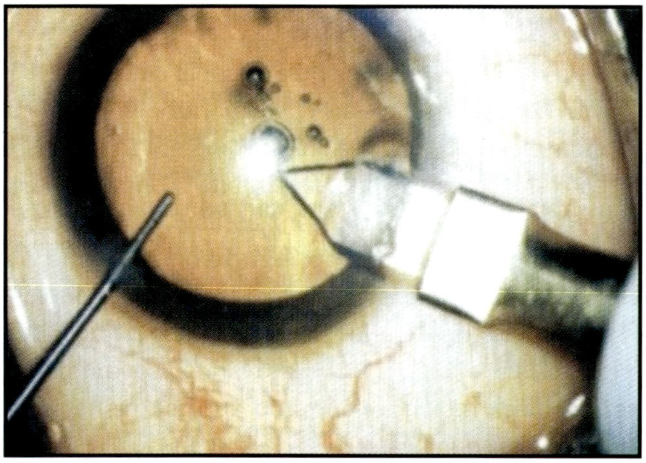

Figure 1.6: The surgeon's right hand making a clear corneal tunnel incision in the temporal quadrant

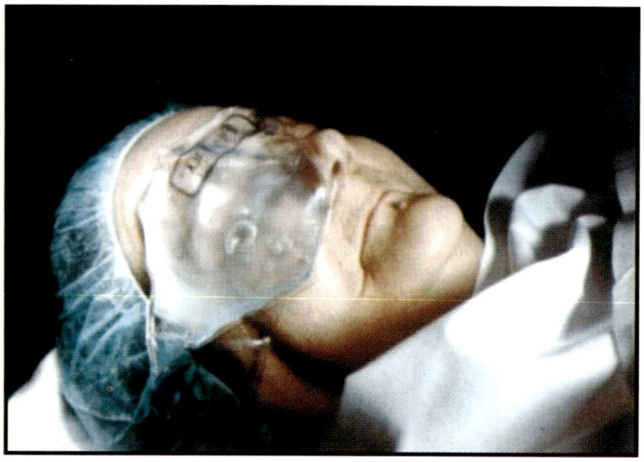

Figure 1.7: A monolateral eye mark of cold gel is placed over the eye before surgery for about 10 minutes

excessive heating of the phaco tip, which in turn can produce pain

- Cortical washing. First, try to remove the subincisional cortex as that is the most difficult
- Viscoelastic injection in the capsular bag and a foldable one-piece plate IOL is implanted
- The viscoelastic is removed from the anterior chamber and the capsular bag by irrigation
- Closure of the corneal incisions by stromal hydration.

The microscope light should begin at the lowest level and gradually increase in intensity. The intensity of the light should increase to normal levels after performing the hidrodissection and the patient should be told to look at the light during surgery.

The skill and experience of the surgeon is one of the most important factors for the No Anesthesia Cataract Surgery. While using this technique, it is important to avoid grasping the conjunctiva or sclera with tooth forceps. The surgeon should use a straight and relatively blunt rod to stabilize the eye during the entire procedure.

As with topical Anesthesia, we should minimize the iris-lens-diaphragm movement and iris manipulations.

No subconjunctival injections should be made following surgery nor should an eyepad be placed.

Microphaco Surgery with Cryoanalgesia

This non-pharmacological Anesthesia technique was designed in 1999 by Francisco J. Gutiérrez-Carmona (Spain). There are no anesthethic drops used, it is a modification of No Anesthesia Cataract Surgery.

Technique

- Before performing the surgery we must tell the patient that he will feel a cold sensation in his eye and that he can move his eyes
- In order to perform the surgery, it is necessary previously to cool all fluids to be used in the operation to around 4 degrees Celsius, except for the povidone drops, which should be at normal temperature for optimum effect
- Before surgery, an eye mask of cold gel (Eyes Pack™ Single) is placed over the eye for about ten minutes (Figure 1.7). This will afford some degree of analgesia to the eyelids, facilitating the insertion of the lid speculum
- Ocular asepsis before surgery is achieved using 5 percent povidone drops. Next, a drop of cold methylcellulose (Celoftal™) is instilled in the eye before placement of the ophthalmic drape to isolate the eyelid. The cold Celoftal™ reduces the stinging sensation of the povidone
- The cornea is previously cooled by continuous irrigation from a flask of cold BSS® in the area in which the paracentesis will be conducted. To perform the paracentesis, the eyeball is held still with a spatula or lens manipulator placed on the corneal periphery

opposite the area where the anterior chamber (AC) is accessed using a paracentesis knife

- Cold viscoelastic material (Viscoat®) is injected through the paracentesis into the anterior chamber, and a lens manipulator is subsequently introduced to stabilize the eyeball
- The cornea is then continuously cooled with BSS® in the area in which the clear corneal incision is to be made. Corneal tunnel incision is performed at 90° to the paracentesis with the help of a a 3.2 mm phaco knife
- Cold Viscoat® is injected into the anterior chamber. Next, the corneal incision is chilled with cold BSS® in order to perform a continuous circular capsulorrhexis with capsular forceps
- The lens nucleus is hydrodissected with cold BSS® irrigation using a Binkhorst, or a straight Rycroft cannula, inserted through the corneal incision
- The process of phacoemulsification is performed with cold fortified BSS® irrigation during linear and pulsed phaco. During phacoemulsification, the cornea must be kept chilled with cold BSS®. When the tip of the phacoemulsifier is inserted into the anterior chamber, the corneal incision is cooled by continuous irrigation from a flask of cold BSS®
- Cortical aspiration is performed with cold fortified BSS® irrigation
- Cold Viscoat® is injected into the capsular bag and the corneal incision is extended to 4.1 mm after chilling. Once the corneal incision is cooled with BSS®, a foldable IOL is implanted
- Closure of the incision is performed by stromal hydration using cold BSS®.

An important point in this technique is the cooling of the incision area before introducing any instrument into the eye.

I have also found it helpful to dim the illumination of the operating microscope initially so that the patient is not startled by the bright light. You can then gradually increase the illumination as needed for visualization intraoperatively. It is also very important that the microscope light is at the lowest intensity level and to tell the patient to fix his gaze at the microscope light. The skill and experience of the surgeon is very important in order to perform this technique.

Xylocaine Jelly

This method of topical anesthesia with 2 percent lidocaine hydrochloride gel (AstraÒ) allows cataract surgeons to eliminate the risks associated with needle injection. The gel helps to keep the cornea moistened and increases contact time with the ocular surface, insuring sustained diffusion and prolonged anesthetic effect . On the other hand, the gel is minimally absorbed by the ocular mucous, reducing the risk of secondary systemic effects.

In preparation for surgery, the patient received three doses of 2 percent xylocaine Jelly (two doses in the holding area, and one before the eye was prepped and draped for the procedure).

The administration of 2 percent xylocaine jelly has demonstrated pain scores similar to those with intracameral anesthesia.

This type of topical anesthesia is used by urologists in urological explorations (cystoscopy, catheterization, exploration by sound and other endourethral operations). Other indications are: nasal and pharyngeal cavities in endoscopic procedures such as gastroscopy and bronchoscopy, proctoscopy and restoscopy and tracheal intubation.

Viscoanesthesia

This a new type of topical intracameral anesthesia by means of a viscoelastic cohesive material which contains an anaesthetic component.

The topical component used pre-operatively, consists of a mixture of 0.3 percent sodium hyaluronate and 2 percent lidocaine hydrochloride, while the intracameral component used per-operatively consists of 1.5 percent sodium hyaluronate and 1 percent lidocaine hydrochloride commercially known as VisThesia™ (CIBA Vision Surgical, Switzerland).

The first step of the viscoanesthesia procedure involves the preoperative application of the topical component of VisThesia™. Once the topical mixture is applied, the patient's eyes are kept closed for approximately 1 minute to allow for optimum diffusion of the mixture. The VisThesia™ intracameral component is then used as a normal viscoelastic, mainly before capsulorrhexis and before IOL implantation.

Preliminary results demonstrate the efficacy and safety of VisThesia™ concept as a viscoanesthetic method for cataract surgery. It provides a longer anesthetic effect when compared with the application of only an aqueous topical anesthetic.

Researchers have evaluated the VisThesia™ intracameral component in an in vitro animal study. Histological evaluation of the retinal and uveal tissues showed no differences between the eyes receiving VisThesia™ injections compared to eyes in the control group receiving balanced salt solution (BSS). There also was no histological evidence of endothelial damage or endothelial cell loss observed.

REFERENCES

1. Agarwal A, Agarwal S, Sachdev MS, et al. No anesthesia cataract surgery with karate chop. In Phacoemulsification Laser Cataract Surgery and Foldable IOLs. Jaypee Brothers, New Delhi, 1998;19:144-54.
2. Arora R, et al. Peribulbar Anesthesia. J Cataract Refract Surg 1991;17:506-8.
3. Assia EI, Pras E, Yehezkel M, et al. Topical anesthesia using lidocaine gel for cataract surgery. J Cataract Refract Surg 1999;25:635-9.
4. Bloomberg L. Administration of periocular Anesthesia. J Cataract Refract Surg 1986;12:677-9.
5. Bloomberg L. Anterior Peribulbar Anesthesia. J Cataract Refract Surg 1991;17:508-11.
6. Davis DB. Posterior peribulbar Anesthesia. J Cataract Refract Surg 1986;12:182-4.
7. Fichman RA. Topical Anesthesia. Saunders DR, Slack 1993; 1661-72.
8. Furuta M, et al. Limbal anesthesia for cataract surgery. Ophthalmic Surg 1990;21:22-5.
9. Garg A: Topical Anesthesia. Current trends in ophthalmology. Jaypee Brothers Publishers 1997;1-5.
10. Gills JP, Cherchio M, Raanan MG. Unpreserved lidocaine to control discomfort during cataract surgery using topical anesthesia. J Cataract Refract Surg 1997;23(4):545-50.
11. Gillow T, Scotcher SM, Deutsch J, While A, Quinlan MP. Efficacy of supplementary intracameral lidocaine in routine phacoemulsification under topical anesthesia. Ophthalmology 1999;106:2173-7.
12. Gutiérrez-Carmona FJ. Phacoemulsification with Cryoanalgesia: A New Approach for Cataract Surgery. In Phacoemulsification, Laser Cataract Surgery and Foldable IOLs. Jaypee Brothers Medical Publishers (2nd ed), New Delhi, 2000;23:226-9.
13. Hay A, et al. Needle perforation of the globe during Retrobulbar and peribulbar injection. Ophthalmology 1991; 98:1017-24.
14. Kimble JA, et al. Globe perforation from peribulbar injection. Arch Ophthalmol 1987;105:749.
15. Koch PS. Efficacy of lidocaine 2 percent jelly as a topical agent in cataract surgery. J Cataract Refract Surg 1999; 25:632-4.
16. Macky TA, Werner L, Apple DJ, et al. Viscoanesthesia Part II: Evaluation of toxicity to intraocular structures after phacoemulsification in a rabbit model. J Cataract Refract Surg 2003;29:556-62.
17. Pandey SK, Werner L, Apple DJ, et al. Viscoanesthesia Part III: Evaluation of the removal time of viscoelastic/viscoanesthetic solutions from capsular bag of human eyes obtained postmortem. J Cataract Refract Surg 2003;29: 563-7.
18. Shriver PA, et al. Effectiveness of retrobulbar and peribulbar Anesthesia. J Cataract Refract Surg 1992;18:162-5.
19. Trivedi RH, Werner L, Apple DJ, et al. Viscoanesthesia Part I: Evaluation of toxicity to corneal endothelial cells in a rabbit model. J Cataract Refract Surg 2003;29:550-5.
20. Zahl K et al. Ophthalmol Clin North Am. Philadelphia, WB Saunders, 1990.
21. Zaragoza-García P. La anestesia en oftalmología. In Monografías de la Sociedad Española de Oftalmología. Madrid, 2000.

2

Bimanual Microincision Phacoemulsification Instrumentation and Techniques

- INCISIONS
- CAPSULORHEXIS
- HYDRODISSECTION AND HYDRODELINEATION
- CHOPPING
- PHACOEMULSIFICATION
- STROMAL HYDRATION AND IOL IMPLANTATION
- BIOMANUAL MICRO-INCISION PHACOEMULSIFICATION

I Howard Fine, Richard S Hoffman, Mark Packer (USA)

INTRODUCTION

The first person to perform bimanual microincision phaco in a way that is reminiscent of what we are currently doing today is Steve Shearing, MD, of Las Vegas. In an article published in the January 1985 issue of the International Journal of Cataract Surgery, the cover story involved the use of this technique (Figure 2.1).[1] Subsequently, Dr Tsutomu Hara from Japan published a paper in 1989 on his experience with bimanual micro-incision phaco.[2] Amar Agarwal, MD, renamed the procedure phakonit in a 1998 publication.[3] Others including Hiroshi Tseunoka, MD[4] from Japan, Randall Olson, MD[5] and David Chang, MD[6] from the United States, Jorge Alio, MD[7] from Spain, and Drs Fine, Hoffman and Packer[8] all have added to the discussion of the value of this technique.

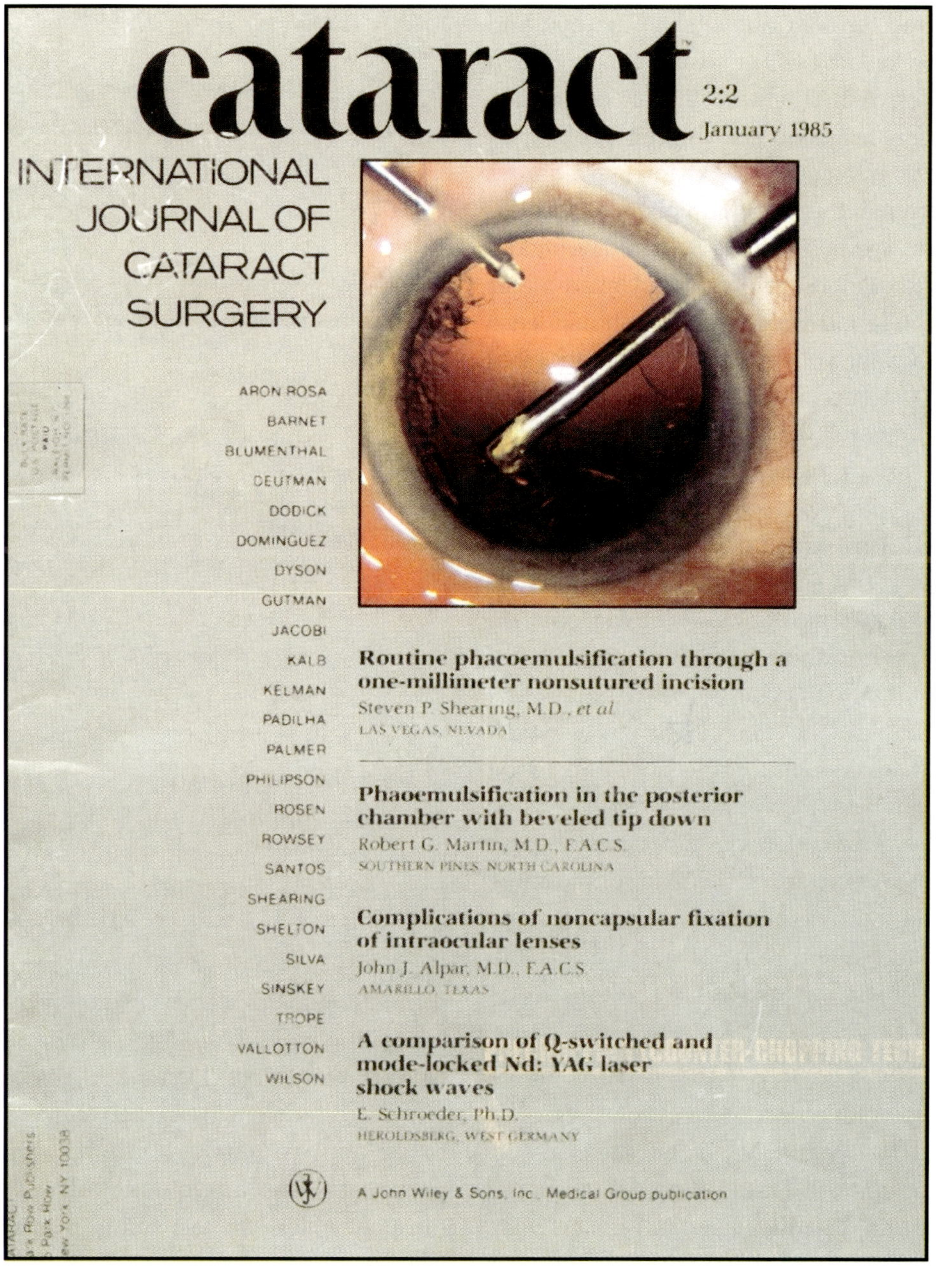

cataract 2:2 January 1985

INTERNATIONAL JOURNAL OF CATARACT SURGERY

ARON ROSA
BARNET
BLUMENTHAL
DEUTMAN
DODICK
DOMINGUEZ
DYSON
GUTMAN
JACOBI
KALB
KELMAN
PADILHA
PALMER
PHILIPSON
ROSEN
ROWSEY
SANTOS
SHEARING
SHELTON
SILVA
SINSKEY
TROPE
VALLOTTON
WILSON

Routine phacoemulsification through a one-millimeter nonsutured incision
Steven P. Shearing, M.D., *et al*
LAS VEGAS, NEVADA

Phacoemulsification in the posterior chamber with beveled tip down
Robert G. Martin, M.D., F.A.C.S.
SOUTHERN PINES, NORTH CAROLINA

Complications of noncapsular fixation of intraocular lenses
John J. Alpar, M.D., F.A.C.S.
AMARILLO, TEXAS

A comparison of Q-switched and mode-locked Nd: YAG laser shock waves
E. Schroeder, Ph.D.
HEROLDSBERG, WEST GERMANY

A John Wiley & Sons, Inc. Medical Group publication

Figure 2.1: Cover page of the January 1985 issue of the journal, Cataract, with picture of Dr Shearing performing early bimanual microincision phacoemulsification

We believe that this technique is better because it involves smaller and quite possibly safer incisions. It is closer to the ideal procedure than coaxial phacoemulsification in that there is dramatic reduction of fluid through the eye and the ideal procedure would be a completely closed system. With bimanual micro-incision phaco we have improved followability, we are able to manipulate tissue with the incoming stream of fluid and we have a much more stable chamber because all of the fluid is entering through one side of the eye and leaving through the other side so we do not have competing currents of fluid around the phaco needle. Of course, bimanual irrigation and aspiration of cortex has been known for a long time to be advantageous.

We began bimanual micro-incision phacoemulsification over two years ago because we were told we would be in the first wave of investigators in the United States on the ThinOptx IOL and we thought we should learn this technique in advance of the commencement of that study. However, we soon recognized that this was a superior procedure and therefore have limited our cataract surgeries and refractive lens exchanges to this technique over the past two years. We are frequently confronted by criticisms saying that it seems to be not worthwhile in that at this time we still have to make an incision between our two micro-incisions for implantation of an IOL. This is reminiscent of the criticism of phacoemulsification in the early 1980s before the availability of foldable IOLs. People felt that it wasn't worthwhile because the phaco incision had to be enlarged to implant an IOL. However, we persisted saying that phacoemulsification was a better procedure than extracapsular cataract extraction and for the same reason – the belief that micro-incision cataract surgery is a better procedure even in the absence of an IOL insertable through these micro-incisions.

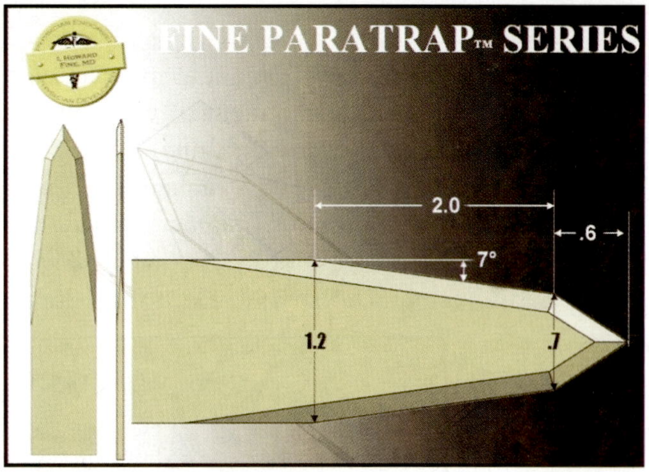

Figure 2.2: Mastel (Rapid City, South Dakota) Fine-Paratrap™ blade

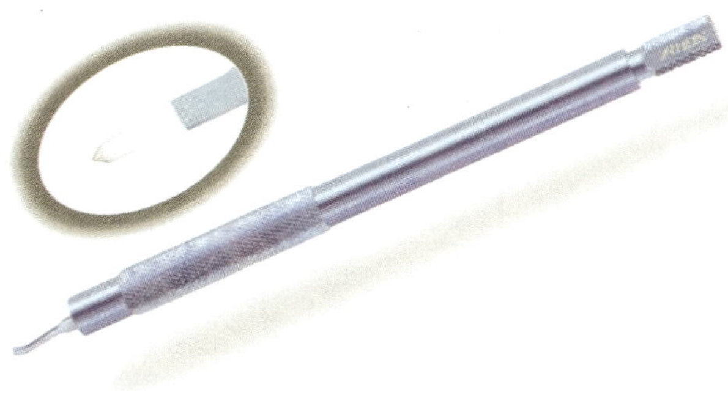

Figure 2.3: Rhein (Tampa, Florida) 3D Blade®, angled handle

INCISIONS

We have a strong preference for diamond knives because they are very reproducible and they do not stretch tissue. Knives we use include the Mastel (Rapid City, South Dakota) Fine-Paratrap™ blade (Figure 2.2), which when inserted to the end of the bevel produces incision sizes of 1.1 to 1.2 mm internally and 1.3 to 1.4 mm externally, the Rhein (Tampa, Florida) 3D Blade® (Figure 2.3) which produces incisions of 1.2 mm internally and 1.4 mm externally and is an excellent blade because it is self directed, the ASICO (Westmont, Illinois) Packer Bimanual Phaco diamond Knife (Figure 2.4), as well as a variety of metal blades including the metal blade from MicroSurgical Technology's (Redmond, Washington) Duet Bimanual set (Figure 2.5). We routinely separate our micro-incisions by 60 to 90 degrees. We like them to be approximately 1.5 mm long and our strong preference for trapezoidal blades is due to the ease through which we can rotate instruments within the incision without being oar-locked.

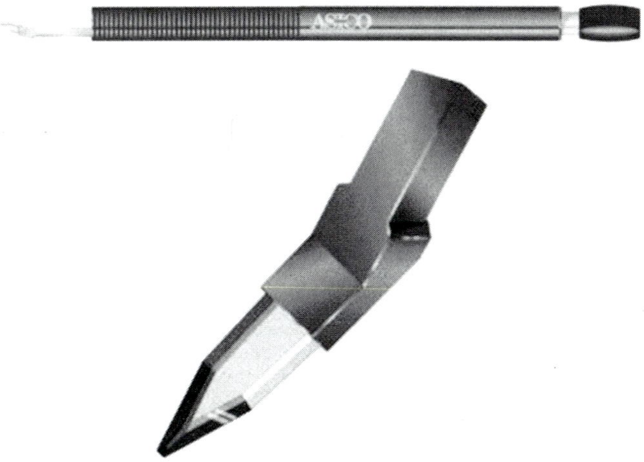

Figure 2.4: ASICO (Westmont, Illinois): Packer bimanual phaco diamond knife

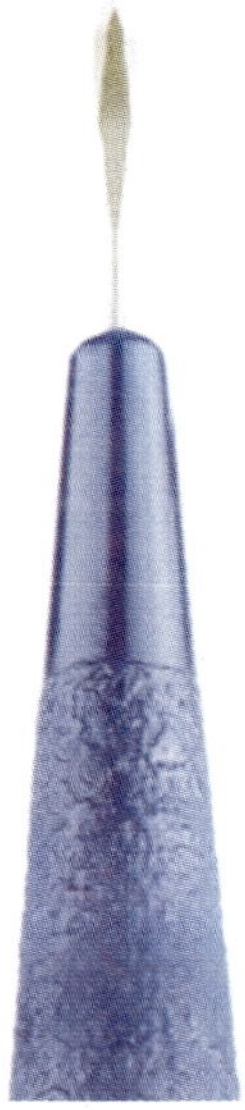

Figure 2.5: MicroSurgical Technology (Redmond, Washington) Duet bimanual metal blade

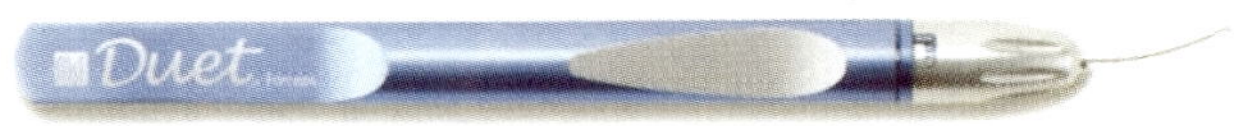

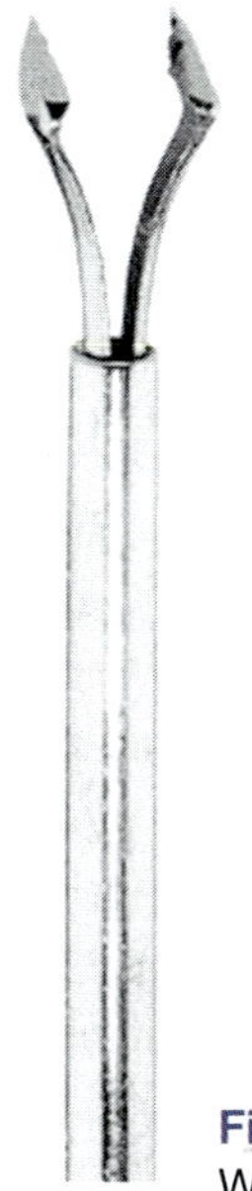

Figure 2.6: MicroSurgical Technology (Redmond, Washington): Fine-Hoffman capsulorhexis forceps

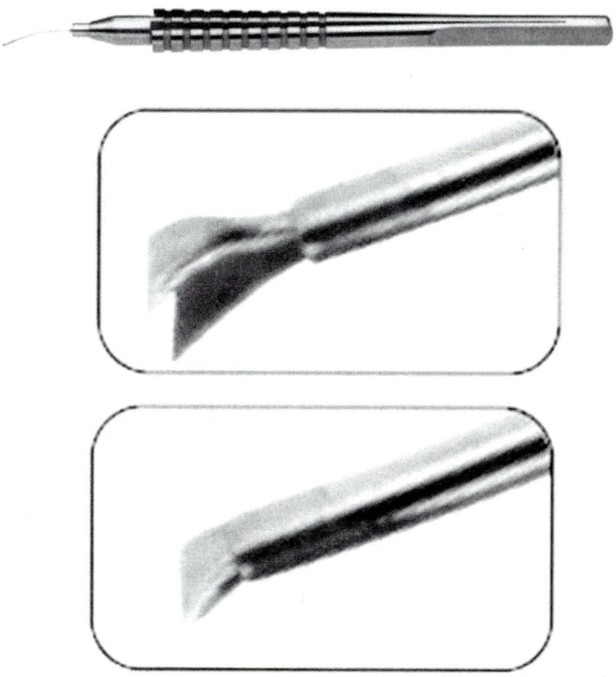

Figure 2.7: ASICO (Westmont, Illinois): Fine-Ikeda forceps

CAPSULORHEXIS

Following incision construction, we exchange aqueous for viscoelastic (Viscoat, Alcon Laboratories, Fort Worth, Texas) by injecting viscoelastic into the distal angle through one of the micro-incisions which allows for extrusion of aqueous and allows us to achieve a stable anterior chamber. We then perform a capsulorhexis utilizing one of several instruments. We have strong preferences for the MicroSurgical Technology (Redmond, Washington) Fine-Hoffman Capsulorhexis forceps (Figure 2.6), the Fine-Ikeda forceps by ASICO (Westmont, Illinois) (Figure 2.7), or the Fine capsulorhexis forceps by Katena (Denville, New Jersey). Each of these allows us to make a very precise capsulorhexis through a 1 mm incision and the MicroSurgical Technology (Redmond, Washington) instrument allows for exchanging the capsulorhexis forceps for intraocular scissors or intraocular tying forceps as each type can snap on and off the same handle.

It is interesting that the size and shape of these capsulorhexes are much more accurate than they were with traditional capsulorhexis forceps through a 2.5 mm incision. We believe this is due to the fact that one cannot use the wrist in making a capsulorhexis through a micro-incision and so we are limited to just finger movements. This is analogous to the accuracy with which we write when we rest our wrist and use only our fingers compared to using both our fingers and wrist in the use of a fountain pen. We aim for a round capsulorhexis sized between 4.5 and 5.5 mm in diameter.

HYDRODISSECTION AND HYDRODELINEATION

We perform cortical cleaving hydrodissection in 100 percent of our cases.[9] One does not have to remove viscoelastic when injecting through these micro-incisions because a little bit of posterior pressure on the incision will allow egress of some of the viscoelastic during the cortical cleaving hydrostep. Following cortical cleaving hydrodissection we spin the lens to be sure that the cortical connections to the capsule have been severed, after which we then do two hydrodelineation injections as we have previously described.[9] We then rock the nucleus from side to side to be sure that we have severed the epinuclear-endonuclear connections.

CHOPPING

We allow for continuous flow throughout the procedure including flow when inserting the chopper. The irrigating chopper is held vertically and the tip is inserted beyond the internal lip of the incision, the handle is rotated horizontally and the open end of the chopper is brought into the eye (Figure 2.8) This prevents snagging of Descemet's membrane. For horizontal chopping maneuvers we have a strong preference for the choppers we designed in conjunction with MicroSurgical Technology (Redmond, Washington), all of which are front irrigating

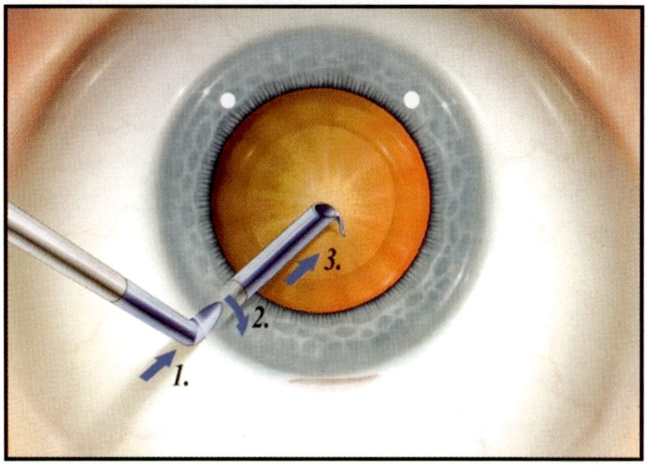

Figure 2.8: Demonstration of vertical chopper being inserted into the eye. Image provided by MicroSurgical Technology (Redmond, Washington)

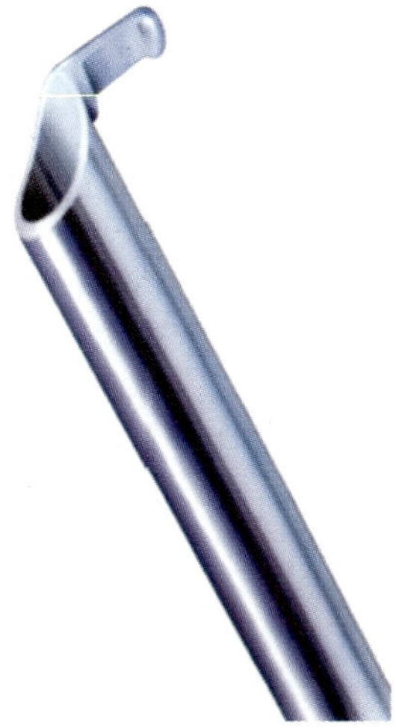
Figure 2.9: MicroSurgical Technology (Redmond, Washington): Fine horizontal chopper

so they deepen the anterior chamber as soon as the open end touches the micro-incision thus avoiding injury to intraocular structures. Also, the irrigation remains constant in direction with rotation of the instrument during the operation. The maneuvers utilized in this technique are exactly the same with an irrigating instrument that we have described previously in our paper on the use of power modulations and the choo-choo chop and flip technique.[10] We utilize horizontal chopping for softer nuclei, grades 1 or 2+ and vertical chopping for nuclei of grades 3 and 4+. We have designed chopping instruments with MicroSurgical Technology (Redmond, Washington) (Figures 2.9 and 2.10), Katena (Denville, New Jersey) (Figure 2.11), Rhein Medical (Tampa, Florida) and ASICO (Westmont,

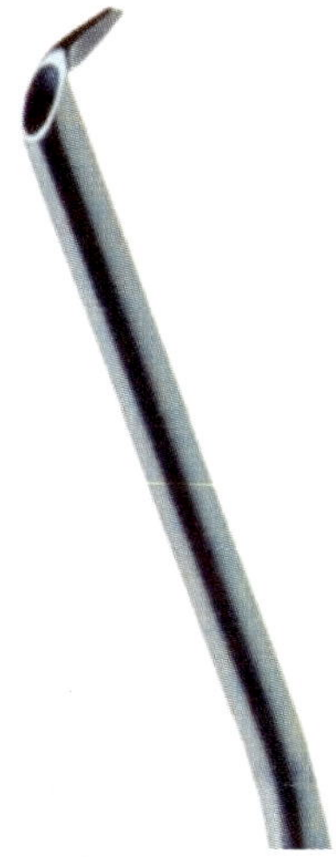

Figure 2.10: MicroSurgical Technology (Redmond, Washington): Fine-Olson vertical chopper

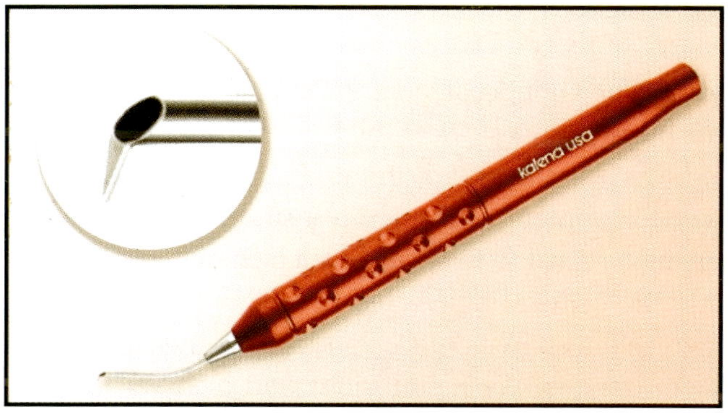

Figure 2.11: Katena (Denville, New Jersey): Irrigating chopper

Illinois). They all work very well. We went through many prototypes in the development of the choppers produced by MicroSurgical Technology (Redmond, Washington). These have some unique advantages in that they are thin-walled and short so that there is a decreased resistance to flow through them and they are bent slightly so that the placement of the micro-incisions, which force us to work over the brow and check, does not necessitate an upward pull on our instrumentation in order to get over the brow or check.

PHACOEMULSIFICATION (PLEASE REVIEW ENCLOSED CD)

We have been able to perform bimanual micro-incision phacoemulsification with most of the machines available in America and Tables 2.1 to 2.5 show the optimized phacoemulsification parameters and power modulations that we prefer.

Table 2.1: I Howard Fine, MD: parameters for bimanual phaco infiniti™

	Chop	*Epinucleus*
Power % linear	35 Linear	15
Flow	36 Fixed	35 Linear
Modulation	50pps, 35% on, Neo: Amp 20 Threshold 5	30pps, 25% No Neo
Vacuum	360 fixed Dynamic Rise 1	300 linear No dynamic rise
Bottle height (cm)	110	110

Table 2.2: I Howard Fine, MD: parameters for bimanual phaco legacy®

	Chop	*Epinucleus*
Power % Linear	40	15
Flow	32	32 (linear)
Modulation	NeoSoniX, 2 pps. Ampl. 80% Threshold 15%	NeoSoniX Burse, 30 msec. Amplitude 40%
Vacuum (mm Hg)	220 (linear)	220
Bottle height (cm)	132	132

Table 2.3: I Howard Fine, MD: parameters for bimanual phaco millennium®

	Chop	*Epinucleus*
Power %	15 Fixed	0-3 Linear
Flow cc/min	46 Fixed	38 Fixed
Modulation (Pulse: pps or burst)	Burst 200 ms	Pulses 3/sec.
Vacuum (mm Hg) linear yaw	220 (linear)	220
Infusion pressure	35	35
Bottle height (cm)	132	132

Table 2.4: I Howard Fine, MD: parameters for bimanual phaco sovereign® with WhiteStar technology

	Chop	*Trim*	*Flip*
Power % linear	40	20	20
Flow Unocc/ occlude (panel except where indicated)	36	22/16	24/16
Modulation WhiteStar	CL	CL	CL
Vacuum (mm Hg) Unocc/ occlude	350 (panel)	200/50 (linear)	200/80 (linear)
Ramp (%)	30	30	30
Bottle height (inches)	38	38	38

Table 2.5: I Howard Fine, MD parameters for bimanual phaco STAAR wave

	Chop	*Trim*	*Flip*
Power %	55 Linear	20 Linear	55
Flow	30	23	26
Modulation	Sonic Random 2	Sonic pulses	Sonic per second
Vacuum (mm Hg)	500	300	200
Bottle height (inches)	45	45	45

The major difference between coaxial phacoemulsification and bimanual micro-incision phacoemulsification resides in the way in which the instruments are coordinated. In coaxial phacoemulsification, we tend to use our second hand instrument, the chopper, very close to the phaco tip, sometimes being a little below it, sometimes a little above, but most frequently just directly in front of it. We have to be very careful in bimanual micro-incision phacoemulsification to not irrigate material purchased at the phaco tip off the tip by the incoming stream of fluid. As a result we tend to work with our phaco tip slightly below and behind the chopper and can approach it from below and behind as we need to use the chopper (Figure 2.12) Our chop maneuvers are those previously described. For horizontal chopping, we touch the center of the endonucleus and with the vertical element of the chop instrument in a vertical orientation, slide it to the distal left periphery until it drops into the golden ring created by hydro delineation. We then lift the endonucleus up and toward the incision and then, using power modulations and high vacuum, we imbed the phaco tip. Once the tip is imbedded, we draw the chop instrument toward the side of the phaco tip and then separate our hands with a little downward force on the chop instrument and an upward force on the phaco tip. This results in a complete division of the endonucleus to hemi-nuclei. We then rotate clockwise and in a similar manner, chop the second hemi-nucleus. At the completion of the second chop, we have a pie-shaped segment that is attached to the phaco tip in its bevel down configuration and we can mobilize it, if it is soft enough, or chop it a second time to reduce the size of the pie-shaped segment.

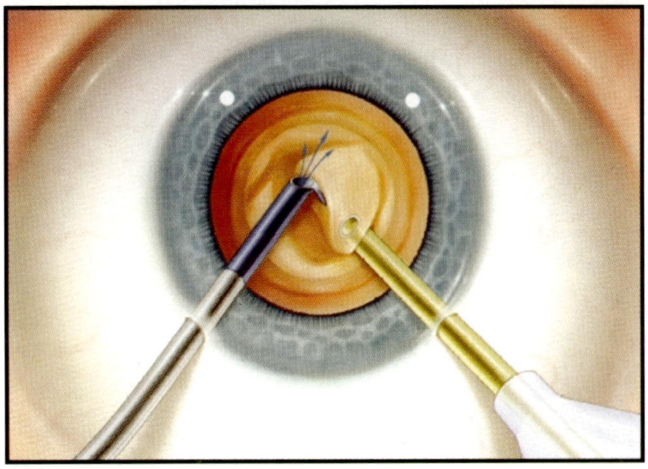

Figure 2.12: Demonstration of working with the phaco tip slightly below and behind the chopper. Image provided by MicroSurgical Technology (Redmond, Washington)

For vertical chopping, we imbed the phaco tip first and then drive the vertical chop instrument diagonally down-ward above the phaco tip and then separate our hands with a little upward movement of the phaco tip and a downward diagonal movement of the chop instrument. This usually results in an immediate division of the endonucleus into two. We then rotate it in such a way as to purchase the largest hemi-nucleus for rechopping and then, once again with the second chop, we have a pie-shaped segment attached to the phaco tip, which can be mobilized or chopped in additional time.

We have not found utilizing the parameters in the above tables that we have had any problems with any of the instrumentation herein described with respect to maintaining a stable anterior chamber. In fact, we have found our chamber to be very much more stable than with coaxial phacoemulsification.

In some instances in which during the procedure we have blown a hole in the posterior capsule with the phaco tip, we have been able to continue the procedure by maintaining irrigation high in the anterior chamber and reaching down into the capsular bag to mobilize nuclear material. This would be impossible with coaxial phacoemulsification because as we brought the phaco tip down, we would be bringing a forceful stream of fluid with fluctuating direction into the capsular bag which would almost certainly extend any pre-existing tear.

We chop the endonucleus as previously described and then mobilize epinucleus at the level of the capsulorhexis. We have a very strong preference for straight, 30 degree phacoemulsification tips used bevel down. The bevel down configuration has several advantages. The approach to the endonucleus through a clear corneal incision is approximately 30 degrees so with the 30 degree bevel down tip, as soon as we touch the endonucleus we can begin to evoke vacuum which helps us bury the tip and to stabilize the nuclear material. Second, all of the energy, both ultrasound and cavitational, is directed toward the nucleus rather than toward the corneal endothelium or the trabecular meshwork. Finally, we can mobilize nuclear material from the level of the capsulorhexis up rather than having to go deeply into the endolenticular space to achieve mobilization of these pie-shaped segments.

When all of the endonucleus has been removed, we then turn the chop element on our chopper horizontally and rotate the phacoemulsification needle to a bevel up position in order to mobilize the epinucleus. This has previously been described.[10] We rotate the epinucleus with the phaco tip in zero foot position, rather than with the chop instrument in order to provide added safety.

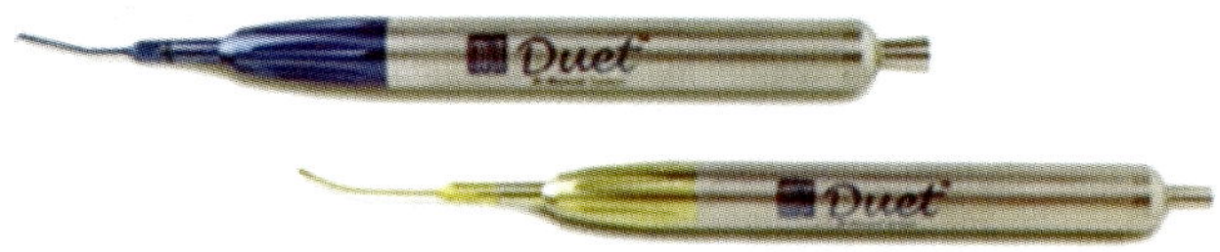

Figure 2.13: MicroSurgical Technology (Redmond, Washington) Duet bimanual irrigation and aspiration instrumentation

This is analogous to the way we rotated nuclear material in the days of one-handed phacoemulsification with the phacoemulsification tip in either foot position zero or foot position one.[10] After we trim and flip the epinucleus, we then will remove our instruments and bring a straight irrigating handpiece through the left incision and an aspirating instrument through the right. We prefer the MicroSurgical Technology (Redmond, Washington) bimanual irrigation and aspiration instrumentation and feel that it is extremely important that the port be highly polished (Figure 2.13). We are aware that those made by Mastel (Rapid City, South Dakota), Rhein Medical (Tampa, Florida), ASICO (Westmont, Illinois), and Katena (Denville, New Jersey) all work very well. We usually use a 0.2 mm aspiration port because following cortical cleaving hydrodissection, most of the cortex is removed and what is left are wispy strands which occlude a 0.2 mm aspiration tip much better than a .3mm aspiration tip. After polishing the posterior capsule and removing residual cortex, we then remove the aspirator and inject viscoelastic prior to removing the irrigator.

STROMAL HYDRATION AND IOL IMPLANTATION

We can then stromally hydrate the two side-port incisions and make an incision between them for the implantation of our IOL. We don't enlarge one of the micro-incisions for IOL implantation because the manipulation through these incisions distorts them somewhat and they seal less well if we enlarge them. For most IOLs we use a 2.7 to 2.8 mm wide incision that is 2 mm long. Some IOLs require larger incisions and we use a trapezoidal knife, the Rhein (Tampa, Florida) 3D diamond blade for all of these incisions. After implantation of the IOL we usually perform coaxial removal of viscoelastic in front of and behind the IOL and then do stromal hydration on both side-port incisions as well as the implantation incision.

Table 2.6: Comparison of outcome results bimanual vs. coaxial data

Percentage of Eyes with Clear Corneas 2-24 Hours Post-op

Chi-Square analyses on all machines indicate no significant differences between coaxial and bimanual phaco in percentage of patients with clear corneas.

Machine	*Coaxial Results*	*Bimanual Results*
Legacy with NeoSoniX	98%	100%
Millennium with Phaco Burst	100%	100%
STAAR Sonic/Ultrasonic Wave	95%	100%
Sovereign with WhiteStar	100%	97%

p > .05 for all comparisons

Table 2.7: Comparison of outcome results bimanual vs. coaxial data

Percentage of Eyes with UCVA of 20/40 or Better 2-24 Hours Post-op

Chi-Square analysis indicates that the STAAR Sonic Wave showed significant improvement in UCVA with bimanual over coaxial phaco.

All other analyses indicate no other significant differences between coaxial and bimanual phaco in percentage of patients with a UCVA of 20/40 or better.

Machine	*Coaxial Results*	*Bimanual Results*
Legacy with NeoSoniX	96%	93%
Millennium with Phaco Burst	100%	95%
STAAR Sonic/Ultrasonic Wave*	**74%**	**100%**
Sovereign with WhiteStar	94%	95%

*p < .01

We continue to test all incisions utilizing fluorescein dye and pressure on the incision to document that sealing has been achieved after stromal hydration and reconstitution of the anterior chamber with Miochol to bring the pupil down and allow for immediate clear vision.

BIMANUAL MICRO-INCISION PHACOEMULSIFICATION

The results of our bimanual compared to coaxial phacoemulsification are seen in tables (Tables 2.6 and 2.7) We see that in all instances they were the same. There was no statistically significant difference in any of these results compared to coaxial phacoemulsification with the possible exception of the STAAR Wave system. This result may have been due to that we combined within these techniques the use of both sonic and ultrasonic depending on the density of the particular portion of the nucleus on which we were working and that combination seems to have advantages over either the ultrasound or sonic system alone.

We believe bimanual micro-incision phacoemulsification represents the future of cataract surgery and refractive lens exchange. We know there will soon be available small incision lenses that will go through these micro-incisions and the full promise of increasingly smaller incisions will be realized.

REFERENCES

1. Shearing SP, Relyea RL, Loaiza A, Shearing RL. Routine phacoemulsification through a one-millimeter non-sutured incision. Cataract 1985;2(2):6-10.
2. Hara T, Hara T. Endocapsular phacoemulsification and aspiration (ECPEA) – recent surgical technique and clinical results. Ophthalmic Surgery 1989; 20(7):469-75.
3. Agarwal A, Agarwal S, Agarwal A. No anesthesia cataract surgery. In Agarwal S, et al. Phacoemulsification, Laser Cataract Surgery, and Foldable IOLs. New Dehli, India, Jaypee Brothers; 1998;144-54.
4. Tseunoka H, Shiba T, Takahashi Y. Feasibility of ultrasound cataract surgery with a 1.4 mm incision. J Cataract Refract Surg 2001;27:934-40.
5. Olson RJ. Microphaco chop. In Chang D, (Ed). Phaco Chop: Mastering Techniques, Optimizing Technology, and Avoiding Complications. Thorofare, NJ, SLACK Inc. 2004;227-37.
6. Chang D. Bimanual phaco chop. In Chang D, (Ed). Phaco Chop: Mastering Techniques, Optimizing Technology, and Avoiding Complications. Thorofare, NJ, SLACK Inc. 2004;239-50.
7. Alio J. What does MICS require. In Alio J. MICS. Panama: Highlights of Ophthalmology; 2004;1.
8. Fine IH, Hoffman RS, Packer M. Optimizing refractive lens exchange with bimanual microincision phacoemulsification. J Cataract Refract Surg 2004;30:550-4.
9. Fine IH, Packer M, Hoffman RS. Hydrodissection and hydrodelineation. In Steinert R, Fine IH, Gimbel HV, Koch DD, Lindstrom RL, Neuhann TF, et al (Eds). Cataract Surgery: Technique, Complications and Management, 2nd edition, Saunders, Philadelphia, PA, 2004.
10. Fine IH, Packer M, Hoffman RS. Use of power modulations in phacoemulsification: Choo-choo chop and flip phacoemulsification. J Cataract Refract Surg February 2001; 27(2):188-97.

3

Minimally Invasive Bimanual Phaco Surgery and Foldable IOL

- **BASIC RESEARCH ON MICROINCISION CATARACT SURGERY USING PHACO MACHINES**
- **CLINICAL RESULTS OF MICROINCISION BIMANUAL PHACO SURGERY**
- **IOL INSERTION THROUGH THE SMALLEST FEASIBLE INCISION**

Hiroshi Tsuneoka (Japan)

INTRODUCTION

The spread of phacoemulsification technique and the advent of foldable intraocular lenses (IOLs) have been accompanied by dramatic advances in the field of cataract surgery. However, a number of problems remain to be resolved. One of these problems involves the need for minimally invasive surgery. At present, cataract surgery can be performed through an incision of 3 to 4 mm, and surgical procedures are under development which will make it possible to not only remove the clouded lens through a micro incision of approximately 1.0 mm, but also to insert the IOL without enlarging that incision.

Regarding lens extraction, considerable attention has been directed in recent years to new emulsification and aspiration techniques using the erbium YAG laser and the neodymium YAG laser. This technology provides numerous advantages, including the absence of heat generated during phacoemulsification and minimal invasiveness of the cornea or the capsular bag, and is expected to drive the next generation of cataract surgery technology.[1] However, it is not yet widely used because it currently takes longer than phacoemulsification for nucleus removal. In contrast to the phaco equipment which is in wide use today, laser phaco machines still have considerable room for improvement before the technology will be fully matured, so we expect that it will be some time yet before these procedures become widely available.

Since 1999 I have been studying the use of ultrasonic phacoemulsification, a mature technology with highly reliable equipment, for lens extraction through a micro incision. I have used this equipment to perform basic research on lens extraction through an incision of 1.4 mm or less.[2] The present article will address micro incision cataract surgery using surgical equipment, surgical techniques, and IOL materials which are widely available today.

BASIC RESEARCH ON MICROINCISION CATARACT SURGERY USING PHACO MACHINES

Use of the Sleeveless Phaco Tip Enables Ultrasmall Incision Cataract Surgery

In ordinary ultrasonic phacoemulsification, the phaco tip is equipped with an infusion sleeve. In order to reduce incision size, it has been necessary to decrease the outer diameter of the infusion sleeve. Phaco machines in current use require an incision of at least 2.6 mm even when using a thin phaco tip. In order to successfully utilize surgical incisions of less than 2.0 mm, the infusion sleeve must be removed to leave the sleeveless phaco tip, with infusion provided through a side port.

In order to use the sleeveless tip safely it is necessary to ensure that adequate infusion is provided through the side port, that the phaco tip does not overheat during emulsification and aspiration, and that there is no deformation of the incision due to movement of the tip.

History of Phacoemulsification Using a Sleeveless Phaco Tip

In 1984, Hara and colleagues began using a sleeveless phaco tip in intracapsular phacoemulsification and aspiration for lens refilling.[3] The technology attracted considerable attention, particularly in the United States, but procedures for lens emulsification and aspiration at that time were quite difficult and no suitable lens refilling material was available, so the method was never widely adopted.

15 years later, in 1999, I began working with bimanual phacoemulsification using a sleeveless phaco tip in order to reduce incision size during cataract surgery. I first performed basic research to make sure that the surgery would be safe, determining the feasibility of bimanual nucleofractis with infusion through a side port, establishing methods for ensuring adequate infusion flow volume, and investigating techniques to prevent thermal burn and deformation at the incision site. I then applied these findings in a clinical setting to develop procedures for lens extraction through a 1.2 to 1.4 mm incision.[2]

Prior to this, in 1998 Agarwal and colleagues reported[4] successful lens extraction through a 0.9 mm incision using the Phakonit method with a sleeveless phaco tip. Under this method thermal burn is avoided by providing external irrigation of the incision through which the ultrasound probe is inserted.

At almost the same time Crozafon reported the successful use of a sleeveless 21-gauge Teflon-coated tip for minimally invasive bimanual phacoemulsification through a 0.9 mm incision. Crozafon felt that thermal burn could be prevented by coating the phaco tip with Teflon, which has poor thermal connectivity.

In 2002 Olson and colleagues reported[5] the feasibility of phacoemulsification through a 1.0 mm incision using the new phaco machine, Sovereign (AMO) with White Star software. They found that tip heating could be minimized by setting the machine for hyper-pulse mode so that ultrasound was generated for extremely short intervals.

In my microincision cataract surgery I use a relatively large incision of 1.2 to 1.4 mm. I find that when the incision is slightly larger than the phaco tip the tip can be cooled by the leakage of infusion solution through the incision, and the extra-space also prevents deformation at the incision site due to tip movement.

Problems Related to Phacoemulsification with a Sleeveless Tip

Major problems when using a sleeveless tip for phacoemulsification include thermal burn at the incision site because of overheating of the phaco tip, and destabilization of the anterior chamber due to inadequate infusion flow. Also, the necessity of providing infusion through the side port means that the traditional nucleofractis hook cannot be used. Many surgeons have been particularly concerned that ultrasound waves through the sleeveless tip could cause a sudden rise in tip temperature, resulting in thermal burn at the incision site, and that the sleeveless phaco tip would therefore be unfeasible for emulsification of hard nuclei where the tip is sometimes fully occluded. To resolve these concerns, my colleagues and I measured incision site temperature in postmortem porcine eyes during phacoemulsification with full occlusion of the phaco tip. Our experiments confirmed the absence of thermal burn when using a 20-gauge sleeveless phaco tip through an incision made by a 19-gauge microvitroretinal (MVR) blade. We also modified a 20-gauge infusion cannula and inserted it through a side port created with a 20-gauge MVR. The cannula modifications ensured adequate infusion flow, stabilizing the anterior chamber, and also made it possible to use the infusion cannula as a nucleofractis hook. This allowed us to safely emulsify and aspirate nuclei with conventional bimanual nucleofractis techniques, and enabled us to confirm the feasibility and safety of phacoemulsification through an incision of 1.2 to 1.4 mm using familiar techniques and widely available surgical equipment.[2]

Avoid Thermal Burn and Injury at the Incision Site: Widen the Incision by 1 gauge

My colleagues and I believed that if the incision was made slightly wider than the outer diameter of the phaco tip, the tip would be satisfactorily cooled by the leakage of infusion solution through the incision, preventing thermal burn at the incision site. To test this hypothesis we measured temperature at the incision site in postmortem porcine eyes during phacoemulsification.

The phacoemulsification device used in our experiments was the Alcon Legacy 20000® with a 20-gauge Kelman phaco tip. Temperature at the incision site was measured with a sheathed thermocouple Model TSC-K0.3 manufactured by Toa Electric Co., Ltd., and a thermometer Model AR5757-F00 manufactured by Chino Co., Ltd.

We created a corneal incision in the postmortem porcine eye using a 19-gauge (1.4 mm) MVR. We also used the MVR to create a tunnel in the cornea above the incision and parallel to it. We inserted the thermocouple electrode of the thermometer through that tunnel, and performed 3 measurements of temperature elevation at the corneal incision during ultrasound oscillation with the phaco tip fully occluded (Figure 3.1). We used a clamp to close the aspiration tube so that aspiration pressure was 0 mmHg during ultrasonic wave generation.

We inserted a sleeveless 20-gauge Kelman phaco tip through the 19-gauge incision and a 20-gauge infusion cannula through the corneal side port. The phaco tip was pressed against the incision, and ultrasound waves were generated continuously for 2 minutes at 80 percent ultrasound power. Our results showed a mean temperature elevation of 8.4°C. At no time during the procedure did the temperature at the incision site exceed 40°C, and no thermal burn was observed (Figure 3.2B).

When the phaco tip is not fully occluded in PEA, the tip lumen and outer wall are bathed in infusion solution, so that even when friction develops there is a sufficient

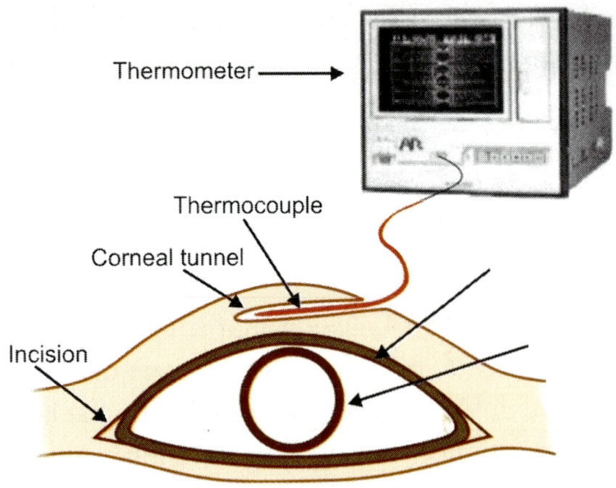

Figure 3.1: Method for measuring temperature at the incision site.

The thermocouple is inserted into a tunnel created in the cornea above the incision site, and temperature at the incision site is measured with ultrasound in operation

flow of infusion solution to cool the tip. However, in phacoemulsification with full occlusion the infusion solution is ordinarily unable to circulate within the phaco tip, so the amount of infusion solution in contact with the outer wall of the tip is limited to the volume of solution passing through the incision site. During fully occluded nucleofractis with a phaco tip equipped with an infusion sleeve, there is a decrease in the volume of infusion solution flowing around the tip. If the tip should press against the incision wall under these circumstances, the infusion solution may not provide sufficient cooling to compensate for the friction heat generated by the tip and sleeve. This can result in the development of thermal burn at the incision site (Figures 3.2A and 3.3A). However, when using a sleeveless phaco tip in an incision which is slightly larger than the tip itself, there is

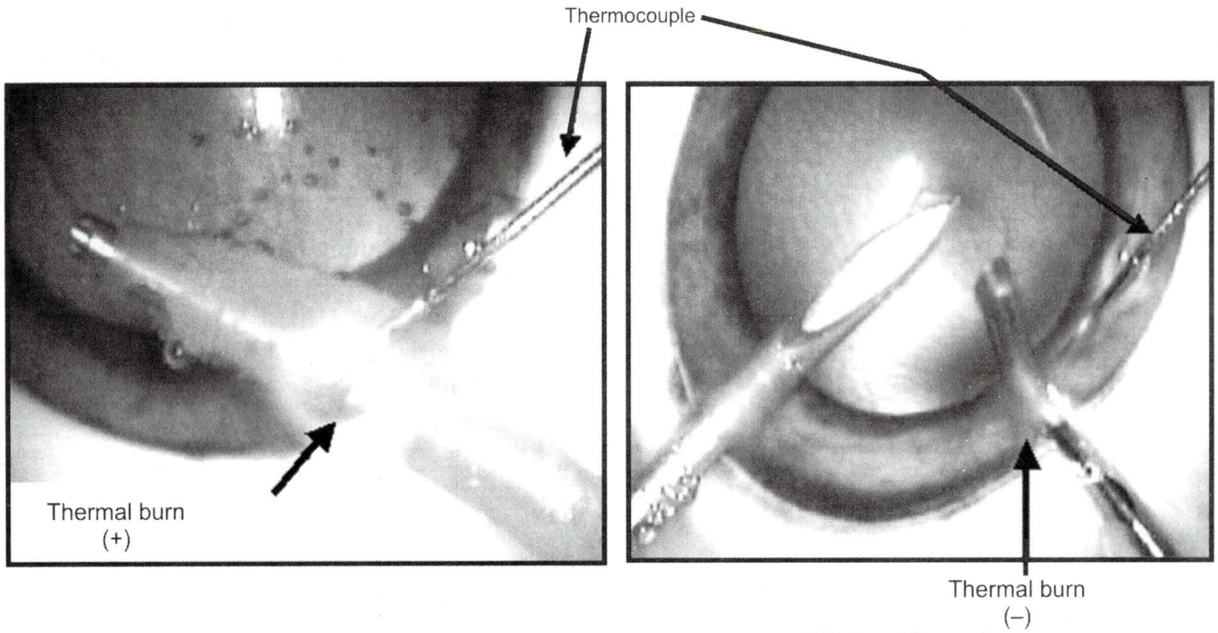

Figures 3.2A and B: Using a thermometer to measure temperature at the incision site in postmortem porcine eyes

Phaco machine setting : Aspiration port occluded (aspiration pressure:0 mm Hg)

US power : 80 percent, Ultrasound duration = 2.0 minutes continuous

A. (Left) A 20-gauge Kelman phaco tip with the infusion sleeve was inserted through a 3.0 mm incision, and ultrasound were operated.

Temperature at the incision site rose only slightly while the tip was kept from pressing on the incision wall. But, once the tip was pressed against the incision wall during ultrasound operation, the temperature at the incision site rose significantly and a thermal burn developed.

B. (Right) A 20-gauge Kelman phaco tip without the infusion sleeve was inserted through a 19-gauge incision, and US were operated.

Temperature did not rise at the incision site even when the tip was pressed against the incision, and no thermal burn developed

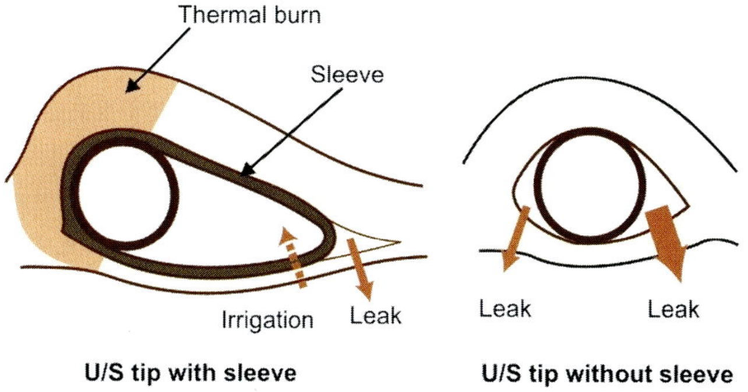

Figures 3.3A and B: Flow dynamics of infusion solution around the phaco tip when the opening of the phaco tip was closed during occlusion mode

A. (Left) Emulsification and aspiration following insertion of a sleeved phaco tip through a 3.0-mm incision.
Because the sleeve is deformed by contact with the incision, leakage volume through the incision is low. During phaco tip fully occluded in phacoemulsification, the flow of infusion solution around the phaco tip within the infusion sleeve is also low.
When the phaco tip pressed against the incision wall, friction heat develops between the phaco tip and the sleeve. Because there is insufficient infusion solution flowing around the tip to provide cooling, the heat is transmitted to tissues at the incision site. Thermal burn develops at the incision.

B. (Right) Emulsification and aspiration following insertion of a sleeveless 20-gauge phaco tip through a 19-gauge (1.4-mm) incision.
Because the phaco tip is not deformed by passage through the incision, there is space between the tip and the incision. Thus the maximum possible volume of infusion solution is available to flow around the tip, providing cooling for any friction between the tip and the incision tissue. No thermal burn develops at the incision site

still considerable leakage of infusion solution through the incision site even during fully occluded phacoemulsification when the tip may be moved in multiple directions and pressed against the incision in order to emulsify the nucleus. This leakage of infusion solution provides sufficient cooling of any friction heat which may develop between the tip and the surrounding tissue, making it possible to emulsify and aspirate the nucleus without the occurrence of thermal burn and without resorting to Teflon-coated phaco tips or ultrasonic wave-control technology (Figure 3.3B). By implementing this technique, thermal burn is less likely to occur when using a sleeveless tip than when using a tip equipped with the infusion sleeve.

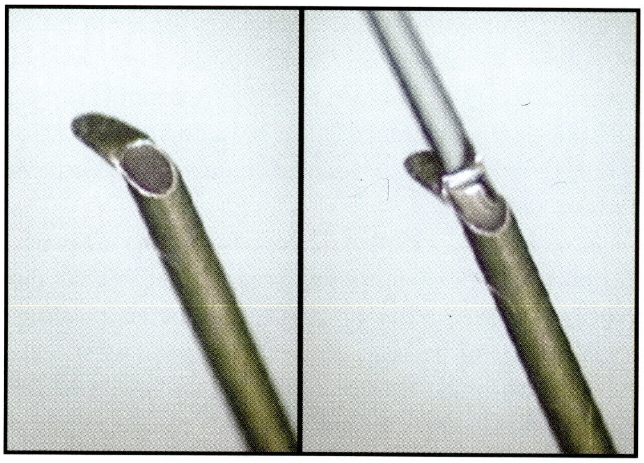

Figure 3.4: The 20-gauge Tsuneoka irrigation chopper from MicroSurgical Technology
My Irrigating Chopper manufactured by MicroSurgical Technology has a large opening at the cannula tip, so we can maintain a sufficient infusion flow with the infusion bottle at 75 cm. Front opening irrigating chopper can avoid the collapse even when the irrigating chopper is pulled back to the insertion site. Also, we can use a strong flow of liquid from the chopper tip to push down the posterior capsule

When we perform bimanual phaco surgery, one of the main points in our surgical technique involves the use of an incision which is 1 gauge larger than the outer diameter of the phaco tip. This means that the incision for a 20-gauge phaco tip is made using a 19-gauge (1.4 mm) MVR, and for a 21-gauge phaco tip we used a 20-gauge (1.2 mm) MVR. The slight space between the phaco tip and the incision wall prevents deformation and injury at the incision site due to movement of the phaco tip.

Tools for Successful Bimanual PEA: the 20-gauge Irrigating Chopper (Figure 3.4)

The goal of bimanual phaco surgery is to remove the nucleus through the smallest feasible incision. In addition, it is desirable to use only a single corneal side port, and to make that port as small as possible also. Creating a third incision for the nucleofractis hook would run counter to the objectives of this surgical technique. With that in mind, we experimented with a bend in the tip of the infusion cannula. This resulted in the production of irrigating chopper having nearly the same shape as conventional nucleofractis hooks. When using the infusion cannula as a chopper, considerations of intraocular operability dictate that instrument size not exceed 20 gauge. However, an ordinary cannula having a 20-gauge outer diameter would have an inner diameter of only 0.6 mm, making it difficult to guarantee adequate infusion volume.

In order to supplement infusion flow using 20-gauge irrigating chopper, surgeons sometimes elevate the infusion bottle to a height of 100 centimeters or more, or pressurize the infusion bottle. However, if we elevate the infusion bottle that high, intraocular pressure will exceed 50 millimeters of mercury. This can damage the optic nerve if surgery is prolonged. Also, higher infusion pressure means greater outflow of liquid through the incision where the phaco tip is inserted. This can cause small nuclear fragments to collect at the phaco tip insertion site, which makes phacoemulsification more troublesome.

In order to maintain infusion flow without elevating intraocular pressure, we need to select an appropriate irrigating chopper. There are now many commercially available options, but only a few provide an adequate and reliable flow of infusion solution. Selecting a suitable irrigating chopper is vital for achieving good results. My Irrigating Choppers from Micro Surgical Technology and ASICO have a large opening at the cannula tip, so I can maintain an infusion flow of more than 45 ml/min with the infusion bottle at 75 centimeters. Also, we can direct a strong flow of liquid from the chopper tip down onto the posterior capsule. This prevents surge-induced capsule rupture.

CLINICAL RESULTS OF MICROINCISION BIMANUAL PHACO SURGERY

Results from our experiments indicated that thermal burn could be prevented by obtaining sufficient leakage through the incision, and that the irrigating chopper can be used to emulsify and aspirate nucleus while maintaining stable anterior chamber depth. In October 1999, I began applying these procedures to micro incision phaco surgery in human patients.

Procedures for Microincision Bimanual Phaco Surgery[6]

After the eye is anesthetized, I make an incision from the temporal clear cornea into the anterior chamber. I use a 1.4 mm keratome or 19-gauge MVR for a 20-gauge phaco tip (Figure 3.5A). The incision is approximately 0.9 mm in length. I also create the infusion side port at a desirable location on the clear cornea, using a same keratome. Sitting at the patient's head, the surgeon positions the side port at eleven o'clock for the left eye or at one o'clock for the right eye.

Injecting a viscoelastic material into the anterior chamber, I use a 26-gauge needle to perform continuous curvilinear capsulorrhexis with a diameter of approximately 5.0 mm, and then initiate hydrodissection. In order to prevent an abrupt rise in anterior chamber pressure, it is important to press the base of the hydrodissection needle firmly against the lower side of the incision so that excess fluid can leak out of the incision while injection is in process.

I insert the Tsuneoka Irrigating Chopper through the side port and the sleeveless phaco tip through the temporal corneal incision, and emulsify and aspirate the lens while using the tip of the cannula for nucleofractis (Figure 3.5B). When I am working on the right eye I hold the irrigating chopper in the left hand and the ultrasound probe in the right hand, and when working on the left eye I do the reverse, with the irrigating chopper in the right hand and the ultrasound probe in the left hand.

In minimally invasive bimanual phaco surgery, I recommend the Trench Divide and Conquer (or Stop and Chop) method for a normal nucleus, and the Crater and Vertical Chop method for a very hard nucleus. With these techniques, phacoemulsification is started without completely occluding the phaco tip in a hard section of the nucleus. So even if we increase the ultrasound power, there is no risk of thermal burn. There is also less dispersion of hard nuclear fragments into the anterior chamber. There is not much movement of the large irrigating chopper. So the procedure is surgeon friendly, and there is less injury at the chopper insertion site.

For a nucleus of ordinary hardness, I usually dig a deep trench and then divide the nucleus (Figure 3.5B). After the nucleus is divided in half, I set the aspiration flow rate at 24 milliliters per minute, maximum aspiration pressure at 160 to 180 millimeters of mercury, and bottle height at 75 centimeters (Figure 3.5C). After the nucleus

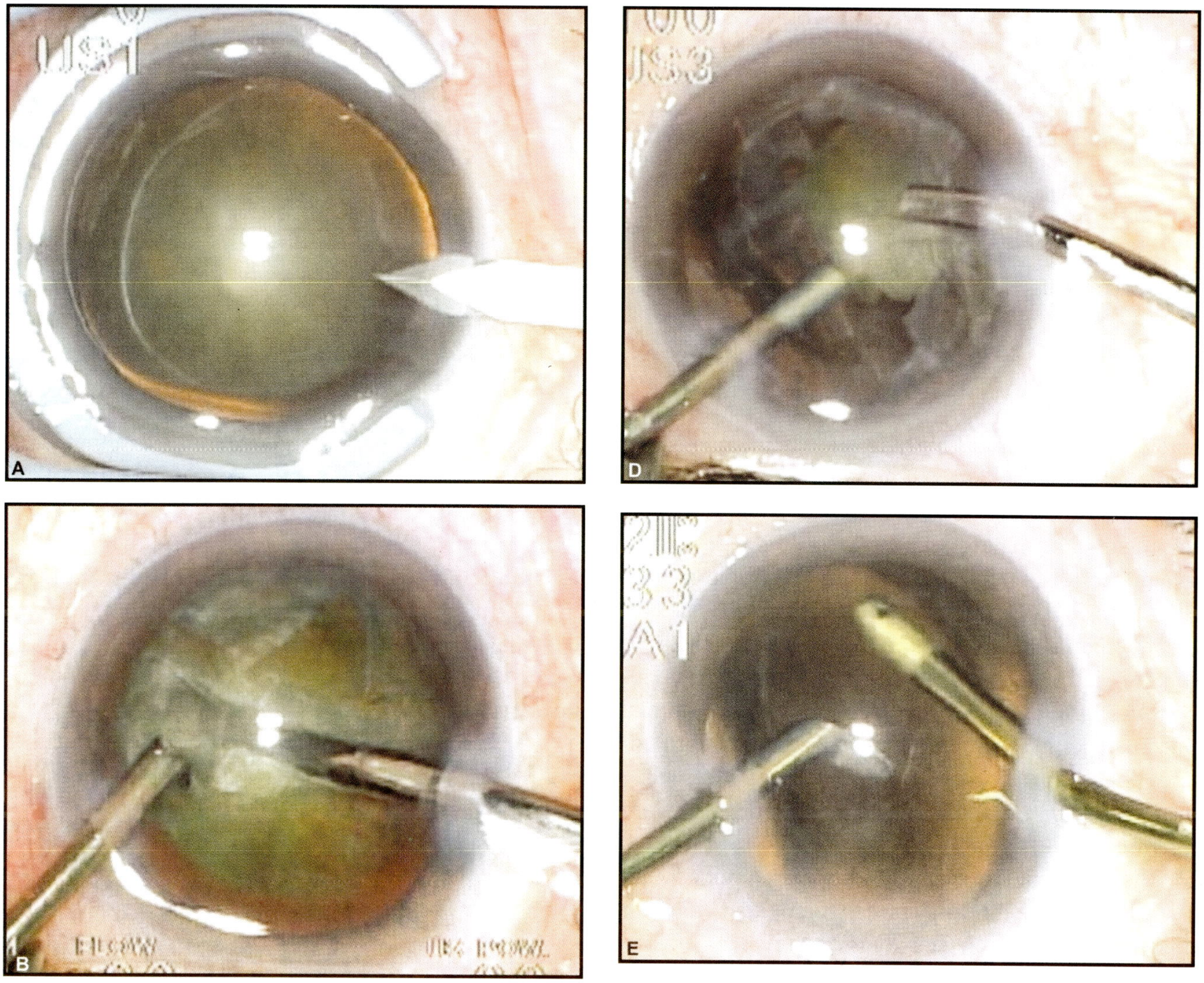

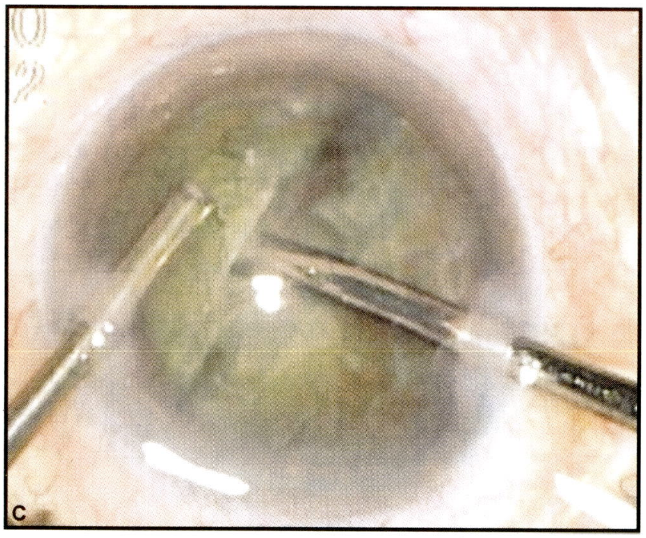

Figures 3.5A to E: Ultrasmall incision (1.4 mm) bimanual phaco surgery

- **A.** A temporal corneal incision is made using a 19-gauge MVR or a 1.4 mm keratome.
- **B.** A 20-gauge sleeveless phaco tip is inserted into the anterior chamber through a 1.4 mm incision and a 20-gauge Tsuneoka irrigating chopper is inserted through a side port. Phacoemulsification is performed using bimanual nucleofractis technique.
- **C.** Vertical chop is performed with mode 2 after the nucleus is divided in half.
- **D.** After the nucleus is divided into quarters and each nuclear fragment can move freely, aspiration pressure is decreased. Strong flow from irrigating chopper can press down the posterior capsule, which prevents surge-induced posterior capsule rupture.
- **E.** Residual cortex is aspirated using a sleeveless I/A tip or 20-gauge bimanual I/A tip through the side port

Table 3.1: Parameters of aspiration in bimanual phaco surgery with 20-gauge phaco tip

[Mode]	Asp. flow rate (ml/min)	Max. asp. pressure (mm Hg)	Bottle height (cm)
Case of ordinary hardness			
1. Trenching	10-20	30-60	75
2. Vertical Chop	24	160-180	75
3. Free nuclear fragments	22	140	75-85
Case of extremely hardness			
1. Crater	10-20	30-60	75
2. Vertical Chop	25	250	75
3. Free nuclear fragments	22	140	80-90

is divided into quarters and the nucleus fragments can move freely, high aspiration pressure is no longer required, so I decrease the aspiration flow rate to 22 millimeters per minute and aspiration pressure to 140 millimeters of mercury, and I raise the bottle slightly (Figure 3.5D). By reducing these settings, we can decrease turbulence in the anterior chamber during surgery, and reduce the risk of surge-induced posterior capsule rupture. I find that aspiration with bimanual phaco surgery is more effective than with standard co-axial phacoemulsification, so surgery time is only slightly increased to 7 to 9 minutes. My aspiration settings are shown in Table 3.1.

The new phaco machines can generate ultrasound by using hyper pulse phaco technology as WhiteStar mode. This not only prevents thermal burn at the incision site, but also prevents the phaco tip from causing nucleus fragment "kick", which can damage the corneal endothelium.

Aspiration of the residual cortex through a micro incision can be performed using a sleeveless I/A tip or a 20-gauge aspiration cannula through the side port (Figure 3.5E). In cases where it is difficult to remove residual cortex below the incision, the positions of the irrigating chopper and the aspiration cannula can be reversed so that this procedure can be performed safely and effectively.

Perioperative and Postoperative Results

Results of Surgery

Since October 1999, I have performed micro incision bimanual phaco surgery on more than 2000 eyes. In recent 500 eyes, mean surgery time is 8 minutes 49 seconds, which is 1 to 2 minutes longer than that of my conventional co-axial phaco surgery. Approximately 80 mL of infusion solution is required per surgery, slightly less than that for conventional procedures. Both operating time and amount of infusion solution increase with greater nucleus hardness.

Incidence of Perioperative Complications

In recent 500 eyes, posterior capsular rupture occurred in 2 eyes (0.4%). No thermal burn developed in any of these cases, even though the use of ultrasound was prolonged.

Postoperative Course

Slight iris injury developed in 24 eyes (1.2%) which showed preoperative shallow anterior chamber and small pupils. There were no other notable postoperative complications.

The rate of endothelial cell loss was 3.0 ± 14.2 percent in 245 eyes with ordinary hard nucleus and 9.8 ± 18.4 percent in 56 eyes with extremely hard nucleus. However, none of these results differed significantly from those for conventional co-axial phaco surgery.

IOL INSERTION THROUGH THE SMALLEST FEASIBLE INCISION[7]

Current bimanual phaco surgery makes it possible to safely remove the lens through an incision of 0.9-1.4 mm, and several companies are developing soft foldable lenses which are thinner than the current commercially available foldable IOLs. In Europe we can see the marketing of IOLs which can be inserted through an incision of 1.5 mm.[8] However, there have been no commercially available IOLs which can be inserted through such a small incision in the United States and Japan, so we have been forced to enlarge the incision to 2.8 to 4.1 mm in order to insert the IOL[3].

Recently, however, I successfully modified a commercially available IOL injector so that the cartridge can insert a soft acrylic lens having an optic diameter of 5.5 mm (AcrySof® SA30AT) through a 2.2 mm incision. This development increases the importance of being able to perform lens extraction through an ultrasmall incision of less than 1.5 mm.

Modified Injector System for Inserting Acrysof SA30AT through a 2.2 mm Incision

I have succeeded in inserting Alcon acrylic foldable lenses having an optic diameter of 5.5 mm (the AcrySof® SA30AT) through a 2.2 mm incision by using a cartridge (Monarch IIC®) and an injector Royal® manufactured by ASICO and modified in my laboratory (Figure 3.6A).

When using the injector Royal, I can operate the plunger with one hand, which leaves my other hand free to stabilize the eyeball. When inserting an IOL, it is necessary to press firmly on the plunger during insertion. However, too much pressure can cause the lens to be inserted too deeply within the eye, which can result in posterior capsular rupture. Because the plunger is a little too long on ASICO's commercially available injector Royal®, I have adjusted the plunger length by placing a rubber ring at the back end of the plunger (Figure 3.6B). This allows me to press firmly on the plunger during insertion without placing the IOL too deeply in the eye, and avoids posterior capsular rupture. Also, since the stopper is made of rubber, after most of the IOL is inserted within the eye I can press slowly on the plunger again to adjust the position of the IOL.

How to Insert the Acrysof SA30AT through a 2.2 mm Opening

After the micro incision of 1.2–1.4 mm is enlarged using a 2.2 mm keratome, I load a single-piece AcrySof SA30AT® (5.5.mm optic) into a Monarch IIC cartridge, which is set in the modified injector Royal®.

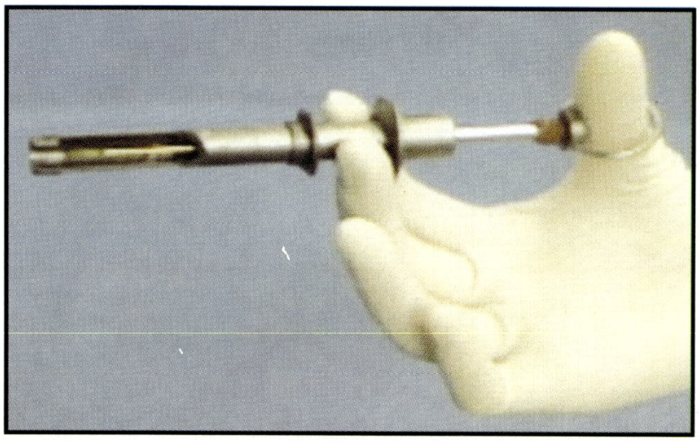

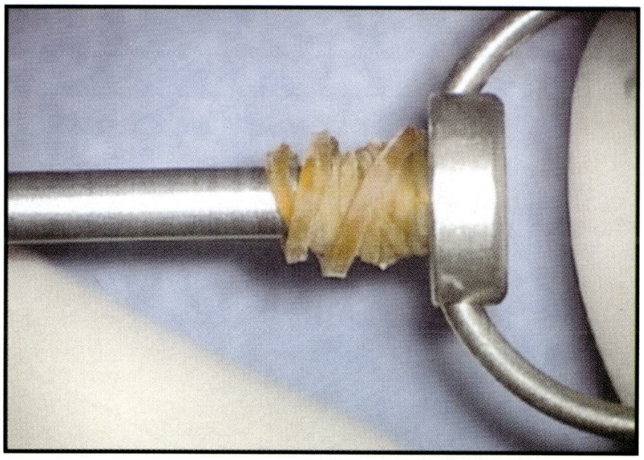

Figures 3.6A and B: Modified injector Royal®
A. Plunger can be operated with one hand when using the injector Royal®
B. The plunger length should be adjusted by placing a rubber ring at the back end of the plunger to avoid the posterior capsule rupture

The injector is positioned so that the front tip of the cartridge tip is pressed against the incision but does not project into the anterior chamber (Figure 3.7A). As the tip of the lens moves through the incision, I insert an appropriate tool, such as a Sinsky hook, through the side port and apply pressure to ensure that the patient's eye is turned toward the incision. After positioning the cartridge tip so that it elevates the inner edge of the corneal incision and presses down on the outer edge, I slowly press the injector plunger forward (Figure 3.7B), without decreasing the pressure of the cartridge on the incision, until the entire optic and the trailing loop are within the anterior chamber (Figure 3.7C). I then use the hook to rotate the lens and to insert the trailing loop into the capsular bag.

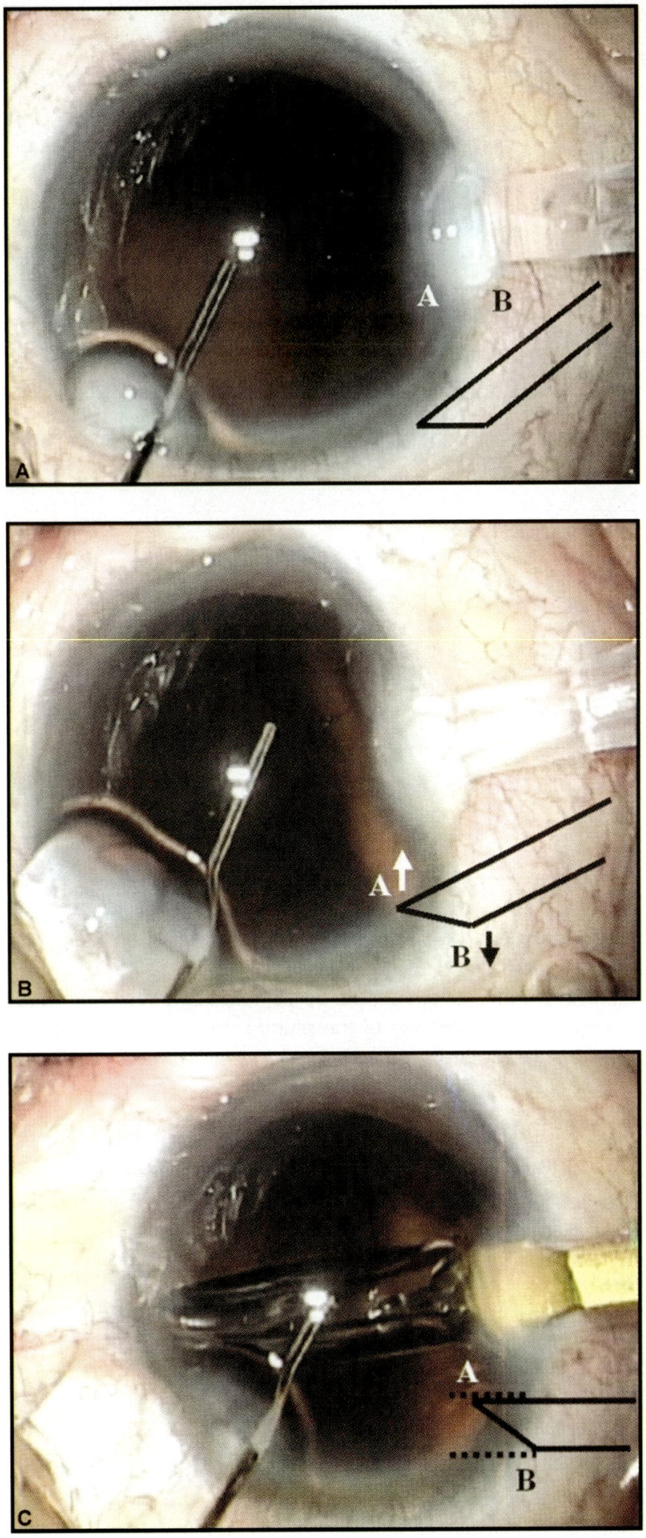

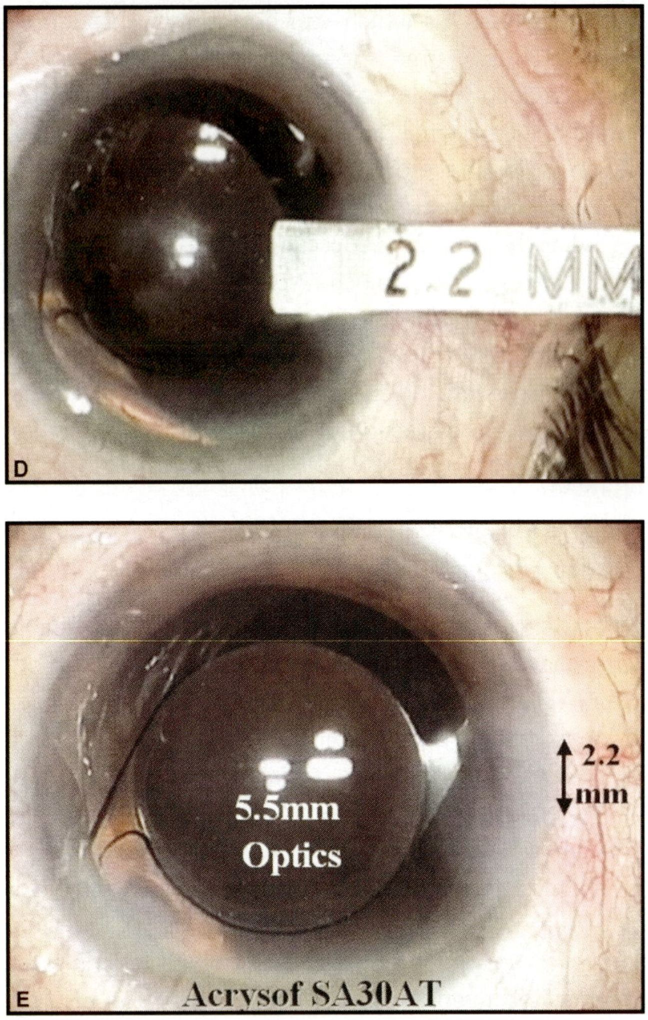

Figures 3.7A to E: How to insert the AcrySof SA30AT® through a 2.2 mm opening

A. The injector is positioned so that the front tip of the cartridge tip is pressed against the incision but does not project into the anterior chamber. As the tip of the lens moves through the incision, an appropriate tool, such as a Sinsky hook, is inserted through the side port to apply pressure to ensure that the patient's eye is turned toward the incision.
B. After positioning the cartridge tip so that it elevates the inner edge of the corneal incision and presses down on the outer edge, the injector plunger is slowly pressed forward.
C. The plunger is pressed without decreasing the pressure of the cartridge on the incision, until the entire optic and the trailing loop are within the anterior chamber.
D. Final incision size is checked with a Tsuneoka micro-incision inner caliper.
E. 5.5 mm optic acrylic IOL is implanted through a 2.2 mm incision

Table 3.2: Final incision in 236 eyes following AcrySof SA30AT implantation

IOL diopter		*Incision before lens insertion (keratome)*		*Incision after lens insertion (internal caliper)*	
< 20 diopter	138 eyes	2.2 mm	138 eyes	2.2 mm	88 eyes
				2.3 mm	45 eyes
				2.4 mm	5 eyes
≥ 20 diopter	98 eyes	2.2 mm	22 eyes	2.2 mm	4 eyes
				2.3 mm	9 eyes
				2.4 mm	9 eyes
		2.4 mm	76 eyes	2.4 mm	76 eyes

Final Incision Size After the IOL Insertion

Immediately after implanting the IOL, I verify the final incision size with a Tsuneoka micro-incision inner caliper manufactured by ASICO (Figure 3.7D).

I have used the AcrySof SA30AT in 236 eyes. In the 138 eyes where I used a lens of less than 20 diopter, it was possible in all cases to insert the lens through an incision of 2.2 mm. However, in 76 out of the 98 eyes for which we used a lens of 20 diopter or greater, we were unable to insert the lens through the 2.2 mm incision, and had to enlarge the incision to 2.4 mm. Of the 160 eyes in which we were able to insert the SA30AT through a 2.2 mm incision, the final incision was 2.2 mm in 92 eyes (57.5%), 2.3 mm in 54 eyes (33.7%), and 2.4 mm in 14 eyes (8.8%) (Table 3.2).

Central positioning of the inserted IOL was satisfactory, and I noted no instances of damage to either the optic or the haptic of the IOL. Following aspiration of the viscoelastic substance, all incisions self sealed. No suturing was required in any of these patients (Figure 3.7E).

Because the central thickness of the AcrySof SA30AT varies depending on lens diopter, it is not possible to insert IOLs of all diopter levels through a 2.2 mm incision. I experienced no problem when using IOLs less than 20 diopter, but it may be safer to use an incision of 2.3 to 2.4 mm for 20 diopter or above.

REFERENCES

1. Kanellopoulos AJ, Dodick JM, Brrauweiler P, Alzner E. Dodick Photolysis for Cataract Surgery. Ophthalmology 1999;106:2197-2202.
2. Tsuneoka H, Shiba T, Takahashi Y. Feasibility of ultrasound cataract surgery with a 1.4 mm incision. J Cataract Refractive Surg 2001;27:934-40.
3. Hara T, Hara T. Clinical results of phacoemulsification and complete in-the-bag fixation. J Cataract Refractive Surg 1987;13:279-86.
4. Agarwal A, Agarwal A, Agarwal S, et.al. Phakonit: lens removal through a 0.9 mm corneal incision. J Cataract Refractive Surg 2001;27:1548-52.
5. Soscia W, Howard JG, Olson RJ. Microphacoemulsification with WhiteStar. A wound-temperature study. J Cataract Refractive Surg 2002;28:1044-6.
6. Tsuneoka H, Shiba T, Takahashi Y. Ultrasonic phacoemulsification using a 1.4 mm incision: clinical results. DJ Cataract Refractive Surg 2002;28:81-6.
7. Tsuneoka H, Hayama A, Takahama M. Ultrasmall-incision bimanual phaco-emulsification and Acrysof SA30AL implantation through a 2.2 mm incision. J Cataract Refractive Surg 2003;29:1070-6.
8. Prats JLR, Alio JL, Galal A. MICS and new intraocular lens technologies. In: Alio JL, et al (Ed): Micro-Incision Cataract Surgery. Highlight of Ophthalmology. Panama, 2004.

4

Air Pump in Phakonit

- AIR PUMP
- HISTORY
- TECHNIQUE
- METHOD
- CONTINUOUS INFUSION
- ADVANTAGES
- TOPICAL OR NO ANESTHESIA CATARACT SURGERY

Amar Agarwal, Sunita Agarwal, Athiya Agarwal, Ashok Garg (India)

AIR PUMP

Various methods have been used to combat surge during phacoemulsification. We describe a simple device that can be used with any phacoemulsification machine to minimize surge during phacoemulsification. An automated air pump is used to push air into the infusion bottle thus increasing the pressure with which the fluid flows into the eye. This increases the steady-state pressure of the eye making the anterior chamber deep and well maintained during the entire procedure. It makes phakonit and phacoemulsification a relatively safe procedure by reducing surge even at high vacuum levels.

HISTORY

The main problem in phakonit we had was the destabilization of the anterior chamber during surgery. We solved it to a certain extent by using an 18-gauge irrigating chopper. Then one of us (S.A.) suggested the use of an antichamber collapser, which injects air into the infusion bottle (Figure 4.1). This pushes more fluid into the eye through the irrigating chopper and also prevents surge. Thus, we were able to use a 20-gauge or 21-gauge irrigating chopper as well as solve the problem of destabilization of the anterior chamber during surgery.

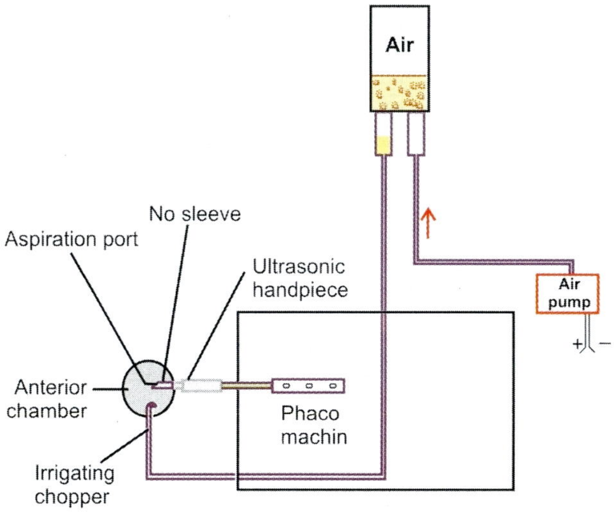

Figure 4.1: Diagrammatic representation of the connection of the air pump to the infusion bottle

INTRODUCTION

Since the introduction of phacoemulsification by Kelman,[1] it has been undergoing revolutionary changes in an attempt to perfect the techniques of extracapsular cataract extraction surgery. Although advantageous in many aspects this technique is not without it's attending complications. A well maintained anterior chamber without intraocular fluctuations is one of the prerequisites for safe phacoemulsification and phakonit.[2]

When an occluded fragment is held by high vacuum and then abruptly aspirated, fluid rushes into the phaco tip to equilibrate the built up vacuum in the aspiration line, causing surge.[3] This leads to shallowing or collapse of the anterior chamber.

Different machines employ a variety of methods to combat surge. These include usage of noncomplaint tubing,[4] small bore aspiration line tubing,[4] microflow tips,[4] aspiration bypass systems,[4] dual linear foot pedal control[4] and incorporation of sophisticated microprocessors[4] to sense the anterior chamber pressure fluctuations.

The surgeon dependent variables to counteract surge include good wound construction with minimal leakage,[5] and selection of appropriate machine parameters depending on the stage of the surgery.[5] An anterior chamber maintainer has also been described in literature to prevent surge, but an extra side port makes it an inconvenient procedure.

We herein describe a simple and effective method to prevent anterior chamber collapse during phacoemulsification and phakonit by increasing the velocity of the fluid inflow into the anterior chamber. This is achieved by an automated air pump which pumps atmospheric air through an air filter into the infusion bottle thereby preventing surge. We stumbled upon this idea when we were operating cases with Phakonit[7] where we wanted more fluid entering the eye, but now also use it in all our phaco cases.

TECHNIQUE

A locally manufactured automated device, used in fish tanks (aquariums) to supply oxygen, is utilized to forcefully pump air into the irrigation bottle. This pump is easily available in aquarium shops. It has an electromagnetic motor which moves a lever attached to a collapsible rubber cap. There is an inlet with a valve, which sucks in atmospheric air as the cap expands. On collapsing, the valve closes and the air is pushed into an intravenous (IV) line connected to the infusion bottle (see Figure 4.1). The lever vibrates at a frequency of approximately 10 oscillations per second. The electromagnetic motor is weak enough to stop once the pressure in the closed system (i.e. the anterior chamber) reaches about 50 mm of Hg. The rubber cap ceases to expand at this pressure level. A micropore air filter is used between the air pump and the infusion bottle so that the air pumped into the bottle is clean of particulate matter.

METHOD

1. First of all, the BSS bottle is taken and put in the IV stand.
2. Now we take an air pump. This air pump is the same air pump, which is used in fish tanks (aquariums) to give oxygen to the fishes. The air pump is plugged on to the electrical connection.
3. An IV set now connects the air pump to the infusion bottle. The tubing passes from the air pump and the end of the tubing is passed into one of the infusion bottles.
4. What happens now is that when the air pump is switched on, it pumps air into the infusion bottle. This air goes to the top of the bottle and because of the pressure, it pumps the fluid down with greater force. With this, the fluid now flows from the infusion bottle to reach the phaco handpiece or irrigating chopper. The amount of fluid now coming out of the hand piece is much more than what would normally come out and with more force (Figures 4.2 and 4.3).
5. An air filter is connected between the air pump and the infusion bottle so that the air which is being pumped into the bottle is sterile.
6. This extra-amount of fluid coming out compensates for the surge which would otherwise occur..

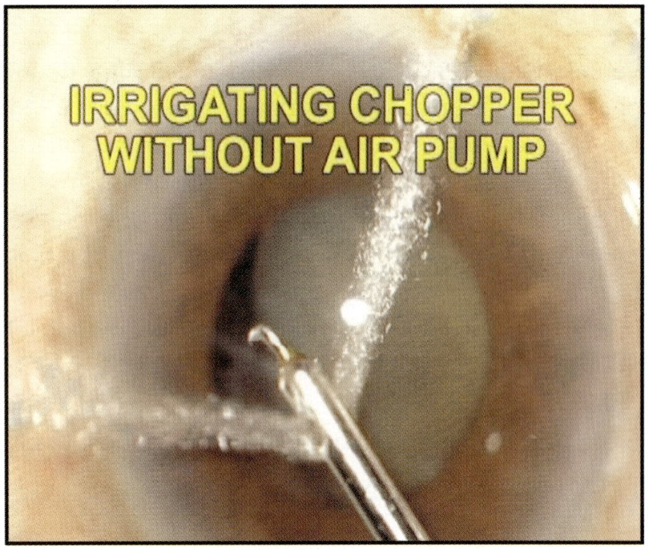

Figure 4.2: Flow of fluid through the irrigating chopper without an air pump

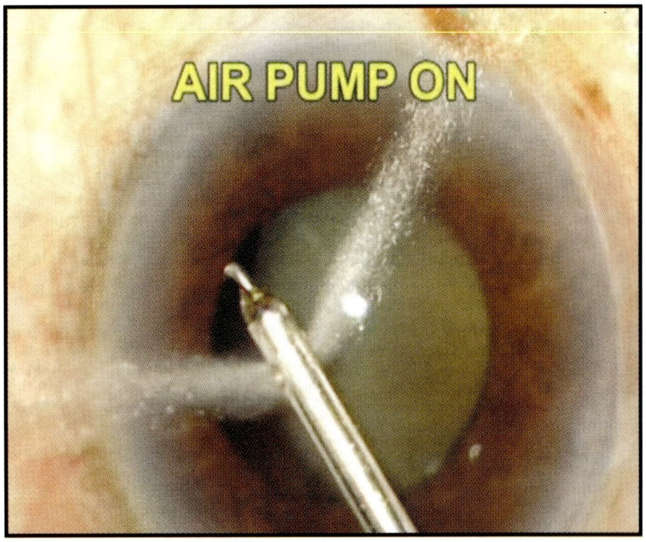

Figure 4.3: Flow of fluid through the irrigating chopper with an air pump. Note when the air pump is on the amount of fluid coming out of the irrigating chopper is much more

CONTINUOUS INFUSION

Before we enter the eye, we fill the eye with viscoelastic. Then once the tip of the phaco handpiece in phaco or irrigating chopper in phakonit is inside the anterior chamber we shift to continuous irrigation. This is very helpful especially for surgeons who are starting phaco or phakonit. This way, the surgeon, never comes to position zero and the anterior chamber never collapses. Even for excellent surgeons this helps a lot.

ADVANTAGES

1. With the air pump, the posterior capsule is pushed back and there is a deep anterior chamber.

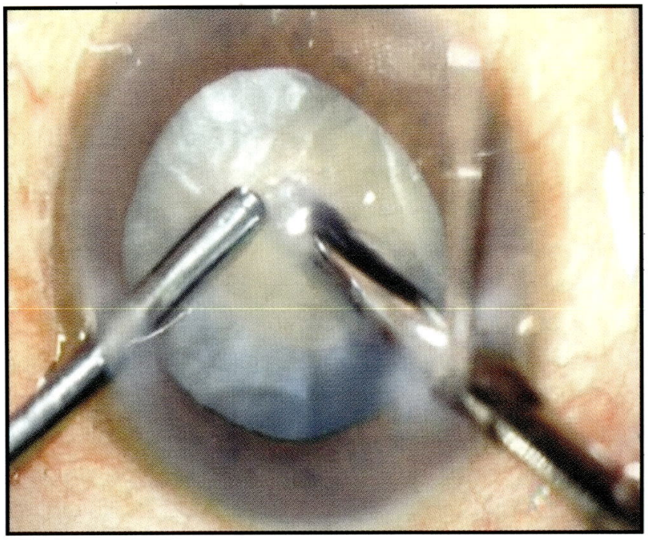

Figure 4.4: Phakonit being performed in a mature brown cataract. Such difficult cases can be operated upon by phakonit because of the air pump. It deepens the chamber and prevents any surge

2. The phenomenon of surge is neutralized. This prevents the unnecessary posterior capsular rupture.
3. Striate keratitis postoperatively is reduced, as there is a deep anterior chamber.
4. One can operate hard cataracts (Figure 4.4) also quite comfortably, as striate keratitis does not occur postoperatively.
5. The surgical time is shorter as one can emulsify the nuclear pieces much faster as surge does not occur.
6. One can easily operate cases with the phakonit technique as quite a lot of fluid now passes into the eye. Thus, the cataract can be removed through a smaller opening.
7. It is quite comfortable to do cases under topical or no anesthesia.

TOPICAL OR NO ANESTHESIA CATARACT SURGERY

When one operates under topical or no anesthesia, the main problem is sometimes the pressure is high especially if the patient squeezes the eye. In such cases, the posterior capsule comes up anteriorly and one can produce a posterior capsular rupture. To solve this problem, surgeons tend to work more anteriorly, performing supracapsular phacoemulsification/phakonit. The disadvantage of this is that striate keratitis tends to occur.

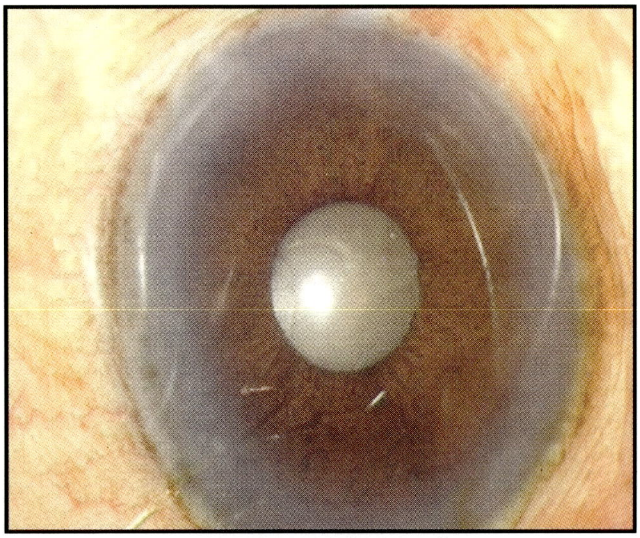

Figure 4.5: Miotic pupil

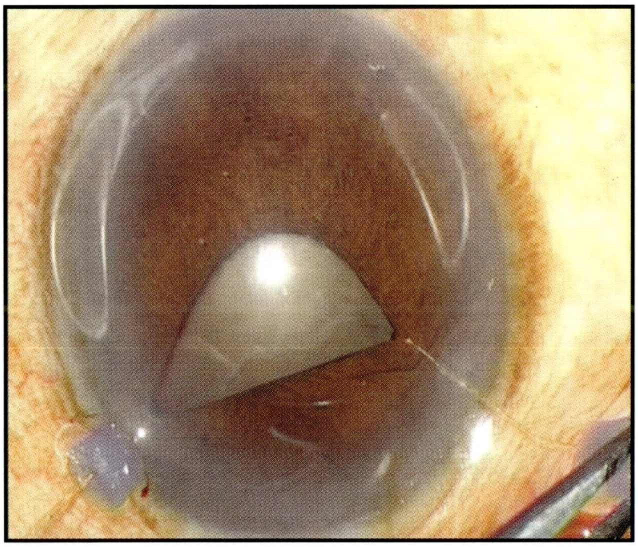

Figure 4.6: Iris hooks used to dilate the pupil

With the air pump, this problem does not occur. When we use the air pump, the posterior capsule is quite back, as if we are operating a patient under a block. In other words, there is a lot of space between the posterior capsule and the cornea, preventing striate keratitis and inadvertent posterior capsular rupture. If one is operating on a patient with a small pupil (Figure 4.5) and shallow anterior chamber once again one can use iris hooks (Figures 4.6 and 4.7) to dilate the pupil and then perform phakonit with the air pump on (Figure 4.8). This will help deepen the chamber and one can complete the

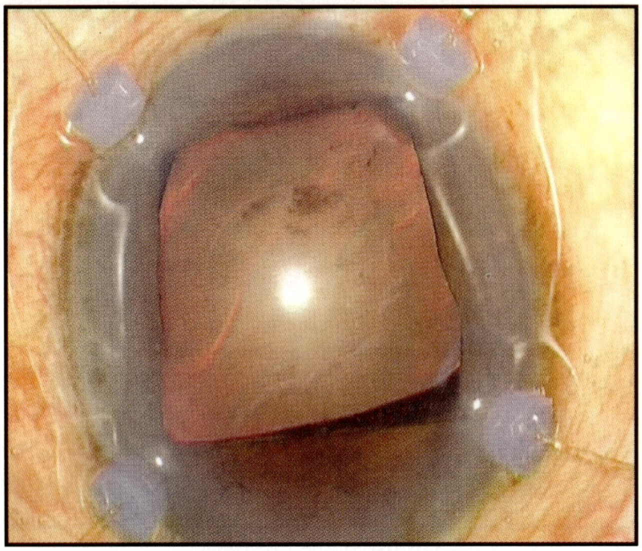

Figure 4.7: Four iris hooks are in place. This way the pupil is well dilated. It is better to do phakonit than phaco in such cases as four areas have already been blocked by the iris hooks. As there is little space left phakonit has an advantage. But one should use the air pump as it makes life easier

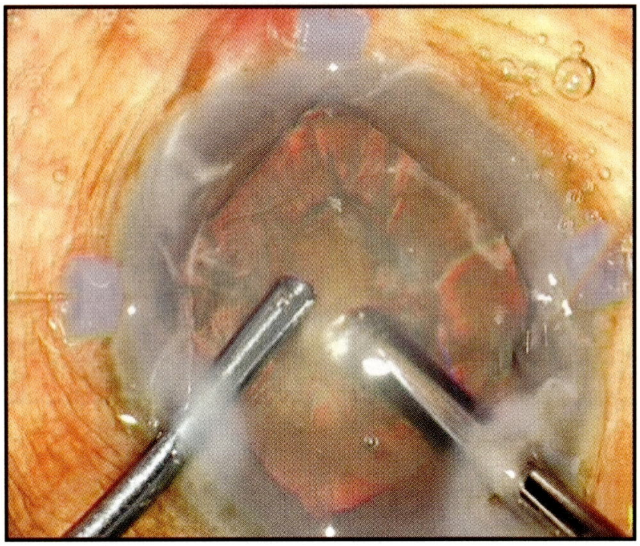

Figure 4.8: Phakonit started. Note the irrigating chopper in the left hand and a sleeveless phaco needle in the right hand

case. Such cases cannot be operated comfortably without the air pump.

DISCUSSION

Surge is defined as the volume of the fluid forced out of the eye into the aspiration line at the instant of occlusion break. When the phacoemulsification handpiece tip is occluded, flow is interrupted and vacuum builds up to its preset values. Additionally the aspiration tubing may collapse in the presence of high vacuum levels. Emulsification of the occluding fragment clears the block and the fluid rushes into the aspiration line to neutralize the pressure difference created between the positive pressure in the anterior chamber and the negative pressure in the aspiration tubing. In addition, if the aspiration line tubing is not reinforced to prevent collapse (tubing compliance), the tubing, constricted during occlusion, then expands on occlusion break. These factors cause a rush of fluid from the anterior chamber into the phaco probe. The fluid in the anterior chamber is not replaced rapidly enough to prevent shallowing of the anterior chamber.

The maintenance of intraocularpressure (steady-state IOP)[2] during the entire procedure depends on the equilibrium between the fluid inflow and outflow. The steady state pressure level is the mean pressure equilibrium between inflow and outflow volumes. In most phacoemulsification machines, fluid inflow is provided by gravitational flow of the fluid from the balanced salt solution (BSS) bottle through the tubing to the anterior chamber. This is determined by the bottle height relative to the patient's eye, the diameter of the tubing and most importantly by the outflow of fluid from the eye through the aspiration tube and leakage from the wounds.[2]

The inflow volume can be increased by either increasing the bottle height or by enlarging the diameter of the inflow tube. The intraocular pressure increases by 10 mm Hg for every 15 centimeters increase in bottle height above the eye.[5]

High steady-state IOPs increase phaco safety by raising the mean IOP level up and away from zero, i.e. by delaying surge related anterior chamber collapse.[2]

Air pump increases the amount of fluid inflow thus making the steady-state IOP high. This deepens the anterior chamber, increasing the surgical space available for maneuvering and thus prevents complications like posterior capsular tears and corneal endothelial damage. The phenomenon of surge is neutralized by rapid inflow of fluid at the time of occlusion break. The recovery to steady-state IOP is so prompt that no surge occurs and this enables the surgeon to remain in foot position 3 through the occlusion break. High vacuum phacoemulsification/phakonit can be safely performed in hard brown cataracts using an air pump. Phacoemulsification or phakonit under topical or no anesthesia[6,7] can be safely done neutralizing the positive vitreous pressure occurring due to squeezing of the eyelids.

SUMMARY

The air pump is a new device, which helps to prevent surge. This prevents posterior capsular rupture, helps deepen the anterior chamber and makes phacoemulsification and phakonit safe procedures even in hard cataracts.

KEY POINTS

1. The air pump is a simple and effective method to prevent anterior chamber collapse during phacoemulsification and phakonit by increasing the velocity of the fluid inflow into the anterior chamber.
2. This is achieved by an automated air pump which pumps atmospheric air through an air filter into the infusion bottle thereby preventing surge.
3. A micropore air filter is used between the air pump and the infusion bottle so that the air pumped into the bottle is clean of particulate matter.
4. Surge is defined as the volume of the fluid forced out of the eye into the aspiration line at the instant of occlusion break.
5. The air pump is a new device, which helps to prevent surge. This prevents posterior capsular rupture, helps deepen the anterior chamber and makes phacoemulsification and phakonit safe procedures even in hard cataracts.

REFERENCES

1. Kelman CD. Phacoemulsification and aspiration; a new technique of cataract removal: a preliminary report. Am J Ophthalmol 1967;64:23-5.
2. Wilbrandt RH. Comparative analysis of the fluidics of the AMO Prestige, Alcon Legacy, and Storz Premiere phacoemulsification systems. J Cataract Refract Surg 1997;23:766-80.
3. Seibel SB. Phacodynamics. Thorofare, NJ, Slack Inc, 1995;54
4. Fishkind WJ. The Phaco Machine: How and why it acts and reacts? In Agarwal's Four volume textbook of Ophthalmology. Jaypee Brothers: New Delhi; 2000. (In print).
5. Seibel SB. The fluidics and physics of phaco. In Agarwal's et al. Phacoemulsification, Laser Cataract Surgery and Foldable IOLs (Second edition). Jaypee Brothers: New Delhi; 2000;45-54.
6. Agarwal et al. No anaesthesia cataract surgery with karate chop; In Agarwal's Phacoemulsification, Laser Cataract Surgery and Foldable IOLs (Second edition). Jaypee Brothers: New Delhi; 2000;217-26.
7. Agarwal et al. Phakonit and laser phakonit. In Agarwal's Phacoemulsification, Laser Cataract Surgery and Foldable IOLs (Second edition). Jaypee Brothers: New Delhi; 2000;204-16.

5

Microphakonit: Cataract Surgery with a 0.7 mm Tip

- HISTORY
- INSTRUMENTATIONS
- TECHNIQUE

Amar Agarwal, Athiya Agarwal, Sunita Agarwal, Ashok Garg (India)

HISTORY

On August 15th 1998 the authors (Amar Agarwal) performed 1 mm cataract surgery by a technique called Phakonit[1-13] (Phako being done with a Needle Incision Technology). Dr Jorge Alio (Spain) coined the term MICS or microincision cataract surgery[14] for all surgeries including laser cataract surgery and phakonit. Dr Randall Olson (USA) first used a 0.8 mm phaco needle and a 21-gauge irrigating chopper and called it Microphaco.[15-18]

On May 21st 2005, for the first time a 0.7 mm phaco needle tip with a 0.7 mm irrigating chopper was used by the authors (Am A) to remove cataracts through the smallest incision possible as of now. This is called Microphakonit.

INSTRUMENTATIONS

Microphakonit (0.7 mm) Needel Tip

When we wanted to go for a 0.7 mm phaco needle the point which we wondered was whether the needle would be able to hold the energy of the ultrasound. We gave this problem to Larry Laks from MST, USA to work on. He then made this special 0.7 mm phaco needle (Figure 5.1). As you will understand if we go smaller from a 0.9 mm phaco needle to a 0.7 mm phaco needle the speed of the surgery would go down. This is because the amount of aspiration flow rate would be less.

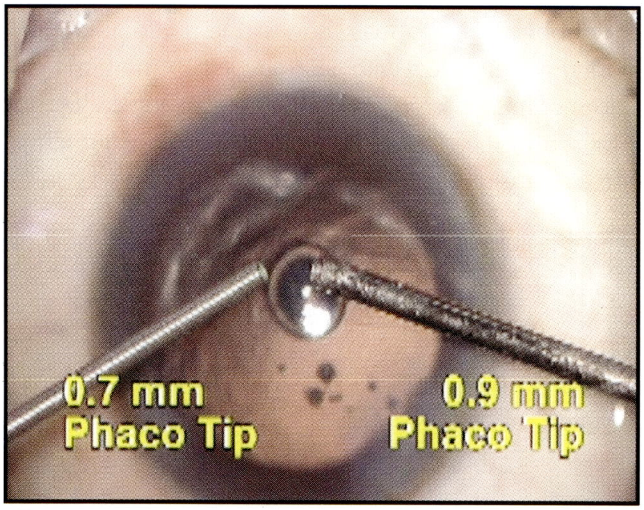

Figure 5.1: 0.7 mm phaco tip (microphakonit) as compared to a 0.9 mm phaco tip (phakonit)

It was decided to solve this problem by working on the wall of the 0.7 mm phaco needle. There is a standard wall thickness for all phaco tips. If we say the outer diameter is a constant, the resultant inner diameter is an area of the outer diameter minus the area of the wall.

The inner diameter will regulate the flow rate/ perceived efficiency (which can be good or bad, depending on how you look at it). In order to increase the allowed aspiration flow rate from what a standard 0.7 mm tip would be, MST (Larry Laks) had the walls made thinner, thus increasing the inner diameter. This would allow a case to go, speed wise, closer to what a 0.9 mm tip would go (not exactly the same, but closer). With the gas forced infusion it would work very well. Finally we decided to go for a 30-degree tip to make it even better.

Microphakonit (0.7 mm) Irrigating Chopper

In Figure 5.2 you will notice two designs of 20-gauge (0.9 mm) irrigating choppers which we designed. On the left is the Agarwal irrigating chopper made by the MST (Microsurgical Technology) company. This is incorporated in the Duet system. The irrigating chopper on the right is made by Geuder, Germany. Notice in the left figure the opening for the fluid is end opening, whereas the one on the right has two openings in the side. Depending on the convenience of the surgeon, the surgeon can decide which design of irrigating chopper

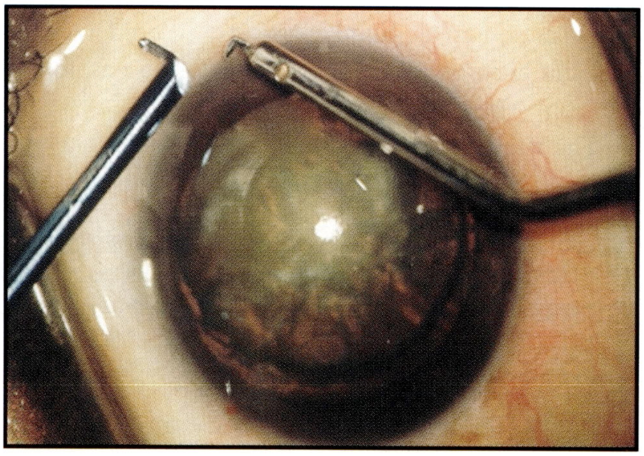

Figure 5.2: Two designs of Agarwal irrigating choppers. The one on the left has an end opening for fluid (microsurgical technology). The one on the right has two openings on the sides (Geuder–Germany)

they would like to use. There are advantages and disadvantages of both types of irrigating choppers. The end opening chopper has an advantage of more fluid coming out of the chopper. The disadvantage is that there is a gush of fluid which might push the nuclear pieces away. The advantage of the side opening irrigating chopper is that there is good control as the nuclear pieces are not pushed away but the disadvantage is that the amount of fluid coming out of it is much less. That is why if one is using the side opening irrigating chopper one should use an air pump or gas forced infusion.

The MST in their irrigating chopper increased flow by removing the flow restrictions incorporated in other irrigating choppers as a bi-product of their attachment method. They also had control of incisional outflow by having all the instruments to be of one size and created a matching knife of the proper size and geometry.

When we decided to go smaller to using a 0.7 mm irrigating chopper (Figure 5.3) we decided to go for an end-opening irrigating chopper. The reason is as the bore of the irrigating chopper was smaller the amount of fluid coming out of it would be less and so an end-opening chopper would maintain the fluidics better. With gas forced infusion we thought we would be able to balance the entry and exit of fluid into the anterior chamber and that is what happened.

We measured the amount of fluid coming out of the various irrigating choppers with and without an air pump (Table 5.1). We also measured the values using the simple aquarium air pump (external gas forced infusion) and the accurus machine giving internal gas forced infusion.

The microphakonit irrigating chopper which we have designed is basically a sharp chopper which has a sharp cutting edge and helps in karate chopping or quick chopping. It can chop any type of cataract.

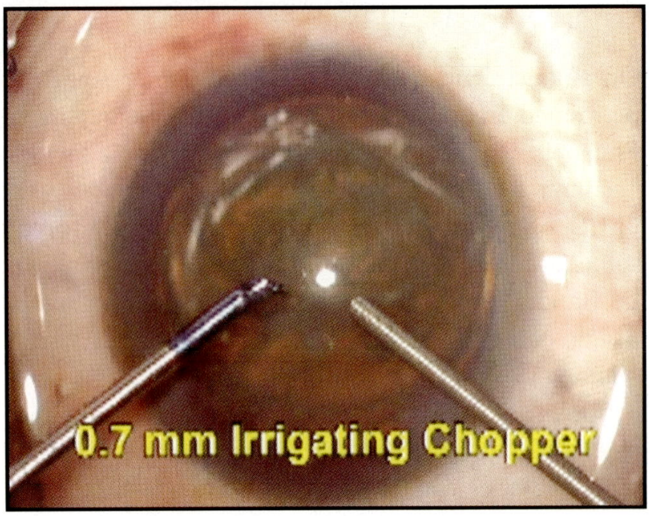

Figure 5.3: 0.7 mm irrigating chopper

Air Pump and Gas Forced Infusion

The main problem in phakonit we had was the destabilization of the anterior chamber during surgery. We solved it to a certain extent by using an 18-gauge irrigating chopper. Then one of us (S.A.) suggested the use of an antichamber collapser,[19] which injects air into the infusion bottle (Figure 5.4). This pushes more fluid into the eye through the irrigating chopper and also prevents surge (Figures 5.5 and 5.6). Thus, we were able to use a 20/21 gauge irrigating chopper as well as solve the problem of destabilization of the anterior chamber during surgery. Now with a 22-gauge (0.7 mm) irrigating chopper it is extremely essential that gas forced infusion be used in the surgery. This is also called external gas forced infusion.

Table 5.1: Fluid exiting from various irrigating choppers (values in ml/minute)

Irrigating chopper	*Without gas forced infusion*	*With gas forced infusion using the accurus machine at 50 mm Hg*	*With gas forced infusion using the accurus machine at 75 mm Hg*	*With gas forced infusion using the accurus machine at 100 mm Hg*	*Air pump with regulator at low*	*Air pump with regulator at low*
0.9 mm side opening	25	36	42	48	37	51
0.9 mm end opening	34	51	57	65	52	68
0.7 mm end opening	27	39	44	51	41	54

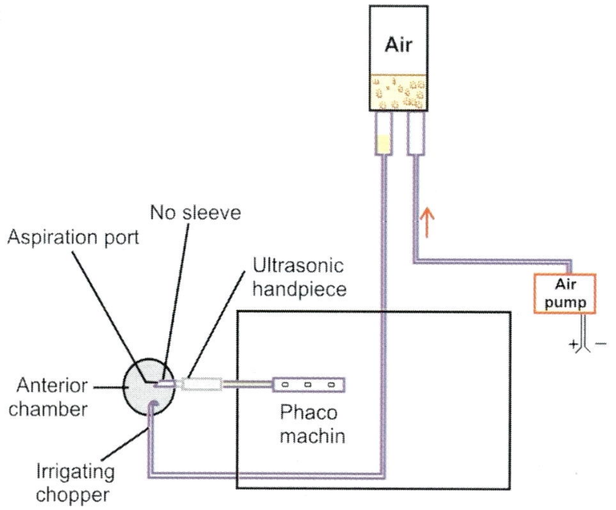

Figure 5.4: Air pump

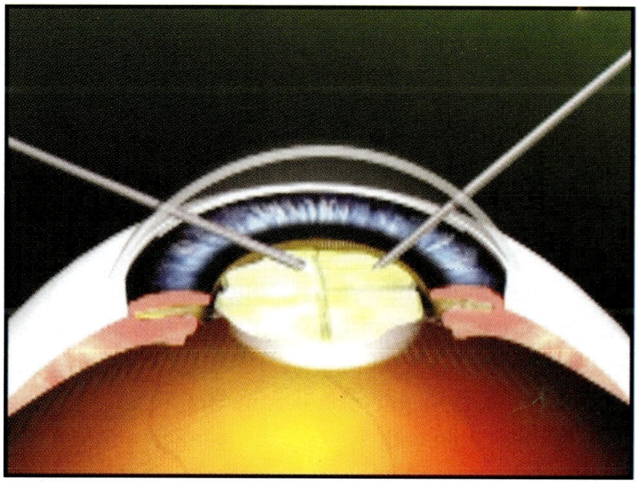

Figure 5.5: Illustration showing normal anterior chamber when case is started. Air pump is not used

When the surgeon uses the air pump contained in the same phaco machine, it is called internal gas forced infusion (IFI). To solve the problem of infection we use a millipore filter connected to the machine. The advantages of the Internal Forced Infusion over the external are:

1. The surgeon doesn't have to incorporate an external air pump to the surgical system to obtain the advantages of the forced infusion.
2. The surgeon can control all the parameters (forced infusion rate, ultrasonic power modulations and vacuum settings) in the same panel of the surgical system he or she is working with.

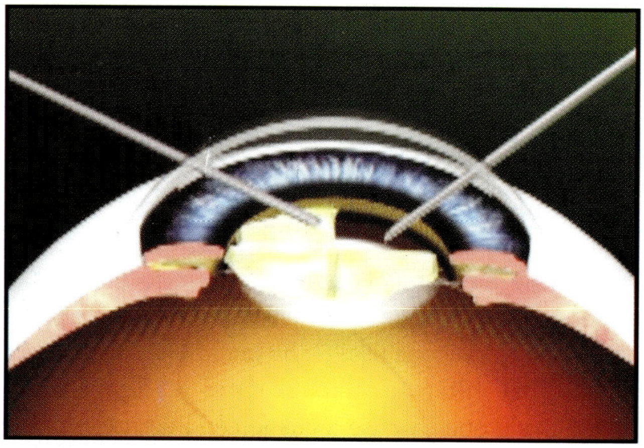

Figure 5.6: Illustration showing surge and chamber collapse when nucleus is being removed. Air pump is not used. Note the chamber depth has come down. When we use the air pump this problem does not occur

3. The forced infusion rate can be actively and digitally controlled during the surgery, adjusting the parameters to the conditions and/or the surgical steps of each individual case.

When we decided to use the 0.7 mm MST Duet set we decided to use the internal gas forced infusion of the accurus machine to measure the pressure of air exactly. This is from Alcon. The advantage by this was that we could regulate the amount of air entering into the infusion bottle and thus titrate the system in such a way that there is no surge or collapse of the anterior chamber. When we are using a 0.7 mm irrigating chopper the problem is that the amount of fluid entering the eye is not enough. To solve this problem gas forced infusion is a must.

The anterior vented gas forced infusion system (AVGFI) of the accurus surgical system helps in the performance of phakonit.This was started by Arturo Pérez-Arteaga from Mexico. The AVGFI is a system incorporated in the Accurus machine that creates a positive infusion pressure inside the eye. It consists of an air pump and a regulator which are inside the machine; then the air is pushed inside the bottle of intraocular solution, and so the fluid is actively pushed inside the eye without raising or lowering the bottle. The control of the air pump is digitally integrated in the Accurus panel. We preset the infusion pump at 100 mm Hg when we are operating microphakonit.

As you will notice in Table 5.1 if we use the air pump at high it is equal to using the accurus machine at about 100 mm Hg pressure and if we use the air pump at low it is equal to using the accurus machine at 50 mm Hg pressure. Some air pumps come with such a regulator so that one can have more air coming out of them. The regulator has a switch for low and high pressure. The cost of the air pump is about US $ 2 to US $ 10/- depending on the country. This can be got from an aquarium shop. If one uses an air pump one can connect a millipore filter to it to prevent any infection. Alternatively one can use a gas forced internal infusion system using the accurus machine. In such a case preset the pump at 100 mm Hg.

Bimanual 0.7 mm Irrigation Aspiration System

Bimanual irrigation aspiration is done with the bimanual irrigation aspiration instruments. These instruments are also designed by Microsurgical Technology (USA). The previous set we used was the 0.9 mm set. Now with microphakonit we use the new 0.7 mm bimanual I/A set (Figures 5.7 and 5.8) so that after the nucleus removal we need not enlarge the incision.

Duet Handles

All these instruments of the 0.7 mm set fit onto the handles of the Duet system. So if a surgeon has already got the handles and is using it for phakonit they need to get only the tips and can use the same handles for microphakonit.

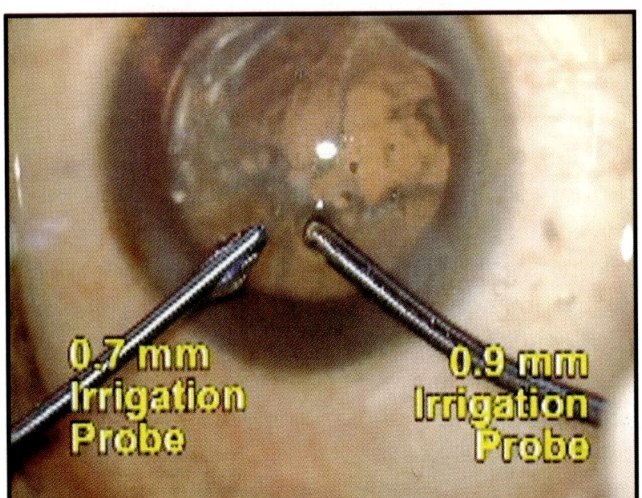

Figure 5.7: 0.7 mm irrigation probe used for bimanual I/A compared to the 0.9 mm irrigation probe

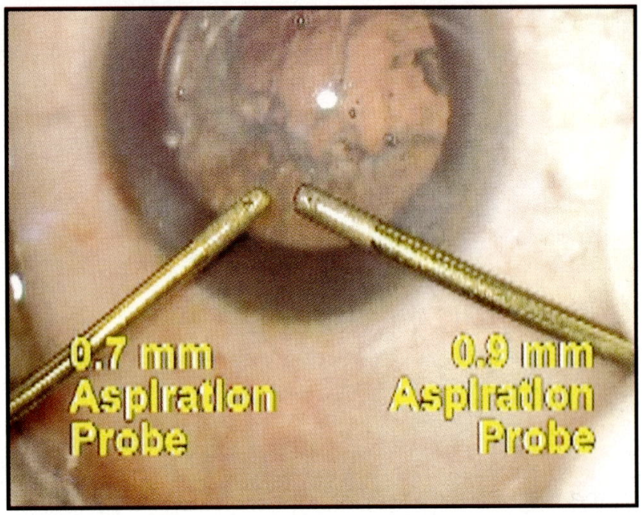

Figure 5.8: 0.7 mm aspiration probe used for bimanual I/A compared to the 0.9 mm aspiration probe

TECHNIQUE

Incision

The incision is made with a keratome. This can be done using a sapphire knife or a stainless steel knife. One should be careful when one is making the incision so that the incision is a bit long as one would be using gas forced infusion in microphakonit. Before making the incision, a needle with viscoelastic is taken and pierced in the eye in the area where the side port has to be made. The viscoelastic is then injected inside the eye. This will distend the eye so that the clear corneal incision can be made easily. Make one clear corneal incision between the lateral rectus and inferior rectus and the other between the lateral rectus and superior rectus. This way one is able to control the movements of the eye during surgery.

Rhexis

The rhexis is then performed of about 5 to 6 mm. This is done with a needle . In the left hand a straight rod is held to stabilize the eye. This is the Globe stabilization rod. The advantage of this is that the movements of the eye can get controlled if one is working without any anesthesia or under topical anesthesia.

Hydrodissection

Hydrodissection is performed and the fluid wave passing under the nucleus checked. Check for rotation of the nucleus. The advantage of microphakonit is that one can do hydrodissection from both incisions so that even the subincisional areas can get easily hydrodissected. The problem is as there is not much escape of fluid one should be careful in hydrodissection as if too much fluid is passed into the eye one can get a complication.

Microphakonit

The 22 (0.7 mm)-gauge irrigating chopper connected to the infusion line of the phaco machine is introduced with foot pedal on position 1. The phaco probe is connected to the aspiration line and the 0.7 mm phaco tip without an infusion sleeve is introduced through the clear corneal incision (Figure 5.9). Using the phaco tip with moderate ultrasound power, the center of the nucleus is directly embedded starting from the superior edge of rhexis with the phaco probe directed obliquely downwards towards the vitreous. The settings at this stage are 50 percent phaco power, flow rate 24 ml/min and 110 mm Hg vacuum. Using the karate chop technique the nucleus is chopped (Figures 5.10A to D). Thus the whole nucleus is removed (Figure 5.11).

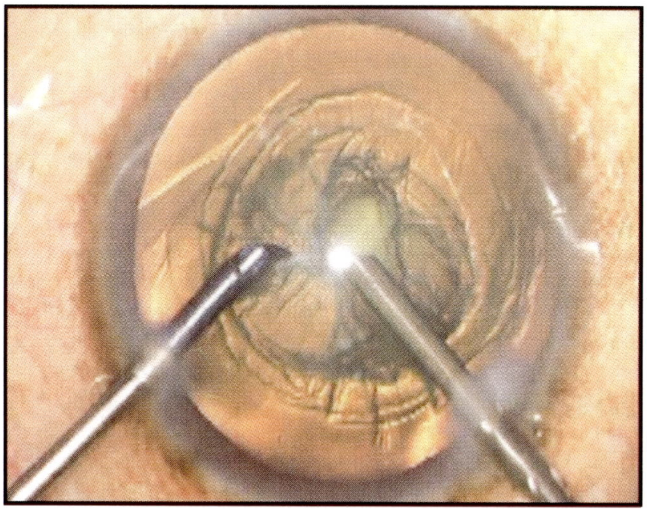

Figure 5.9: Microphakonit started. 0.7 mm irrigating chopper and 0.7 mm phako tip without the sleeve inside the eye. All instruments are made by MST, USA. The assistant continuously irrigates the phaco probe area from outside to prevent corneal burns

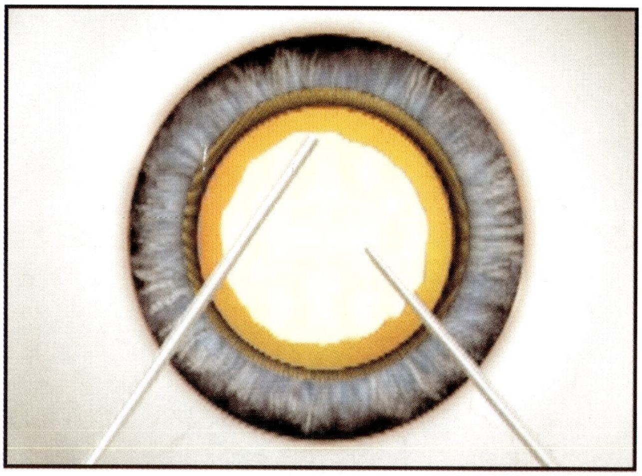

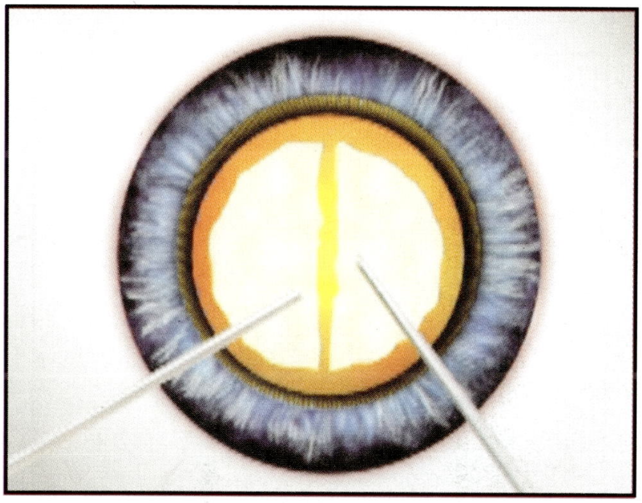

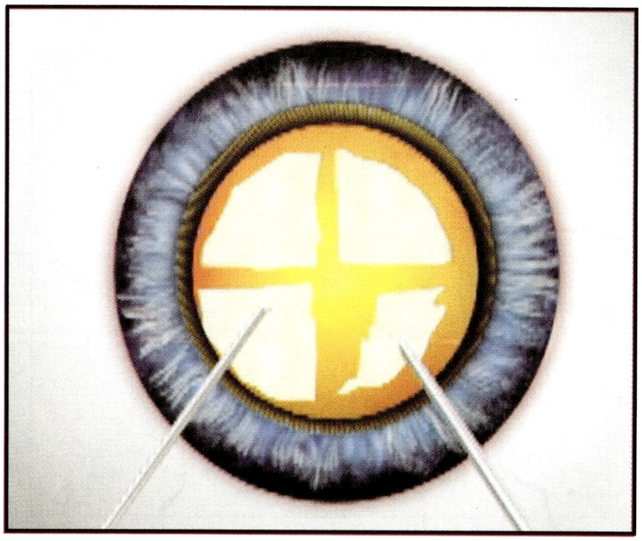

Figures 5.10A to C

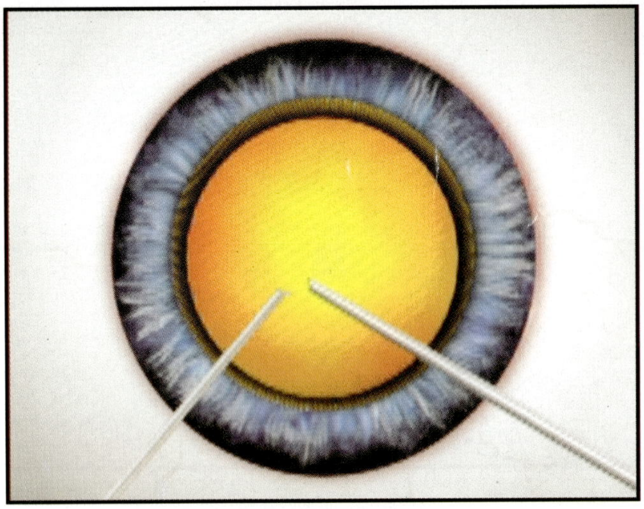

Figures 5.10A to D: Illustration showing the nucleus removal

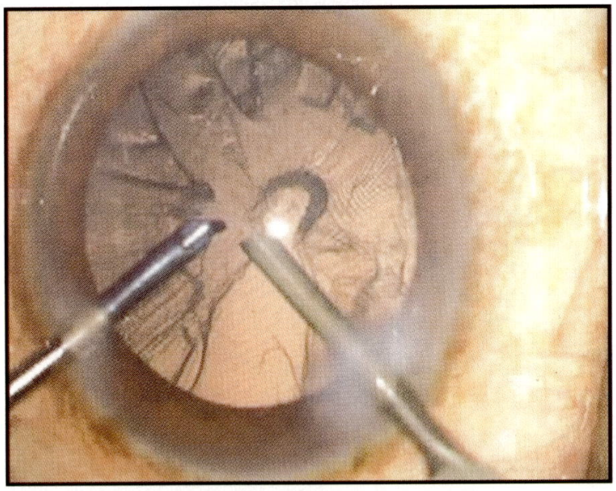

Figure 5.11: Microphakonit completed. The nucleus has been removed

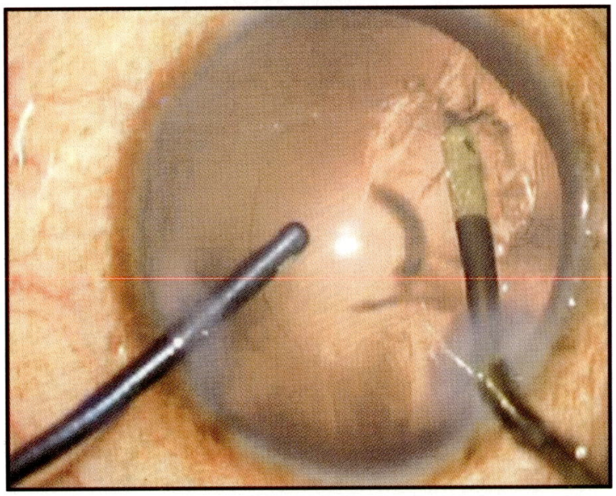

Figure 5.12: Bimanual irrigation aspiration started with the 0.7 mm set

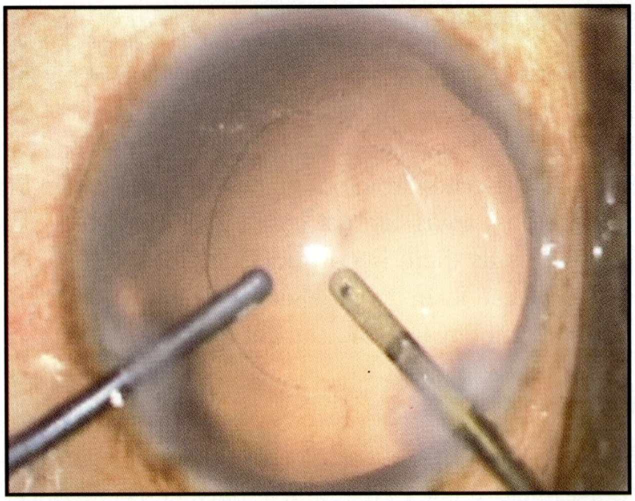

Figure 5.13: Bimanual irrigation aspiration completed

Table 5.2: Differences between phakonit and microphakonit

Features	*Phakonit*	*Microphakonit*
Irrigating chopper	0.9 mm	0.7 mm
Phaco needle	0.9 mm	0.7 mm
Control in surgery	Good	Better control
Valve construction	Extremely important	Not very important as incision is much smaller
Iris prolapse	Can occur if valve is bad	Very rare
Intraoperative floppy iris syndrome	Can be managed	Much better to manage as incision is much smaller and there is better control
Hydrodissection	Can be done from both incisions	To be careful as very little space is there for escape of fluid
Air pump (gas forced infusion GFI)	Can be done without it though better with it	Mandatory. 0.7 mm irrigating choppers even with higher end machines need GFI
Flow rate	Can keep any value	Do not keep it very high. 20-24 ml/min
Bimanual I/A	0.9 mm	0.7 mm

Cortical wash-up is then done with the bimanual irrigation aspiration (0.7 mm set) technique (Figures 5.12 and 5.13). During this whole procedure of microphakonit gas forced infusion is used.

SUMMARY

With microphakonit a 0.7 mm set is used to remove the cataract. At present this is the smallest one can use for cataract surgery. With time one would be able to go smaller with better and better instruments and devices. The problem at present is the IOL. We have to get good quality IOL's going through sub 1mm cataract surgical incisions so that the real benefit of microphakonit can be given to the patient (Table 5.2).

REFERENCES

1. Agarwal A, Agarwal S, Agarwal A. No anesthesia Cataract surgery. In Agarwal, et al (Eds): Textbook Phacoemulsification, Laser Cataract Surgery and Foldable IOL's, (First edition). Jaypee, India 1998;144-54.
2. Pandey S, Wener L, Agarwal A, Agarwal S, Agarwal At, Apple D. No anesthesia Cataract surgery. J Cataract and Refractive Surgery 2001;28:1710.
3. Agarwal A, Agarwal S, Agarwal At. Phakonit: A new technique of removing cataracts through a 0.9 mm incision. In Agarwal et al (Eds): Textbook Phacoemulsification, Laser Cataract Surgery and Foldable IOL's, (First edition). Jaypee, India 1998;139-43.
4. Agarwal A, Agarwal S, Agarwal At. Phakonit and laser phakonit: Lens surgery through a 0.9 mm incision. In Agarwal et al (Eds): Textbook Phacoemulsification, Laser Cataract Surgery and Foldable IOL's, (Second edition). Jaypee, India 2000;204-16.
5. Agarwal A, Agarwal S, Agarwal At. Phakonit. In Agarwal et al (Eds): Textbook Phacoemulsification, Laser Cataract Surgery and Foldable IOL's, (Third edition). Jaypee, India 2003;317-29.
6. Agarwal A, Agarwal S, Agarwal At. Phakonit and laser phakonit. In Boyd/Agarwal et al (Eds): Textbook Lasik and Beyond Lasik, Higlights of Ophthalmology, Panama 2000; 463-68.
7. Agarwal A, Agarwal S, Agarwal At. Phakonit and Laser Phakonit- Cataract Surgery through a 0.9 mm Incision. In Boyd/Agarwal et al (Eds): Textbook Phako, Phakonit and Laser Phako, Higlights of Ophthalmology, Panama, 2000; 327-34.
8. Agarwal A, Agarwal S, Agarwal At. The Phakonit Thinoptx IOL. In Agarwals textbook Presbyopia. Slack, USA, 2002; 187-94.
9. Agarwal A, Agarwal S, Agarwal At. Antichamber collapser; J Cataract and Refractive Surgery 2002;28:1085.
10. Pandey S, Wener L, Agarwal A, Agarwal S, Agarwal At, Hoyos J. Phakonit: Cataract removal through a sub 1.0 mm incision with implantation of the Thinoptx rollable IOL. J Cataract and Refractive Surgery 2002;28:1710.
11. Agarwal A, Agarwal S, Agarwal At. Phakonit: phacoemulsification through a 0.9 mm incision. J Cataract and Refractive Surgery 2001;27:1548-52.
12. Agarwal A, Agarwal S, Agarwal At. Phakonit with an acritec IOL. J Cataract and Refractive Surgery 2003;29:854-5.
13. Agarwal S, Agarwal A, Agarwal At. Phakonit with Acritec IOL. Highlights of Ophthalmology 2000.
14. Jorge Alio. What does MICS require in Alios textbook MICS; Highlights of Ophthalmology 2004;1-4.
15. Soscia W, Howard JG, Olson RJ. Microphacoemulsification with Whitestar. A wound-temperature study. J Cataract and Refractive Surgery 2002;28;1044-6.
16. Soscia W, Howard JG, Olson RJ. Bimanual phacoemulsification through two stab incisions. A wound-temperature study; J Cataract and Refractive Surgery 2002;28:1039-43.
17. Randall Olson. Microphaco chop in David Changs textbook on Phaco Chop. Slack, USA 2004;227-37.
18. David Chang. Bimanual phaco chop in David Changs textbook on Phaco Chop; Slack , USA 2004;239-50.
19. Agarwal A. Air pump in Agarwal's textbook on Bimanual phaco: Mastering the phakonit/MICS Technique; Slack , USA 2005.

6

Microincision Cataract Surgery

- INDICATIONS AND PATIENT SELECTION
- ANESTHESIA
- MICS SURGICAL INSTRUMENTS
- INCISIONS
- PRECHOPPING (COUNTER CHOPPING TECHNIQUE)
- LOW ULTRASOUND (LUS)—MICS SURGICAL STEPS
- RESULTS OF LUS—MICS
- MICS PROS AND ADVANTAGES

Jorge L Alio, Jose-Luis Rodriguez Prats, Ahmed Galal (Spain)

INTRODUCTION

Cornea incisions performed at the beginning of the surgery are one of the most important elements in cataract surgery today. Incision size has progressive reduced from 10 mm in the intracapsular era to 7 mm in extracapsular cases and finally from 3.4 mm to 2.8 mm, which was the minimum incision performed before the recent era of MICS (Figure 6.1). Such a microincision has a great advantage in reducing the induced astigmatism developing after the surgery, which affected the refractive results of the procedure. Cataract surgery nowadays, in addition to being considered a therapeutic procedure to cure the cataract, is also considered as a refractive surgery. The need to reduce the incision to the minimum possible for the sack of astigmatic reduction that may reach up to 3.00 D with conventional techniques. Another essential factor is reduction of the amount of energy being liberated inside the eye when using U/S emulsification. Until now the amount of energy being liberated or the power used to operate a cataract inside the eye has not yet been determined. As it is a source of mechanical, waveshock, constitutional and thermal damage, this energy and power delivered inside the eye has an effect on the ocular structures. The intraocular structures, endothelial cells, corneal stroma, and incisions are all affected by the liberated thermal effects of this energy. By definition Microincision Cataract Surgery (MICS) is the surgery performed through incisions of 1.5 mm or less. Understanding this global concept implies that it is not only about achieving a smaller incision size but about making a global transformation of the surgical procedure towards minimal aggressiveness. Protection of the intraocular structures and ensuring a safe surgery with no complications is another aim for modern cataract surgery. Lowering the energy levels as achieved in MICS surgery is considered an important step in this technique. Lower energy levels cause no burns at the incision sites in addition to the other biophysical effects with reduced loss of endothelial cells and less intraocular tissue trauma.

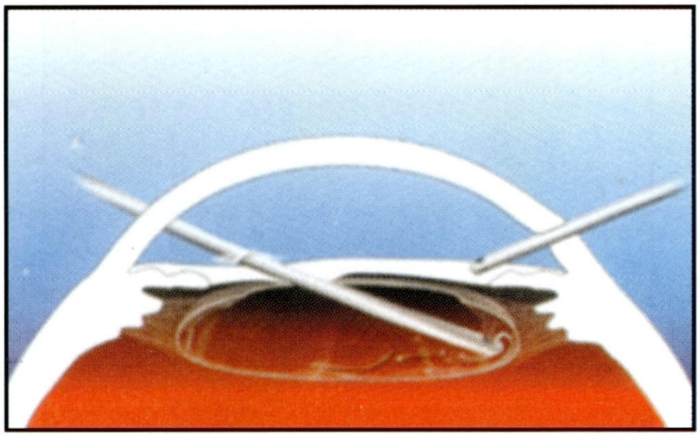

Figure 6.1: Bimanuality in MICS

INDICATIONS AND PATIENT SELECTION

The application of MICS in cataract surgery is unlimited with regards to cataract density or hardness as this technique is able to treat all grades of cataract density according to the nuclear density scale. The authors have found that an optimal elective indication nowadays of MICS is "lens refractive surgery." Considering the delicate working technique, MICS can also be indicated for subluxated cataractus lenses and posttraumatic cataracts of grade I or II, zonular laxity and finally congenital cataracts. The classification of cataract grading should be done based on "lens opacities classification system III" (LOCS III classification) (Figure 6.2). Soft and moderately hard nuclei up to +2 hardness can be easily emulsified by using low ultrasound MICS (LUS-MICS) and prechopping will shorten the time of surgery and the energy delivered inside the eye. Hard nuclei of grade 3 or over are more amenable to LUS-MICS, which is capable of emulsifying hard nuclei of any density.

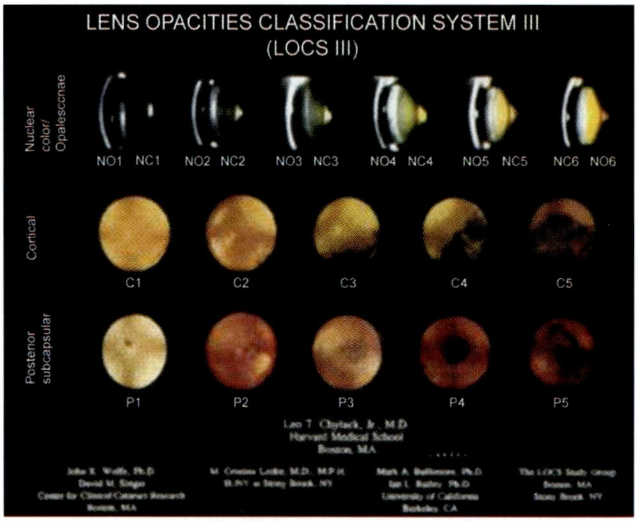

Figure 6.2: Alio's MICS microblade

ANESTHESIA

Generally MICS can be done using topical anesthesia 0.75 percent Bupivacaine plus 2 percent Lidocaine by instillation of 2 drops every 5 minutes before surgery, with supplemental intra-cameral preservative-free 1 percent Lidocaine diluted 1:1 in BSS in considered sufficient.

MICS SURGICAL INSTRUMENTS

Bimanuality is becoming an important fact for modern surgeon. He need to use is both hands with equal efficiency in addition to the new concept of separation of functions and using the irrigation as an instrument in the surgery, the new MICS instruments were developed.

The instruments were designed to be finger-friendly and each has its own function. These instruments will be a new extension of the surgeons' fingers inside the eye.[1]

MICS Microblade

To create a trapezoidal incision from 1.2 to 1.4 mm micro blade (Katena Inc, Denville, NJ, USA) (Figure 6.3): Made of diamond or stainless steel. The anterior tapering tip is 1.2 mm and the base is 1.4 mm. This design is essential to perform incisions with an internal diameter smaller than the external diameter. This incision design enables the surgeon to move his instruments freely inside the anterior chamber without performing any stress on the incision lips thus avoiding tissue distortion and induced astigmatism.[1]

MICS Capsulorhexis Forceps (Katena Inc, Denville, NJ, USA) (Figure 6.4)

No more worries about how you are going to perform your rhexis because through the smallest incision the delicate body of this instrument can pass even through a paracentesis incision. This extremely delicate forceps, was designed to function efficiently through a side port incision enabling the surgeon to have precise control of the capsulorhexis maneuver. It has micro-triangular tips that can be used to puncture and grasp the capsule to perform the capsulorhexis with a single instrument. Besides that you can use it for other intraocular maneuvers such as grasping the iris to perform small

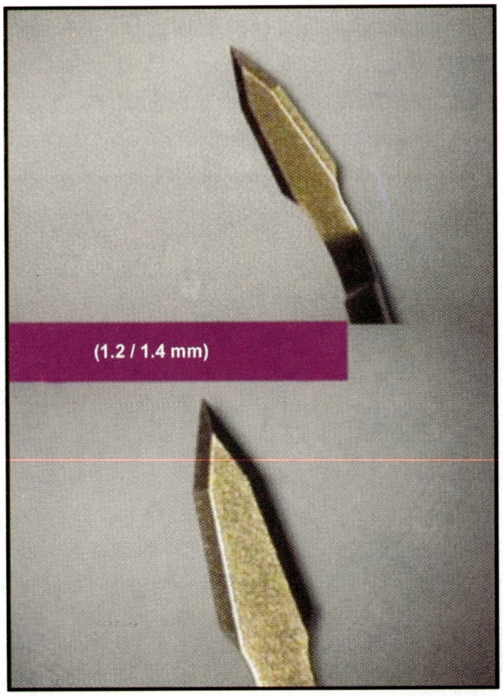

Figure 6.3: Alio's MICS capsulorhexis forceps

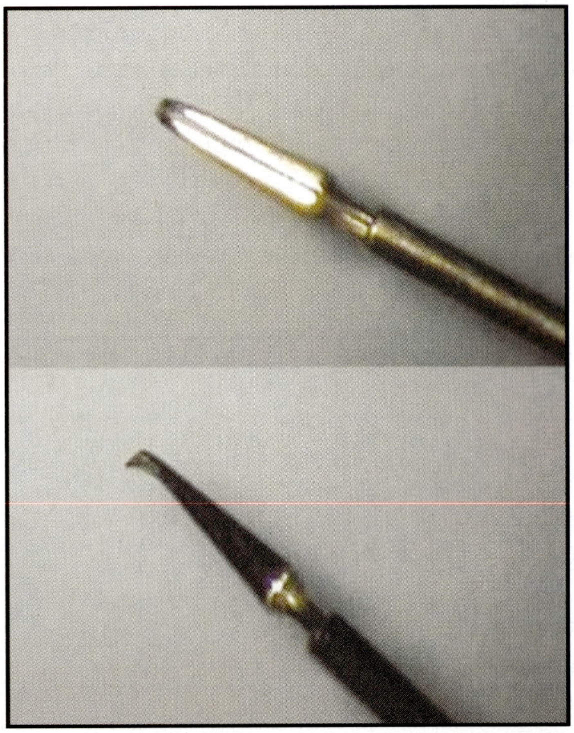

Figure 6.4: Alio's MICS hydromanipulator irrigating fingernail

iridotomies or to cut pre-existing synechia in the anterior or posterior chambers. [1]

Alió MICS Prechoppers

These two twin instruments are an essential step of the procedure. They have been designed with the idea of cutting the cataract with counter chopping technique without the induction of zonular stress. They are to be used bimanually and, as opposed to the single handed pre-chopping technique, can be used in all types of cataracts regardless of the hardness. The tip has a blunted square hook that should be introduced gently underneath the anterior capsular rim, one instrument opposite to the other. The two advancing sides of the instruments have a cutting edge so the instrument sharply cuts the cataract as it progresses from the periphery towards the center. When the instruments reach the center of the nucleus both sides pass the deep central most posterior part of the nucleus to divide it into two hemispherical parts. One of the choppers should be kept in position to protect one hemisphere from moving forward and then the second chopper is taken to the periphery again underneath the anterior capsular rim, 90° degrees apart from the created groove, thus making the dissection of one of the parts and then the same maneuver is performed again with the other. Another alternative in to rotate the two hemispherical fragments and to repeat the initial maneuver 90° apart from the initial one. In both cases, four quadrants are created. This allows for a sharp decrease in the use of the ultrasonic energy and makes the whole procedure faster. Ultrasound (or laser) energy is no longer necessary to cut a cataract but to emulsify cataract fragments instead.[1]

MICS Hydrodissector or Irrigating-Fingernail (Katena Inc, Denville, NJ, USA) (Figure 6.5)

Naturally, you are aware of the basic characteristic of this instrument but this is not all. It makes manipulation of the nucleus fragments easy as well functioning as an irrigating instrument. This can also be useful to further divide the nuclear fragments. With soft to medium density cataracts there are no problems at all but you should use it with care for further segment dissection as

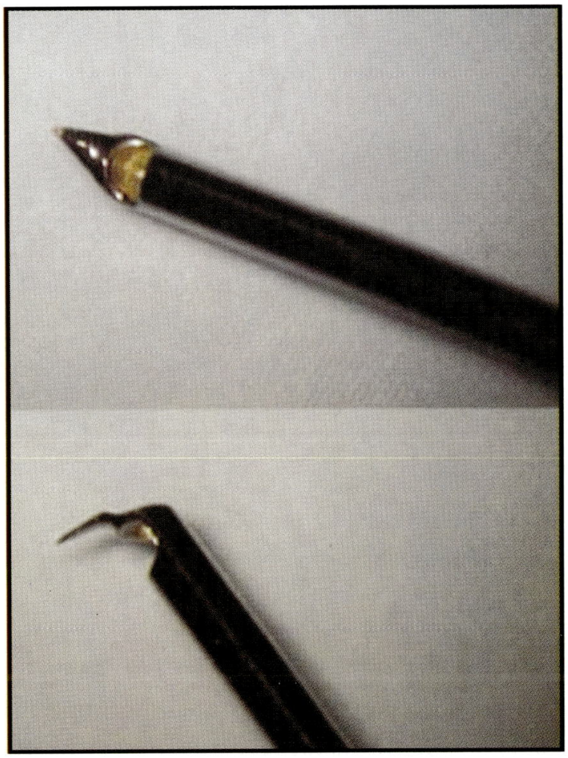

Figure 6.5: Alio's MICS chopper

cataract density increases. The forward directed pointing tip is a fingernail-like, hence its name, which has a highly blunt point-like end. The irrigating fluid exits through a large port (1 mm) directed under the tip. This feature helps pushing away the posterior capsule to obtain stable fluidic control in the anterior chamber when combined with phaco or MICS aspirating tip. The flow rate or the free irrigation flow of this instrument is 72 cc/min, which is considered the highest flow compared to other instruments performing the same function in the market. This generates the anterior chamber stability regardless of the level of the high vacuum in MICS.[1]

Another point is the rate of endothelial cell loss associated with the conventional phacoemulsification, which is related to the fluidics. The problem is that the side ports are situated on the lateral sides of the phaco tip and are small in diameter giving exit to the fluids under high pressure. Bearing in mind the position of the phaco tip inside the anterior chamber during the process, we will notice that if the side ports are horizontally oriented and at a higher level than the iris plane, the

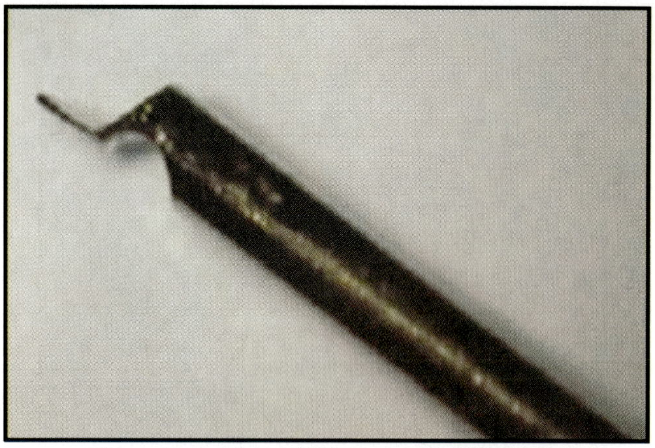

Figure 6.6: Alio's MICS aspiration handpiece

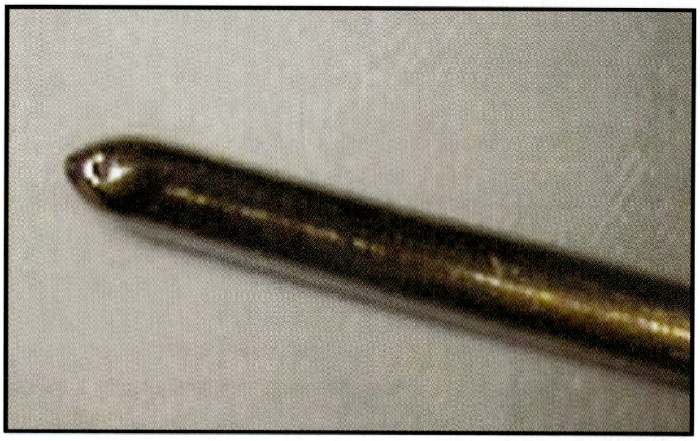

Figure 6.7: Alio's MICS manipulator

irrigating fluids directly reduce endothelial cell numbers. In addition to severe turbulence in the anterior chamber with direct effect on the endothelial cells. This never happens in case of our MICS hydrodissector as the irrigating port is deep inside the posterior chamber and facing the posterior capsule, stabilizing the anterior chamber more, cleaning the posterior capsule of the cortical cells and protecting the endothelium. Irrigating instruments in MICS are designed to function through sealed incisions to guarantee the anterior chamber stability.[1]

MICS irrigating Chopper (Katena Inc, Denville, NJ, USA) (Figure 6.6)

This instrument was designed to chop medium to hard cataract if prechopping has not been performed. It has a sharp pointed triangular shaped tip which is angled downward to "chop" off segments of the nucleus. The irrigating fluid exits through a large port (1 mm) directed under the tip of the instrument. This feature helps to push away the posterior capsule to obtain stable fluidic control in the anterior chamber when combined with phaco or MICS aspirating tip.[1]

MICS Aspiration Handpiece (Katena Inc, Denville, NJ, USA) (Figure 6.7)

The bullet shaped tip is designed for easy entry through a paracentesis incision and has a 0.3 mm diameter aspirating port close to the tip in the interior part of the curvature. This design works to maintain the fluid balance in the anterior chamber when used with the MICS irrigating fingernail, MICS chopper and while aspirating the residual cortex. Is to be used in combination with the other irrigating instruments to keep an adequate balance of the fluidics in MICS. [1]

Intraocular Manipulator (Katena Inc, Denville, NJ, USA) (Figure 6.8)

The manipulator is multifunctional. It provides efficient help in iridolenticular synechia dissection, IOL manipulation and other intraocular maneuvers such as vitreous knuckles or stabilization of the IOL. It moves safely and effectively with a very delicate blunt tip of its conical shaped design. The base is wide enough to seal the incision, maintaining the stability of the anterior chamber, preventing as much trauma as possible to the intraocular structures. The conical base is the same diameter as the

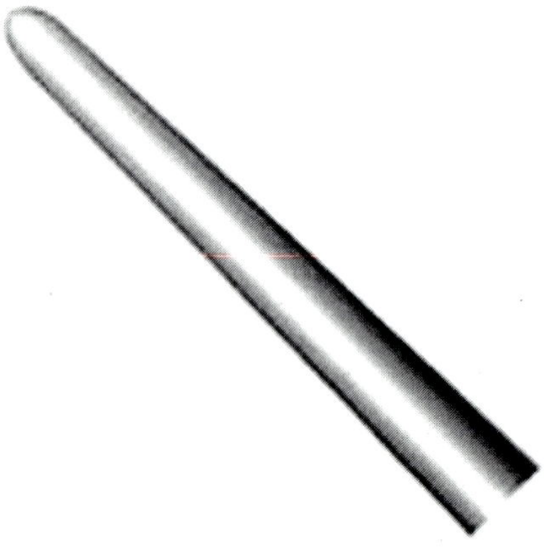

Figure 6.8: Alio's MICS scissors

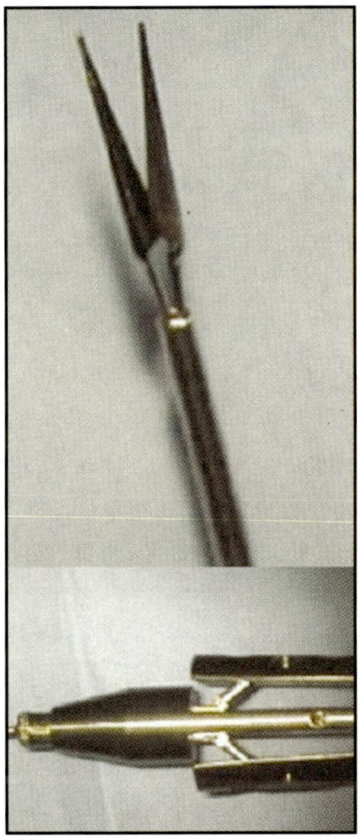

Figure 6.9: LOCS III classification

internal MICS incision in order to keep the anterior chamber stability thus preventing outflow of the viscoelastic.[1]

MICS scissors (Katena Inc, Denville, NJ, USA) (Figure 6.9)

The handling of any membranes even delicate ones, synechia or fibrosed capsules is made easy by using these unique scissors. The design has a 23 gauge (0.6-mm) shaft, making it fit exactly through a very small paracentesis. It has extremely delicate blunt tipped blades, which are ideal for cutting synechia and capsular fibrosis and membranes as well as for performing small iridotomies.[1]

INCISIONS

After the surgical field is isolated and an adjustable eye speculum (Duckworth and Kent) England is inserted, the positive corneal meridian is marked (Figure 6.10) and 2 trapezoidal incisions of 1.2 mm internally and 1.4 mm externally are performed using the Alio corneal keratome (Katena) (Figure 6.11). With this, an external incision of 1.4 mm will be adequate for better instrument manipulation. The two incisions are performed in clear cornea

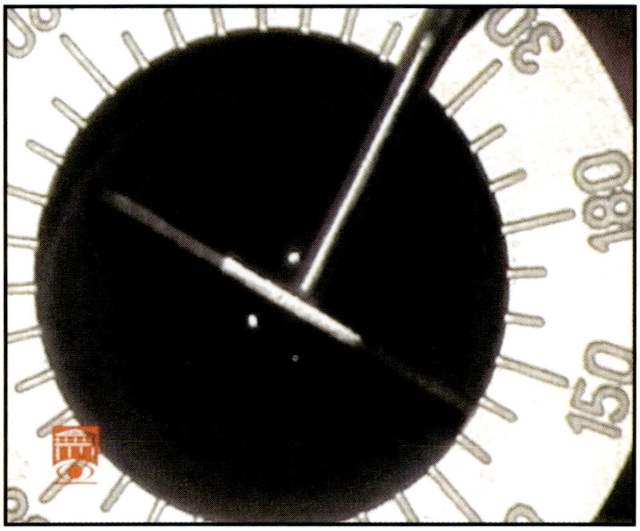

Figure 6.10: Marking of the corneal principle incision at the positive corneal meridian

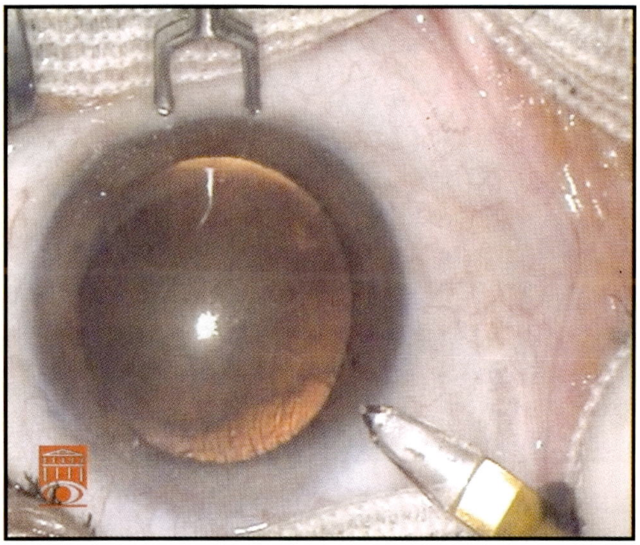

Figure 6.11: MICS is performed through corneal incisions

90° apart, at 10 and 2 o'clock (Figures 6.12A and B) followed by the injection of 1 percent Lidocaine preservative free diluted 1:1 in BSS.

PRECHOPPING (COUNTER-CHOPPING TECHNIQUE)

After performing the capsulorhexis using Alio's capsulorhexis forceps (Figure 6.13), the prechopping is performed. This is a bimanual technique requiring the use of both hands with the same efficiency. This technique allows manual cut division of the nucleus, without creating any grooves prior to the MICS

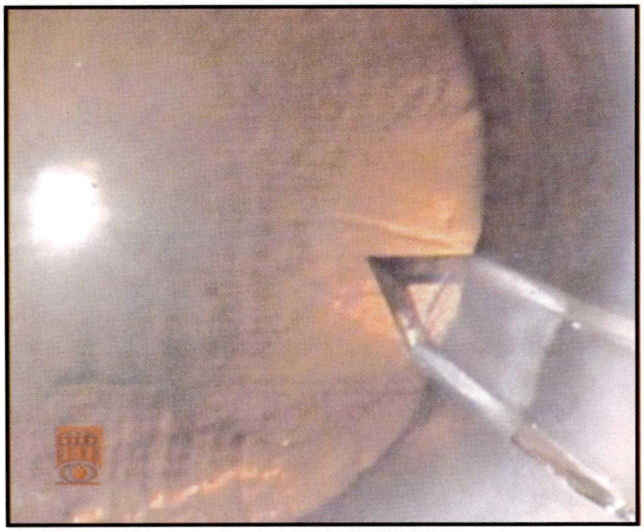

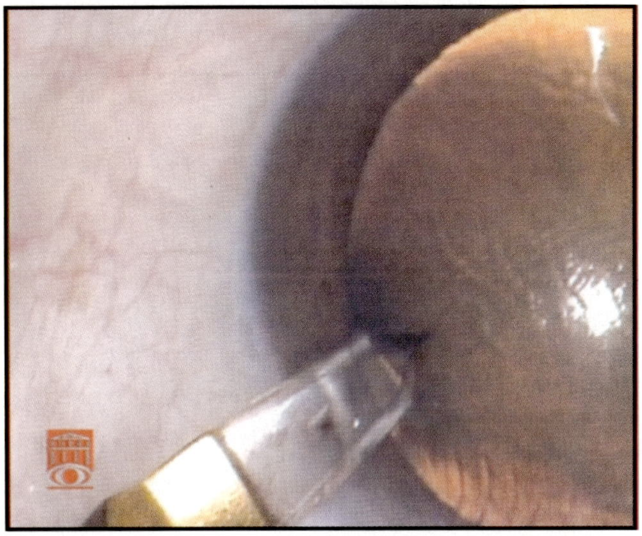

Figures 6.12A and B: The 2 clear corneal incisions are 90° apart

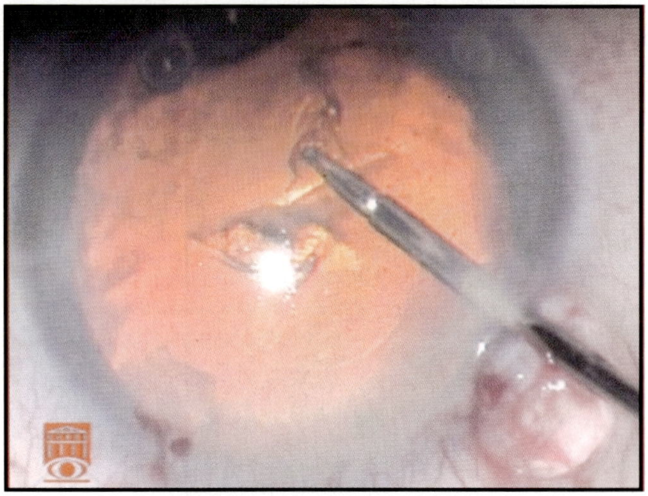

Figure 6.13: CCC using Alio's capsulorhexis forceps

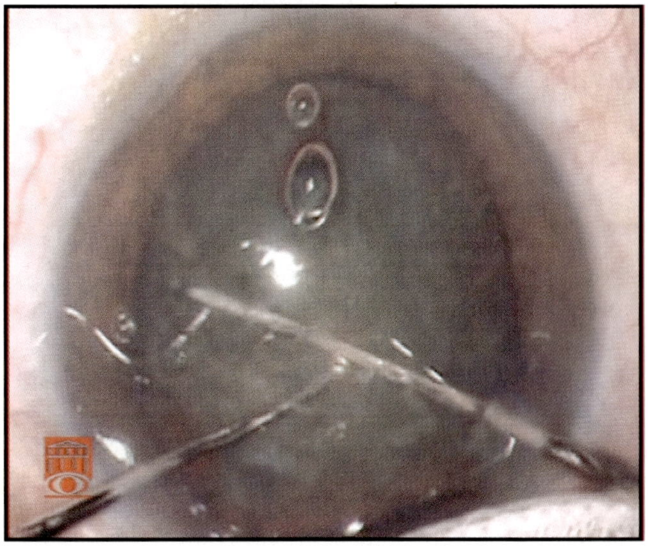

Figure 6.14: Prechopping

procedure. In order to protect the endothelium and to perform an adequate counter-chopping technique, more dispersive or cohesive viscoelastic material is injected. The technique of counter prechopping could be applied to all surgical grades of cataract density (up to grade +5). A chopper is introduced through one of the 2 incisions depending on the surgeon's preference. Through the other incision a nuclear manipulator is introduced to decrease the stress on the capsule and zonules being inserted beneath the anterior capsulorhexis edge and the rounded microball tip of the nuclear manipulator will protect the posterior capsule during the prechopping procedure. The tips of the nuclear manipulator and the chopper should be aligned on the same axis together with the hardest point of the nucleus along the direction of the lens fibers then appropriate force is applied between the two instruments (Figure 6.14). After cracking the nucleus into the fragments, the nucleus is rotated and the maneuver is repeated on the other axis to crack the nucleus into 4 quadrants. To avoid damaging the zonules, a nucleus sustainer could be used as introduced through the second incision and inserted below the anterior capsule at the equator of the lens. Such sustainer is not recommended in our technique as well as other authors, adding more risks for the zonules and complexity to the procedure. The procedure is short, safe and

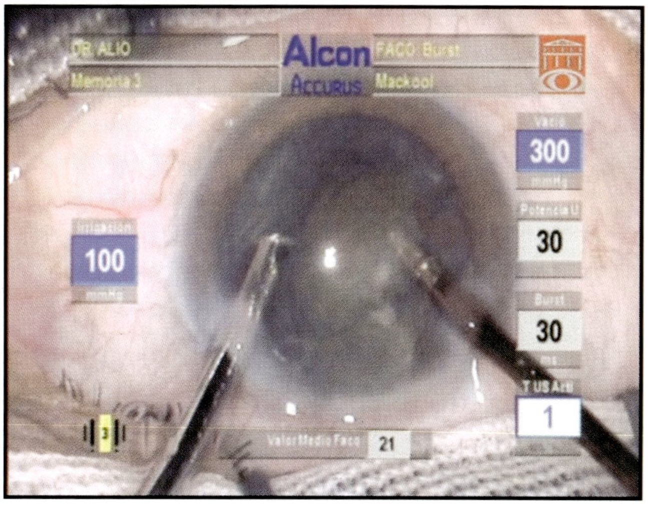

Figure 6.15: Separating the quadrants to begin MICS

could be done in few seconds but with the advantages of cutting down the surgical time and minimizing the energy used during nucleus emulsification. Once the fragments have been obtained, the MICS tip and Alio hydromanipulator fingernail are introduced to manipulate and emulsify the fragments. [1]

LOW ULTRASOUND (LUS)-MICS SURGICAL STEPS

The MICS technique could be performed using phacoemulsification which is termed low ultrasound MICS (LUS-MICS) and by using laser which is termed laser-MICS. After termination of pre-chopping the Accurus machine is adjusted according to the previous described settings. MICS Mackool tip and Alio's hydromanipulator fingernail are introduced through the 2 incisions and an inferior segment is mobilized and brought in contact with the MICS tip assisted with Alio's hydromanipulator in order to be emulsified (Figure 6.15). After the elimination of the fist hemi-nucleus, the second pre-chopped hemi-nucleus is rotated to the distal portion of the bag and Alio's hydromanipulator is used to mobilize the segments making them easy to be emulsified. Using this technique reduces the tendency for the nuclear material to come up into the anterior chamber during the procedure maintaining its position within the epinuclear cover (Figures 6.16A and B). Following the emulsification of all the nuclear segments, the epinuclear rim is trimmed in the different quadrants

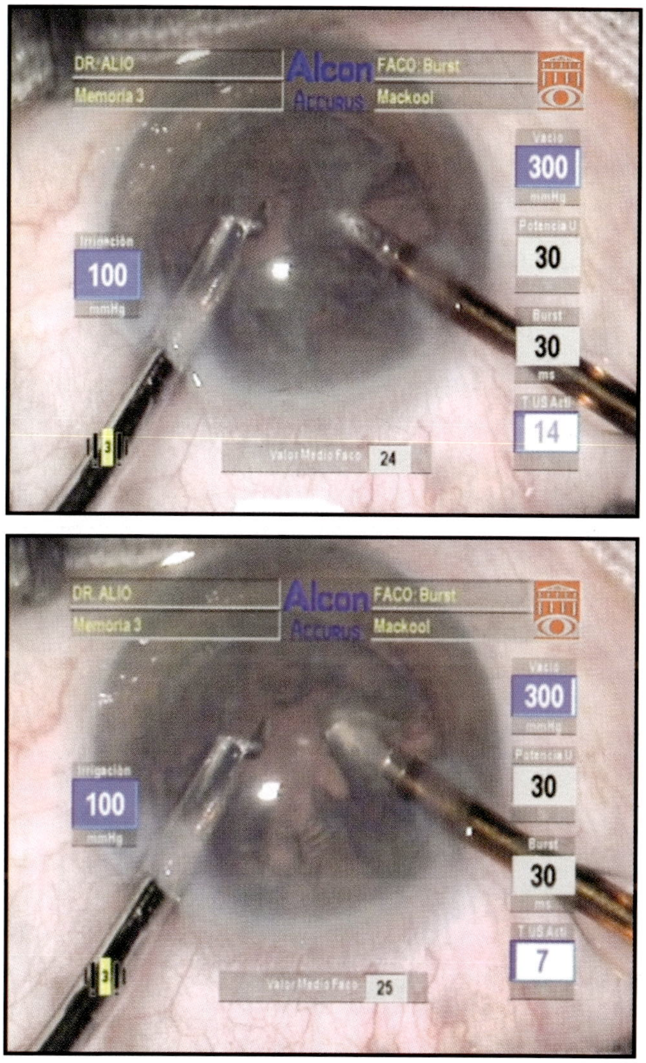

Figures 6.16A and B: The 4 quadrants of the nucleus being emulsified using MICS surgery

in such way to remove all the cortical material remaining in the capsular bag (Figure 6.17). An adequate OVD is injected deep in the capsular bag to reform the bag and prepare it for IOL implantation and helps to force the Viscoat anteriorly facilitating its removal to prevent post-operative rise of IOP.[1]

RESULTS OF LUS-MICS

MICS surgery using ultrasound energy as accurus machine (Figure 6.18), offer the advantage of being having a superior biological effect on the ocular structures more than conventional phaco procedures. Studying the

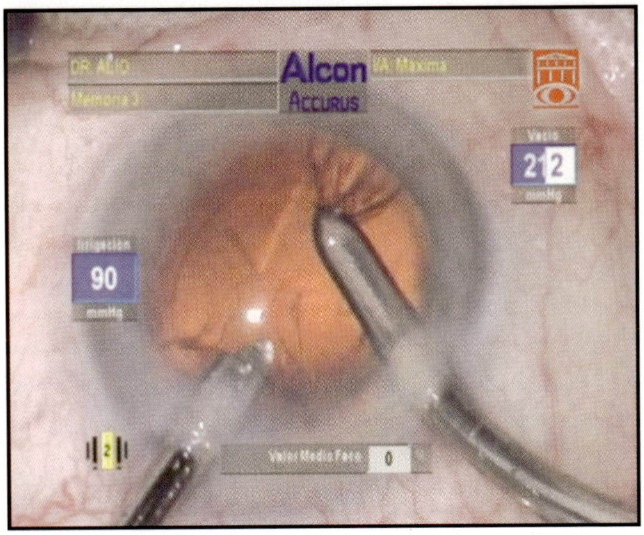

Figure 6.17: Complete removal of the cortex

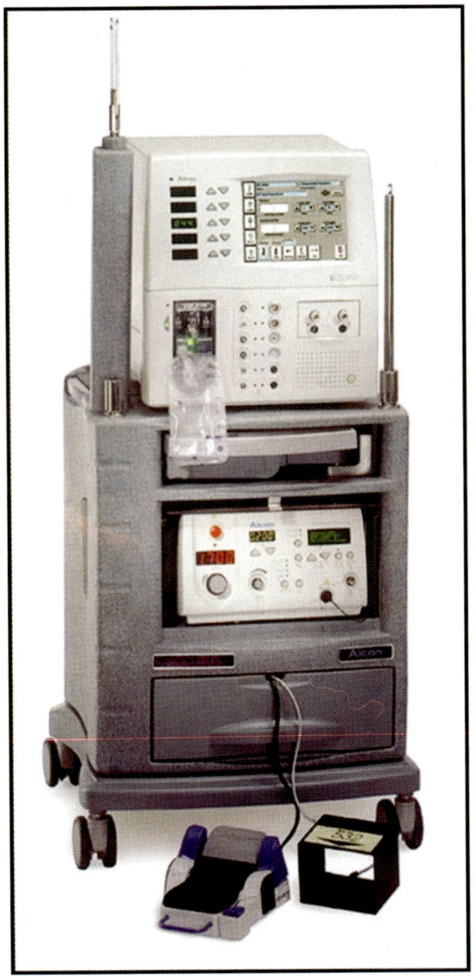

Figure 6.18: Accurus phacoemulsificator

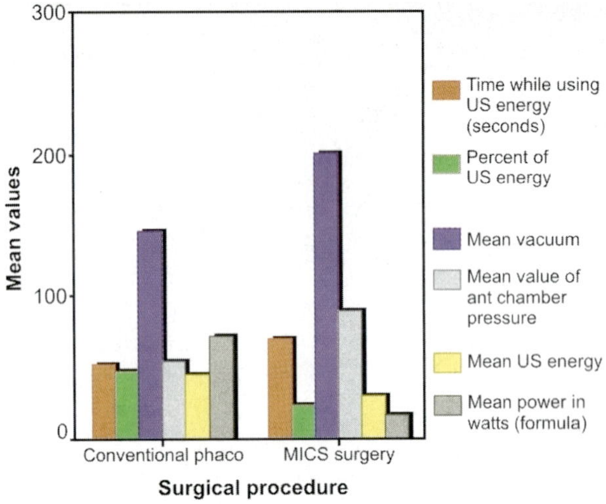

Figure 6.19: Bar graph showing the difference parameters used in both MICS and conventional phacoemulsification

parameters that controls the procedure in both technique the following was found:

Concerning the pressure of anterior chamber (AC), working in closed compartment is the character of MICS surgery while operating through the microincisions, and because of that it was fundamental to find the pressure of AC higher in MICS surgery rather that in conventional phaco (Figure 6.19).

Concerning the vacuum used during surgery it was found to be higher in MICS surgery, which is essential in performing MICS surgery .

The percent of phaco used with different machines differed according to the machine used. The grade of cataract operated with different machines was compared as illustrated. Less percent of phaco was performed when Accurus machine using the MacKool while using burst 30 and 300, but Burst 300 mode offered less power delivered to the ocular tissue when the power was calculated.

Study of endothelial cell count and inflammatory reaction:

MICS surgery offers the advantage of lowering the percent of cell loss during the procedure. As well as the flare developing after the procedure was found to be much lower in MICS surgery.

MICS PROS AND ADVANTAGES

Performing small incision in cataract surgery has a number of theoretical advantages:

- Fast visual recovery and improved visual outcome
- Decrease in post-operative astigmatism
- Reduction in the anatomical healing time
- Less rate of complications.
- IOL insertion through microincision is now possible.
- Reduction in the operating time with.

MICS could be performed using laser power as safe as US power. The use of either source of energy permits:

- Visual acuity improvement the first day post-operative
- Reduction of the inflammatory reaction post-operatively
- Reduction of the endothelial cell damage.

Improving both techniques will open the way to emulsify all grades of nucleus density and this could be achieved by improving the safety and the fluidity of the low US phaco and laser, with the possibility of obtaining greater aspiration and more vacuum and to maintain continuous contact between the crystalline to be removed and the laser aperture.

REFERENCES

1. Alio JL, Rodriguez-Prats JL, Galal A. Micro-incision cataract surgery. Highlights of Ophthalomology International. Miami USA, 2004.
2. Tsuneoka H, Hayama A, Takahama M: Ultrasmall-incision bimanual phacoemulsification and AcrySof SA30AL implantation through a 2.2 mm incision. J Cataract Refract Surg 2003;29:1070-6.
3. Tsuneoka H, Shiba T, Takahashi Y. Ultrasonic phacoemulsification using a 1.4 mm incision: clinical results. J Cataract Refract Surg 2002;28:81-6.
4. Chylack, LT, Wolfe JK, Singer DM, et al. lens opacities classification system III. Arch Ophthalmol 1993;111:831-3.

7

Sealed Capsule Irrigation Device and Phakonit

- HISTORY
- PRINCIPLE
- PERFECT CAPSULE
- SURGICAL TECHNIQUE
- RESEARCH

Amar Agarwal, Anthony Maloof, Sunita Agarwal,
Athiya Agarwal, Ashok Garg (India)

HISTORY

One of the real bugbears in cataract surgery is posterior capsule opacification. It has not been possible to effectively isolate and specifically target lens epithelial cells following phacoemulsification. Dr Anthony Maloof from Australia developed and designed a disposable instrument (Figure 7.1) called the "perfect capsule" (Milvella Pty. Ltd, Sydney, Australia) which helps selective targeting of the lens epithelial cells with a new technique called the sealed capsule irrigation (SCI) device. This device has been used in human eyes by many surgeons since then . On 11th July 2003 the first live surgery in a conference showing the SCI after phakonit cataract surgery under no anesthesia[1-3] was telecast in the Indian Intraocular Implant and Refractive surgery conference at Chennai, India by one of us (Am A).

PRINCIPLE

Using an injection-moulded (Figure 7.2) silicone device, sealed capsule irrigation[4,5] isolates the internal lens capsule, including residual lens epithelial cells, from the rest of the eye. The basic idea is to seal the rhexis (Figure 7.3) and then irrigate the capsular bag with an irrigating solution (Figure 7.4) which would prevent posterior capsular opacification. The main point here is that the sealing of the capsule should be perfect so that the

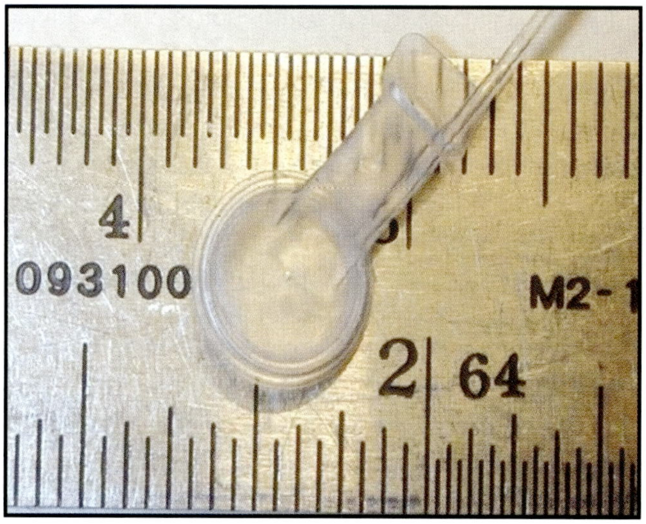

Figure 7.1: Perfect capsule

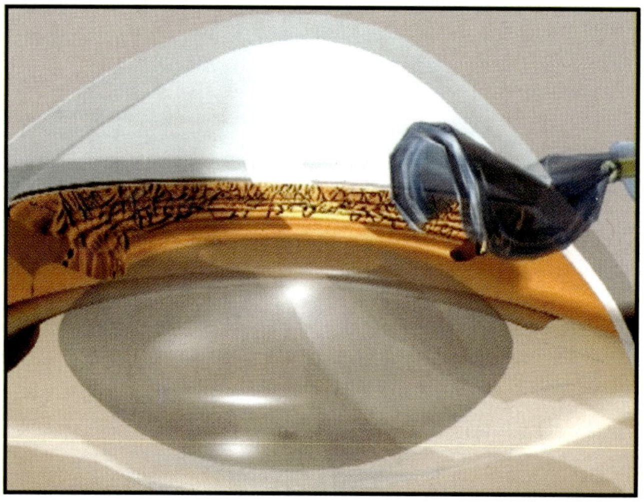

Figure 7.2: Perfect capsule is easy to fold and insert through a 3 mm incision

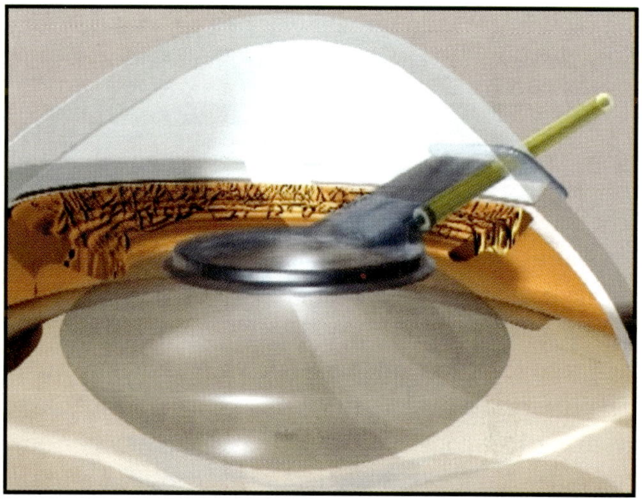

Figure 7.3: Perfect capsule is placed onto the capsular bag and vacuum activated by a syringe

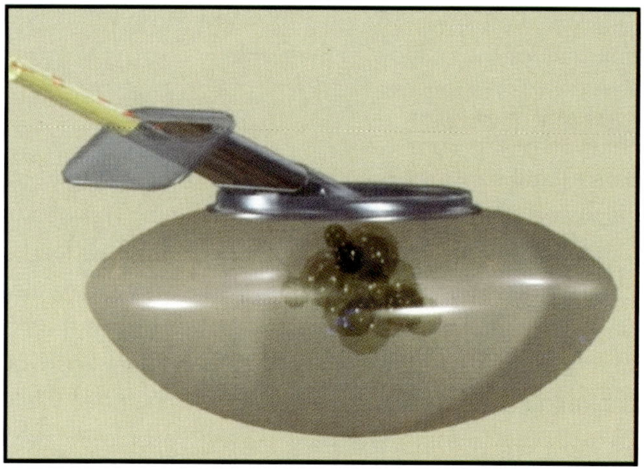

Figure 7.4: Irrigation of the capsular bag is done

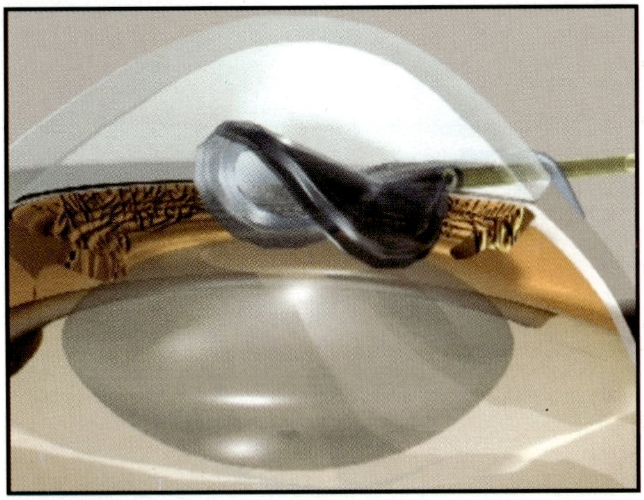

Figure 7.5: Perfect capsule is removed from the eye

surgeon can irrigate the capsular bag without it leaking into the anterior chamber. Then finally the device is removed from the eye (Figure 7.5).

PERFECT CAPSULE

The sealed capsule irrigation device (see Figure 7.1) known as perfect capsule (Milvella, Australia) is made of medical grade silicone. It has an overall diameter of 7 mm and an inner diameter of 5 mm. It has been designed to temporarily seal a rhexis of less than 5 mm. The device utilizes a vacuum ring (similiar to that used to fixate the globe during Lasik), which attaches onto the outer surface of the anterior lens capsule and seals around the rhexis. There is a separate channel through which one can pass an irrigating solution into the capsular bag and through that same area there is a channel for the outflow of the fluid.

SURGICAL TECHNIQUE

The tunnel construction is very important—it should be short and steep, pointing towards the rhexis. This allows especially in high myopic eyes where the AC is deep a proper placement of the perfect capsule on the capsular bag. The next step is to perform a rhexis of less than 5 mm (Figure 7.6). After removing the nucleus and cortical aspiration (Figure 7.7) one should fill the chamber a little bit with viscoelastic. Then the perfect capsule is taken out of its sterile package. The perfect capsule is held with a forceps (Figure 7.8) and as it is soft it can be folded (Figure 7.9) and passed through a 3.2 mm incision (Figure 7.10). If one has done phakonit the 1 mm incision has to be increased. Once folded the forceps is passed into the anterior chamber with the perfect capsule (Figure 7.11). The perfect capsule then unfolds inside the anterior chamber. Using the left hand with a globe stabilization rod one should press gently on the perfect capsule so that it touches the anterior capsule (Figure 7.12) . Once done then the assistant is told to pull the syringe connected to the perfect capsule and lock it. This syringe creates a suction so that the perfect capsule seals the rhexis margin (Figure 7.13). One should be careful that the iris does not get stuck in between the capsule and the perfect capsule.

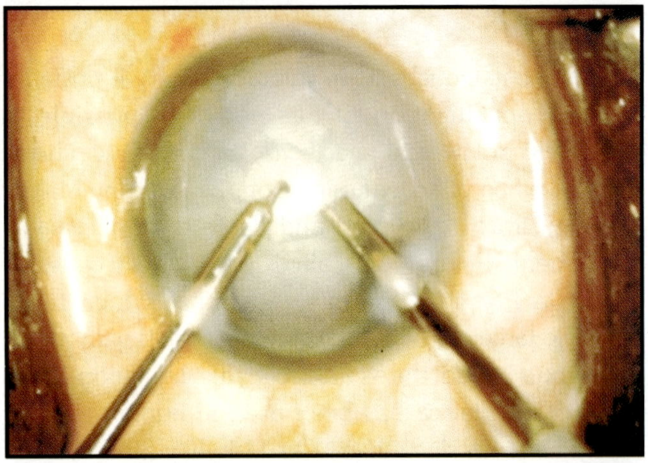

Figure 7.6: Phakonit started after rhexis performed of under 5 mm

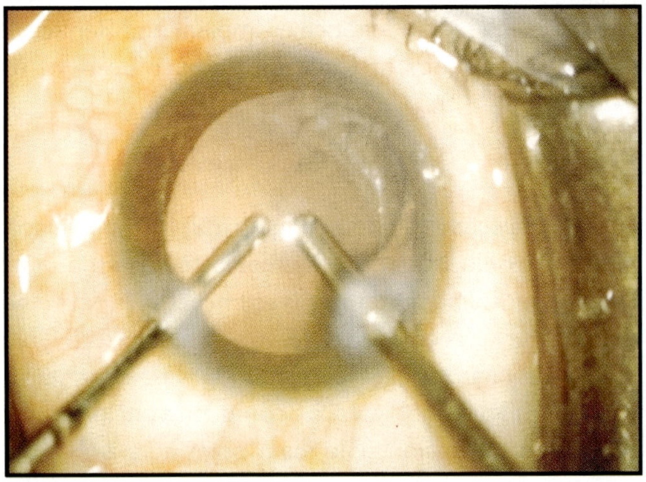

Figure 7.7: Bimanual irrigation aspiration

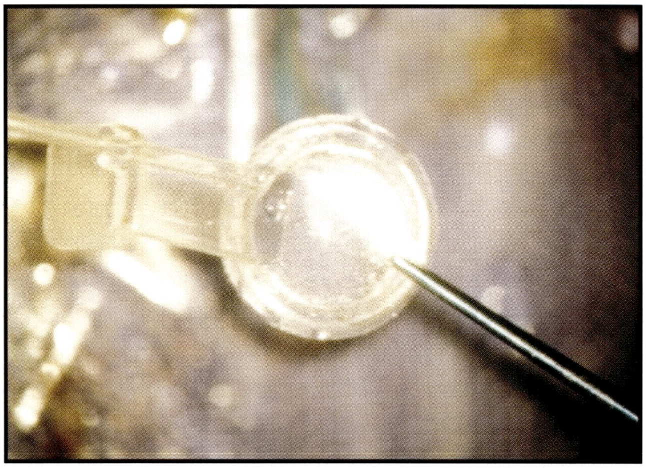

Figure 7.8: Perfect capsule held with a forceps

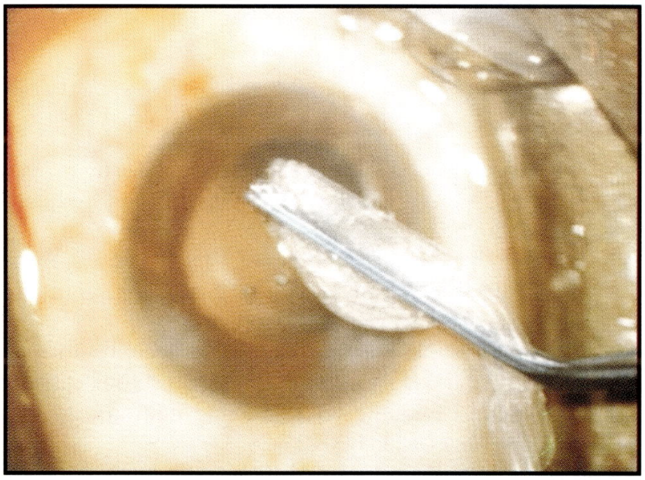

Figure 7.9: Perfect capsule folded

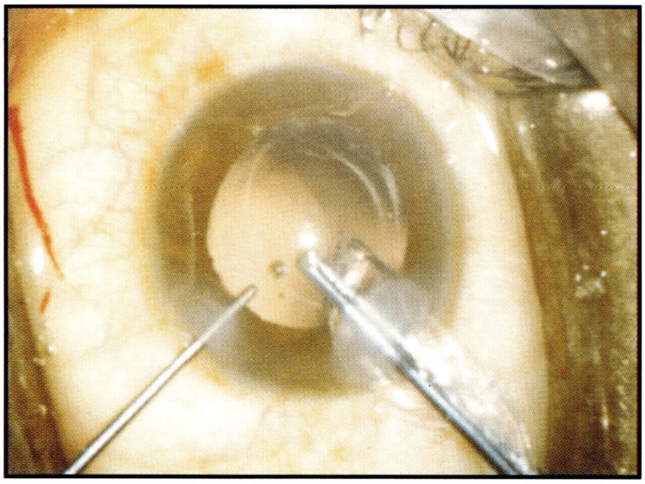

Figure 7.10: Perfect capsule passed into the eye

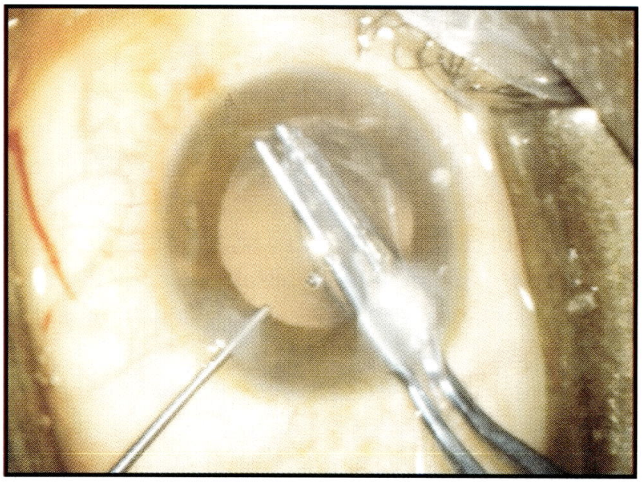

Figure 7.11: Perfect capsule placed over the rhexis

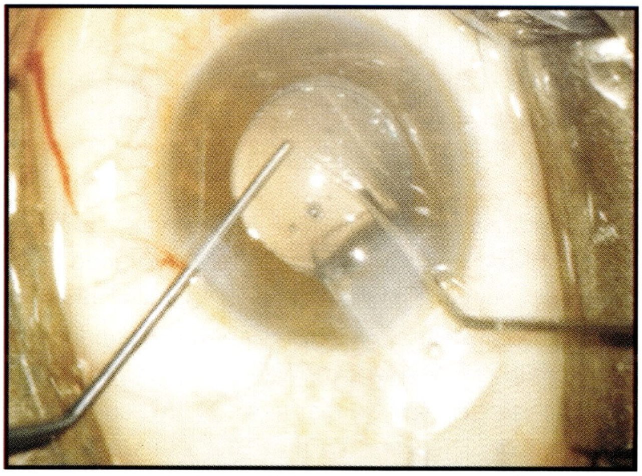

Figure 7.12: Perfect capsule locks over the rhexis

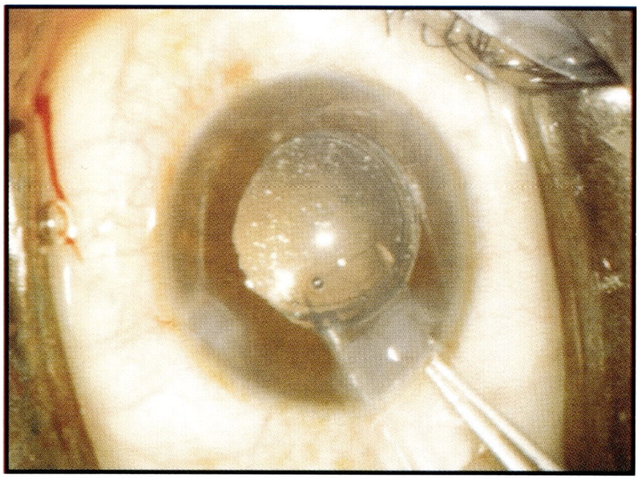

Figure 7.13: Once the perfect capsule is in place irrigation of the capsular bag is done with distilled water and then finally the perfect capsule is removed

Once the sealing has been done one can inject trypan blue (Blurhex, Dr Agarwal's Pharma) via a cannula through the opening in the perfect capsule meant for irrigation. The Blurhex will not leak into the anterior chamber. This indicates the sealing is perfect. Then the capsular bag is irrigated with distilled water. The distilled water will not come into contact with any other structures as it passes in and out of the capsular bag. We used the air pump in the irrigation to make the flow through the cannula better.

Once done the next step is top remove the perfect capsule. For this the assistant disengages the lock in the syringe so that the suction is broken. Then gradually viscoelastic is injected inside the eye. Then the perfect capsule is disengaged from the capsule with the globe stabilization rod. Once it is free in the anterior chamber the perfect capsule is pulled out of the eye. As it is soft it comes out quite comfortably.

RESEARCH

Further research has to be done to use cytotoxic drugs which will prevent posterior capsule opacification. This is just the beginning and not the end. Today we are able to seal the capsular bag effectively and this can lead in the future to many more uses. We are now trying to work on the perfect capsule so that it can be passed through a sub 1.5 mm incision so that one can use it after phakonit. The point here is that then the microlenses will not need a sharp optic to reduce the posterior capsular opacification.

The SCI was started off with focusing on prevention of PCO, however today with all the feedback from surgeons who have seen and used it SCI will be widened in its positioning. SCI is targeted to maintain a clear capsular bag and through this provide long term quality of vision. This is immediately relevant for (a) any lens-based refractive procedure (accommodating lenses, clear lens extraction/multifocal lenses, piggybag lenses); (b) cataract surgery where in the future one can implant IOLs without sharp edges—and using lens materials which today are seen as inferior (e.g. hydrophilic, silicone etc.)—so introduce optically improved materials with improved techniques like phakonit; and (c) mid term relevance for retinal surgeons who benefit from clear capsules when doing a vitrectomy.

REFERENCES

1. Sunita Agarwal, Athiya Agarwal, Mahipal S Sachdev, Keiki R Mehta, I Howard Fine, et al. Phacoemulsification, Laser Cataract Surgery and Foldable IOL's; (Second edition) Jaypee Brothers; Delhi, India 2000.
2. Benjamin F Boyd, Sunita Agarwal, Athiya Agarwal, Amar Agarwal. Lasik and Beyond Lasik. Highlights of Ophthalmology; Panama 2000.
3. Agarwal et al. No anesthesia cataract surgery with karate chop; In Agarwal's Phacoemulsification, Laser cataract surgery and foldable IOLs (Second edition). Jaypee Brothers: New Delhi 2000;217-26.
4. Anthony Maloof. Sealed lens capsule irrigation. Cataract and Refractive Surgery Today; 2002.
5. Sean Henahan, Anthony Maloof. Sealed capsule irrigation device could cut PCO after cataract; Eurotimes 2002;8(5).

8

ThinOptx Rollable IOL

Jairo E Hoyos, Melania Cigales, Jairo Hoyos-Chacón (Spain)

INTRODUCTION

The current surgical option of choice for the treatment of cataract is phacoemulsification and the implant of an intraocular lens (IOL) in the capsular bag. Although there was a time when the success of cataract surgery was based solely on a good anatomical result and improved visual acuity, today, we strive to obtain a good refractive outcome and rapid visual recovery in addition to these initial goals. Moreover, cataract surgery is performed ever more early when the patient still has an acceptable visual acuity. Since the onset of cataract surgery, the problem of incision-induced astigmatism has been known. This occurs when the corneal meridian at the point of incision is flattened.[1] The spread of the use of phacoemulsification and flexible IOLs has allowed a reduction in incision size, diminishing astigmatism and promoting the quick recovery of vision. Despite the demonstration by some authors[2] that incisions smaller than 3 mm (scleral tunnel incisions or self-sealing corneal incisions) do not provoke significant changes in the patient's preexisting astigmatism, recent technical advances in phacoemulsification machines have meant that surgery can now be performed through incisions as small as 1 mm using bimanual microinsertion techniques (Phakonit).[3] The emergence of these microincision techniques has forced industry to design lenses that do not require the extension of the incision for their insertion in the eye.

PROPERTIES OF THE THINOPTX LENS

The ultrathin ThinOptx lens was designed for microincisional surgery and was implanted for the first time in 2001 by J Hoyos and O. Asís (Spain).[4,5] The ThinOptx rollable IOL is manufactured by ThinOptx Inc. (Abingdon, VA, USA) and is presently undergoing clinical trials in Europe and U.S.A for the U.S. Food and Drug Administration.

The ThinOptx rollable IOL is a monoblock lens of plate design, manufactured in a hydrophilic acrylic material with a water content of 18 percent. Its dimensions: length 11.2 mm, optical zone 5.5 mm and thickness 50 to 400 μm, enable this lens to be implanted through a clear cornea incision of 1.5 mm.[4] The lens haptics have two teardrop-shaped orifices that indicate the correct positioning of the lens when these point in a clockwise direction. The haptics have four small flaps (one at each corner) to confer the lens stability when implanted in the capsular bag (Figure 8.1).

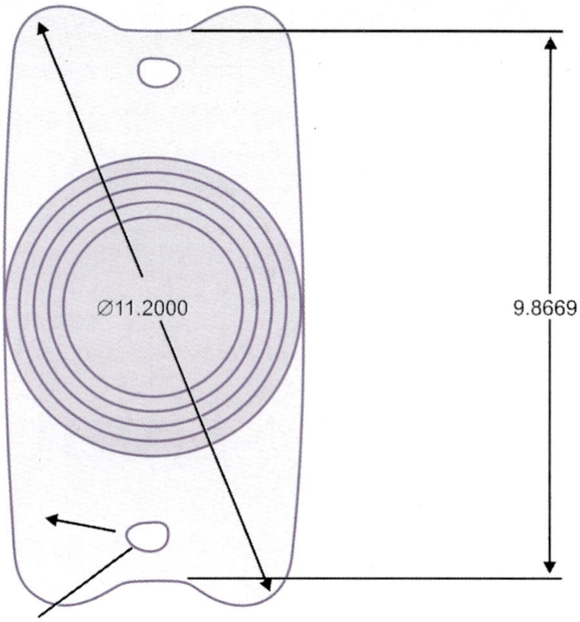

Figure 8.1: ThinOptx rollable IOL

The ultrathin nature of the ThinOptx lens is attributable to its refractive rather than diffractive optic design. The anterior surface of the lens has a number of concentric rings (3 to 5), which provide its dioptric power, and the posterior surface is smooth and parallel to the anterior surface (Figure 8.2). The anterior surface thus has an escalated perimeter comprised of steps 50 μm high similar to a Fresnel design (Figure 8.3). However, the ThinOptx design should not be compared to a Fresnel design, which is diffractive and each step is a prism that focuses light by bringing it to several points of focus. In contrast, the optical steps of the ThinOptx have a radius of curvature that brings each point of light to a single focus point (Figure 8.4). Further properties of the ThinOptx are its pliability and memory, allowing it to regain its original shape after handling.

The dioptric power of the lens ranges from +15.0 D to +25.0 D, with an A constant of 118.94.

IMPLANT TECHNIQUES

The ThinOptx lens is supplied immersed in a balanced solution in a sterile sealed vial. The lens is carefully transferred using non-toothed forceps to a vessel

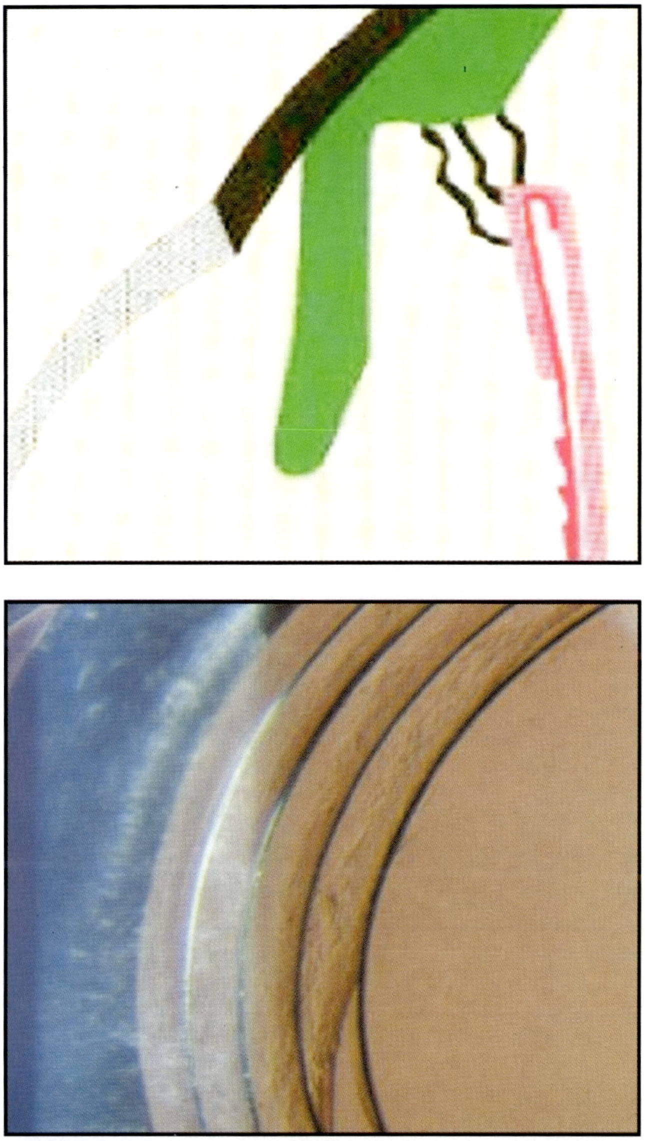

Figures 8.2A and B: The anterior surface of the ThinOptx rollable IOL has steps and the posterior surface is smooth and parallel to the anterior surface

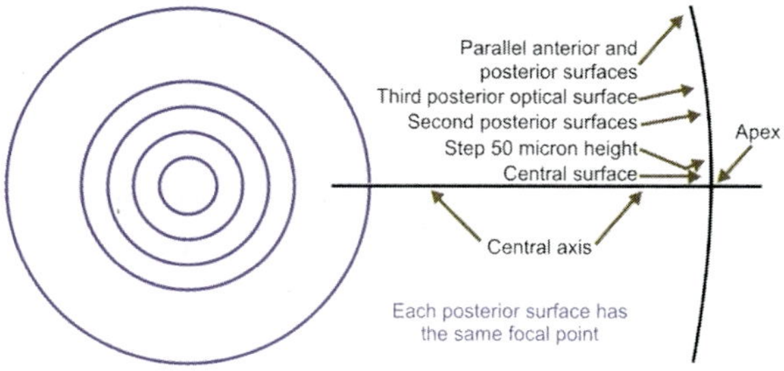

Figure 8.3: Optics design of the ThinOptx

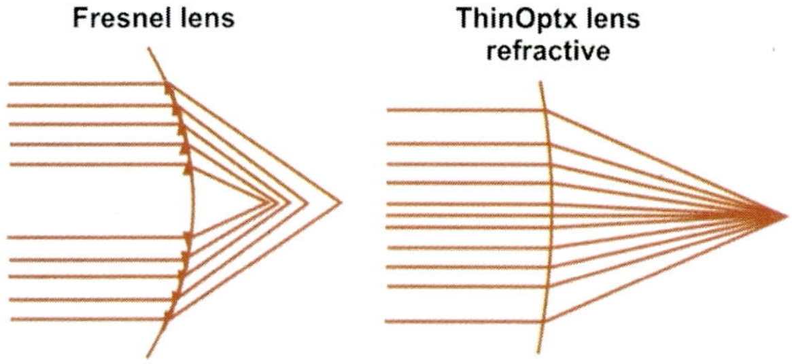

Figure 8.4: The Fresnel design is a defractive lens, and each step is a prism that focuses light at several points of focus. In contrast, the ThinOptx is a refractive lens that acts by bringing each point of light to a single point of focus

containing balanced saline solution (BSS) at 37°C to soften the lens before it is rolled before its insertion in the eye. The lens can be easily warmed by holding the vial in the surgeon's hands for a few minutes before insertion. The first lenses were implanted by manually rolling into the shape of a cigarette, and different injectors were specifically developed for this lens design.

Manual Rolling Technique

The prewarmed, softened lens, is removed from the BSS using forceps and placed on the tip of the index finger. The lens is then grasped using the forceps along the right longitudinal border such that the teardrop orifices in the haptics point in a clockwise direction. The forceps tip is turned inwards to start the rolling maneuver and withdrawn to continue rolling between the index finger and thumb as if rolling a cigarette. Thus, in a few seconds, the lens will have taken on the shape of a cylinder with a pointed end, and being at room temperature, will also have hardened. With the help of the forceps, the pointed end of the lens can now be introduced through the incision into the capsular bag, which is previously filled with viscoelastic (Figure 8.5). Once the lens is inside of the eye, the natural body temperature will cause the lens to soften again and unroll in 15 to 20 seconds. The unrolling process can be assisted by inserting an instrument through the paracentesis to make sure it adopts a good position in the capsular bag. The manual rolling procedure is technically challenging and handling the lens with the fingers could introduce foreign particles in the eye, possibly inducing an inflammatory reaction.

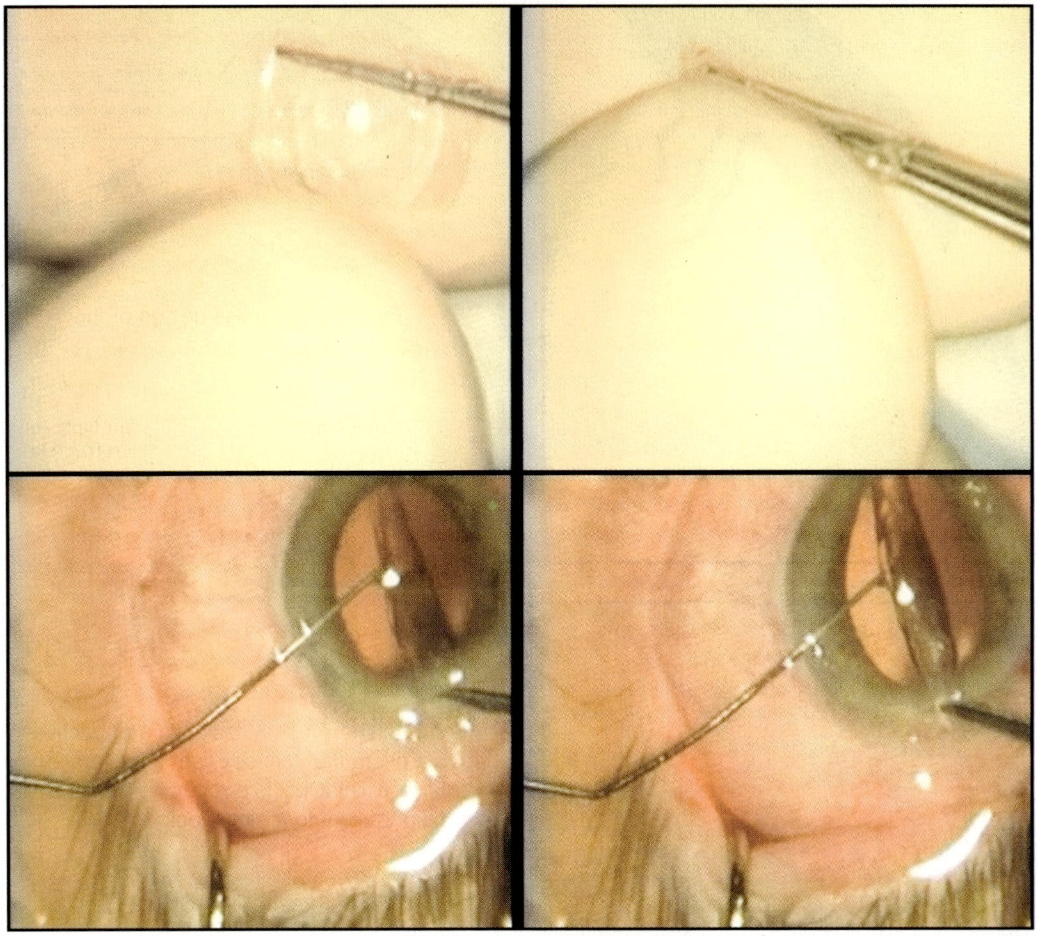

Figure 8.5: Manual rolling technique

Use of the First Injector Design

The first injector developed is metallic and has a reusable plastic cartridge at the tip (Figure 8.6). The ThinOptx IOL is removed from the storage solution and is grasped with the forceps as described above. Then, with the teardrops correctly aligned, the lens is placed in the slit of the cartridge previously filled with BSS. The IOL is then rolled on the cartridge as it is being introduced. When already rolled-up inside the cartridge, the forceps are used to push it until the lens tip emerges through the opposite end. The cartridge is then fitted to the injector and the insertion procedure initiated by placing the injector at the edge of the corneal incision. By carefully squeezing the plunger, we can aim the IOL towards the capsular bag filled with viscoelastic (Figure 8.7). When the lens has been fully introduced, with the help of an instrument, the lens is unrolled and the implant completed. The advent of this injector simplified the insertion technique but rolling the lens in the cartridge still poses technical difficulties.

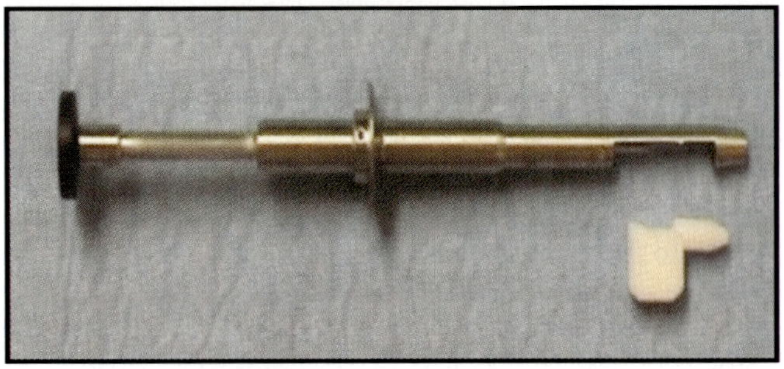

Figure 8.6: The first injector developed is metallic and has a reusable plastic cartridge at the tip

Use of the Inserter

The inserter is made of reusable plastic and is also used to roll the IOL. It comprises two pieces that fit together,

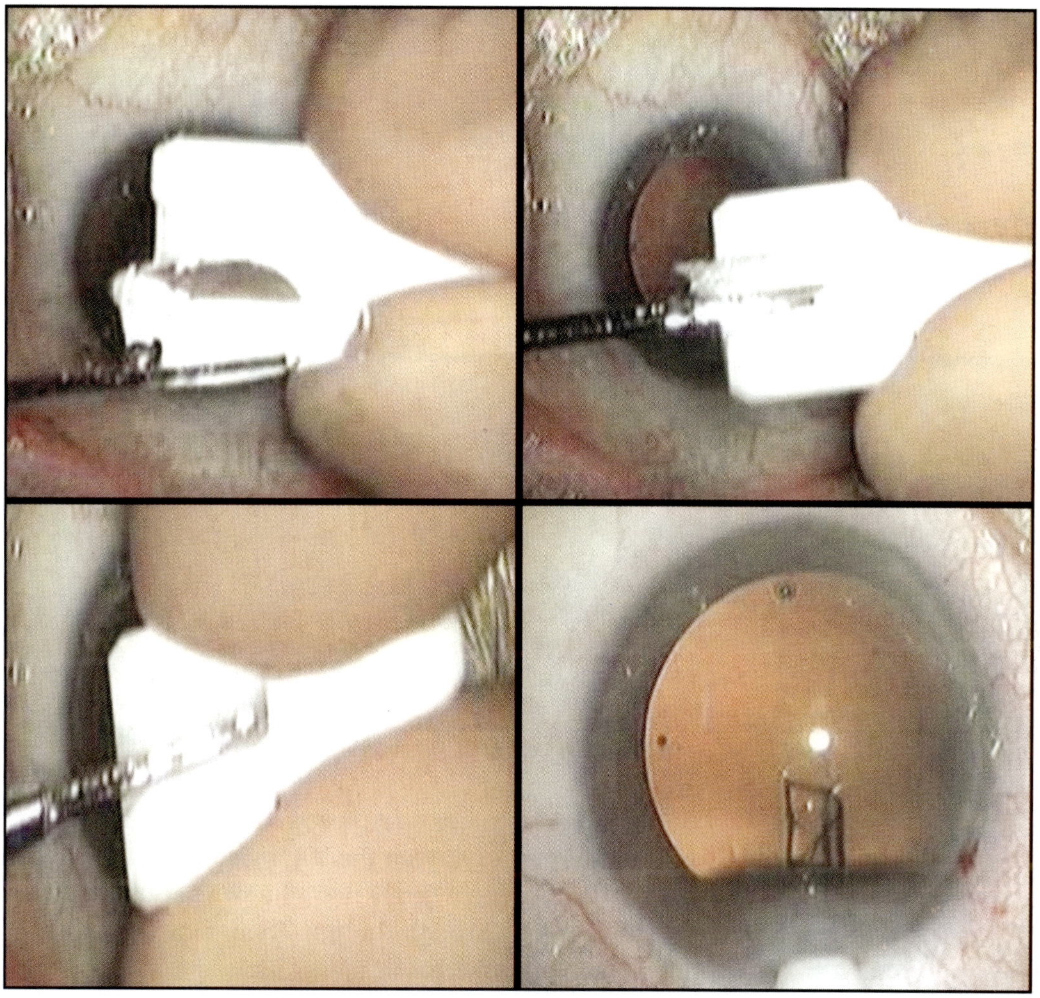

Figure 8.7: Use of the initial injector design

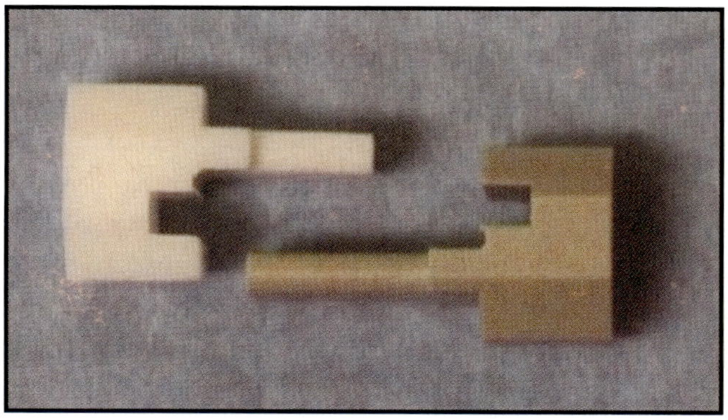

Figure 8.8: The inserter comprises two pieces that fit together and is also used to roll the IOL

one brown and the other white (Figure 8.8). The prewarmed lens is positioned transversally on the platform of the brown section with its teardrop orifices pointing clockwise. Next, the white section is fitted by slowly sliding into place as it rolls the lens. Once this manoeuvre is complete, a small 1 mm gap remains between the two inserter pieces which is where we find the rolled-up lens. Now that the lens has been rolled, the inserter is placed in BSS at room temperature so that the IOL hardens. At the time of implant, the inserter is removed from the solution and its two sections separated to find the IOL rolled-up in the center (Figure 8.9). We can then introduce the lens through the corneal incision using forceps as described in the manual rolling section. The inserter has helped the IOL rolling procedure but introducing the lens using forceps is still difficult, especially since as it touches the eye, the lens becomes soft.

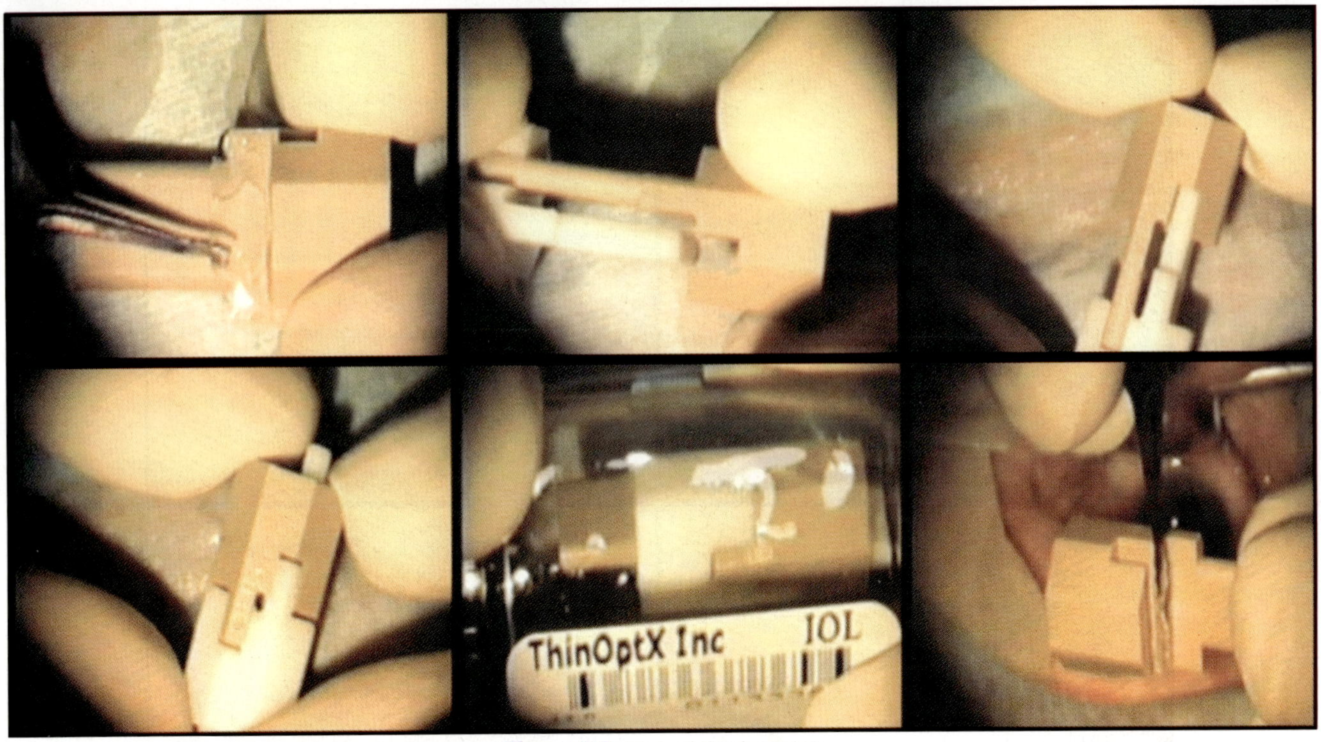

Figure 8.9: Use of the inserter

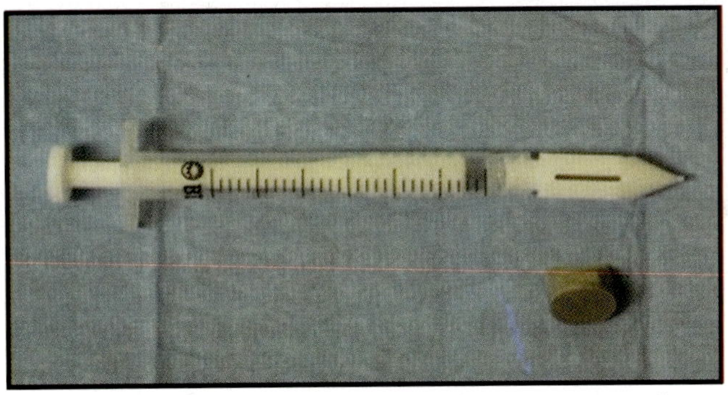

Figure 8.10: The new injector has the appearance of a syringe with a rolling/injecting piece at the tip

Use of the New Injector

The new injector design is exclusively made of plastic and has the appearance of a syringe (Figure 8.10). It has a rolling/injecting piece at the tip, with a slit through which the lens is longitudinally introduced, making sure the teardrops point clockwise. Before introducing the lens in this piece, it has to be refilled with BSS and it has to be checked that the injector plunger has been drawn back. With the lens in the slit, the rolling piece is introduced by intermittent small compressions until a surge is felt, followed by a sustained firm push until the end. With the IOL rolled-up inside the injector, we can now gently push the plunger until the haptic protrudes through the tip. Then, simply placing the tip of the injector in the incision, the lens is expelled using the plunger into the capsular bag (Figure 8.11). This new design simplifies the lens rolling procedure, and its injection system facilitates lens insertion.

TECHNICAL COMPLICATIONS

Lens Fragility and Rolling

It has to be borne in mind that we are working with an ultrafine lens that can easily tear. The IOL becomes soft and foldable when warm and it is very important to only handle the lens when it is in this state. At room temperature, the lens quickly hardens and the rolling process should therefore be rapidly and precisely undertaken.

If the incision is too small, or the lens is not perfectly rolled, it will be difficult to insert through a microincision. As the lens touches the incision, the body temperature will cause it to soften and unroll making it practically

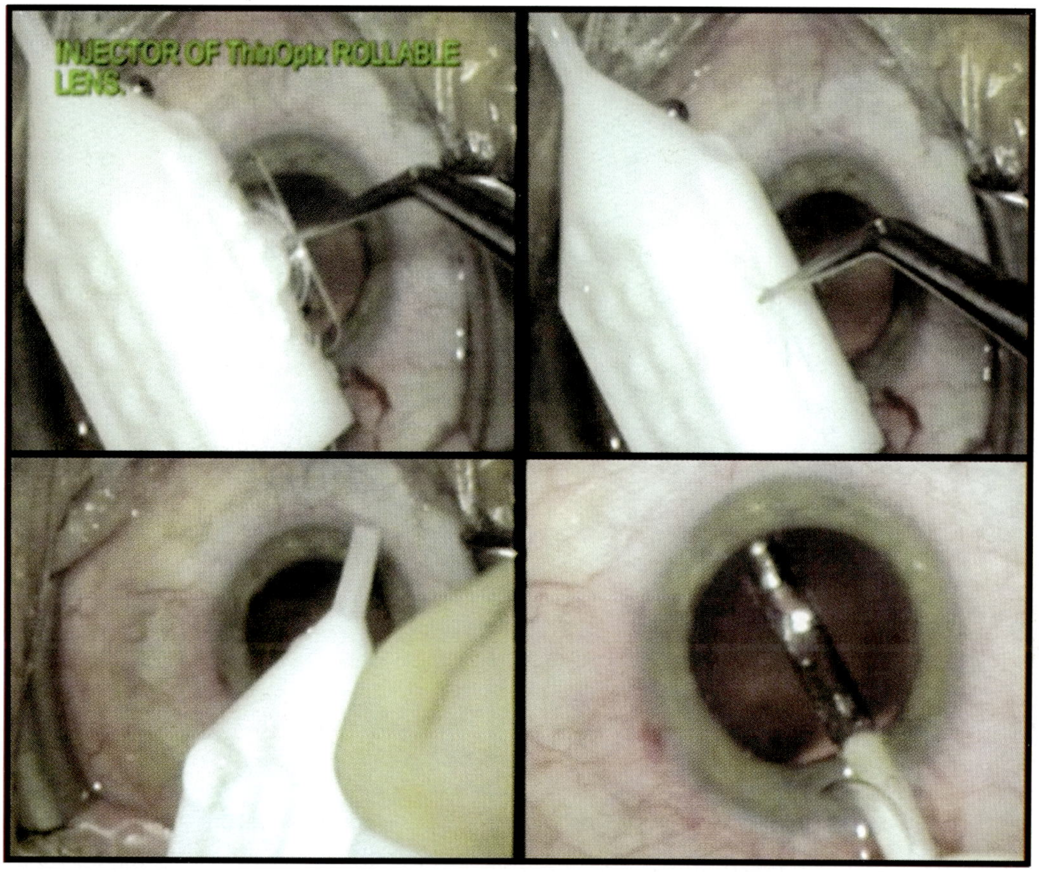

Figure 8.11: Use of the new injector design

impossible to implant. This is a common problem when using forceps to insert the lens rather than an injector.

On the other hand, if we exert excessive pressure on the plunger when using the injector to introduce the lens, it could break. Some authors[4] have managed to implant the ThinOptx lens through corneal incisions of 1 to 1.5 mm, while others[5] prefer 2 mm incisions. There have even been reports[6] of making the incision in the shape of a cone with the inner part 1.5 mm and external part 3.0 mm, so that the lens can be inserted in a less traumatic manner and thus avoid tearing.

Correct Positioning of the Lens

When describing the ThinOptx lens in this report, we highlighted the fact that it has an escalated anterior surface and smooth posterior surface. The implant should be performed with the surfaces in this position. To help distinguish the two sides, the lens haptics have teardrop-shaped fenestrations, which have to be pointing in a clockwise direction. This position should be borne in mind from the time we start to roll the lens to insert it in the eye in the correct position. If when we introduce the lens we find the teardrops point anticlockwise, then the lens has to be flipped over. To do this, the eye is packed with viscoelastic to protect the capsule and endothelium, and with the help of two instruments we can turn the soft, unfolded lens through the paracenteses (Figure 8.12). This maneuver is not difficult, but care must be taken not to rupture the capsule.

Capsular Rupture

The ThinOptx lens was designed to be implanted in the capsular back so that if the capsule is ruptured during phacoemulsification, another type of lens has to be used.

It should be emphasized that the lens is hard when injected in the eye. Hence if we push the plunger too

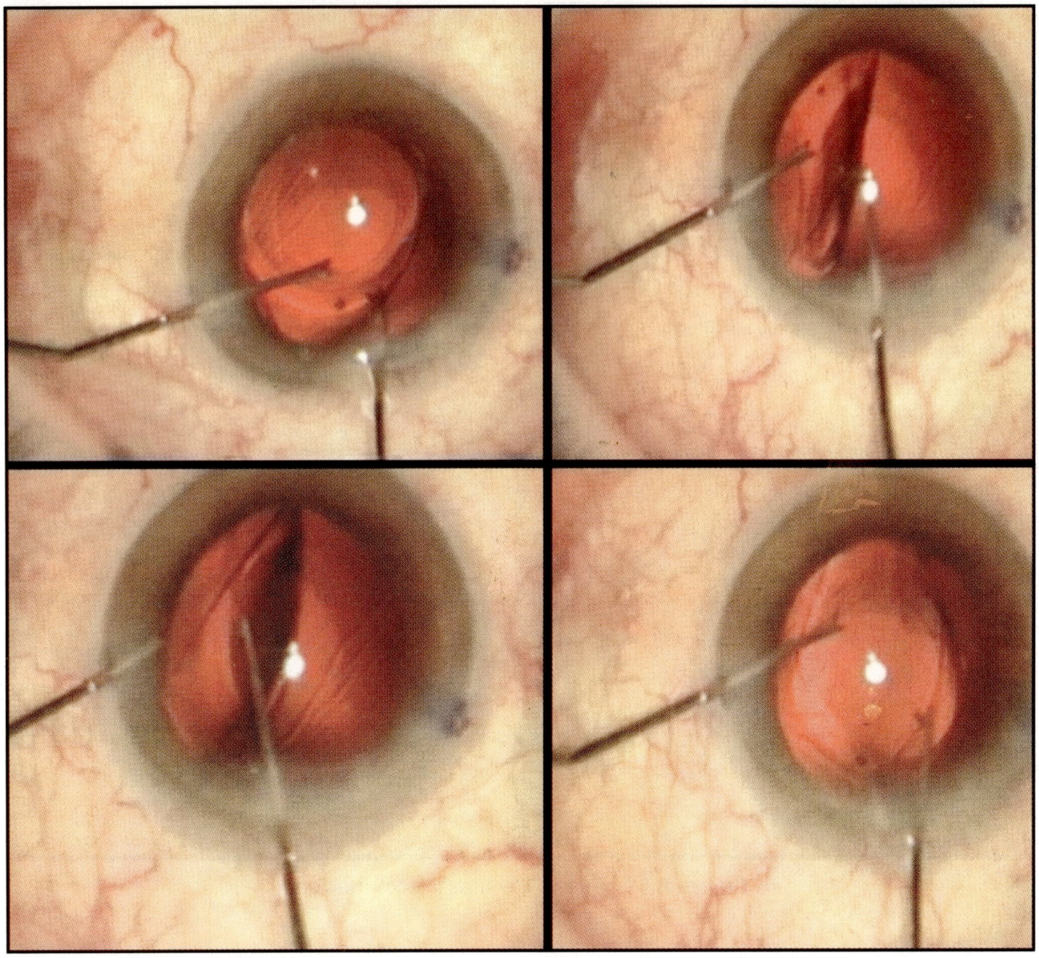

Figure 8.12: Flipping over an incorrectly implanted IOL

quickly, the lens could be abruptly expelled and penetrate the posterior capsule. Indeed, we suffered this complication in one of our first implants using the injector.

RESULTS

A prospective study was performed on 8 patients (3 men, 5 women) with cataracts in whom we implanted a ThinOptx rollable lens in one eye. The contralateral eye was implanted with a different IOL model so that we could compare the outcomes. The follow-up period was 1.5 to 3 years. The mean age of the patients was 68 years (range 55 to 84). Surgery was performed at the Instituto Oftalmológico Hoyos (Barcelona, Spain). All patients underwent a thorough ophthalmologic examination prior to surgery. The indication for surgery was an operable cataract of the crystalline lens with a potential postoperative best corrected visual acuity of 20/40 or better. Written informed consent was obtained from each patient before surgery.

At the follow-up visits we determined visual acuity (UCVA and BCVA), refraction, intraocular pressure, and performed a slit lamp examination. The preoperative mean BCVA was 20/80 (range 20/400 to 20/30). After surgery, mean UCVA was 20/50 (range 20/80 to 20/25) and mean BCVA was 20/20 (range 20/30 to 20/15). Table 8.1 shows pre- and postoperative visual acuity values for this series.

The mean power of the lenses implanted was +23.5 D (range from +16.5 to +24.0 D). The postoperative refractive outcome expressed as the spherical equivalent (SE) was –0.65 (SD 0.89). The lens powers implanted and refractive outcomes are provided in Table 8.2.

Table 8.1: Visual acuity pre- and post-surgery

Pre- BCVA	Post- UCVA	Post-BCVA
20/400	20/25	20/20
20/80	20/40	20/30
20/100	20/50	20/15
20/200	20/80	20/30
20/30	20/60	20/25
20/80	20/30	20/20
20/80	20/80	20/15
20/200	20/80	20/20

Table 8.2: Implanted lens powers and postoperative refractive outcomes (SE= Spherical equivalent)

IOL Power	Refraction	SE
+23.0	–0.75 x 60°	–0.30
+16.5	–1.00 x 180°	–0.50
+24.0	+1.00 –2.00 x 165°	0
+21.0	–0.5 –0.75 x 120°	–0.80
+21.0	–1.00 x 155°	–0.50
+22.0	+1.50 –1.75 x 80°	+0.75
+20.0	–1,50 –1.00 x 100°	–2.00
+24.0	–1.25 –1.00 x 105°	–1.75

Since some of our patients showed good near visual acuity using their correction for distance vision, we decided to measure the accommodation range. To do this, negative lenses were added to the patient's prescription for near vision until one line of visual acuity was lost. The accommodation range determined in this way was between 0.5 and 1 D.

Intraoperative complications were generally related to difficulties in rolling the lens. In one eye, the posterior capsule was ruptured as the lens was expelled from the injector. After retrieving the lens, we replaced it with a sulcus lens. This case is not included in this study.

In every case, the lens remained well-centred in the immediate postoperative period and during the entire follow-up (Figure 8.13).

In 2 eyes, we noted an inflammatory reaction in the anterior chamber, which presented one week after surgery with pain, tyndall and a red eye. These twc lenses had been implanted using the manual rolling procedure and we think the cause may have been a foreign particle entering the eye due to handling the lens (e.g. talc). After treatment with corticosteroids, the complication was solved within a month in both cases. As sequelae, both eyes showed posterior sinechia,

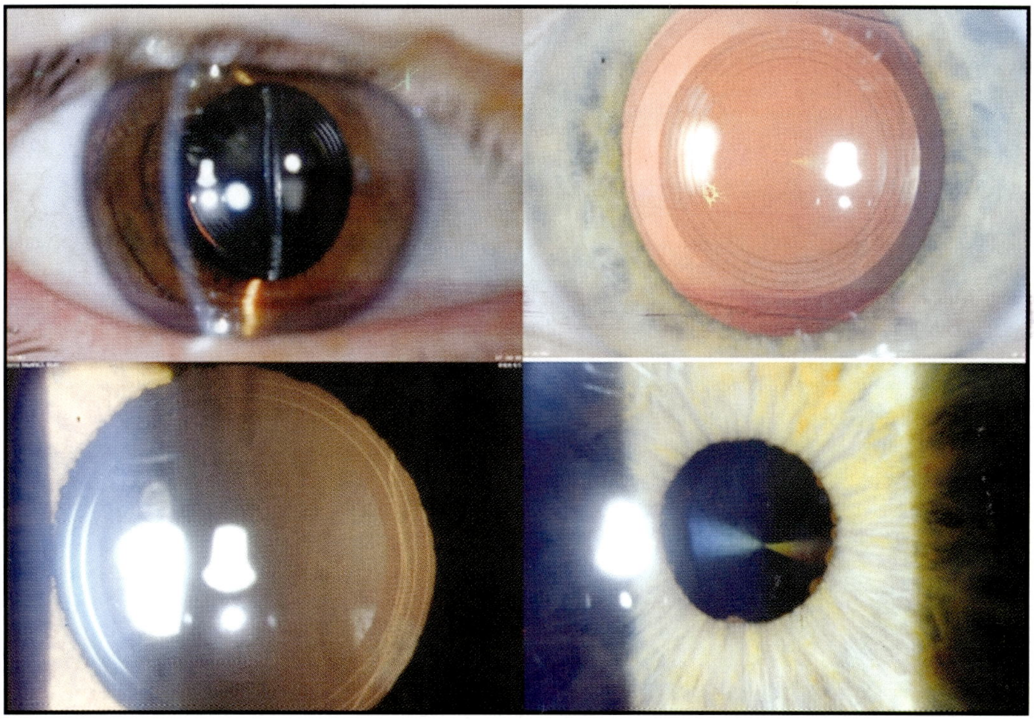

Figure 8.13: Panoramic views of implanted ThinOptx lenses

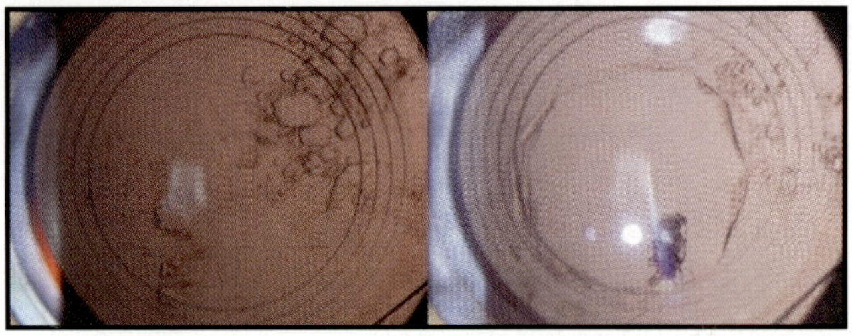

Figure 8.14: Capsular opacification observed 1 year after implant and the same case after Yag laser capsulotomy

slightly deforming the pupil, although visual acuity was unaffected.

Three of the eight cases required a posterior Yag laser capsulotomy because of capsular opacification (one at 1 year and two at 2 years post-surgery). No complications arose after the capsulotomy (Figure 8.14).

CONCLUSIONS

- The rollable ThinOptx is an ultrathin IOL that can be introduced through a microincision
- The optics design of this lens is refractive and unlike diffractive lenses (Fresnel prisms), it induces no optical aberrations resulting in a good quality of vision
- In some cases, we have observed some degree of accommodation
- The use of an injector helps the insertion procedure and reduces complications.

REFERENCES

1. Matsumoto Y, Hara T, Chiba K, Chikuda M. Optimal incision sites to obtain an astigmatism-free cornea after cataract surgery with a 3.2 mm sutureless incision. J Cataract Refract Surg 2001;27(10):1615-9.
2. Merriam JC, Zheng L, Urbanowicz J, Zaider M. Change on the horizontal and vertical meridians of the cornea after cataract surgery. Trans Am Ophthalmol Soc 2001;99:187-95; discussion 195-7.
3. A Agarwal, S Agarwal, A Agarwal. Phakonit and laser phakonit: lens removal through a 0.9 mm incision. In Agarwal S, Agarwal A, Apple SJ, Buratto L, Alió JL, Pandey SK, et al (Eds): Textbook of Ophthalmology. New Delhi, Jaypee Brothers Medical Publishers 2002;3:1829-40.
4. Pandey SK, Werner L, Agarwal A, Agarwal S, Agarwal A, Lal V, et al. Phakonit: cataract removal through a sub-1.0 mm incision and implantation of the ThinOptX rollable intraocular lens. J Cataract Refract Surg 2002;28(9):1710-3.
5. Centurion V, Caballero JC, Cezar-Lacava A, Argento C. Diseño microincisional – Lente ThinOptx. In Soler FL, Lorente R, Asis O (Eds): Cirugia microincisonal de la catarata. Sociedad Española de Cirugia Implanto-Refractiva 2004;5:223-8.
6. Centurion V, Lacava C, Caballero JC. A lente intraocular dobravel: cirurgia de catarata por micro-incisoes. In: Padilha MA (Ed). Catarata. Rio de Janeiro, Cultura Medica 2003: 297-318.

9

Refractive Lens Exchange

- TECHNIQUE
- RESULTS
- DISCUSSION

I Howard Fine, Richard S Hoffman, Mark Packer (USA)

SYNOPSIS

Refractive lens exchange with bimanual microincision extraction offers a potentially safer and more controlled method of crystalline lens extraction. Future lens technology will permit refractive lens exchanges through two microincisions.

ABSTRACT

Bimanual microincision phacoemulsification entails the removal of the crystalline lens through two 1.2 mm incisions. Infusion is provided through a separate irrigating handpiece and phacoemulsification and aspiration are performed through a sleeveless phacoemulsification needle. We describe herein a technique for refractive lens exchange utilizing bimanual microincision phacoemulsification. Capsulorhexis formation, cortical cleaving hydrodissection, lens extraction in the iris plane, and residual cortex removal are all performed through these microincisions. The technique offers the advantages of improved surgeon control throughout these steps of the procedure and added safety by maintaining continuous pressurization of the eye while removing the lens distant from the posterior capsule.

INTRODUCTION

The notion of removing the crystalline lens through two microincisions is not a new concept and has been attempted with varying degrees of success and failure since the 1970s.[1-6] With the development of new phacoemulsification technology and power modulations,[7] we are now able to emulsify and fragment lens material without the generation of significant thermal energy. Thus removal of the cooling irrigation sleeve and separation of infusion and emulsification/aspiration through two separate incisions is now a viable alternative to traditional coaxial phacoemulsification. Machines such as the AMO WhiteStar, Staar Sonic Wave, Alcon NeoSoniX, Bausch and Lomb Medennium (with burst mode), and Dodick Nd:YAG Laser Photolysis systems offer the potential of relatively "cold" lens removal capabilities and the capacity for bimanual lens surgery.[8-11]

With advances in multifocal and accommodative lens technology, removal of the crystalline lens as a form of refractive surgery (refractive lens exchange) should become a more popular procedure. We believe bimanual microincision phacoemulsification has several independent advantages that make it a procedure of choice for refractive lens exchange. The following is our current technique for refractive lens exchange utilizing bimanual microincision phacoemulsification.

TECHNIQUE

The procedure is performed under topical anesthesia after appropriate informed consent, preoperative measurements for IOL determination, and preoperative dilation and antibiotics. A Mastel Paratrap diamond keratome (Mastel Precision Surgical Instruments, Rapid City, SD) is utilized to create two 1.2 mm clear corneal incisions 30 to 45° from the temporal limbus (60-90° from each other) (Figure 9.1). One-half cc of non-preserved lidocaine 1 percent is instilled into the anterior chamber followed by complete expansion of the anterior chamber with Viscoat®. A straight 25-gauge needle is then inserted through the right-handed microincision to perforate the central anterior lens capsule while simultaneously lifting a flap edge to begin a capsulorhexis (Figure 9.2). Needles routinely bent at the tip for conventional capsulorhexis initiation have been found to lacerate the roof of the microincision during withdrawl of the needle. The straight unaltered 25-gauge needle is less likely to result in this complication. After removal of the needle, a capsulorhexis forceps, specially designed to fit and function through a 1 mm incision is then inserted through the same incision and used to complete a 5 to 6 mm rhexis (Figure 9.3).

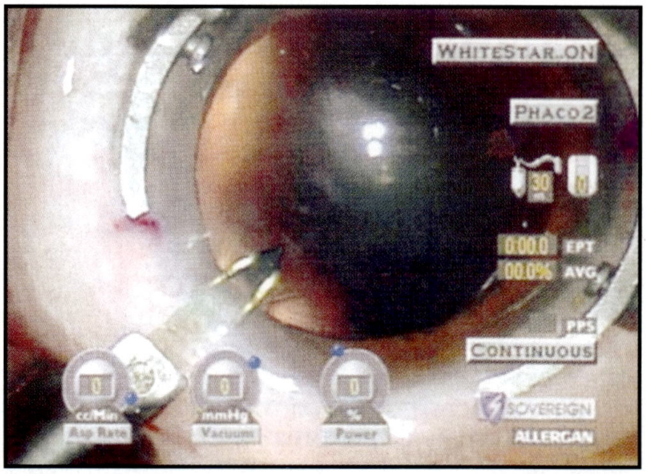

Figure 9.1: Left-handed 1.2 mm clear corneal microincision placed 45° from the temporal limbus utilizing a Mastel Paratrap diamond knife

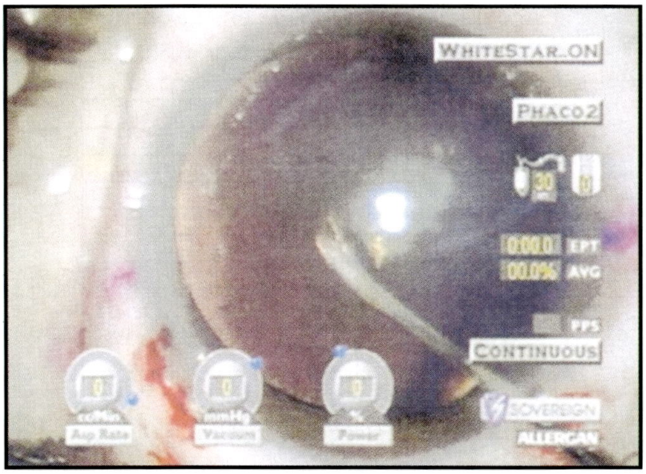

Figure 9.2: A straight 25-gauge needle begins the capsulorhexis by perforating the central anterior lens capsule while simultaneously lifting a flap edge

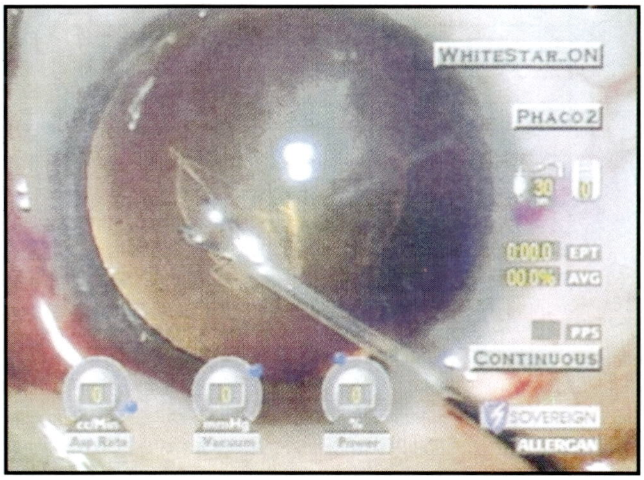

Figure 9.3: Capsulorhexis formation utilizing an ASICO microincision capsulorhexis forceps

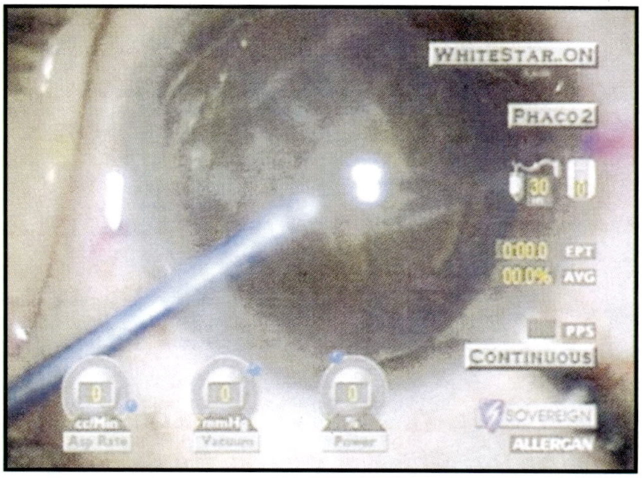

Figure 9.4: The Duet System (MST Microsurgical Technology) beveled irrigating handpiece within the left-handed microincision

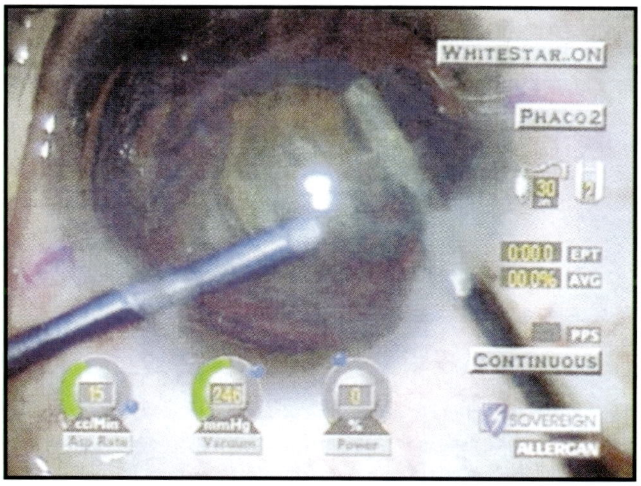

Figure 9.5: The soft lens is carouselled in the iris plane and consumed utilizing high vacuum levels. Forward movement of the lens is prevented with the irrigating handpiece

Cortical cleaving hydrodissection[12] with decompression is then performed in two separate distal quadrants followed by a third round of hydrodissection to prolapse the entire lens or at least one-half of the lens out of the capsular bag. The microincision irrigating handpiece (Figure 9.4) is placed in the left-hand incision and the unsleaved phaco needle is inserted through the right-hand incision. Lens extraction is then performed in most cases without phaco power, utilizing high levels of vacuum while carouselling the relatively soft lens in the plane of the iris until it is consumed (Figure 9.5). Small amounts of ultrasound energy can be utilized when needed. Care should be taken to avoid directing the infusion flow towards the phaco needle tip so as to prevent dislodging nuclear material from the tip. While maintaining infusion with the irrigating handpiece, the phaco needle is removed and the aspiration handpiece is inserted to remove residual cortex and polish the posterior capsule. If subincisional cortex is difficult to extract, the I/A handpieces can be alternated between the two incisions in order to gain easier access to the subincisional capsular fornix (Figure 9.6).

Once all cortex has been removed, the aspiration handpiece is removed and viscoelastic is injected into the

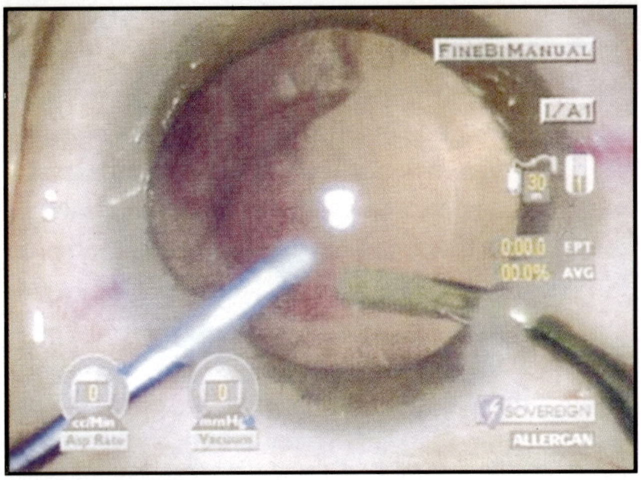

Figure 9.6: Subincisional cortex is easily removed using the Duet System (MST) bimanual irrigation and aspiration handpieces. (Note the Effective Phaco Time EPT = 0 and Average Percent Phaco Power AVG = 0 following lens removal)

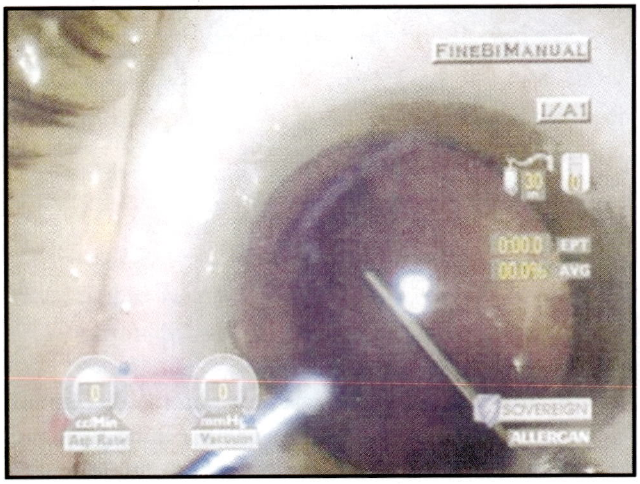

Figure 9.7: Viscoelastic is injected into the capsular bag while maintaining infusion with the irrigating handpiece

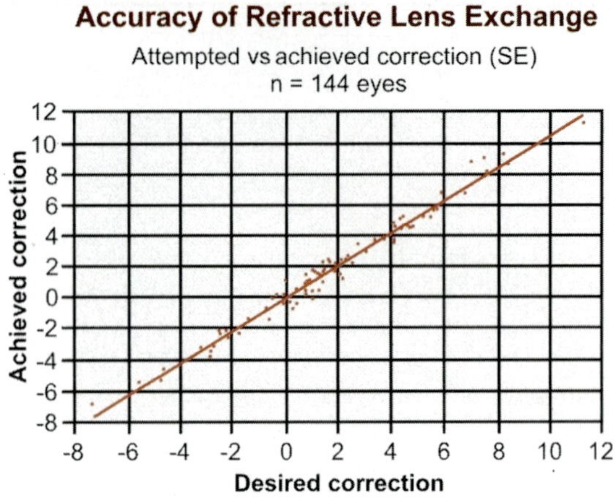

Figure 9.8: Attempted versus achieved spherical equivalent correction for the Array Multifocal IOL

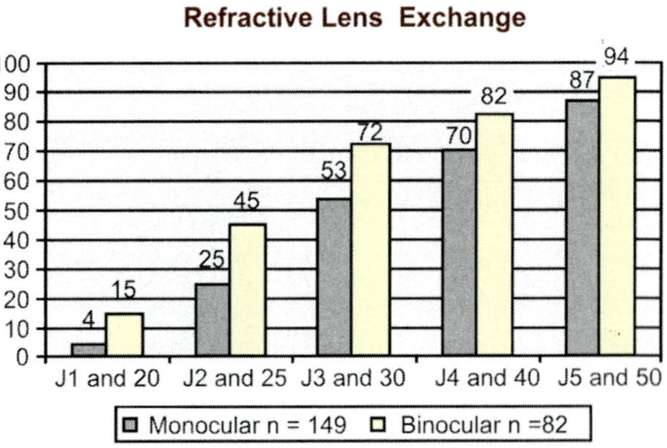

Figure 9.9: Refractive lens exchange results using the Array multifocal IOL

capsular bag and anterior chamber while withdrawing the irrigating handpiece (Figure 9.7). Following this, the viscoelastic cannula is removed from the eye and a new 2.5 mm clear corneal incision is placed between the two microincisions for IOL insertion. After IOL insertion, stromal hydration of the 2.5 mm incision is performed to assist in its self-sealing. Bimanual I/A is performed to remove all viscoelastic. The aspiration handpiece is then removed and irrigation of the anterior chamber maintained. Stromal hydration of the empty incision is performed to assist in closure of the microincision. The irrigation handpiece is then removed followed by stromal hydration of that incision. In this manner, the eye is fully formed and pressurized throughout the procedure avoiding hypotony and shallowing of the anterior chamber.

RESULTS

We achieved excellent results utilizing the Array multifocal foldable IOL. Almost all of our achieved spherical equivalents were within .5 diopters of our target spherical equivalent values (Figure 9.8) Our visual acuity results were also very good with approximately 44 percent of our patients achieving almost complete spectacle independence and a second 44 percent receiving near spectacle independence with some exceptions, most notably prolonged reading or driving at night[13] (Figure 9.9).

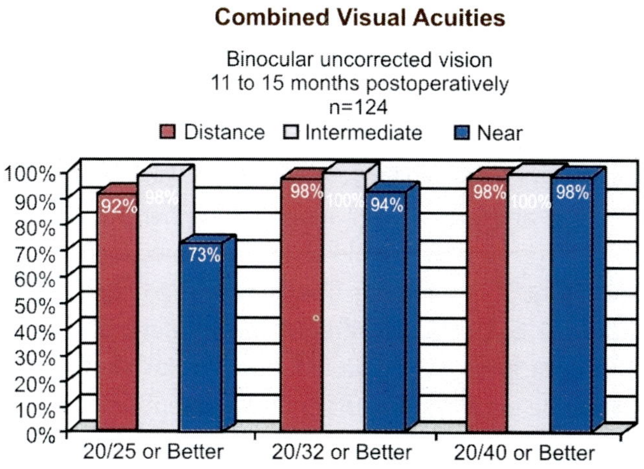

Figure 9.10: Combined visual acuity results in refractive lens exchange for the crystalens accommodative IOL

Bilateral Satisfaction (n = 130)

Do not wear spectacles	25.8 %
Wear almost none of the time	47.7
	73.5 %
Wear some of the time	15.6
Wear most of the time	6.3
Wear almost all the time	4.7

Figure 9.11: Quality of life data for crystalens refractive lens exchange patients

The results that we achieved with the eyeonics crystalens are seen in Figures 9.10 and 9.11. We see that 73 percent of the patients achieved distance, near and intermediate visual acuities of 20/25 or better and that corresponds extremely well with the percentage of patients who believe themselves to be totally spectacle independent (Figure 9.11).

DISCUSSION

Bimanual microincision phacoemulsification offers advantages over current traditional phacoemulsification techniques for both routine cataract extraction and refractive lens exchanges. While it is true that coaxial phaco is an excellent procedure with low amounts of induced astigmatism,[14] bimanual phaco offers the potential for truly astigmatic neutral incisions. In addition, these microincisions should behave similar to a paracentesis incision with less likelihood for leakage and, theoretically, a lower incidence of endophthalmitis.

The major advantage we have seen from bimanual microincisions has been an improvement in control of most of the steps involved in endocapsular surgery. Since viscoelastics do not leave the eye easily through these small incisions, the anterior chamber is more stable during capsulorhexis construction and there is much less likelihood for an errant rhexis to develop. Hydrodelineation and hydrodissection can be performed more efficiently by virtue of a higher level of pressure building in the anterior chamber prior to eventual prolapse of viscoelastic through the microincisions. In addition, separation of irrigation from the aspirating phaco needle allows for improved followability by avoiding competing currents at the tip of the needle. In some instances, the irrigation flow from the second handpiece can be used as an adjunctive surgical device-flushing nuclear pieces from the angle or loosening epinuclear or cortical material from the capsular bag. Perhaps the greatest advantage of the bimanual technique lies in its ability to remove subincisional cortex without difficulty. As originally described by Brauweiler,[15] by switching infusion and aspiration handpieces between two microincisions, 360° of the capsular fornices are easily reached and cortical clean-up can be performed quickly and safely.

The disadvantages of bimanual phacoemusification are real but easy to overcome. Maneuvering through 1.2 mm incisions can be awkward early in the learning curve.

Also, additional equipment is necessary in the form of small incision keratomes, rhexis forceps, irrigating choppers (for dense nucleii), and bimanual I/A handpieces. All of the major instrument companies are currently working on irrigating choppers and other microincision adjunctive devices for microincision surgery. For refractive lens exchanges, irrigation can be accomplished with the bimanual irrigation handpiece that can also function as the second "side-port" instrument negating the need for an irrigating chopper.

The greatest criticism of bimanual phaco lies in the fluidics and the current limitations in intraocular lens technology that could be utilized through these micro-incisions. By nature of the size of these incisions, less fluid flows into the eye than occurs with coaxial techniques. Most current irrigating choppers integrate a 20-gauge lumen that limits fluid inflow. This can result in significant chamber instability when high vacuum levels are utilized and occlusion from nuclear material at the phaco tip is cleared. Thus, infusion needs to be maximized by placing the infusion bottle on a separate IV pole that is set as high as possible. Also, vacuum levels usually need to be lowered below 350 mm Hg to avoid significant surge flow.

At the conclusion of bimanual phaco, perhaps the greatest disappointment is the need to place a relatively large 2.5 mm incision between the two microincisions in order to implant a foldable IOL. An analogy to the days when phaco was performed through 3.0 mm incisions that required widening to 6.0 mm for PMMA IOL implantation is clear. It was not until the development of foldable IOLs that we could truly take full advantage of small incision phaco. Similarly, we believe the advantages of bimanual phaco will prompt many surgeons to try this technique, with the realization that microincision lenses will ultimately catch up with technique. Although these lenses are currently not available in the US, many companies are developing lens technologies that will be able to employ these tiny incisions.

Medennium is developing its Smart Lens™—a thermodynamic accommodating IOL. It is a hydrophobic acrylic rod that can be inserted through a 2 mm incision and expands to the dimensions of the natural crystalline lens (9.5 mm × 3.5 mm). A 1 mm version of this lens is also being developed. ThinOptX fresnel lenses will soon be under investigation in the US and will be implantable through 1.5 mm incisions. Finally, injectable polymer lenses are being researched by both Pharmacia and Calhoun Vision.[16,17] If viable, the Calhoun Vision injectable polymer offers the possibility of injecting a light-adjustable-lens through a 1 mm incision that can then be fine-tuned postoperatively to eliminate both lower order and higher order optical aberrations.

Utilization of bimanual microphacoemulsification as we have described for refractive lens exchange and routine cataract surgery offers an enormous advantage of maintaining a more stable intraocular environment during lens removal. This may be especially important in high myopes who are at a greater risk for retinal detachment following lens extraction.[18-20] By maintaining a formed and pressurized anterior chamber throughout the procedure, there should be less tendency for anterior movement of the vitreous body with a theoretical lower incidence of posterior vitreous detachment occurring from intraoperative manipulations. Future studies will need to be performed in order to document a significant reduction in posterior segment mobidity utilizing this method of lens removal.

We have found this technique to be simple, efficacious, and safe since most of the lens extraction is occurring in the plane of the iris, away from the posterior capsule and the corneal endothelium.

REFERENCES

1. Girard LJ. Ultrasonic fragmentation for cataract extraction and cataract complications. Adv Ophthalmol 1978;37:127-35.
2. Shearing SP, Relyea RL, Loaiza A, Shearing RL. Routine phacoemulsification through a one-millimeter non-sutured incision. Cataract 1985;2:6-10.
3. Hara T, Hara T. Endocapsular phacoemulsification and aspiration (ECPEA)—recent surgical technique and clinical results. Ophthalmic Surgery 1989;20(7):469-75.
4. Tsuneoka H, Shiba T, Takahashi Y. Feasibility of ultrasound cataract surgery with a 1.4 mm incision. J Cataract Refract Surg 2001;27:934-40.
5. Tsuneoka H, Shiba T, Takahashi Y. Ultrasonic phacoemulsification using a 1.4 mm incision: clinical results. J Cataract Refract Surg 2002;28:81-6.
6. Agarwal A, Agarwal A, Agarwal S, Narang P, Narang S. Phakonit: phacoemulsification through a 0.9 mm corneal incision. J Cataract Refract Surg 2001;27:1548-52.
7. Fine IH, Packer M, Hoffman RS. The use of power modulations in phacoemulsification: Choo choo chop and flip phacoemulsification. J Cataract Refract Surg 2001;27:188-97.
8. Soscia W, Howard JG, Olson RJ. Microphacoemulsification with WhiteStar. A wound temperature study. J Cataract Refract Surg 2002;28:1044-6.
9. Hoffman RS, Fine IH, Packer M, Brown LK. Comparison of sonic and ultrasonic phacoemulsification utilizing the Staar Sonic Wave phacoemulsification system. J Cataract Refract Surg 2002;28:1581-4.
10. Fine IH, Packer M, Hoffman RS. New phacoemulsification technology. J Cataract Refract Surg 2002;28:1054-60.

11. Alzner E, Grabner G. Dodick laser photolysis: thermal effects. J Cataract Refract Surg 1999;25:800-3.
12. Fine IH. Cortical cleaving hydrodissection. J Cataract Refract Surg 1992;18:508-12.
13. Fine IH, Packer M, Hoffman RS. Power modulations in new technology: Improved outcomes. J Cataract Refract Surg, 2004;30:1014-9.
14. Masket S, Tennen DG. Astigmatic stabilization of 3.0 mm temporal clear corneal cataract incisions. J Cataract Refract Surg 1996 22:1451-5.
15. Brauweiler P. Bimanual irrigation/aspiration. J Cataract Refract Surg 1996;22:1013-6.
16. de Groot JH, van Beijma FJ, Haitjema HJ, et al. Injectable intraocular lens material based upon hydrogels. Biomacromolecules 2001;2:628-34.
17. Hoffman RS, Fine IH, Packer M. Light adjustable lens. In Agarwal S, Agarwal A, Sachdev MS, Mehta KR, Fine IH, Agarwal A (Eds): Phacoemulsification, Laser Cataract Surgery, and Foldable IOLs (3rd edition). Thorofare, NJ, Slack, Inc. (In press).
18. Rodriguez A, Gutierrez E, Alvira G. Complications of clear lens extraction in axial myopia. Arch Ophthalmol 1987; 105:1522-3.
19. Ripandelli G, Billi B, Fedeli R, Stirpe M. Retinal detachment after clear lens extraction in 41 eyes with axial myopia. Retina 1996;16:3-6.
20. Colin J, Robinet A, Cochener B. Retinal detachment after clear lens extraction for high myopia: seven-year follow-up. Ophthalmology 1999;106:2281-84.

10

Futuristic IOLs for Bimanual Microincision Phaco

- INJECTABLE POLYMERS
- SMART IOL

I Howard Fine, Richard S Hoffman, Mark Packer (USA)

INTRODUCTION

Although the Acri.Tec (Berlin, Germany) and the ThinOptx (Abingdon, VA) IOLs have both been utilized in clinical trials in Europe and Asia, their results are still uncertain with respect to stability of refraction and possible deformation of these lenses under the forces of capsular bag constriction. However, there is on the horizon new technology that may be very promising.

Calhoun Vision (Pasadena, CA), which has produced the Light Adjustable IOL, is capable of providing an injectable polymer with light adjustable technology. This is one of several companies that are working with injectable technology (Figure 10.1). The problem with these efforts resides in the fact that it requires a lens extraction through an approximately 1 mm capsulorhexis, and this indeed is very difficult to do. Although the Advantecs (cataract system) was tested by Bausch and Lomb (San Dimas, CA) and was capable of clear lens exchange through such small incisions that technology is currently on hold. We have experimented in our own surgery center on 1mm capsulorhexis clear lens extractions in cadaver eyes and have found it to be technically extremely formidable and unpredictable. However, the promise of light adjustability, allowing sequential adjustments, for which Calhoun holds the patents, would make this type of approach extremely appealing. The problems of posterior capsule opacification also will have to be addressed since fluid injectable polymers would leak into the vitreous chamber if a posterior YAG laser was necessary.

Injectable Polymers

- AMO/Groningen/pharmacia
- Calhoun vision
- Vision science reserch cooperative

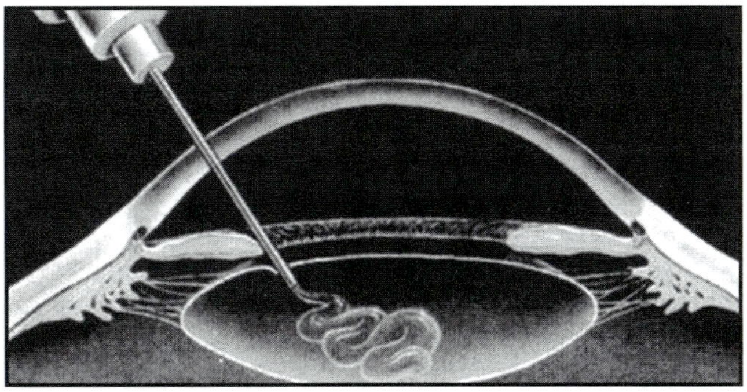

Figure 10.1: Companies currently working on injectable polymer IOLs

SmartIOL™, US and World Patent Pending

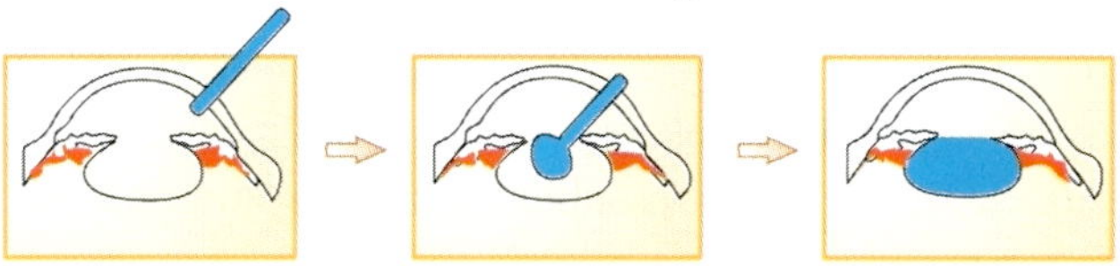

Figure 10.2: Schematic rendering of insertion of a Smart IOL

SmartIOL™

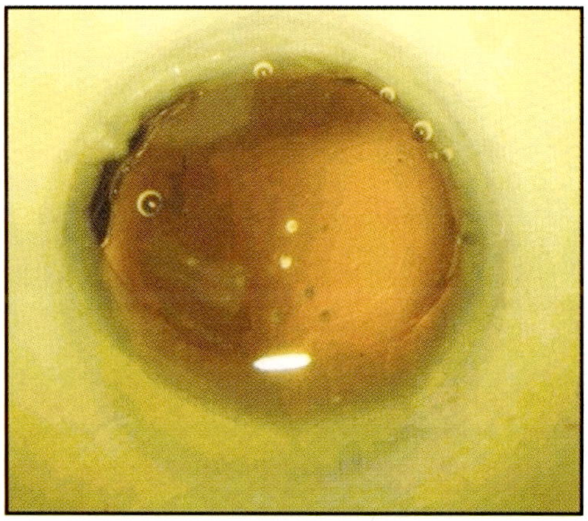

Figure 10.3: Smart IOL in a cadaver eye, completely filling the capsular bag once fully reconstituted

Another model of a futuristic IOL that offers perhaps even more promise is the Smart IOL by Medennium (Irvine, CA). The SmartIOL is a thermodynamic hydrophobic acrylic IOL that is designed to completely fill the capsular bag, but is convertible at room temperature to a thin rod, which can be injected through a very small incision. Under the influence of body temperature, the lens reconstitutes to its initial size, shape and imprinted dioptric power (Figure 10.2). This lens would not only fill the capsular bag but become adherent to it because it is a hydrophobic acrylic, which becomes covered, soon after implantation, with fibronectin, a naturally occurring bio-adhesive (Figure 10.3). We think that because of its high refractive index and its stable gel configuration at body temperatures, this is an extremely desirable technology. With its high refractive index, minute changes in the shape of the lens would result in large amplitudes of accommodation. Also of importance is that it could include light adjustable technology which would give us the ability for sequential adjustment over time as subtle changes in the patient's refractive error occur.

The future for micro-incision IOLs is extremely bright and I think although at this time we can only look at extensions of existing technology, I believe break through technology will be on the horizon very soon.

11

PCO Prevention and Management in Microphaco

- BLOCK LEC MIGRATION
- EPCO RESULTS
- KILL THE LEC

Frederic Hehn (France)

INTRODUCTION

None can prevent posterior capsule opacification (PCO), which results from the proliferation of the lens epithelial cells (LEC), that remain in the lens bag, especially in the equatorial region. Depending on the length of the follow-up,[15] the PCO occurs and has been reported in up to 80 percent of eyes having a cataract extraction with an IOL implantation.

Albert Galand[6] developed in 1996 the concept of a systematic posterior continuous curvilinear capsulorhexis (PCCC), but there is some risks of retinal detachment, and the learning curve of this technique is hard.[8] Marie-josé Tassignon[17] developed the concept of 'the bag in the lens ' to avoid the PCO, but the stability of the lens and the realization of this difficult technique are in concern. The square[1] edge IOL design provides a lower rate of PCO, but does not eradicate it.

With MICS (microincision cataract surgery), bimanual technique consisting in separate irrigation and aspiration; It allows micro-incision of 1.5 mm width for entirely procedure from corneal incision until IOL implantation . But in regard of PCO the problem is the same that it was in conventional 3.2 incision cataract surgery.

The well known preventing factors of a PCO are: no IOL decentration, a 360° IOL overlapping of capsulorhexis, an ablation of viscoelastic behind the optic, a reduction of the retro-optical space, no folds on posterior capsule the speed of the capsular bend formation,[13] the adhesion between the optic and posterior capsule by fibronectin, IOL materials, and of course Square Edge IOL design. But only a total cleaning of anterior and equatorial LEC could be efficient to avoid the PCO.

The LEC give always anterior or posterior capsular bag opacification in the shape of fibrosis or pearls and sometimes shrinkage with IOL displacement (Figure 11.1).

The problem of PCO is not only the cost and the morbidity of Nd:yag capsulotomy, but the real challenge is to keep a soft capsular bag. With a soft capsular bag, LEC free, it will be possible to restore accommodation in pseudophakic eyes with the "phacoersatz" and avoid to practice anterior vitrectomy and PCCC in children's cataract surgery.

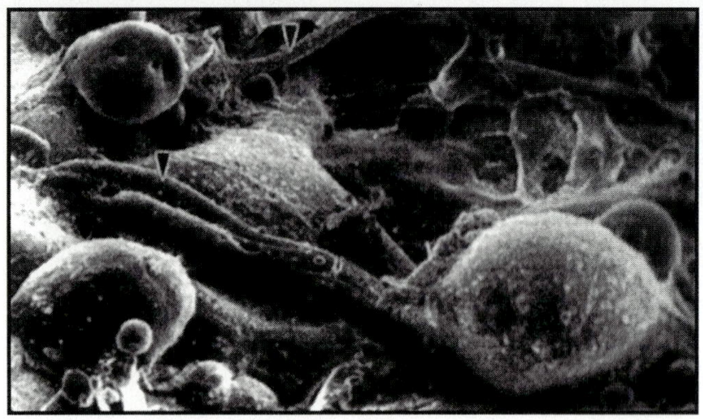

Figure 11.1: "Fibroblast like": At time of pearls and fibrosis game is over

There are only two ways to avoid PCO, Block LEC migration, or kill the LEC.

BLOCK LEC MIGRATION

There are two possibilities to block cell migration; the first is to block them by IOL shape "the square edge", the second is to block LEC in equatorial region with a capsular ring.

Square Edge

What are we speaking about? We are speaking about cell. The LEC become 'fibroblast like'[8] from 10 μm diameter << IOL' optic diameter (500 μ or more). 'Fibroblasts like' have got *'arms and legs and hands and feet'* and they try to conquer the retro-optical space. Be sure that 'Fibroblast like' are not afraid of a SE IOL design and that they can pass it round. Obviously the square edge shape concept does not exist at the cellular scale ; because the fibroblast like cells are not at all cubic, and they have got three-dimensional coordinates. Secondly, the IOL itself at the cellular scale of 10 μm is not smooth at all and it is not perfectly polished but rough and porous[5] (Figures 11.2 and 11.3).

At the scale of 10 μm the IOL optic material, seems to be porous and rough, and the SE sharp of the IOL becomes a very academic point of view. That the reason why some authors[3] demonstrate a failure of discontinuous bend to prevent LEC migration in vitro (Figures 11.4 and 11.5).

But is there nothing right at all about a SE IOL design effect? Some studies show there is a SE effect on the

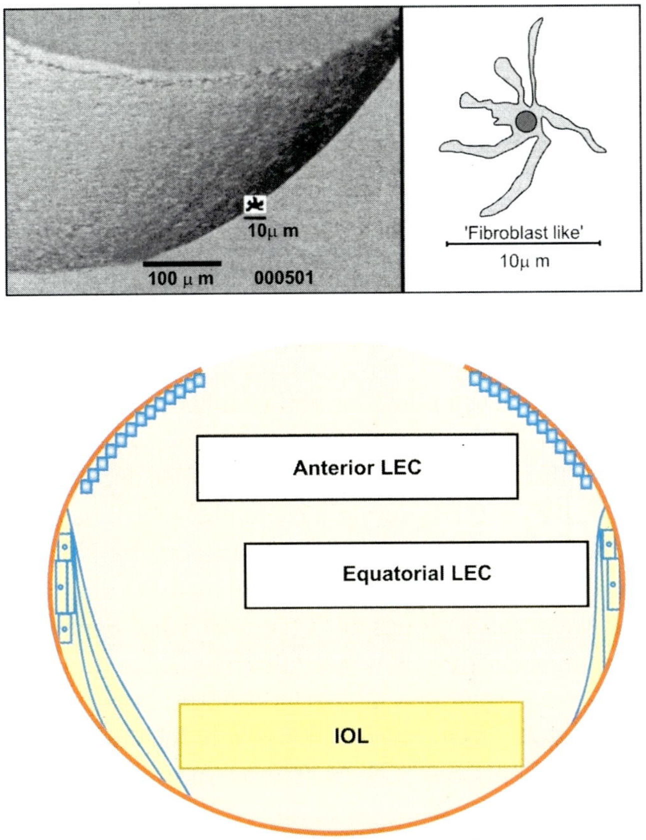

Figures 11.2 and 11.3: (Escobar-Gomez)[5] a SEM of the SA30AL at the scale of 100 μm
(On this figure a virtual 'fibroblast like' wide of 10 μm has been drawn by the author)

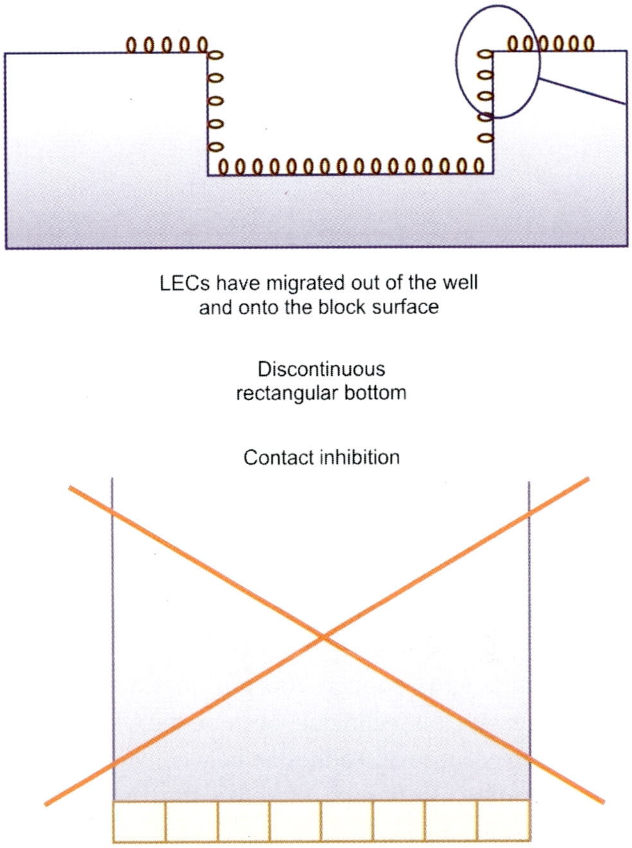

Figures 11.4 and 11.5: Failure of discontinuous bend to prevent LEC migration in vitro Bhermi GS, Spalton DJ[3]

PCO regardless of the type of IOL material. Other studies show that the difference in terms of PCO rate is due to the IOL material, and not statistically due to the SE effect. Obviously both factors, SE IOL design and type of IOL's material, influence the PCO rate .We now know that, of course, there is a SE effect but it is not a contact cellular inhibition, but it is a mechanical tension effect. **Boyce, Bhermi and Spalton**[2,3] have shown, by a mathematical model, that in fact a SE IOL design exerts twice more pressure than a round edge at the point p. This 'p' point is the contact between the corner of the edge and the posterior capsule. This high pressure blocks the LEC migration (Figure 11.6).

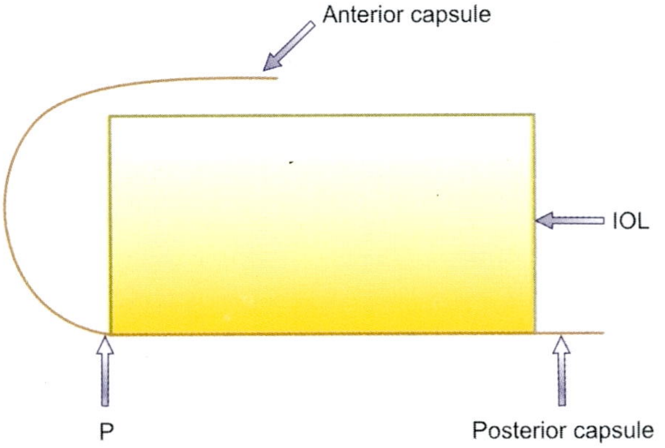

Figure 11.6: A square edge exerts twice more pressure on posterior capsule than a round edge

Capsular Rings: CBR and CTR Respective Actions Against PCO

Many other systems failed to completely clean the capsular bag without any risk for the zonula, the endothelium or the posterior capsule. Only a ring is able to go to the equatorial region, to try to mechanically block the LEC, or to block it by a disposable drug delivery system like 5FU[4] and so on...

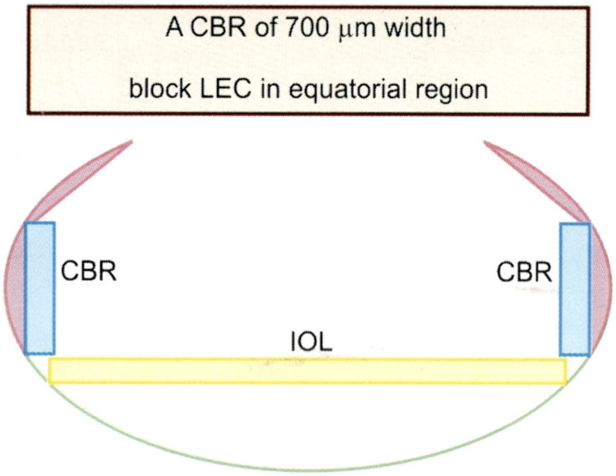

Figure 11.7: Capsular bending ring inside the capsular bag

CBR

There are two methods with rings; the first is to block LEC in equatorial region by a CBR: capsular bending ring which is large enough 700 µm, that the study of NISHI, but with this technique, because the CBR is large it avoid the collapse and adhesion between anterior and posterior capsule (which increase the risk of LEC migration) (Figure 11.7).

Nishi O, Nishi K study[14] HEMA IOL HM60 STORZ + 13 mm CTR PMMA square edge not polished 0.7 mm width and 0.2 mm thickness One eye IOL + CTR Second eye only IOL 2 years follow-up.

84 eyes of 42 patients EPCO computer image analysis

Rate of Nd: YAG casulotomy	5%	ring
	20%	without
Folds post-cap	0%	ring
	25%	without

CTR

HEHN F. clinical trial[9] At the contrary we explore the way of classical CTR which increases the speed of the adhesion between anterior and post capsule. We have analyzed 415 eyes with 24 months follow-up (Table 11.1). Two groups of patients with (n = 310) and without (n = 105) a CTR, during the months after a cataract surgery and we have compared the rate of Nd yag capsulotomy and EPCO grading for evaluate the PCO. We have got 3 groups of 3 kinds of IOL's materials. Hydrophilic acrylic (Stabibag Ioltech), silicone (Clariflex AMO) and hydrophobic acrylic (SA60AT Alcon). The CTR was simply a choice from the same laboratory than the IOL: Tensiobag Ioltech, Reform Alcon, Injectoring AMO (Figure 11.8).

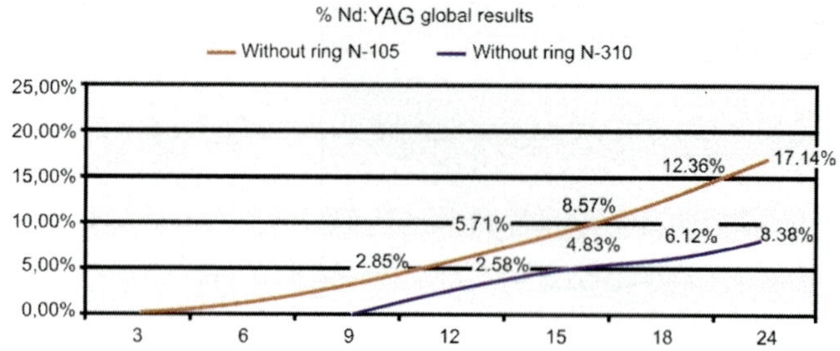

Figure 11.8: Global mean results percent Nd: YAG for PCO 24 months follow-up

EPCO RESULTS

Globally EPCO score index is less with CTR: 0.254 than without: 0.396 $p < 0.01$ (Table 11.2).

When the ring is inside the bag, it exerts a tangential tension of the posterior capsule all around 360°. Therefore a CTR increases the pressure at the 'p' point and then the SE tension effect of IOL, to mechanically block the LEC migration. That is the most fundamental effect of a CTR against the PCO but it is not the only one (Figures 11.9 and 11.10).

Previous research, by Rupert **Menapace**[7,14,16] suggested that capsular tension rings prevent the PCO through more than one mechanism. First, the ring causes posterior capsule stretching, which reduces the IOL

Table 11.1: Rate percent of Nd: YAG for PCO at 24 months follow-up

Hydrophobic	without CTR	n = 41	12.19%[5]	with CTR	n = 96	5,20%[5]	$p<0.01$
Hydrophilic	without CTR	n = 33	21.21%[7]	with CTR	n = 106	10,37%[11]	$p<0.001$
Silicone	without CTR	n = 31	19.35%[6]	with CTR	n = 108	9,25%[10]	$p<0.01$

Table 11.2: At one year follow-up in 23 eyes EPCO score is less with CTR than without

Hydrophobic	without CTR	N = 3	0,229	With CTR	N = 5	0,107	p<0,01
Hydrophilic	without CTR	N = 2	0,523	With CTR	N = 4	0,360	p<0,01
Silicone	without CTR	N = 4	0,459	With CTR	N = 5	0,317	p<0,01

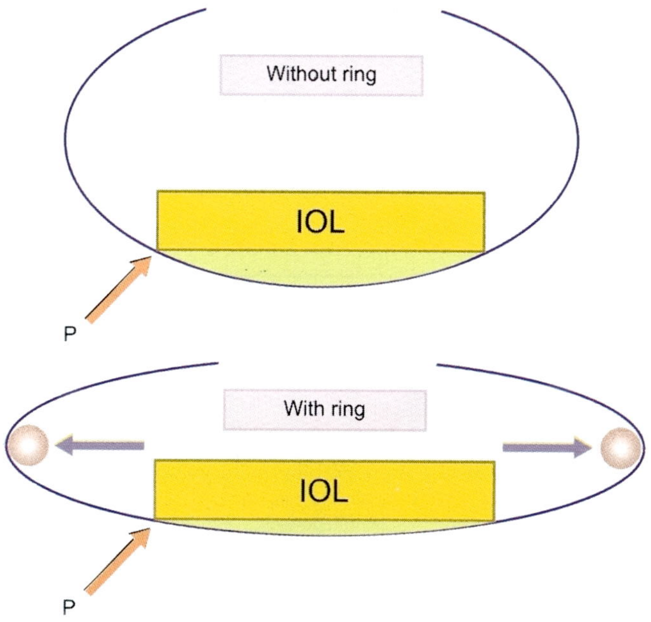

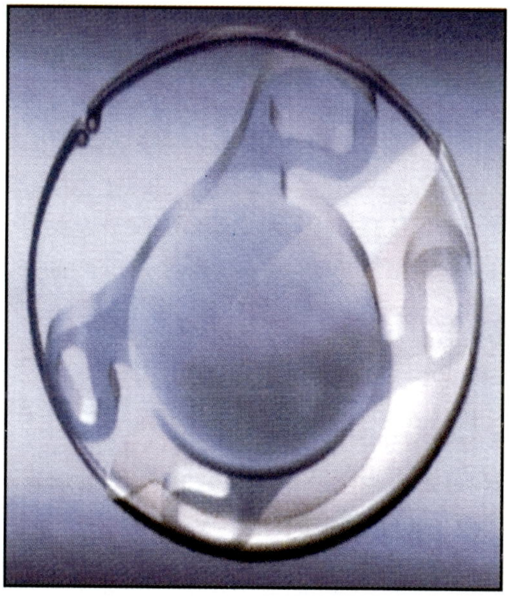

Figures 11.9 and 11.10: Effect of a capsular tension ring inside the bag

capsule distance. The well tension of the capsular bag reduces the retro-optical space: the CTR increases the 'no space no cell' theory. The immediate well tension of the bag with the ring (before the natural retraction of the capsular bag), increases the speed of the capsular bend formation, before the LEC get enough time to conquer the retro-optical space: the CTR increases the CBI (Capsular bending index),[13] which is fundamental, to avoid the LEC migration. The instantaneous tension of the bag by the ring facilitates the capsular adhesion between the posterior capsule and the IOL optic by fibronectin, laminin or collagen type IV, which are present on capsular or on LEC surface, and so on, are free to absorb the IOL surface after the break of the blood aqueous barrier: the CTR increases the 'sandwich' theory.[10]

I expect so that a CTR would probably increase the LEC destruction by a direct cell compression. Other well known properties of the ring can be combined to reduce the PCO rate, like the better long terms centration for all lens with a CTR. CTR facilitates the equatorial LEC removal by an IOL rotation inside the capsular bag without any risk for the zonula, it facilitates the retro-optical viscoelastic ablation too, according to the 'no space no cell' theory, it facilitates the anterior capsular bag cleaning to prevent capsular shrinkage. Eventually, a CTR decreases capsular fold of posterior capsule and then it avoids the LEC migration along the folds.

The 10 Specific CTR Preventing PCO Factors

01 : the CTR increases the pressure at the 'p' point and then the SE IOL design tension effect

02 : the CTR reduces the retro-optical space too, according to the 'no space, no cell ' theory

03 : the CTR increases the speed of the capsular bend formation

04 : the CRT facilitates the adhesion between the capsule and the IOL according to the 'sandwich' theory.

05 : the CTR probably makes some equatorial LEC destruction by direct cell compression.

06 : the CTR prevents IOL decentration, deformation and tilting with soft IOL

07 : the CTR facilitates the equatorial LEC removal by an IOL rotation inside the capsular bag

08 : the CTR facilitates the retro-optical viscoelastic ablation too, according to the 'no space no cell' theory.

09 : the CTR facilitates the anterior capsular bag cleaning to prevent capsular shrinkage.

10 : the CTR decreases the capsular folds of posterior capsule.

KILL THE LEC

1. **Perfect Capsule**™[11] This system, which is able to kill the LEC by hypo-osmolarity. But is there some risk for endothelium if the suction leaks ? Actually perfect casule device is not available for MICS because it needs a 3.2 mm width cornea incision (Figures 11.11 and 11.12).
2. **Aqualase®**[12] an hot hydrojet, able to hydrolyse the nucleus of the crystalline. Is there any possibilities to hydrolyse the LEC in equatorial region? Actually aqualase is compatible with bimanual technique, but not with MICS because the needle of aqualase handpiece needs of 3.2 incision, the next generation of aqualase certainly will be compatible with MICS (Figures 11.13).
3. **Phaco-laser** (the Dodick photolysis) is compatible with MICS, recently at ARVO 2004 meeting, it has been shown the possibility of direct LEC destruction by Nd yag laser on anterior capsule (Figures 11.14).
4. **CBJ Cleanbagjet®** is a new phaco handpiece, which produce a micro hydrojet able to clean the LEC even in equatorial region, developed by Ioltech laboratories, first clinical results are expected at ASCRS 2005 congress (Figures 11.15 to 11.17).

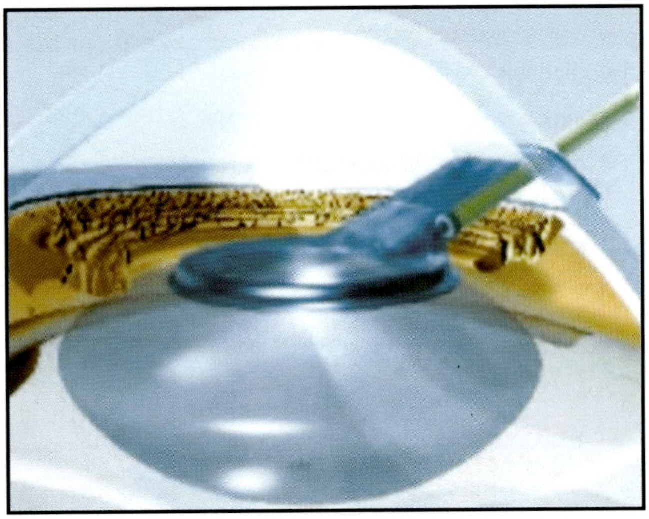

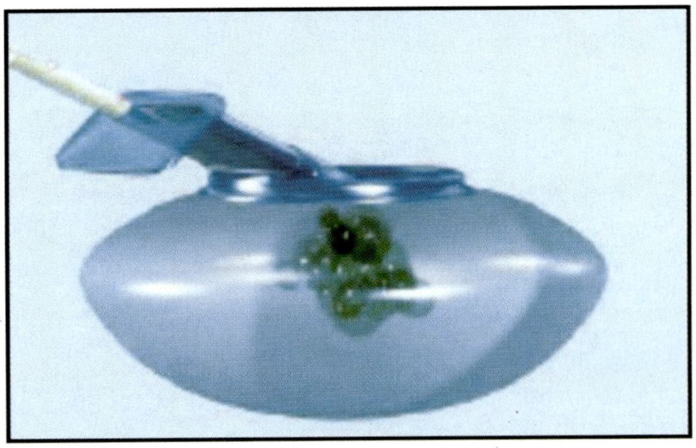

Figures 11.11 and 11.12: Perfect capsule™ system

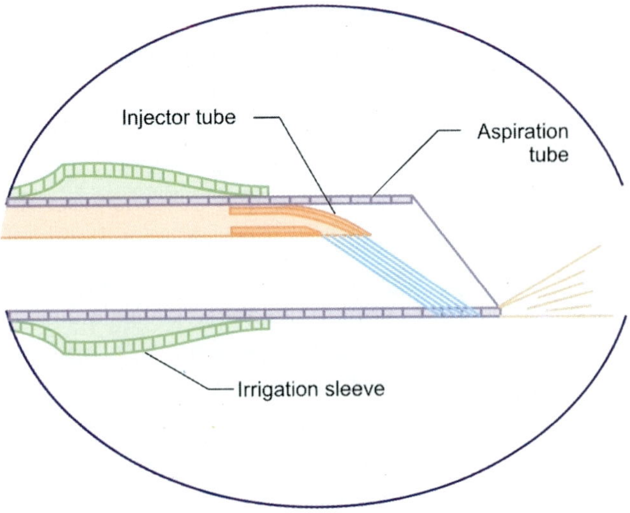

Figure 11.13: Aqualase®

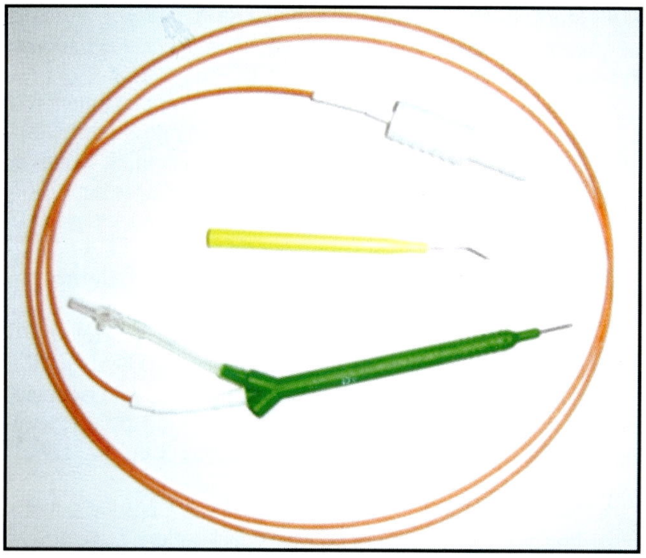

Figure 11.14: Phaco laser (the Dodick photolysis)

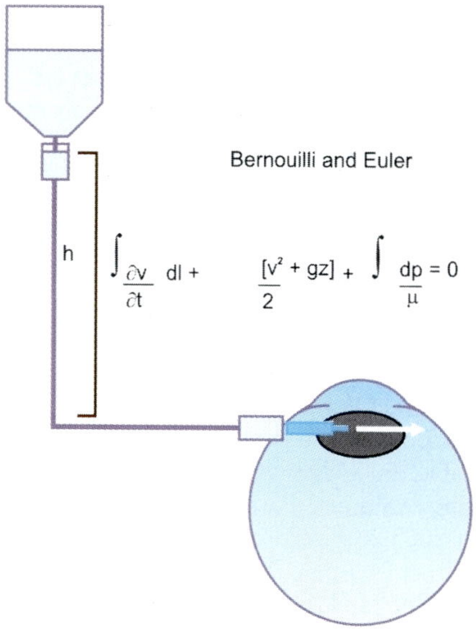

Figure 11.16

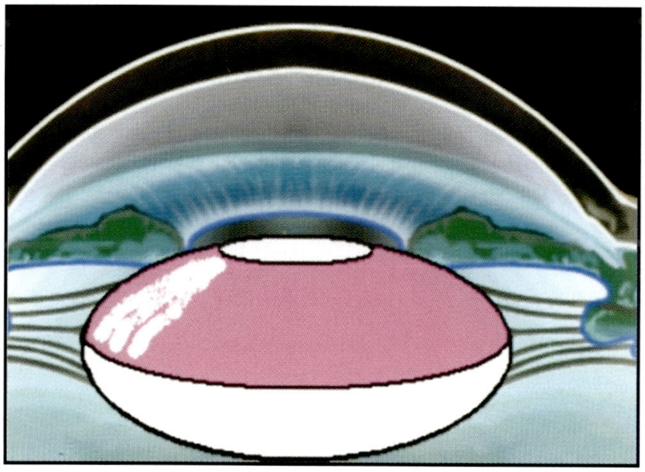

Figure 11.15

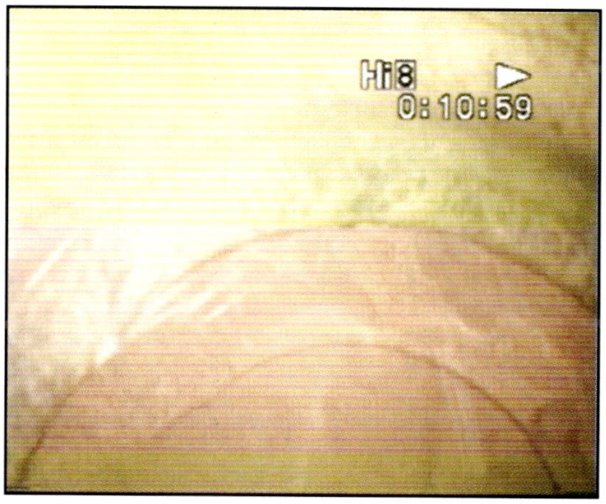

Figures 11.15 to 11.17: Cleanbag jet®

CONCLUSION

With MICS or not, PCO remains the really final frontier in cataract surgery. Until we will be not able to take off or kill entirely the equatorial LEC, PCO occurs irreversibly from month to month after cataract surgery. The more IOL becomes softer smaller and thinner CTR will take a greater place especially against PCO. without PCO it will be possible to treat accommodation in pseudophakic eye and perform cataract surgery as easily in children than in adult without anterior vitrectomy nor PCCC (Figure 11.18).

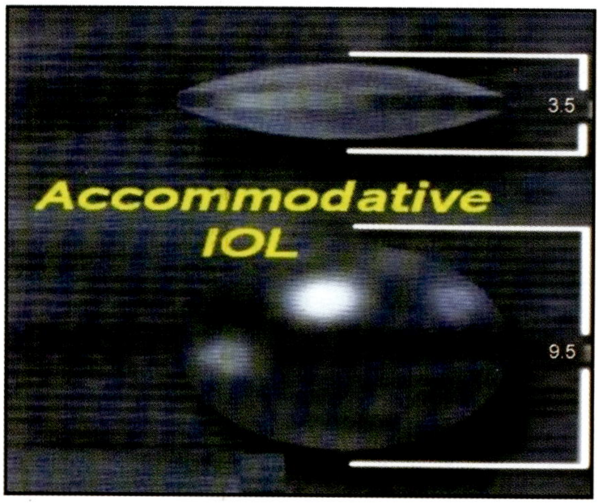

Figure 11.18: Phacoersatz: Accommodative IOL

REFERENCES

1. Auffarth GU, Golescu A, Becker KA, Volcker HE. Quantification of posterior capsule opacification with round and sharp edge intraocular lenses. Ophthalmology 2003; 110(4):772-80.
2. Boyce JF, Bhermi GS, Spalton DJ, El-Osta AR. Mathematical modeling of the forces between an intraocular lens and the capsule. J Cataract Refract Surg 2002;28(10):1853-9.
3. Bhermi GS, Spalton DJ, El-Osta AA, Marshall J. Failure of a discontinuous bend to prevent lens epithelial cell migration in vitro. J Cataract Refract Surg 2002;28(7):1256-61.
4. Cochener B, Bougaran R, Pandey S, Apple D, Colin J. [Non-biodegradable drug-sustained capsular ring for prevention of secondary cataract. Part I: In vitro evaluation] J Fr Ophtalmol 2003;26(3):223-31.
5. Escobar-Gomez M, Apple DJ, Vargas LG, Werner L, Arthur SN, Pandey SK, et al. Scanning electron microscopic and histologic evaluation of the AcrySof SA30AL acrylic intraocular lens. Manufacturing quality and morphology in the capsularbag. J Cataract Refract Surg 2003;29(1):164-9.
6. Galand A, Van Cauwenberge F, Moosavi J. Posterior capsulorhexis in adult eyes with intact and clear capsules. J Cataract Refract Surg 1996;22:458-61.
7. Georgopoulos M, Menapace R, Findl O. After-cataract in adults with primary posterior capsulorhexis. J Cataract Refract Surg 2003;29:955-60.
8. Hara T, Azuma N, Chiba K, Ueda Y, Hara T. Anterior capsular opacification after endocapsular cataract surgery. Ophthalmic Surg 1992;23(2):94-8.
9. HEHN F. Update on capsular tension ring implantation to prevent PCO Advance in Ophthalmology (2nd edn). 2004.
10. Linnola RJ, Sund M, Ylonen R, Pihlajaniemi T. Adhesion of soluble fibronectin, vitronectin, and collagen type IV to intraocular lens materials. J Cataract Refract Surg 2003; 29(1):146-52.
11. Malouf A. Sealed lens capsule irrigation. Cataract and Refractive Surgery Today 2002.
12. Mackool RJ, Brint SF. Aqualase: a new technology for cataract extraction. Curr Opin Ophtalmol 2004;15:40-3.
13. Nishi O, Nishi K, Akura J. Speed of capsular bend formation at the optic edge of acrylic, silicone, and poly (methyl methacrylate) lenses. J Cataract Refract Surg 2002;28(3): 431-7.
14. Nishi O, Nishi K, Menapace R, Akura J. Capsular bending ring to prevent posterior capsule opacification: 2 year follow-up. J Cataract Refract Surg 2001;27(9):1359-65.
15. Ohadi C, Moreira H, Mc Donnell P. Posterior capsule opacification. Curr Opin Ophtalmol 1991;2:46-52.
16. Strenn K, Menapace R, Vass C. Capsular bag shrinkage after implantation of an open-loop silicone lens and a poly(methyl methacrylate) capsule tension ring. J Cataract Refract Surg 1997;23(10):1543-7.
17. Tassignon MJ, De Groot V, Vrensen GF. Bag-in-the-lens implantation of intraocular lenses. J Cataract Refract Surg. 2002;28(7):1182-8.

12

Bimanual Microincisional Phaco for Complicated Cases

- ADVANTAGES OF BIMANUAL IRRIGATION-ASPIRATION
- BIMANUAL MICROINCISIONAL PHACO FOR CATARACTS WITH LARGE ZONULAR DEFECTS
- BIMANUAL MICROINCISIONAL PHACO FOR RESIDUAL NUCLEUS FOLLOWING POSTERIOR CAPSULE RUPTURE
- BIMANUAL MICROINCISIONAL PHACO FOR INTRAOPERTIVE FLOPPY IRIS SYNDROME

David F Chang (USA)

INTRODUCTION

While many surgeons have found bimanual microincisional phaco to be advantageous for their routine cases, others still consider standard coaxial phaco to be the superior technique. I believe that bimanual microincisional phaco does offer unique advantages for several complicated surgical situations. For this reason, even surgeons who prefer coaxial phaco may benefit from adding the bimanual microincisional phaco technique to their surgical armamentarium.

ADVANTAGES OF BIMANUAL IRRIGATION-ASPIRATION

Like many surgeons, I generally prefer a coaxial irrigation-aspiration (IA) handpiece for routine cortical cleanup. This instrumentation utilizes the same phaco incision, and does not require the two additional smaller incisions on either side. 21-gauge bimanual IA instruments also require a larger paracentesis incision than that typically made for the chopper. However, there are several difficult surgical situations where a bimanual IA technique can be extremely helpful (Figures 12.1C]. These include the presence of weak zonules, a zonular dialysis, difficulty with the sub-incisional cortex, and cortical cleanup in the presence of a posterior capsule defect.[1]

In the case of subincisional cortex, bimanual handpieces allow the surgeon to approach the subphaco incisional area from the side. In addition, the aspirating handpiece can be switched to the opposite incision to access what was previously the "subincisional" location. This is particularly helpful in the presence of a smaller capsulorhexis diameter. While nuclear disassembly techniques, such as phaco chop, can remove the nucleus through a small capsulotomy, the latter significantly impedes coaxial IA access to the subincisional area.

A second benefit of having more than one port for the aspirating handpiece is that the 0.3 mm opening can always be kept oriented away from the posterior capsule. With coaxial IA, the aspirating opening must be rotated sideways toward the capsular fornices as one approaches the subincisional quadrant of cortex. In the subincisional area, the port must momentarily aim posteriorly. The risk of aspirating the posterior capsule is further increased if either the capsule is lax, as with weak zonules, or if the chamber is repeatedly shallowing due to poorly balanced fluidics. In contrast, with bimanual IA, the surgeon never has to aspirate beneath the instrument shaft, thereby eliminating the need to rotate the port sideways or posteriorly. This is extremely beneficial if a lax posterior capsule is repeatedly trampolining toward the tip, of if the posterior capsule has ruptured.

If the cross-sectional diameter of the coaxial IA tip is too small, the phaco incision will leak excessively during surgery. This is a disadvantage of using an all-metal sleeve, as opposed to the bulkier silicone infusion sleeve. With appropriately tight paracentesis incisions, bimanual IA instrumentation provides excellent chamber fluidic stability. In addition, there is a less rapid irrigation inflow rate with this system. This reduces the posteriorly directed hydrostatic infusion force, and the total volume of irrigation passing through the eye. Surge is generally less of a problem with cortical cleanup than with phaco due to the small 0.3 mm size of the aspirating port.

Separating the irrigating and aspirating functions onto different instruments allows one to distance these openings further apart. Dissociating the two is advantageous if there is a posterior capsule rent or zonular dialysis, and one specifically wants to aim the infusion away from the problem area. Finally, there are ergonomic advantages to using a more slender aspirating instrument. Without the constraint of the bulky silicone irrigation sleeve, the aspirating tip can more easily reach the peripheral-most fornices of the capsular bag. This is particularly advantageous when one is trying to avoid aspirating lax posterior capsular folds or exposed vitreous. By initiating aspiration only when the tip is buried more peripherally within the cortex, one assures that the cortex will immediately block capsule or vitreous from entering the tip.

As an alternative to coaxial phaco, bimanual microincisional phaco offers many of the same advantages as bimanual IA in complicated surgical settings. The beneficial principles behind separating the coaxial fluidic functions into two instruments remain the same.

BIMANUAL MICROINCISIONAL PHACO FOR CATARACTS WITH LARGE ZONULAR DEFECTS

In 2003, I first reported the use of bimanual microincisional phaco for cataracts with large zonular defects (Figures 12.1A to C and 12.2A to C).[2,3] Phaco of the nucleus is challenging in such cases for several reasons. The deficient zonular support increases the risk of posterior capsule rupture and vitreous loss. When the anterior capsule is not taut, creation of a capsulorhexis is more difficult to control, and the nucleus may not rotate because the bag lacks sufficient torsional stability. The normal hydrostatic infusion pressure may further stretch and unzip the damaged zonules, and fluid may be misdirected through the zonular defect where it can hydrate the vitreous and shallow the anterior chamber. Finally, if vitreous prolapses anteriorly, it will follow the exiting fluid currents and prolapse to the phaco incision.

I recommend several helpful strategies in these eyes. First, I err on the side of making a slightly smaller capsulorhexis than usual to assure its successful completion This improves control of the flap being torn, and allows more opportunity to rescue an escaping tear. I employ Mackool disposable capsule retractors (FCI ophthalmic) to act as artificial zonules.[4,5] Unlike capsular tension rings, these PMMA hooks anchor the capsular bag to the limbus. This provides bag support in the anterior-posterior direction, torsional stability, and can re-center a slightly subluxated bag. The retractors are designed to

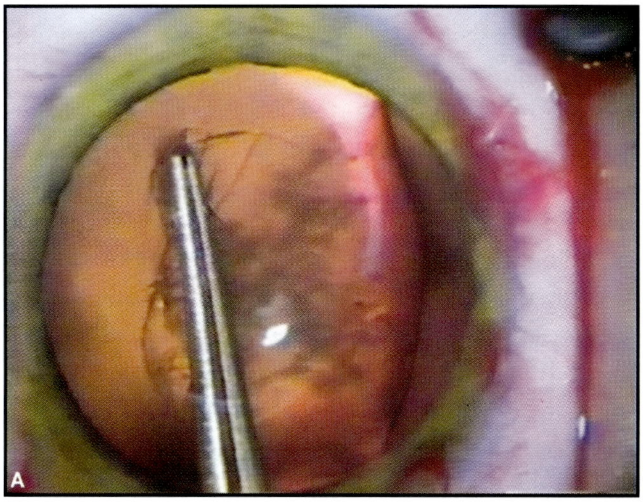

Figure 12.1A: Capsulorhexis creation in a traumatic cataract with a large zonular dialysis

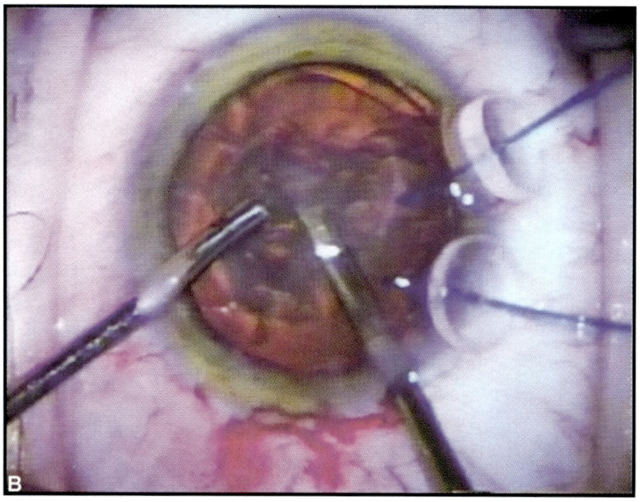

Figure 12.1B: Mackool disposable capsule retractors (FCI Ophthalmics) anchor capsular bag to the limbus. Bimanual phaco performed through two 1.2 mm incisions

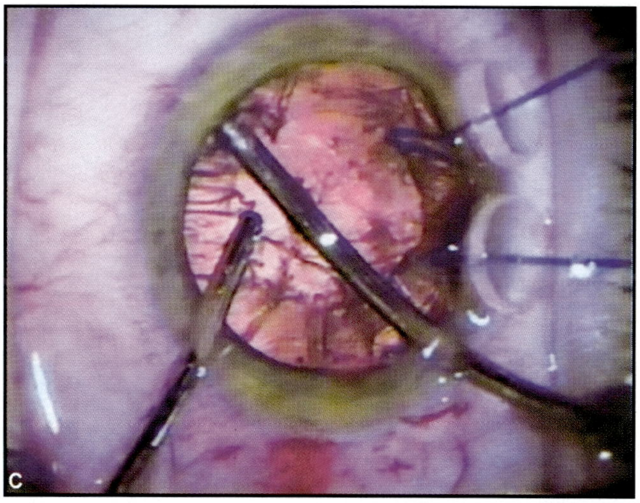

Figure 12.1C: Cortex removed with bimanual irrigation-aspiration handpieces

wrap around a small diameter capsulorhexis, and will not impede cortical cleanup. While many surgeons utilize nylon iris hooks for this purpose, they principally support the capsulorhexis edge. Iris retractors are too short to bolster the equatorial region of the bag, which is where the needed zonular support is missing.

Bimanual microincisional phaco helps to overcome many of the fluidic challenges of these cases. I use a side-irrigating chopper to intentionally reduce irrigation inflow and hydrostatic pressure, relative to front-irrigating choppers or to a coaxial infusion sleeve. This lessens the risk of fluid misdirection syndrome. To avoid post-

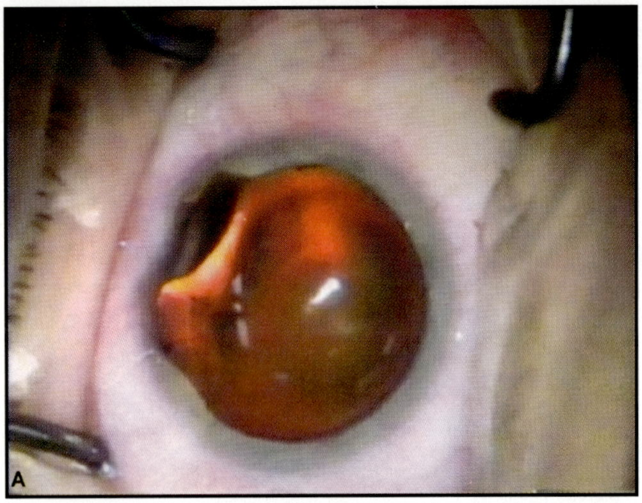

Figure 12.2A: Traumatic cataract with zonular and iridodialysis

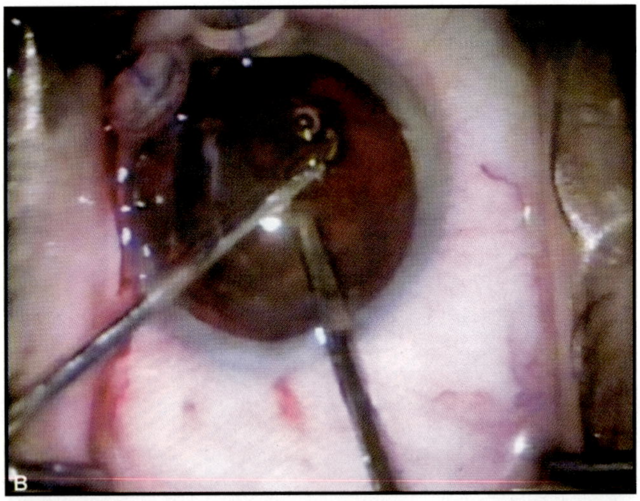

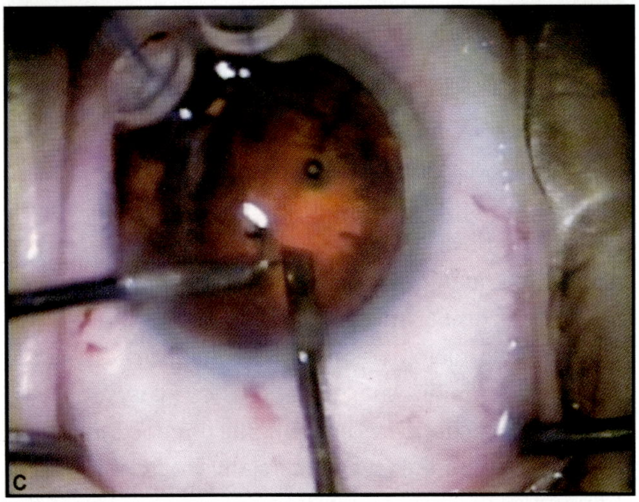

Figures 12.2B and C: Bimanual phaco performed with Mackool disposable capsule retractors

occlusion surge associated with reduced irrigation inflow, I reduce the aspiration flow rate to 20 to 26 cc/min, and the vacuum limit to 125 to 175 mm Hg. I also employ Staar Surgical's Cruise Control device, which is a disposable flow-restricting device to decrease surge.[6] For 20-gauge bimanual IA instrumentation, 1.2 mm incisions produce a near watertight fit. By minimizing incisional fluid leak, this reduces the total volume of irrigation circulating throughout the case, and limits the opportunity for exposed vitreous to prolapse to the incisions. The ability to separate the aspiration and irrigation ports means that the infusion source can be aimed away from the zonular or capsular defect. Finally, the slender bimanual instrument profiles are advantageous in the presence of multiple capsule retractors in the eye.

I have performed a consecutive series of 10 cases using this technique for cataracts with large zonular defects. By combining the use of Mackool capsule retractors with bimanual microincisional phaco, vitreous loss and posterior capsule rupture were avoided in all 10 cases.

BIMANUAL MICROINCISIONAL PHACO FOR RESIDUAL NUCLEUS FOLLOWING POSTERIOR CAPSULE RUPTURE

Following posterior capsular rupture, the surgeon's first priority becomes removing any remaining lens material–in particular, the nucleus.[1] Dr Richard Packard and I have reported our clinical results in using the Viscoat posterior assisted levitation (PAL) technique to levitate a partially descended nucleus into the anterior chamber via a pars plana sclerotomy.[7] The sclerotomy is made with an MVR blade inserted 3.5 mm posterior to the limbus. The levitated nucleus can then be removed by either resuming phaco, or by manual extraction via a larger extracapsular cataract incision. In deciding which extraction method to use, one must consider the size and density of the nucleus, the size of the capsular defect, the presence of vitreous prolapse, other complicating surgical factors, and the individual surgeon's level of comfort with either alternative.[1]

If a decision is made to continue phaco, a trimmed Sheet's glide, as described by Marc Michelson, should be inserted through the phaco incision.[8] By spanning the pupil, the plastic glide should help prevent descent of small lens particles, and may block vitreous from being drawn to the phaco tip. Typically, the coaxial phaco tip is inserted above and alongside the glide, which can create two problems. First, the incision must be enlarged to accommodate the glide. Secondly, as one maneuvers the phaco tip within the anterior chamber, the glide is displaced along with it, potentially damaging intraocular structures.

As an alternative, I would employ bimanual micro-incisional phaco through separate limbal incisions after first positioning the Sheet's glide through the phaco incision (Figures 12.3A and B).[3] This avoids displacing

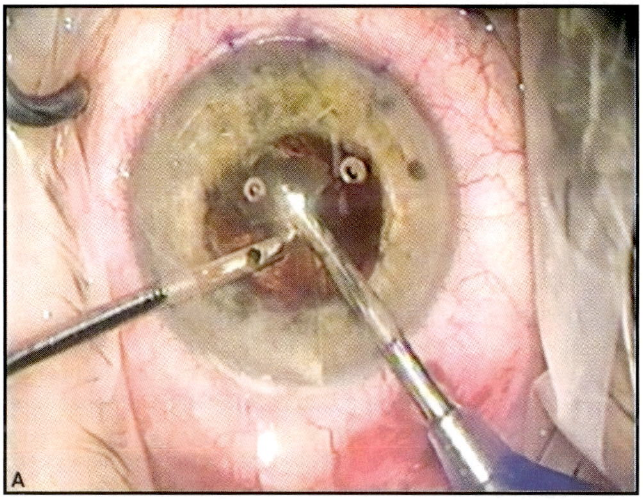

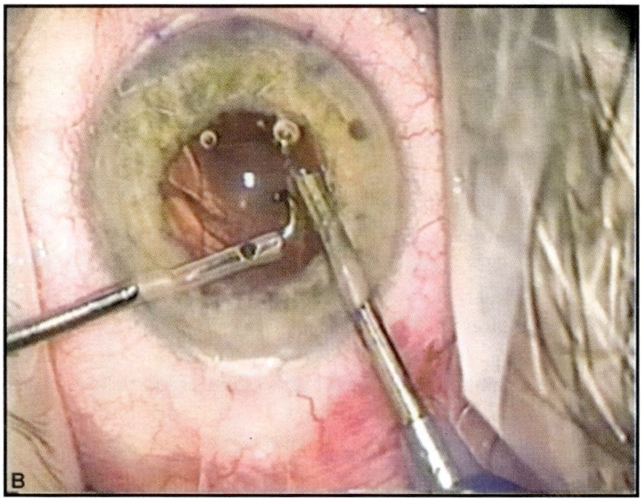

Figures 12.3A and B: Removal of residual nuclear fragments following ruptured posterior capsule. Trimmed Sheet's glide inserted through the clear corneal phaco incision. Bimanual phaco performed through separate 1.2 mm incisions, employing low aspiration flow and vacuum settings

the glide with movement of the phaco tip. The most important advantage is dissociating the irrigation and aspiration openings. By avoiding the competing irrigation-aspiration countercurrents of a coaxial design, one can work at much lower and safer aspiration flow and vacuum settings. One can direct the irrigation inflow away from the nuclear fragments being aspirated. This can minimize fluid turbulence in the anterior chamber, which might flush fragments posteriorly through a capsular defect.

BIMANUAL MICROINCISIONAL PHACO FOR INTRAOPERATIVE FLOPPY IRIS SYNDROME

At the 2005 ASCRS Annual Meeting, John Campbell, MD and I presented a newly described small pupil syndrome, the intraoperative floppy iris syndrome (IFIS).[9] This syndrome is characterized by repetitive incisional prolapse of a floppy, billowing iris, and progressive intraoperative miosis. In addition to poor preoperative pupil dilation, we also determined that mechanical stretching and sphincterotomies do not prevent the IFIS. We also noted a higher incidence of posterior capsule rupture with IFIS.

Following both a retrospective and a prospective study, we discovered that the cause of this syndrome is tamsulosin (Flomax ®), a systemic alpha-1 blocker that is the most commonly prescribed medication for benign prostatic hypertrophy (BPH). Alpha-1 sympathetic receptor blockade relaxes the smooth muscle in the prostate and bladder neck, thereby improving the urinary retention symptoms associated with BPH. We postulate that tamsulosin also blocks the iris dilator smooth muscle, as the same alpha-1A receptor subtype for which this drug is specific also predominates in the iris smooth muscle. We believe that the floppy behavior is due to loss of normal iris dilator muscle tone that provides the stromal rigidity usually observed intraoperatively.

In addition to employing iris retractors or pupil expansion rings,[10] I have found bimanual microincisional phaco to be helpful in these cases (Figures 12.4A and B). Snug incisions sized to minimize fluid leak can prevent the floppy iris from prolapsing. In addition, the irrigation currents can more consistently be kept circulating within the anterior chamber. This reduces the

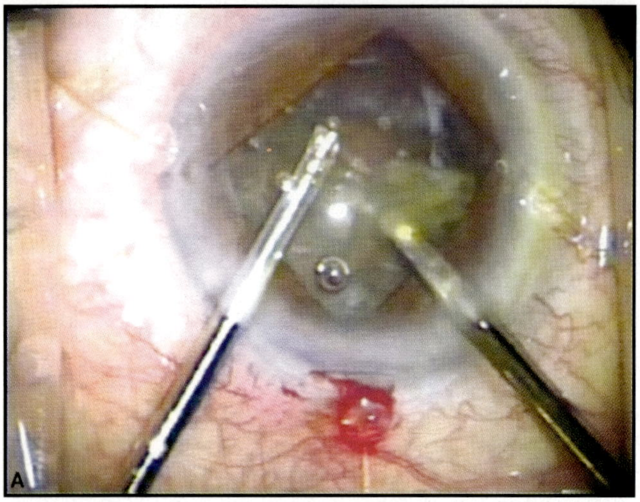

Figure 12.4A: Bimanual phaco employed in a case with intraoperative floppy iris syndrome due to Flomax ®. Four iris retractors maintain pupil expansion

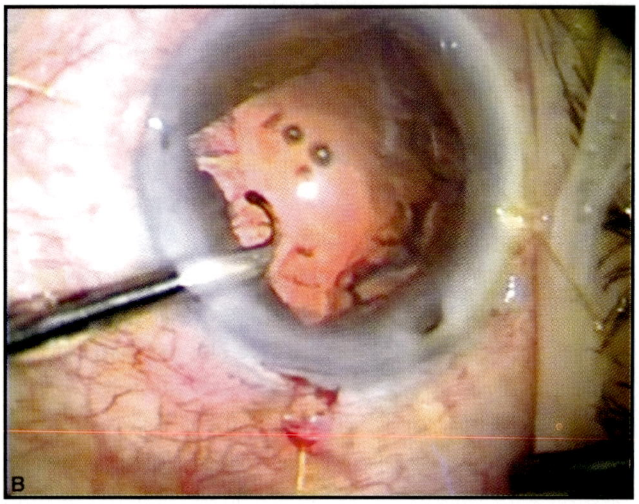

Figure 12.4B: Iris immediately prolapses upon withdrawl of phaco tip despite iris retractors

billowing caused by coaxial irrigation flow alternatively passing both above and then behind the pupil plane. It is the mechanical stimulation from the repetitive billowing and iris prolapse that produces the progressive intraoperative miosis that is so problematic in these eyes.

In conclusion, just as with cortical IA removal, bimanual and coaxial phaco represent two varying but excellent alternatives for removing the nucleus. The decision will generally reflect surgeon preference and IOL size requirements. However, just as there are special circumstances during which bimanual IA provides particular advantages, the same is true for bimanual microincisional phaco. Surgeons already skilled in the latter technique can take advantage of these benefits in challenging situations such as with capsular rupture, zonular dialysis, and IFIS.

REFERENCES

1. Chang DF. Managing residual lens material after posterior capsule rupture. Techniques in Ophthalmology 2003;1(4): 201-6.
2. Chang DF. Bimanual phaco for cataracts with zonular defects. Video Presentation, AAO Annual Meeting, Anaheim, CA, 2003.
3. Chang DF. Chapter 19. Bimanual Phaco Chop for Capsular or Zonular Defects. In Chang DF. Phaco Chop: Mastering Techniques, Optimizing Technology, and Avoiding Complications. Thorofare, NJ, Slack, 2004.
4. Chang DF. Chapter 14. Phaco Strategies for Complicated Cataracts. In Chang DF. Phaco Chop: Mastering Techniques, Optimizing Technology, and Avoiding Complications. Thorofare, NJ, Slack, 2004.
5. Mackool RJ. Capsule stabilization for phacoemulsification (letter). J Cataract Refract Surg 2000;26:629.
6. Chang DF, 400 mmHg High-vacuum bimanual phaco attainable with the Staar Cruise Control device. J Cataract Refract Surg 2004;30:932-3.
7. Chang DF, Packard RB. Posterior assisted levitation for nucleus retrieval using Viscoat after posterior capsule rupture. J Cataract Refract Surg 2003;29:1860-5.
8. Michelson MA. Use of a Sheets' glide as a pseudoposterior capsule in phacoemulsification complicated by posterior capsule rupture. Eur J Implant Surg 1993;570-2.
9. Chang DF, Cambell JR. Intraoperative floppy iris syndrome (IFIS) due to Flomax ®. Presented Annual Meeting, ASCRS, Washington DC 2005.
10. Akman A, Yilmaz G, Oto S, Akova Y. Comparison of various pupil dilatation methods for phacoemulsification in eyes with a small pupil secondary to psueudoexfolication. Ophthalmology 2004;111:1693-8.

13

Update on Various Nucleus Delivery Techniques in Manual Small Incision Cataract Surgery

- DELIVERY OF NUCLEUS INTO THE ANTERIOR CHAMBERS
- REMOVAL OF NUCLEUS OUT OF THE WOUND (VARIOUS TECHNIQUES)

Ashok Garg, Arif Adenwala (India)

INTRODUCTION

Manual Small Incision Cataract Surgery has emerged as the first practical alternative to phacoemulsification especially in developing countries as it is low cost and can achieve rapid postoperative recovery with minimal surgery related complications.

Manual Small Incision Cataract Surgery (MSICS) is a good alternative to expensive technique of phacoemulsification. It can be performed in almost all types of cataract.

This technique has almost all the advantages of phaco surgery. Important steps involved in SICS are:

a. Wound construction: Scleral tunnel is usually preferred.
b. Nucleus management: This includes:
   - Prolapsing of nucleus in AC
   - Removal of nucleus out of the wound.

     There are different methods for removal of nucleus out of the wound.
c. Implantation of intraocular lens.

   Nucleus management consists of:

   a. Delivery of nucleus into the anterior chamber
   b. Removal of nucleus out of the wound.

DELIVERY OF NUCLEUS INTO THE ANTERIOR CHAMBERS

After construction of good adequate capsulorhexis and hydrodissection, nucleus is prolapsed in the anterior chamber. This is done either by hydrodissection, viscoexpression or with use of Sinskey's hook by rotating the nucleus.

REMOVAL OF NUCLEUS OUT OF THE WOUND[6] (VARIOUS TECHNIQUES)

This is very important part of SICS. There are different methods available for it:

1. The Blumenthal technique.
2. Use of irrigating vectis.
3. Viscoexpression.
4. Phacofracture.
5. Manual phacofracture Cardona's technique.
6. Phaco sandwich technique.
7. Manual multiple phacofragmentation.
8. Prechop manual phacofragmentation.
9. Quarter's extraction technique.
10. Chopsticks technique.
11. Use of claw vectis.
12. Plain wire vectis.
13. Fish hook technique.
14. Phaco-punch technique.
15. Hybrid technique.
16. Slider pincer technique.
17. Double wire snare splitter technique.
18. Manual phacocracking.

The preliminary step in almost all the methods is prolapse of nucleus into the anterior chamber:

The Blumenthal Technique[6]

The important feature of nucleus delivery by this technique is hydrodissection of the nucleus followed by its hydrodynamic expression. This technique was indicated by Dr Michael Blumenthal.

Method Initial step is fixing of anterior chamber maintainer. It is usually inserted from the temporal side. The tube is attached to BSS bottle which is held 50 to 60 cm from patient's eye. The height can be adjusted. The next step is to engage the nucleus into the wound. The delivery of nucleus occurs by hydropressure generated by AC maintainer.

Lens glide is passed below the nucleus and with slight pressure over the scleral lip, the nucleus is removed. Instead of lens glide we can also apply pressure with needle over the scleral lip.

If the AC is shallow you can increase the height of bottle and vice versa.

Advantages[18]

- AC is formed at all the times
- The procedure is not dependent on viscoelastics
- No sophisticated instruments are required
- It can be used for all types of cataract and capsulotomy.

Disadvantages[18]

- Failure to manipulate the nucleus in the anterior chamber can cause zonular dialysis

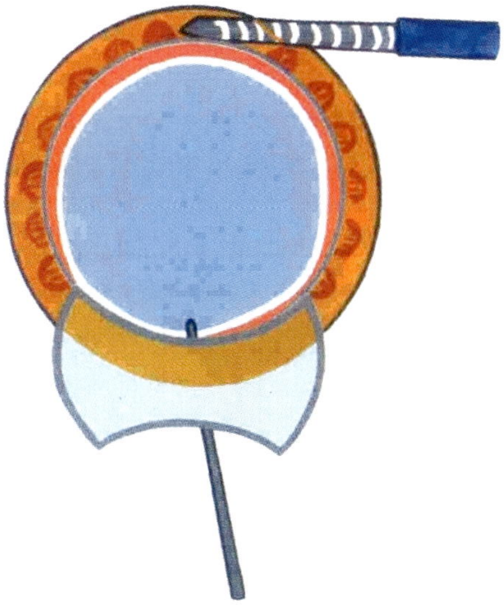

Figure 13.1: Nuclear prolapse:Sinskey's hook placed behind the superior pole of nucleus (Courtesy: Dr KPS Malik and Dr Ruchi Goel)

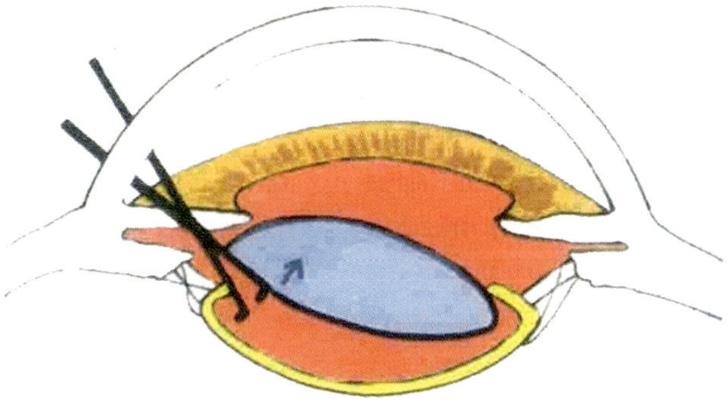

Figure 13.2: Nuclear prolapse out of the bag:Superior pole is lifted up using Sinskey's hook as a crowbar (Courtesy: Dr KPS Malik and Dr Ruchi Goel)

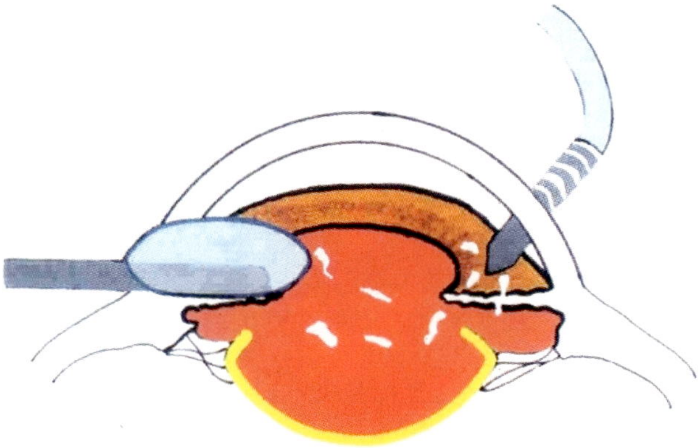

Figure 13.3: Modified Blumenthal technique: Nucleus engaged in the section (Courtesy: Dr KPS Malik and Dr Ruchi Goel)

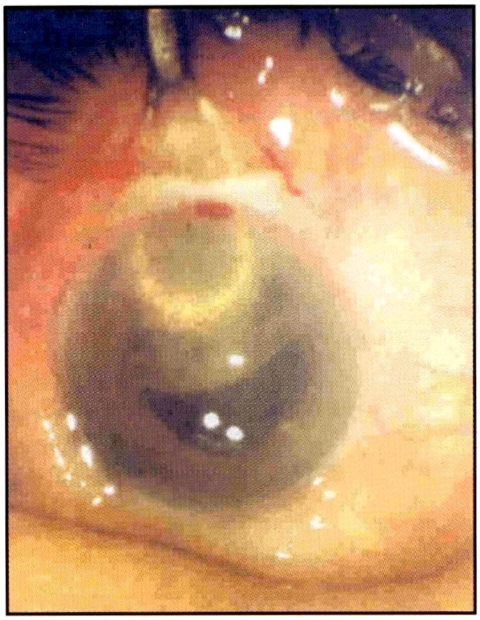

Figure 13.4: Use of irrigating vectis (Courtesy: Dr KPS Malik and Dr Ruchi Goel)

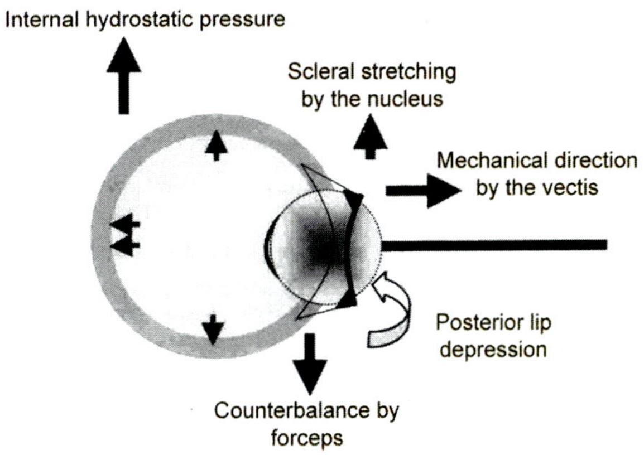

Figure 13.5: Mechanism of nucleus delivery with irrigating vectis (Courtesy: Dr KPS Malik and Dr Ruchi Goel)

- Keeping the bottle at adequate height is important; otherwise it may lead to frequent changes in the depth of the anterior chamber
- Traumatic delivery can damage the corneal endothelium.

Nucleus Removal using Irrigating Wire Vectis[7]

Irrigating Wire Vectis is use to deliver the nucleus either by hydroexpression or by viscoexpression.

Instruments

Various sizes of vectis are available. It has two surfaces, viz. anterior concave surface and posterior surface. The anterior end had three 0.3 mm openings. The posterior end is attached to syringe or infusion set.

Technique

Delivery of nucleus in the anterior chamber. Push the viscoelastic and insinuate the irrigating vectis below the nucleus. Apply counter pressure by holding superior rectus forceps. Now start the irrigation and pull the vectis out of the wound. Give pressure over the scleral lip posteriorly.

Pressure must be built up in the anterior chamber before pulling the nucleus out. Posterior lip depresssion is important part of nucleus delivery.

Mechanism of Nucleus Delivery[7]

It includes:

a. Mechanical pull by irrigating vectis
b. Internal hydrostatic pressure
c. Scleral stretching by the nucleus
d. Posterior scleral lip depression
e. Counter balance force by superior rectus forceps.

Advantages

- Anterior chamber is maintained after the nucleus delivery
- Damage to corneal endothelium is minimal.

Problem Associated

i. *Damage to iris:* Iris trauma can occur while insinuating the irrigating vectis below the nucleus. This can be prevented by pushing the viscoelastic above and below the nucleus. This pushes the iris posteriorly. Insert the vectis below the nucleus and deliver out the nucleus.
ii. *Posterior capsular tears:* It is quite rare with every irrigating vectis.

Viscoexpression[6]

This is another technique of removal of nucleus out of the wound. It is a common technique which is used by many surgeons due to its added advantages.

Technique

The preliminary step is to prolapse the nucleus out into the anterior chamber. Before this a good hydrodissection and hydrodelineation is very important. Now push viscoelastic into the anterior chamber. While pushing the viscoelastic engage the nucleus into scleral lip and then apply pressure over the posterior scleral lip and deliver the nucleus out. Viscoelastic is continuously pushed while removing the nucleus.

Advantages

- Viscoelastic material acts as a cushion or support to the corneal endothelium and so chances of its damage is minimal
- Anterior chamber is always maintained
- Damage to iris tissue is less
- Incidence of posterior capsule tear is also less.

Disadvantages

- Large quality of viscoelastic is required. This becomes expensive
- If viscoelastic material is not removed completely, there is increase incidence of postoperative uveitis and secondary glaucoma
- Not suitable for black cataracts.

Phacofracture[3]

This technique was described by Peter Kansas.[14,17]

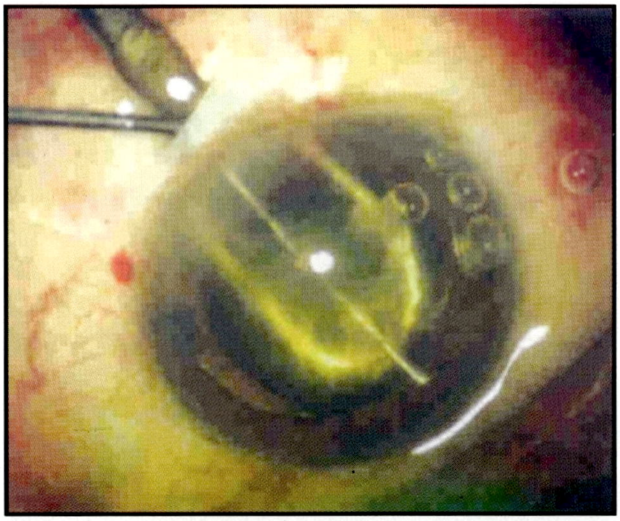

Figure 13.6: Phacofracture technique using Sinskey's hook and wire vectis (Courtesy: Dr KPS Malik and Dr Ruchi Goel)

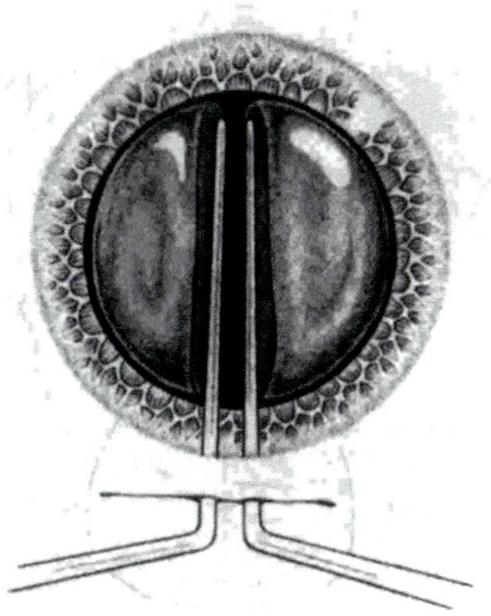

Figure 13.7: Separation of the nuclear fragments (Courtesy: Rozakis alternative to small incision cataract surgery)

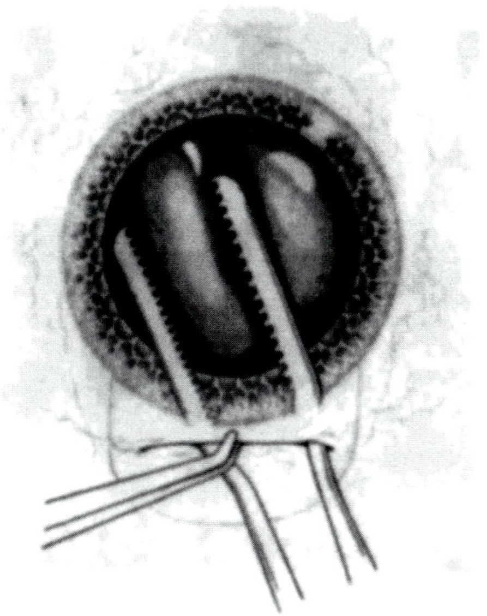

Figure 13.8: Removal of the nuclear fragment (Courtesy: Rozakis alternative to small incision cataract surgery)

Technique

The initial step is to prolapse the nucleus out of the bag. Viscoelastic is pushed both above and below the nucleus in the anterior chamber.

The solid curved vectis is insinuated under the nucleus and the nucleotome is positioned on the anterior surface of nucleus. Both instruments are brought close to each other. This will lead to splitting of the nucleus in to two halves.

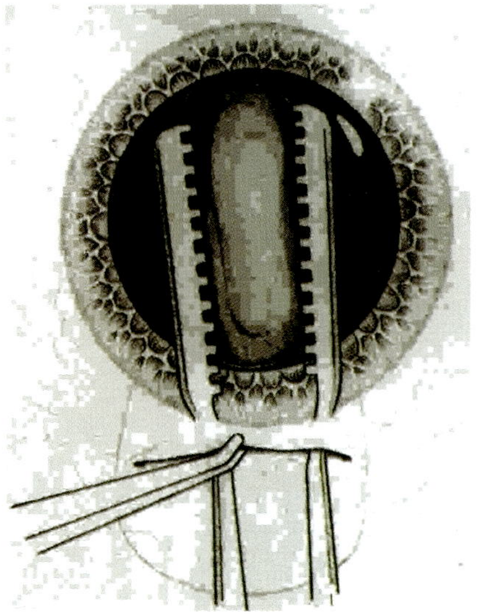

Figure 13.9: Removal of the last piece of the nucleus (Courtesy: Rozakis alternative to small incision cataract surgery)

Both the halves are separated and each half is removed with nuclear forceps or by pushing viscoelastic inside the AC.

Modification

This technique involves the use of Sinskey's hook and wire vectis to sandwich the nucleus and removing it out of the wound.

The anterior chamber should always be deep throughout the surgery.

Advantages

Manual phacofracture is a easy way that eliminates the hazards of the phacomachine with the ability to perform small incision with less expenses.

Complications

a. *Damage to iris tissue and superior iridodialysis* can occur during fragment extraction. This can be prevented by using lens glide or by pushing the iris posteriorly by pushing viscoelastic.
b. *Capsular disruption* can occur.
c. *Corneal endothelium damage:* This can occur due to passage of 2 instruments in AC and the maneuvering required to sandwich the nucleus and removing it out of the wound.

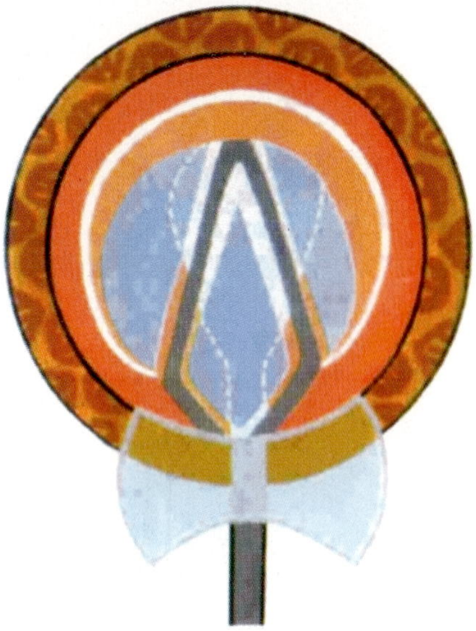

Figure 13.10: Phacofracture using trisector (Courtesy: Dr KPS Malik and Dr Ruchi Goel)

The other techniques for phacofracture includes:

A. *Bisector Technique*[6]*:* This requires the use of bisector. It is type of modification of phacofracture method. The preliminary step is to insinuate the wire vectis behind the nucleus and the bisector is passed on the anterior surface of the nucleus.

   The two instruments are maneuvered toward each other: leading to cleavage of nucleus into two halves. Constant pressure on bisector on vectis splits the nucleus into two halves. Both the halves are separated and removed by using nucleus holding forceps with vectis or by using viscoelastic material.

B. *Using Trisector*[13]*:* It is similar technique of phacofracture in which bisector is used thus dividing the nucleus into three pieces.

   The trisector consists of 2 longitudinal limits which are sharp in the posterior end. The bisector is passed under the nucleus and pressed toward the nucleus. This divides the nucleus into 3 pieces. Each piece is then removed with serrated forceps.

   Advantages
   - Safer delivery of nucleus
   - Less dependence on assistant personnel
   - The elimination of phacomachine and
   - The cost-effectiveness.

C. *Phacosalute and fracture*[6]*:* The nucleus is prolapsed into the AC. Inject the viscoelastic material. The superior portion of the nucleus is then amputated or pinched off using a capsular forceps and expressed using a irrigating vectis.

   Disadvantages
   - Corneal endothelial damage: Since two instruments are used simultaneously, the chance of endothelial damage is more. This can be prevented by injecting viscoelastic above and below the nucleus.

D. *Use of snare (Wire Loop):* This technique was introduced by Gerard Keener in 1983. He made a snare using 18 to 19 G blunt tipped needle and 32 G steel wire.

   Technique: Nucleus is prolapsed in AC and viscoelastic material is pushed above and below the nucleus. The lens loop/snare is passed below the nucleus. The lens is shifted into vertical position and brought across the nucleus. The loop is constructed by pulling posteriorly on the coil. This leads in the division of nucleus into the halves.

   The two halves are then separated by injecting viscoelastic material. Each halve is removed with fine toothed forceps.

Advantages
- Fragmentation of the nucleus is safe an non–expensive technique
- It can be used for hard cataract where phaco is difficult
- It can also be used in cases of zonular dehisences
- It is safe, smooth, cost-effective and easy to use technique.

Disadvantages
- Difficult in small pupils
- Difficult in soft nuclei and subluxated lens
- It can cause some damage to the corneal endothelium.

Manual Phacofracture Cardona's Technique

In order to perform the manual bisection of the nucleus according to Cardona's technique, it is important to dislocate the crystalline nucleus in the anterior chamber.

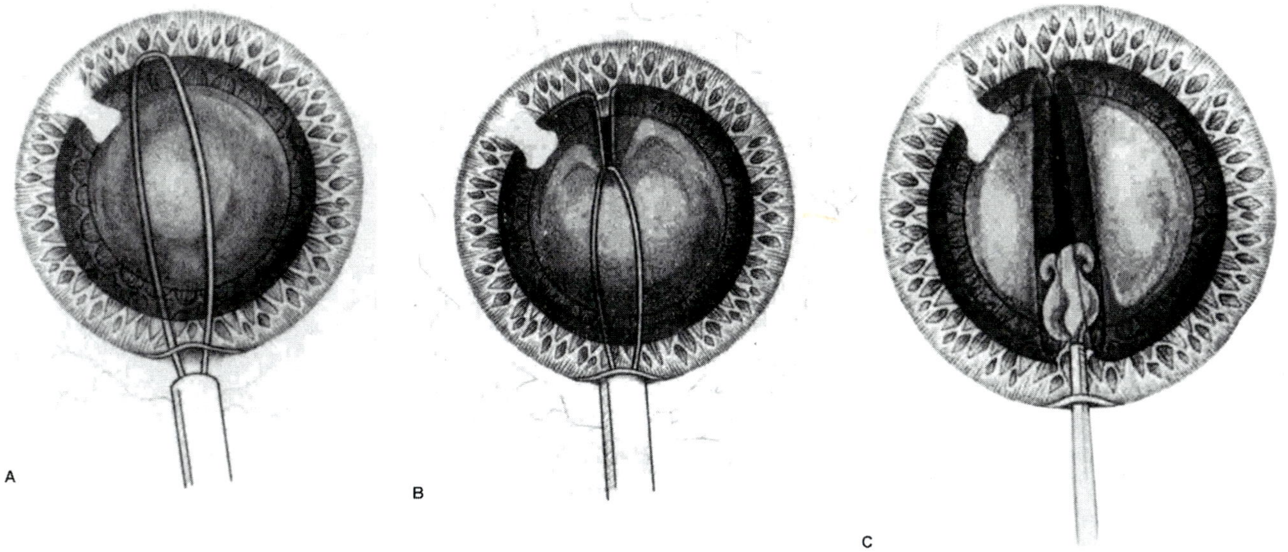

Figures 13.11A to C: Use of snare (Courtesy: Rozakis alternative to small incision cataract surgery)

Technique

Scleral tunnel of about 5 mm is made. After capsulorhexis and hydroprocedures, nucleus is prolapsed in the anterior chamber.

Through the tunnel incision, vectis is inserted under the nucleus and bisector is placed onto the nucleus. Nucleus is supported by the non-slipping vectis and fragmented into two with the sawing movement of bisector. The nuclear pieces are then removed out of the scleral tunnel wound.

Phaco Sandwich Technique[4,11]

This technique was introduced by Luther L Fry. This procedure require 7.5 mm opening for most of the nuclei and large incision for harder cataract.

Technique

Tipping up of the nucleus is very important step. The capsule and iris are hold with iris spatula and the nucleus is nudged toward 6 o'clock with hook. The superior pole of nucleus is then caught with spatula and tipped up.

The viscoelastic is placed between superior pole of nucleus and posterior capsule. The iris is pushed posteriorly with viscoelastic and the nucleus is elevated with the spatula. The lens loop is paced beneath the nucleus and spatula is placed on top of nucleus. Both instruments are approximated leading to sandwiching of the nucleus.

Thus with two handed technique the nucleus is removed.

Advantages

- This technique can be used for all pupil sizes and almost all types of nucleus
- It can be used with large can opener capsulotomy
- Safe and easy technique which does not require expensive instrumentation.

Disadvantages

- Large amount of viscoelastic material is required
- Not suitable for very soft cataract
- Relative contraindication for subluxated cataract
- Large capsulorhexis is required
- Increase chance of damage to the posterior capsule
- Iridodialysis—Iris may get caught when both the instruments are approximated and removed.

Complications

The most common complication seen in one study done are:

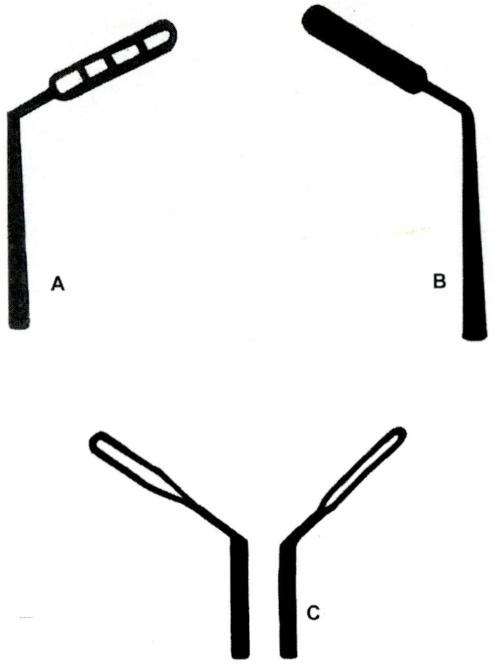

Figure 13.12: Instruments used for phacofragmentation. A. Nucleotome, B. Spatula and C. Manipulators (Courtesy: Dr KPS Malik and Dr Ruchi Goel)

a. Posterior capsular rupture.
b. Loss of vitreous.
c. Transient corneal edema.

Modifications[6]

In this technique, the lens loop and spatula is not used. The instruments used are plain wire vectis and visco-cannula.

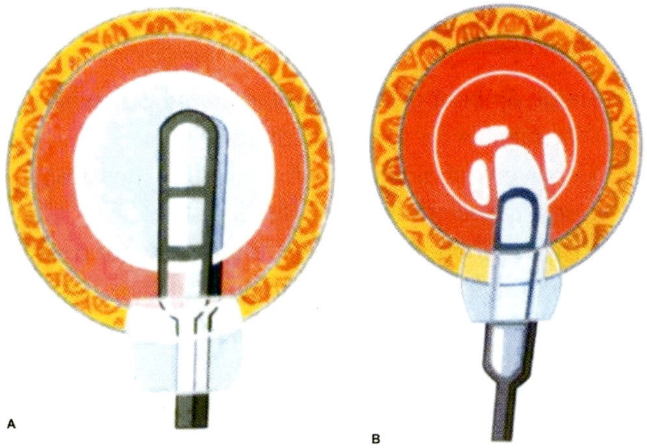

Figures 13.13A and B: Manual multiphacofragmentation (Courtesy: Dr KPS Malik and Dr Ruchi Goel)

The plain wire vectis is insinuated below the nucleus and viscoelastic is pushed above and below the nucleus. The viscocannula is placed in front of the nucleus. The nucleus is sandwich with these instruments and removed. The viscoelastic is injected, while the nucleus is brought out.

Sinskey hook can also be used instead of cannula.

Manual Multiple Phacofragmentation[6]

It is technique of manual SICS in which the nucleus is fragmented into multiple pieces and then removed.

Technique

In this procedure special instruments are required.

Instruments

a. *Nucleotome:* It is racquet shaped instrument of length 8 mm and width 2 mm. It is divided by 3 transverse bars. It is held at 45° to long handle.
b. *Spatula:* The shape of spatula should be same as nucleotome.
c. *Manipulators:* Used to collect the nuclear fragments in to center.

Procedure

The initial steps remain the same. The spatula is passed below the nucleus present in the anterior chamber and the nucleotome is placed over the nucleus.

Viscoelastic should be sufficient to keep the AC deep. Both the instruments are then brought close to each other. This causes fragmentation of large nucleus into small pieces.

The manipulators are used to remove the lens fragments from scleral lip into center of wound. The small pieces are then removed either by using viscoelastic or with the help of nucleus holding forceps.

Advantages

- Hard cataracts can be removed through the small wound by making small nuclear pieces.

Disadvantages

- Damage to corneal endothelium is quite high as two instruments are passed in the anterior chamber

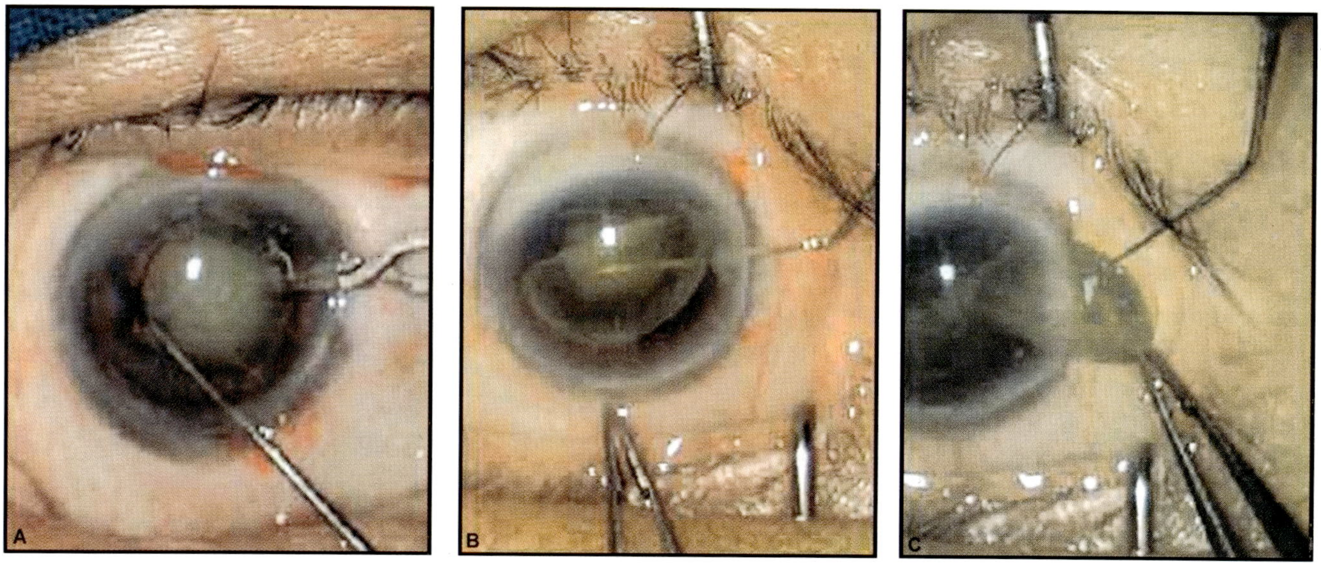

Figures 13.14A to C: Technique of prechop manual phacofragmentation (Courtesy: Dr Pipat Kongsap)

- Damage to iris tissue is also seen. This is seen both while inserting and removing the instrument
- Use of special instruments like nucleotome which may not be available everywhere.

Prechop Manual Phacofragmentation[12]

In this technique of cataract surgery, the nucleus is manually split into 2 fragments with prechopper forceps and then removed.

Technique

After good rhexis and hydroprocedures viscoelastic is injected into the anterior chamber. The sinskey hook is passed through side port to stabilize the nucleus. The prechop forceps is inserted through the wound and passed into center of nucleus core. Opening the forceps will cause splitting of nucleus into 2 pieces. Complete division of nucleus should occur otherwise, the steps are repeated. Each piece is prolapsed into anterior chamber and then removed using viscoelastics or serrated with the help of nucleus forceps.

Advantages

- This technique of phacofragmentation is done in the bag and not in anterior chambers and so cause less damage to corneal endothelium.
- Does not require expensive instruments.
- Visual recovery is rapid.

Disadvantages

- Not suitable for hard/black cataracts
- Also not suitable for subluxated cataract
- Initial learning curve for nucleus fragmentation is very important.

Quarters Extraction Technique for Manual Phacofragmentation[9]

Technique

In this procedure the nucleus is manually split and fragments removed. After capsulorhexis, hydrodissection, hydrodelineation and the surface cortex aspiration, the edge of the nucleus is prolapsed into the AC.

The front quarter of the nucleus is cut and removed with nuclear punches. A corner of the remaining three quarter of nucleus is wedged into the wound and rotated out with a claw vectis.

Disadvantages

- This technique is not suitable for very hard/large nucleus
- It requires learning curve for fragmentation of the nucleus.

Chop Bisector/Chop Trisector and Chopsticks Technique for Extraction of the Nuclear Fragments

It is alternative form of manual phacofragmentation in which chop bisection/chop trisection or chop multisection is done.

Technique

The division of the nucleus is carried out by slipping a phacochopper from 6 o'clock to 12 o'clock and applying counter chopper with another manipulator introduced below the nucleus. The extraction of the nuclear fragments is carried out by viscoexpression with the help of vectis or by picking the fragments with the spatula and the chopper. The extraction of nuclear fragments with the Chinese chopsticks technique allows a better adjustment of the final size of the incision to the size of the nuclear fragments.

Use of Claw Vectis[10]

It is simpler one handed technique using a claw vectis. It is a vectis with a claw placed on its tip.

Technique Nucleus is delivered into anterior chamber. Viscoelastic is injected in the anterior chamber. When the nucleus is pulled through the scleral tunnel, it is fixed by the claw and then removed. Viscoelastic is injected while removing the nucleus, so that the corneal endothelium damage is less.

Advantage

- It is better than two handed sandwich technique which may be difficult for many surgeons.

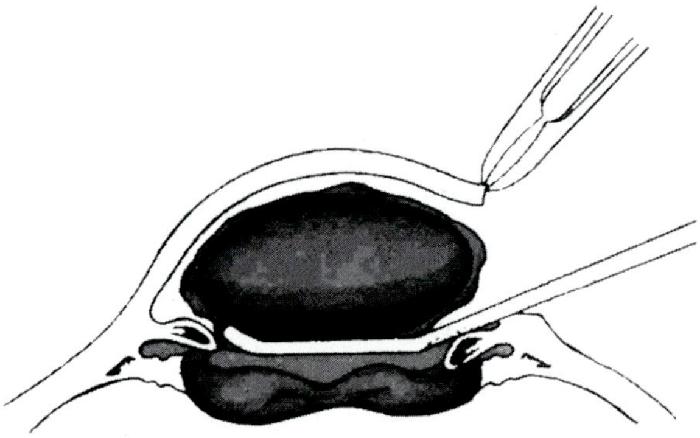

Figure 13.15: Use of wire vectis (Courtesy: Rozakis alternative to small incision cataract surgery)

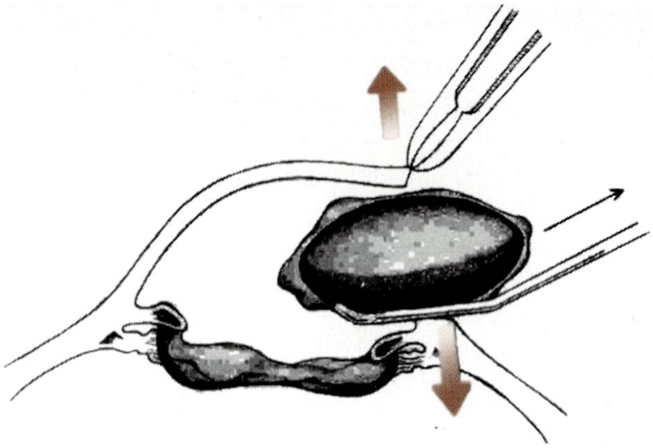

Figure 13.16: Delivery of nucleus using wire vectis (Courtesy: Rozakis Alternative to small incision cataract surgery)

Disadvantages

- Special instruments (claw vectis) are required
- Damage to iris tissue.

Using of Plain Wire Vectis[6]

Technique The Preliminary step is the delivery of nucleus into the AC. Push viscoelastic above and below the nucleus. This will prevent the damage of corneal endothelium. Then judge the size of tunnel depending on grade of nucleus.

Pass the wire vectis below the nucleus, so that the nucleus lies in concavity of vectis. Remove the vectis out with simultaneous pressure over the scleral lip posteriorly. The pressure over scleral lip will open the scleral wound and will help in delivery of nucleus.

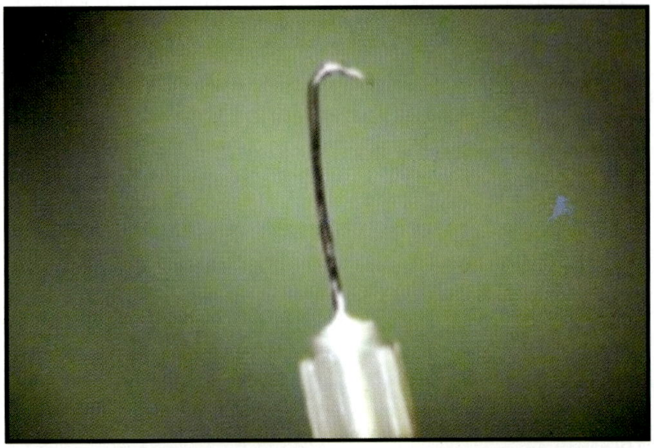

Figure 13.17: Fish hook showing the bent top of the 30 G ½ inch needle (Courtesy: Dr A Hennig, Nepal)

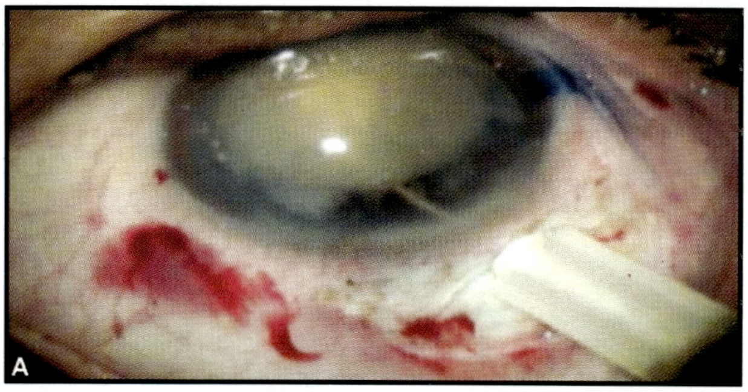

Figure 13.18A: Insertion of the hook between nucleus and posterior capsule (Courtesy: Dr A Hennig, Nepal)

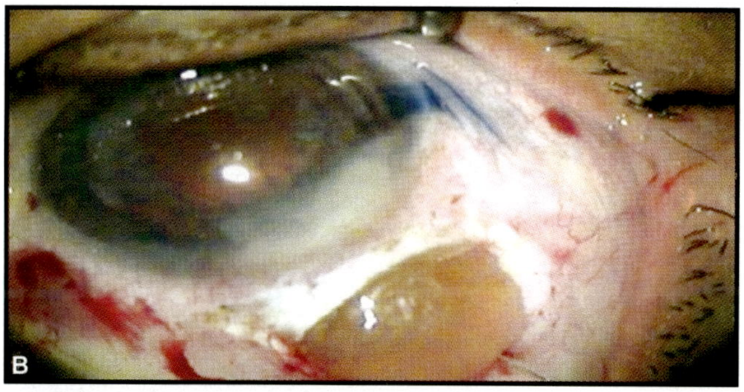

Figure 13.18B: Hook extraction of the nucleus out of the capsular bag (Courtesy: Dr A Hennig, Nepal)

Advantages

- Use of single instrument and so less chance of damage to surrounding structures
- Less expensive technique.

Disadvantages

- Increase chance of iridodialysis, common at the 6 o'clock position.
- Anterior chamber becomes shallow after delivery of the nucleus.

Fish Hook Technique[8]

In 1997 Dr Albrecht Hennig used a small hook for nucleus extraction instead of anterior chamber maintainer and hydro-expression of the nucleus. It is named as Hennig technique or Fish hook technique.

Technique

Fish hook is made of a 30 G ½ inch needle, bending it with fine pliers or a needle older. There are two bends:

1. The tip of the needle which wil insert in the central nucleus.
2. A slight bend between the tip and the plastic mount to assure an easy insertion between the lower part of the nucleus and the posterior capsule.

The hook is mounted on a 1 ml tuberculin syringe and can be reautoclaved.

After completing the rhexis and hydroprocedures, viscoelastic is injected between nucleus and posterior capsule and into the anterior chamber. The bent 30 G needle hook is inserted between nucleus and posterior capsule with the sharp needle tip pointing to the right slide. Then hook is turned and slightly pulled back so that the needle tip is engaged into the central lower portion of the nucleus.

Without lifting, the nucleus is pulled out of the capsular bag and through the tunnel. Cortex remains in the anterior chamber, acts as a cushion and thus protects the endothelium from any contact with the nucleus. Once the tip of the hook is correctly inserted into the nucleus, there is no risk to damage any part of the eye.

Advantages

- It is less expensive
- Sophisticated instruments are not required
- Easy to learn
- It can be widely used in case of high volume camps where large numbers of cataract surgery are to be done in short time.

Disadvantages

- Insertion of Fish hook is important. The tip should not touch the corneal endothelium or the Descemet's membrane should not get detached
- May not be useful in all cases of hard cataract.

Phaco-punch Technique

This technique requires the use of phaco-punch which was designed by Dr Bidaye.

Instruments

It consists of irrigating vectis with a plate in the base and ridge at its distal rim. The three irrigating ports allows viscoexpression, the ridge allow fracture of nucleus and plate help in sandwiching the nucleus between it and scleral corneal lip.

Technique

The irrigating phaco-punch is connected to HPMC syringe and is passed below the nucleus. Corneal endothelium is protected by cushion of HPMC. By injecting HPMC pressure is slowly built into the anterior chamber. The increased pressure will push the nucleus out of the wound gape, along the path guide by the punch by depressing the scleral wound with the punch.

The small ridge at distal end prevents the nucleus sliding back into the eye and creates cleavage line for short bite of nucleus. The plate prevents iris prolapse and serves as sandwich plate.

The combined effect removes small bit of the nucleus and converts the round nucleus into bean shaped nucleus. The nucleus is then rotated to align it in vertical direction along its long axis and is removed by injecting viscoelastic material

Hybrid Technique[18]

In the hybrid technique the nucleus is first sculpted with the phacoemulsification. The nucleus is then prolapsed into the anterior chamber and removed by any methods of nucleus delivery.

This technique is mainly useful for beginners who have started learning phacoemulsification. The technique of phacoemulsification is practiced step by step till the surgeon gain confidence in emulsifying the entire nucleus.

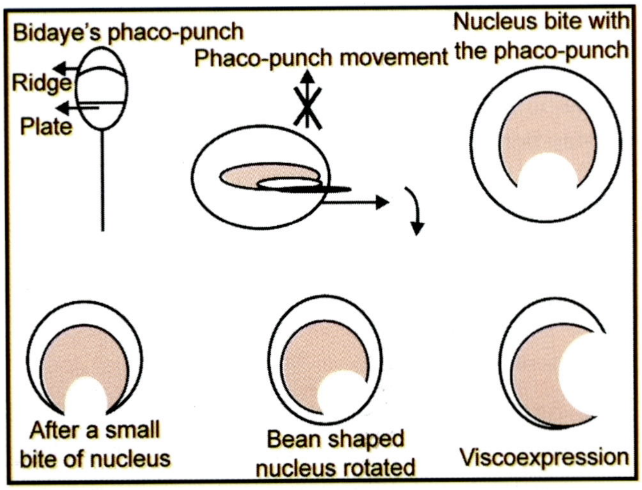

Figure 13.19: Technique showing the use of Bidaye's phaco-punch (Courtesy: Dr Vilas Bidaye)

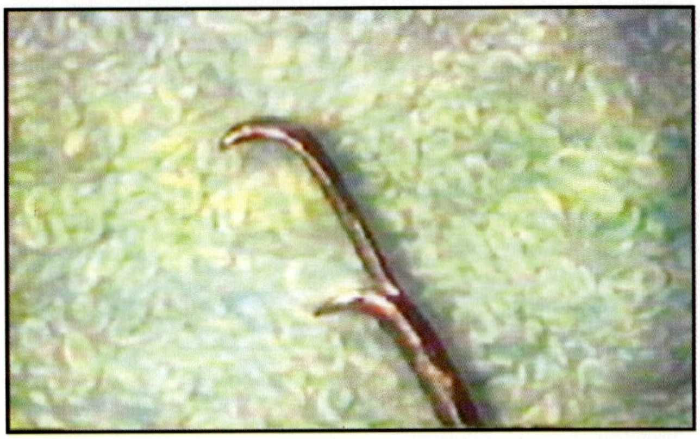

Figure 13.20: The slider pincer instrument. Note the inner part of the upper slider is sharp while the lower part is flat to prevent it shipping off the nucleus held

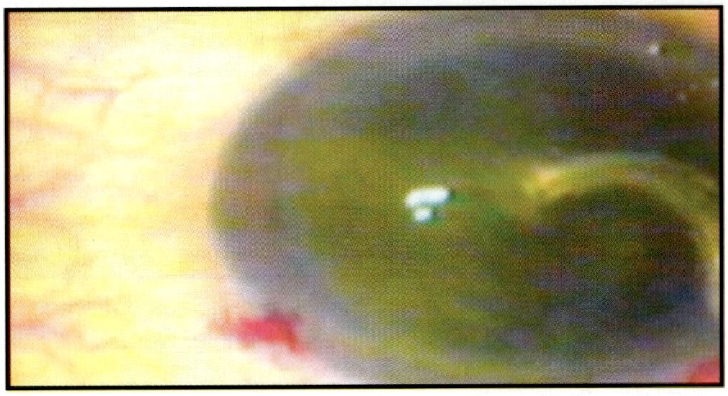

Figure 13.21: Once the nucleus is in the anterior chamber, the jaws is inserted via the 3.2 mm incision on the surface of the nucleus

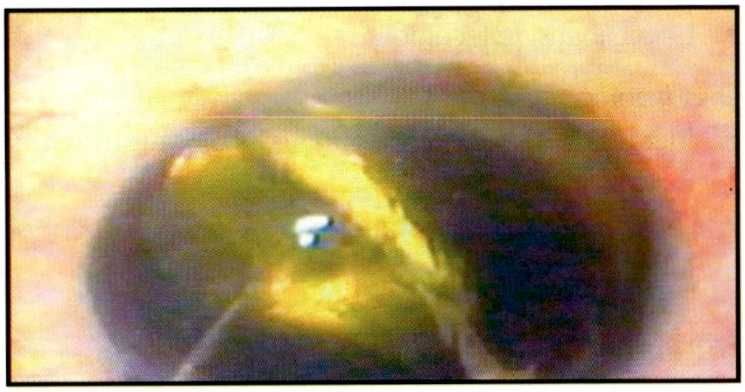

Figure 13.22: As the slider is approximated it immediately slices through the nucleus. Literally with this instrument no resistance is noted even with the hardest nucleus

Advantages of Nucleus Division over Phacoemulsification

- It is easier to learn
- It is not machine dependent
- It is less expensive

- The time for removal of nucleus is not time dependent. In phaco the removal of nucleus depends on grade of nucleus
- High learning curve in phacoemulsification.

Precaution to be Taken in Nucleus Division

a. Initially always attempt the procedures on widely dilated eyes.
b. Approach each care with a mindset that will allow ready conversion to standard extracapsular cataract extraction, if there is difficulty in prolapsing the nucleus in the AC.
c. Initially the size of incision should be more.
d. While inserting the lens loop beneath the nucleus, it should be directed at an angle toward right edge of nucleus. This will ease in process of learning the ıoop onto position.
e. Do not fight to extract the nucleus half.

Jaws Slider Pincer Technique

This technique has been developed by Dr Keiki Mehta (India) for small incision, nonphaco Cataract Surgery. All existing techniques at present are dependent on the lens lying flat with a hard nucleus being sheared off or chopped off with the nucleus lying horizontally flat abutting the posterior capsule. Risk factors involved with these techniques is that the dome of the cornea may be damaged with endothelial cell loss leading to corneal decompensation.

Instrument

The jaw slider Pincer forcep is a especially designed instrument to cut even the hardest cataract into the longitudinal slices. It has a tip designed as a beak of a bird and properly rounded to permit its easy entry into the eye. The jaws are made of hardened tungsten steel to prevent any whiplash on handling hard cataracts. The tips of the pincer forceps are designed with the part placed at 12 o' clock being blunt while the 6 o' clock placement is made curved and sharp to permit easy slicing.

Technique

A good capsulorhexis and hydrodissection is done. Once the lens is made to rotate out. Out of the capsular bag, pincer forcep is introduced via the incision. It is introduced in its closed form, sideways and than gradually opened up to encompass the width of the nucleus. Once it is properly positioned, the jaws are closed which automatically sections the nucleus into two parts. In case of suprahard cataracts, it is necessary to cut the cataract into three or four slices. Always remember to cut the pieces longitudinally as cross cutting makes it more troublesome to remove. With the help of non-apposing curved forceps, the pieces can be easily removed in their entirety.

Advantages

- There is no stress on the incision which does not shear and lead to troublesome irregular astigmatism
- It prevents the development of extensive endothelial cell loss
- Simple effective technique which can be done easily with minimal risks.

The Double Wire Snare Splitter Technique

This technique has also been developed by Dr Keiki Mehta (India) for small incision non-phaco cataract surgery. Many splitting techniques are being used by Ophthalmologists to guillotine the nucleus. Single strands of wire, nylon or polypropylene have been used but the problem is that using a single looped snare does not efficiently work as holding the lens eccentrically leads invariably to the nucleus being irregular cut.

Instrument

A disposable splitter was designed using two strands of wire and a disposable needle. A 20-gauge needle is cut off at the tip and the edges are rounded but maintaining a slight bevel as it permits easier entry into the eye. It is made by using two strands of 28-gauge flexible stainless steel wire threaded through a 20-gauge blunted Disposable needle. Of the two loops of wire, one leg of each is entwined around the other. Thus the two loops are now converted to three strands. Such a dual splitter work simultaneously leaving three fragments of nucleus, each of which is smaller than 4.00 mm (Figure 13.23).

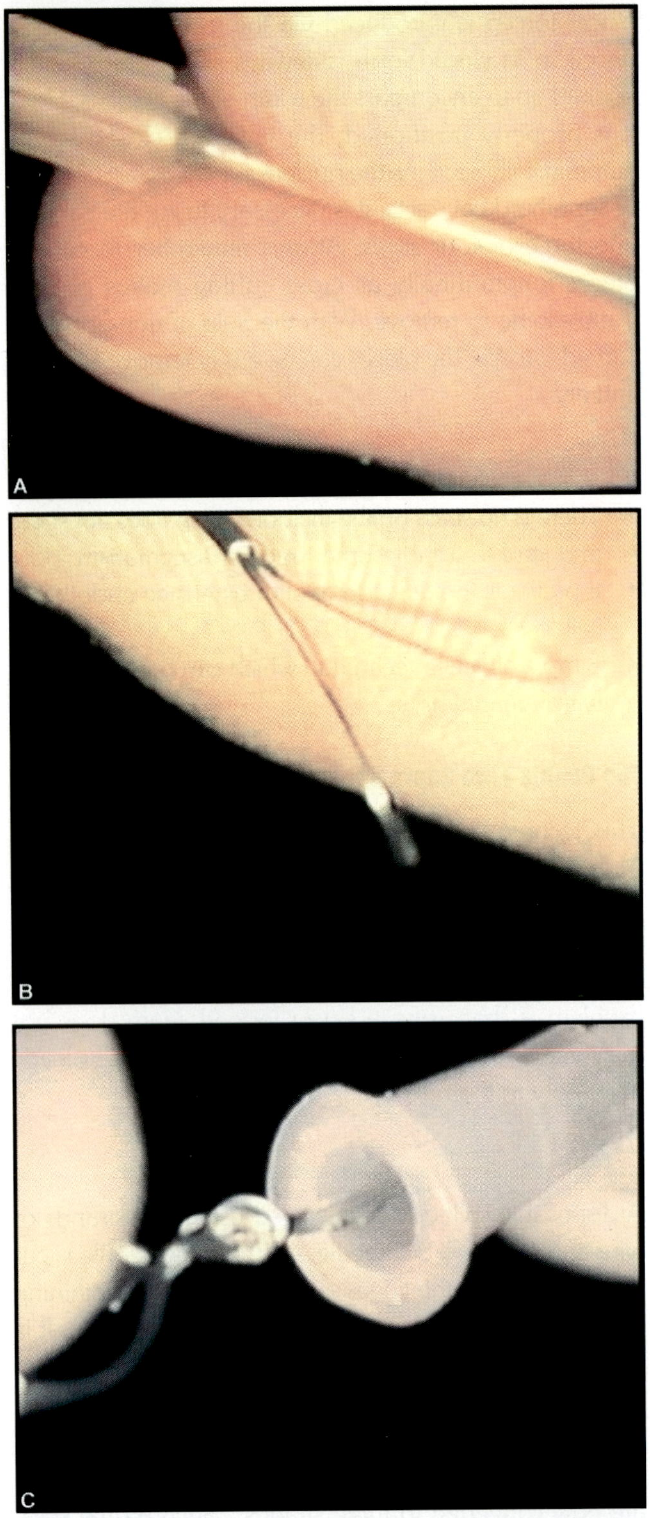

Figures 13.23A to C: Dual splitter: Manner of construction: (A) Standard 20-gauge, 1" length disposable needle selected, (B) Loops extended. Note divergence, (C) The four wires are knotted together and made into a small loop

Surgical Technique

After excellent workup of sclerocorneal tunnel incision, wound construction and capsulorhexis, viscoelastic is placed in the anterior chamber and a blunt rotator is placed on the opposite pole of the slightly prolapsed nucleus to get it rolls over on itself into the anterior chamber. Now wire loop is inserted into the anterior chamber first horizontally and then gradually turned till they sweep over the edge of the nucleus and then snugly hold it. Following the trisection of the nucleus, usually the middle portion often simply slips out at the time of the wire loop removal. With the specially designed forceps which has special recurved tracks grooved into the jaws through a 4.00 mm incision individual fragments are held and simply removed in the single stroke (Figures 13.24 to 13.26).

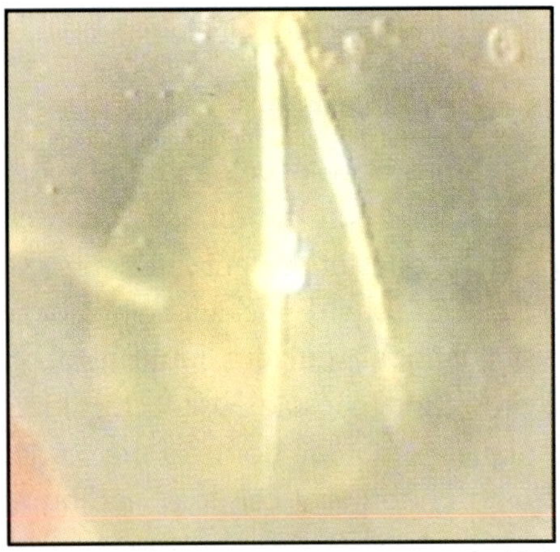

Figure 13.24: Pull the loops snug to hold the nucleus. Note the spread of the wire loops

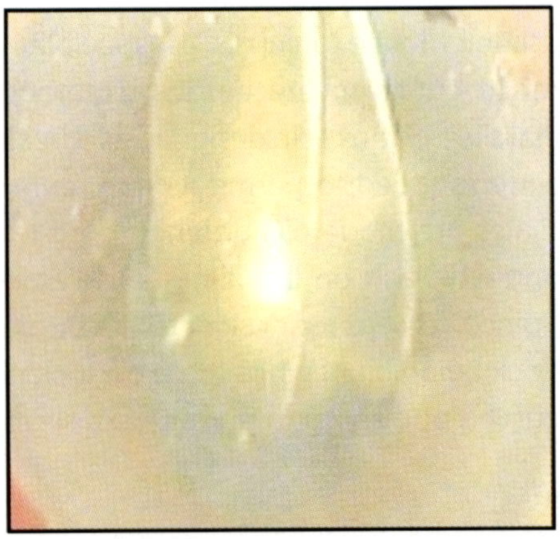

Figure 13.25: Note how snuggly the nucleus is held. It remains immobile

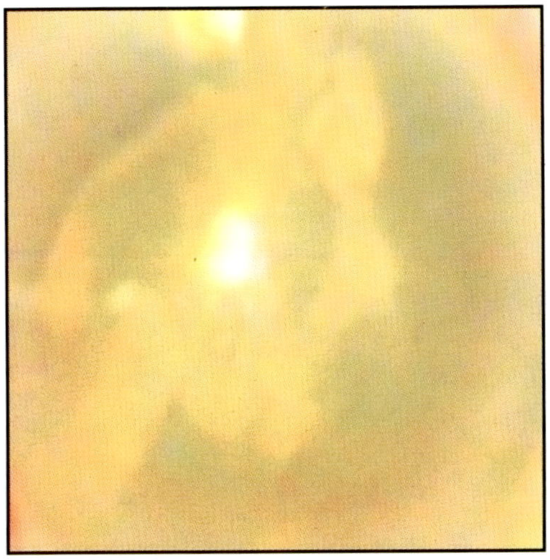

Figure 13.26: The nucleus is sliced into three parts

Advantages

- The eye is exceptionally quieter
- Harder the nucleus, the easier the trisector works which is the hallmark of this procedure
- It is an exceptional technique not only for MSICS but also for the phaco surgeon who often face hard cataracts usually coupled with compromised endothelium
- The advantage of splitting the nucleus into three parts permits easier removal of the smaller fragments through small incisions hence less iatrogenic astigmatism.

Manual Phacocracking

The principles of manual phacocracking is adapted from tunnel cracking in phacoemulsification. The needle no.21 is bent in the same way as capsulotomy needle and is stabbed into a lens about half thickness of the lens to the center of the lens. The sinskey hook is embedded above the needle to crack lens into 2 pieces.

Surgical Techniques

The 15° blade is used to do paracenthesis at 12 o'clock and 7 o'clock (in the right eye). The paracenthesis at 7 o'clock is larger than 12 o'clock to insert needle no. 21 via this route. Temporal clear corneal incision is done by keratome 3.2 millimeters. Viscoelastics are injected into anterior chamber. Capsulorhexis forcep is used to do capsulorhexis about 7-8 millemeters. Hydrodissection and hydrodelamination are performed to slightly tilt lens into anterior chamber. Viscoelastics are injected in front of the lens and behind the lens to protect the endothelium cell and posterior capsule. A needle no. 21 is bent in the same way as capsulotomy needle and its bevel is down (Figure 13.27A). The needle no. 21 is stapped into lens about half thickness of the lens to the center of the lens (Figure 13.27B). A sinskey hook is embedded above the needle to crack lens into 2 pieces (Figure 13.27C). If the lens is not separated completely, the spatula is used with the sinskey hook to separate lens completely (Figure 13.27D). The viscoelastics are injected in anterior chamber again to protect endothelium cell and posterior capsule. The incision is enlarged to 6 millimeters. The sinskey hook is used to pull each pieced of the lens out of the eye while the spatula is inserting under the lens to guide lens into the incision (Figure 13.27E). The lens cortexs are irrigated and aspirated out by Simcoe cannula. An intraocular lens is implanted into posterior chamber. The viscoelastics are irrigated and aspirated out by Simcoe cannula. The incision is sutured with 10-0 nylon 1 stitch. The anterior chamber is formed by balanced salt solutions.

Complications

The most common complication in the small incision cataract extraction by manual phacocracking is corneal edema (11 eyes in 108 eyes) that it is transient. The corneal edema resolves a few days postoperatively. It occures in the case that have a hard nuclear sclerosis. I suggest that this technique is done in the case of mild to moderate nuclear sclerosis. The other complications are posterior capsule ruptured (2 eyes in 108 eyes).

Visual Outcomes

Postoperative visual acuity is good and stable in few weeks postoperatively. The visual acuity is better than 20/40 in about 83.39 percent of the cases that nearly similar to phacoemulsification group.

CONCLUSION

Thus there are different techniques for the removal of nucleus out of the wound. Each method has its

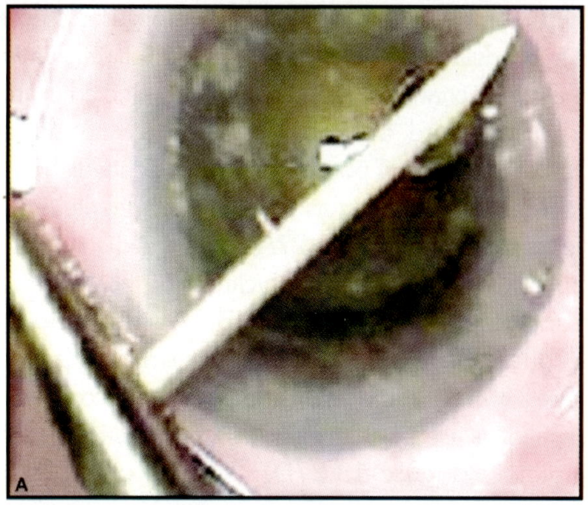

Figure 13.27A: The 21-gauge needle is bent

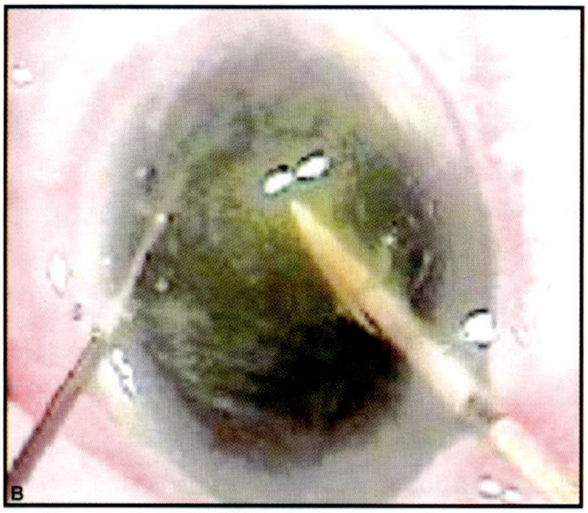

Figure 13.27B: The needle penetrates the lens

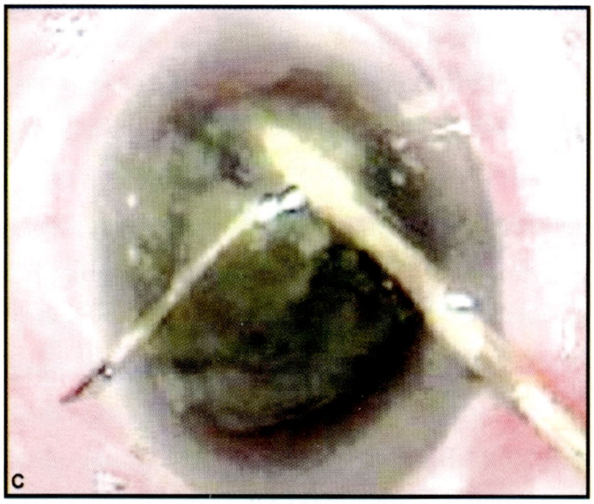

Figure 13.27C: The needle and a second instrument are used to crack the lens

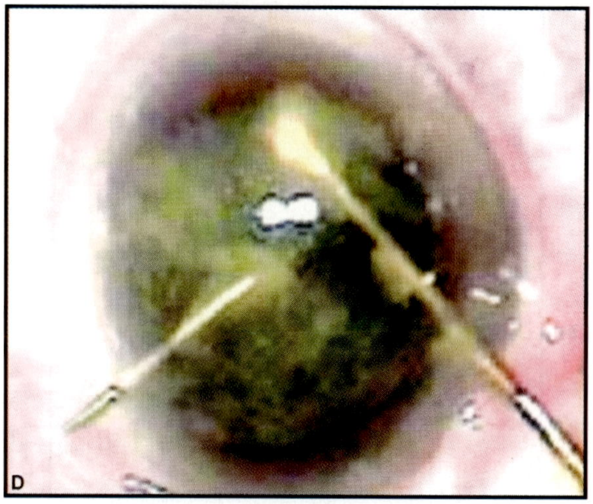

Figure 13.27D: The spatula and Sinskey hook are used to separate the lens pieces

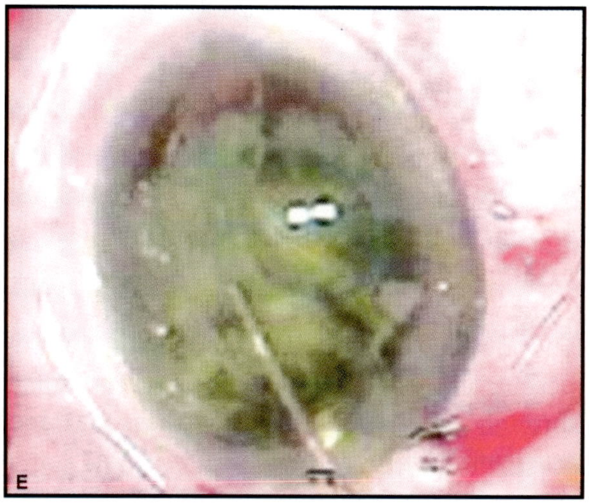

Figure 13.27E: The lens pieces are removed with the Sinskey hook and spatula

advantages and disadvantages, which depends on the experience of the operating surgeon. The technique followed should be comfortable to the doctor and should give good postoperative visual results.

BIBLIOGRAPHY

1. Band BF. The small incision phacosection planned extracapsular manual technique. Highlights Ophthalmology 1997; 25:15-25.
2. Bayramlar H, Cekic O, Totan Y. Manual tunnel incision extracapsular cataract extraction using sandwich technique. JCRS 1999;25(3): 312-5.
3. Beirouty ZA, Barker NH, Shanmugam NS. Sutureless one-handed small incision cataract surgery by manual

nucleosuction: A new technique for cataract extraction. Eur J Implant Ref Surg 1995;7:295-8.

4. Bidaye V. Nucleus management in small incision cataract surgery. Ophthalmology on the Web-Cyber lectures.
5. Blumenthal M, Ashkenazi, Assia E, Cahane M. Small incision manual cataract surgery. Using Selective Hydrodissection.
6. Bucher P. Manual Phaco Fragmentation. A small incision cataract operation technique. Basel: University Eye Hospital; 1992.
7. Gerald T, Keener Jr. The Nuclear Division Technique for Small Incision Cataract Extraction. In Rozakis cataract surgery: Alternative small incision techniques, NJ Slack 1990;163-91.
8. Guliani BP, Ag OP. Our technique of SICS, Fish hook method. Manual of Small Incision Cataract Surgery 2002; 1153-6.
9. Hepsen IF, Cekic O, Bayramlar H, Totan Y: Small incision extracapsular cataract surgery with phacotrisection. JCRS 2000;26(7);1048-51.
10. Junsuke Akkura, Shuzo Kaneda, Ishihara M, Matsura K. Quarters extraction technique for manual phaco fragmentation. JCRS 2000;26.
11. Junsuke Akkura, Shuzo Kaneda, Shiro Hatta, Kazuki Matsura. Manual Sutureless Cataract Surgery using Claw Vectis. JCRS 2000;26.
12. Kansas PG. Phacosection.Manual small incision cataract surgery. Albany: International Ophthalmology Seminar 1994;1-158.
13. Kongrap P. Prechop manual phaco fragmentation: Cataract surgery without a phacoemulsification machine. Asian Journal of Ophthalmology 2002;4(4):7-9.
14. Luther L Fry. The Phacosandwich Technique. In: Rozakis Cataract surgery: Alternative small incision techniques. NJ Slack 1990;71-110.
15. Malik KPS, Ruchi Goel. Nuclear management. Manual of small incision cataract Surgery 2002;39-58.
16. Moustafa Kamal Nassar. Manual phacofracture, small incision cataract surgery. Bull Egyptian Ophthalmology Society 2001; 94(2).
17. Peter Kansas. Phacofracture. In: Rozakis cataract surgery: Alternative small incision techniques. NJ Slack 1990;45-70.
18. Ravi Thomas, A BMS, Challa JK, George T. Methods of Nucleus Extraction. IJO 1993;4(4):202-6.
19. Samas Basak. My technique of SICS using irrigating vectis. Manual of Small Incision Cataract Surgery 2002;138-45.

14

Catarefractive Surgery: A Next Step to Phaconit

HISTORY

Jerome Jean Bovet (Switzerland)

INTRODUCTION

Concept

Removal of the crystalline lens before the vision decrease because of opacity offer many advantage to any refractive surgery or clear lens extraction.The concept of catarefractive surgery is different to refractive lens exchange because you wait that you can see a touch of cataract.The advantage that you can prepare your patient of different technique like monovision, multifocale lens, correction of the astigmatism or induce an astigmatism because the overall spherical aberration of the human eye increase with advancing age, this is the result of increasing lenticular aberration. This implies that if you correct high order aberration by corneal surgery, you will lose this effect at a later date by cataract surgery. Once the patient developed a cataracte it is more difficulte to test the patient, if it will be a good candidate for a catarefractive surgery and the surgery will be more approximative

Bimanual Microphaco

Why should we carry out phakonit bimanual microsurgery instead of conventional 3 mm phacosurgery? When starting work on a new procedure, it is always difficult to decide, when problems arise, whether to stop or to continue. First, to do a microincision without a special lens is of little use because you will need to enlarge your incision to 3 mm or do another incision. The interest in starting to work with microincision phaco at the moment arises from the fact that a new, foldable lens has been developed that can be inserted into an incision between 1.5 to 1.7 mm. Also, the benefit of using such a small incision is that we can be sure that there will be no shift to astigmatism later. When we examine the results of cases up to now, we see shifts of at least one diopter after cataract surgery. If this shift can be avoided, we will have better results with multifocal lenses, because we need less than one dioptre to maximise and utilise all their potentials.

HISTORY

Bimanual Phaco

To know who start the bimanual procedure we have to come back quit late the first which work with bimanual was de Dardenne in Bonn Germany he has the first the idea to take out the crystalline of a baby with a bimanual aspiration irrigation, Brauweiller[1] come back with the technique with phaco and bimanual aspiration irrigation which is far more easier than with the monocannula. 1982 Steven P Shearing[2] start to do phacoemulsification bimanual with a sleeweless tip. Amar Agrawal[3] in India and Stunoeka[4] in japan restart the technique of bimanual microphaco, the reason the technique start this time that we found new lens wich can be insert under an incision of less than 2.8 mm.

Astigmatism Keratotomy

About history of refractive surgery Fiedorov in 1970 give to ophtalmologist, the radial keratotomy technique because of the continuous hyperhopic shift the method stop to be the major method for refractive correction but the Astigmatism keratotomy is still used because this method stay stable overtime and it is a good compromise to correct little astigmatism[5] till 3 diopters without any problem, with the development of the excimer the radial keratotomy disapear leaving the astigmatism keratotomy

Catarefractive Surgery

Cataract and refractive surgery[6] englobe all the different previous notion that we work with. We have 3 main subjects: cataract, accomodation,and refractive surgery. All this concept we need to achieve the catarefractive surgery for exemple if you don't use an astigmatism correction like AK or LASIK your multifocal lens will never work and so you will loose your pseudoaccommodation correction,the catarefractive surgery concept is larger than prelex because you have to integrate more notion to obtain your goal. Catarefractive surgery integrate fully the notion of bimanual microphaco because to correct and to assure no astigmatism in the long-term you have to do your catarefractive surgery with a bimanual micro- incision of less of 3 mm. Catarefractive surgery is used at any age for hypermetropique eye more than 3 diopters, after the age of 50 all the emmetropic and miopic eye (Flow charts 14.1 and 14.2).

Preoperative Examinations

To start the concept of catarefractive surgery we have to do routinely an refraction with and without cycloplegia

Flow chart 14.1: Catarefractive diagram (i)

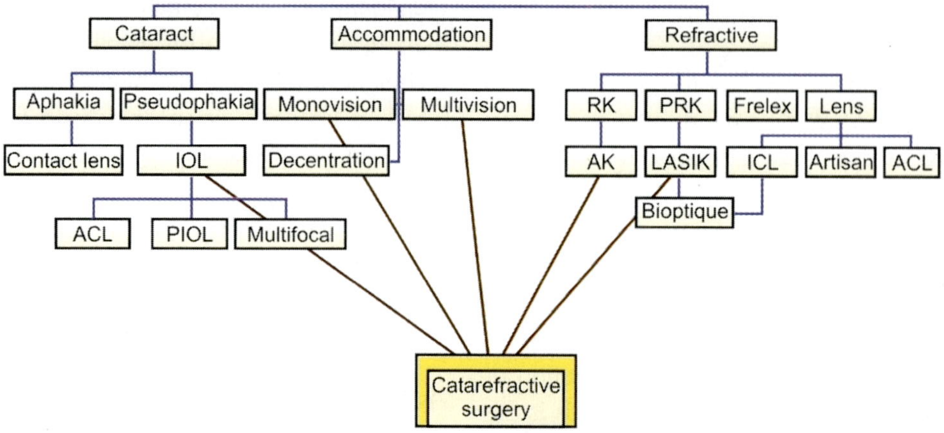

Flow chart 14.2: Catarefractive diagram (ii)

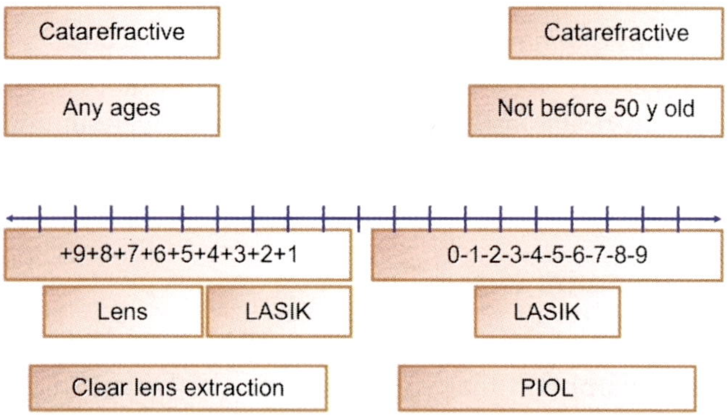

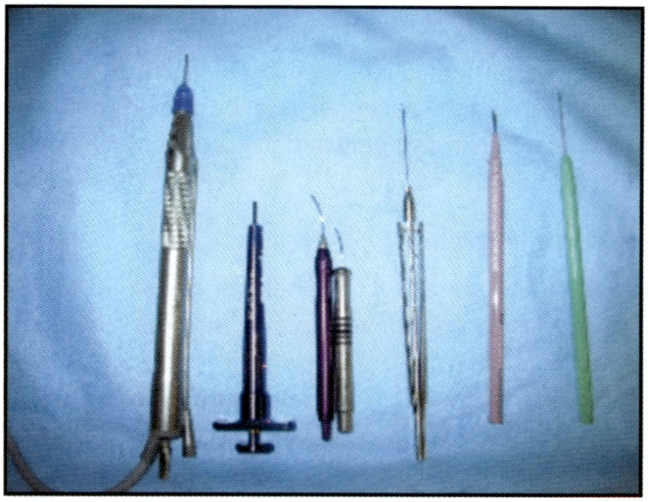

Figure 14.1: Instruments

even the patient is older than 50 to be sure to find all the residual ammetropia.

To test[7] if the patient will support a monovision correction it is very easy to try if the patient will able to support a +1.5 diopters of one eye

It is very important to use an accurate system of Biometry if you don't use the Zeiss IOL master we strongly suggest to use your ultrason tip with the prägershell added.

Pachymetry is important if we want to finish the procedure with a lasik.

And at the end topography to be shure that you have not a frust keratoconus.

Bimanual Microphacoemulsification Technique (Figure 14.1)

The technique we general use for a right eye is under topical anesthesia with the Gills[8,9] technique we do a 1 mm paracentesis at 4 O'clock and a 1, 2 mm incision with a flat knive at 2 O'clock we will enlarge later on for the lens we always control the width of the incision we always have to remember that the diameter is not the circumference and the relation is $C=2\ \pi r$ with this relation more the diameter come little more the constant in relation is big $\pi = 3.14$ for a diameter of 1 mm the circumference is 3.14 mm and the cornea is not extensible like the scleral tissue.

Injection of acid hyaluronic, and capsulorhexis with a double curve forceps (Figure 14.2). You have to try many different forceps to find your cup of tea the most rigid, straight on used for vitrectomies are the worst, my best choice are the dobble curve first from the top (Figure 14.4) The difference with a conventional phaco

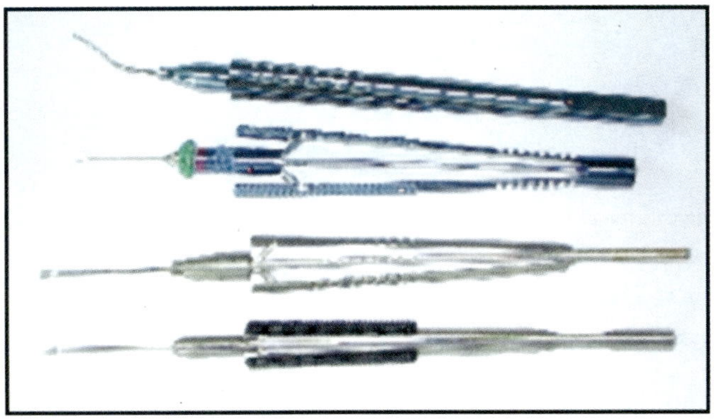

Figure 14.2: Capsulorhexis forceps

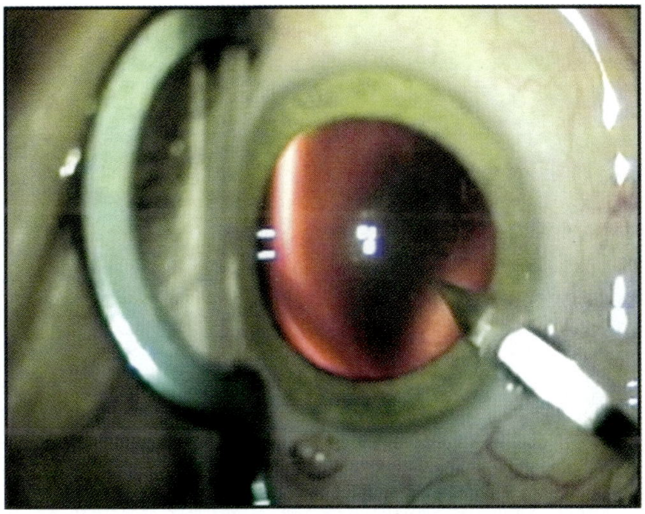

Figure 14.3: Paracentesis 1.2 mm for the phacotip

is the sleveless tip, the diameter of the bimanual irrigation-aspiration and the injector with a new catridge which permit to inject the lens without going inside the anterior chamber with the cartridge.

Bimanual microphaco technique change with the hardness of the cataracte we use most of the time for a 2+cataract a irragating Nagahara chopper and we use a phacochop technique.[10, 11]

To succed to your bimanual microphaco[12] (Figure 14.5) you have to change your fluidic systeme you have to change the diameter of your irrigation from 20-gauge to a 19-gauge to increase the input in the anterior chamber the flow rate of the output as to be increase to 38 to 40 cc/min to cool down the phacotip, the paracentesis have to be 1 mm and for the phaco tip of 1, 2 mm (Figure 14.3). To have the same efficacy during

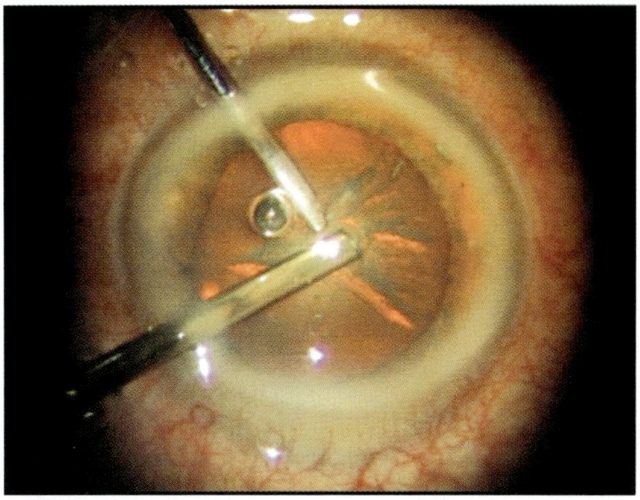

Figure 14.4: Bimanual microphaco (i)

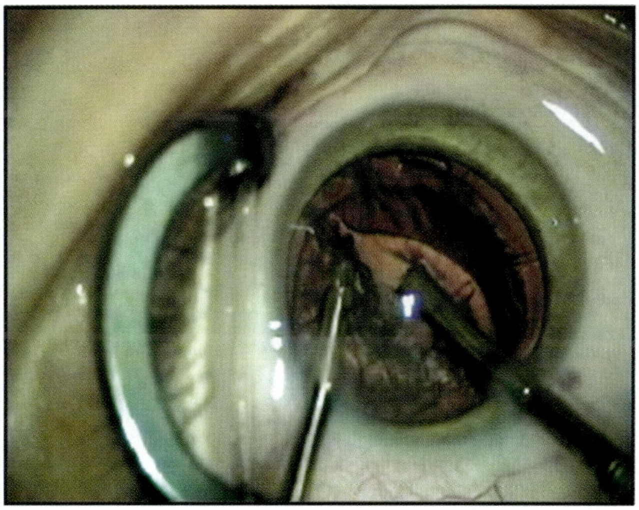

Figure 14.5: Bimanual microphaco (ii)

the phacotime we have to increase the vacuum to a level of 300 to 500 mm Hg.

You have to play with the pedal like with the pedal of a piano not to give to much and to longer phacopower if you don't want to burn your cornea.

To increase momentally the flow which facilitate the aspiration of fragment of the nucleus you can use an air pump connected to your BSS bottle to increase the pressure which increase the flow.[13]

Only a few lens[14-16] can be injected through an incision less than 2mm (Figure 14.6) for this purpose you have to put end to end the catridge and the corneal incision,then we have to shoot the lens like suppository

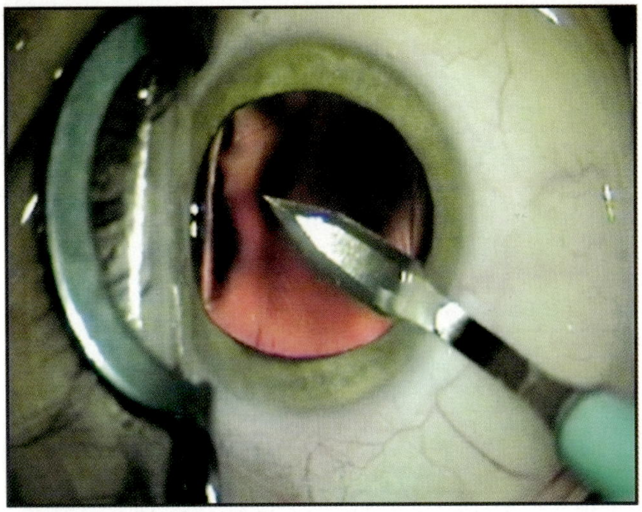

Figure 14.6: Enlarge to 1.7 mm

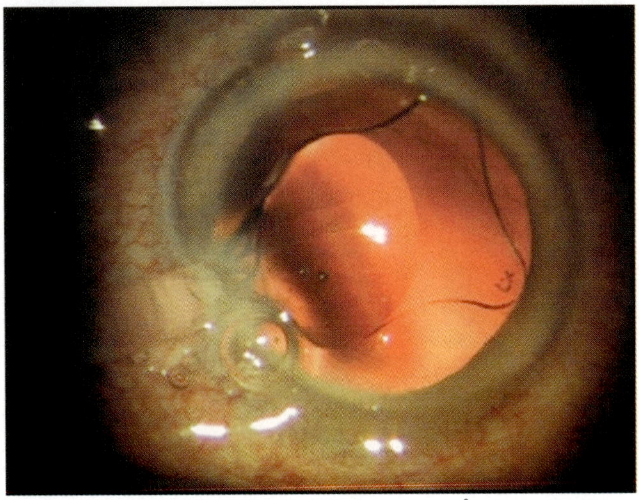

Figure 14.7: Insertion of an AcriSmart 36 Å the Cartridge stay outside

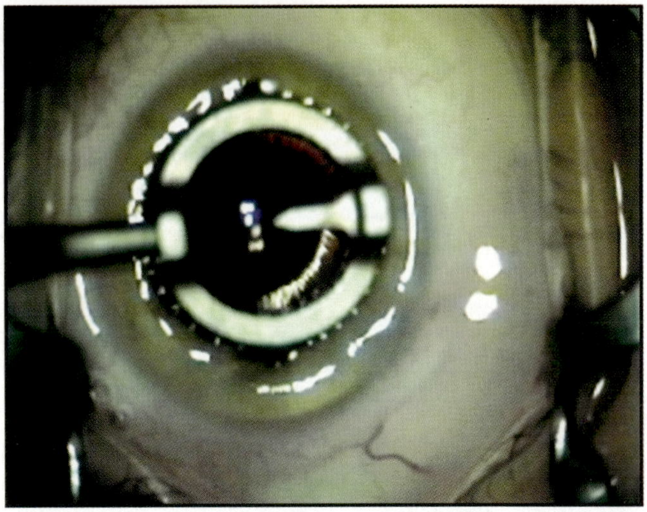

Figure 14.8: Mark before the AK4

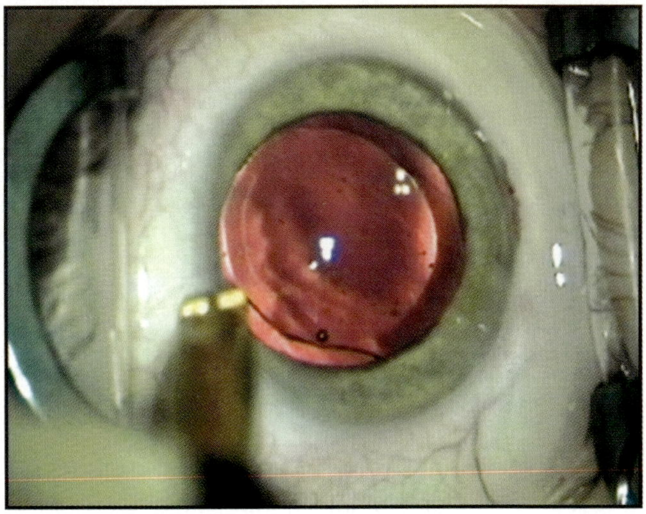

Figure 14.9: AK with a diamond knife 600 micron depth

inside the anterior chamber, we use most of the time the AcriSmart 36 or 48 because of is stability and is accurancy with our biometry.The lens acrismart from Acritec is a acrylic hydrophilic-coated hydrophobic platelette lens . This lens has a very good reaction and the placement inside the bag is optimal (Figure 14.7).

Astigmatism Keratotomy

Once we have finish the cataract operation, we correct the astigmatism with an AK astigmatism keratotomy.[6] We use the Gill's normogram at the steepest meridian with a diamond knive of deepest of 600 micron. To correct 1 diopties of astigmatism we do a two incisions at the limbus of 6 mm at the steepest meridian (Figures 14.8 and 14.9).

Monovision versus Multifocal

To correct the presbyopia[17,18] the only technique we have to test the patient before the operation is the monovision which can also be a "multifocal vision with two eyes" the visual brain has to choose which image is treated the one for near or the one for distance and the selection of the patient is very easy. We just have to add from one eye or the other an addition of +1.5 to know if the patient is a true alternate he will have no pain or no disagreement the other patient cannot be correct with this technique.

To have more confort during night we have to prefer the lens which are prolate or aberrated corrected. At the end if we didn't reach the goal we can do a lasik[7] after a delay of 3 monthes to be shure that the vision is stabilize.

Example Case Report

W female 54-yr old

BCVA RE 07 -2.5-0.5/0 LE 0.5 -3.5 -1.5/160

Intervention catarefractive surgery

Bimanual microphaco insertion incision 1.7 mm

+AK 2 incision at the limbus 5 mm arcuate

RE AcriSmart 36 A 16.5 D LE Acrismart 36A 15.5D+AK.

Result :

UCVA RE 0.4 LE 0.8

BCVA RE 1.0 -1 -05/0 LE 1.0 -0.5/0

Binoculare vision UCVA 0.8

Binoculare vision for near 0.5 Birkhauser at 20 cm.

CONCLUSION

Bimanual Microphaco

Remember your physics for your incision $2\pi R = C$

Select your right instruments: for your 2 paracentesis, for your irrigating choper, phacotip as to be 0.9 mm diameter.

Increase irrigation 36 mm/min + air pump

Reduced ultrasound with your foot pedal

Take your time, time consuming.

Catarefractive Surgery

In conclusion to use the catarefractive technique you have to carefully select your patient.

You can take out the crystalline of any hypermetropic patient with more than 3 diopters after the age of 20 years old.

You can use this technique with the myopic patient older than 45 years old and with more than 4 diopters. You have to test the monovision before you do the procedure and if you want to have a full success you have to correct the astigmatime.

To be very accurate wait 3 weeks before to do the second eye.

REFERENCES

1. Brauweiler P. Bimanual irrigation/aspiration. J Cataract Refract Surg. 1996;22(8):1013-6.
2. Sharing SP, Releya RL, Loiza A, Shearing RL. Routine phacoemulsification through a one-millimeter non sutured incision. Cataract 1985;2:6-10.
3. Agarwal A, Agarwal A, Agarwal S, Narang P, Narang S. Phakonit: phacoemulsification through a 0.9 mm corneal incision. Journal of Cataract and Refractive Surgery. 2001; 27(10):1548-52.
4. Tsuneoka H, Shiba T, Takahashi Y. Feasibility of ultrasound cataract surgery with a 1.4 mm incision. Journal of Cataract and Refractive Surgery. 2001;27(6):934-40.
5. Gills JP, van Der Karr M, Cherchio M. Combined toric intraocular lens implantation and relaxing incisions to reduce high preexisting astigmatism. Journal of Cataract and Refractive Surgery 2002;28(9):1585-8.
6. Bovet J. Cataract in clear cornea by phacoemulsification and correction of astigmatism by AK. Indian Academy of Ophthalmology Advances in ophthalmology. Mumbai 1998
7. Bovet J, Chiou A, de Courten C, Rabineau P, Achard O. Bioptic. ESOPES, KSMG, Tunis life 2000.
8. Bovet J, Baumgartner JM, Bruckner JC, Ilic V, Achard O. L'anesthésie topique en chirurgie oculaire et sa préparation. In: Safran AB, Landis T, Dayer P (Eds): Les Dimensions de la douleur en ophtalmologie. Paris Masson, 1998;166-73.
9. Fenzl RE, Gills JP. Intracameral lidocaine in routine phacoemulsification. Ophthalmology 2000;107(10):1803-4.
10. Sullivan BR. Phaco chop: Mastering techniques, optimizing technology, and avoiding complications. American Journal of Ophthalmology 2004;138(4):707.
11. Metha KR. The new phaco cleaves techniques for hard cataracts. J Intraocular Implant and Refractive Society India 1996;1:74-5.
12. Bovet J, Achard O, Baumgartner JM, Chiou A, de Courten C, Rabineau P. Bimanual Phaco Trick and Track ASCRS-ASOA Film San Diego 2004;1-5.
13. Vejarano LF, Tello A, Vejarano A. Phakonit: Incisions and use of a pressurized inflow system. Journal of Cataract and Refractive Surgery 2004;30(5):939.
14. Bovet J, Achard O, Baumgartner JM, Chiou A, de Courten C, Rabineau P. 0.9 mm Incision Bimanual Phacoand IOL Insertion Through a 1.7 mm Incision Symposium on cataract, IOL and refractive surgery abst ASCRS-ASOA San Francisco 2003;12-6.
15. Agarwal A, Agarwal S, Agarwal A. Phakonit with an AcriTec IOL. Journal of Cataract and Refractive Surgery 2003;29(4):854-5.
16. Dogru M, Honda R, Omoto M, Fujishima H, Yagi Y, Tsubota K. Early visual results with the rollable ThinOptX intraocular lens. Journal of Cataract and Refractive Surgery 2004;30(3):558-65.
17. Chiou AGY, de Courten C, Bovet J. Pseudophakic ametropia managed with a phakic posterior chamber intraocular lens. J Cataract Refract Surg 2001;27:1516-8.
18. Steinert RF, Post CT, Brint SF, Fritch CD, Hall DL, Wilder LW, et al. Ophthalmology 1992;99(12):1752/PMID: 1480385.

Section 2

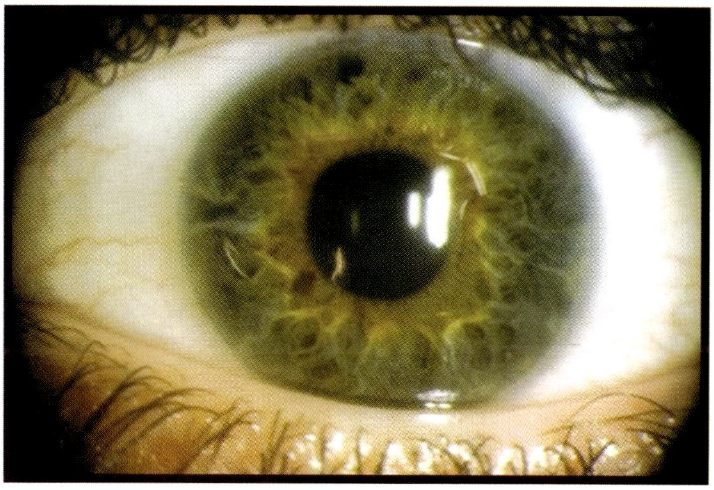

Refractive Surgery Technologies (Presbyopia, Lenticular and Corneal-based Refractive Techniques)

15

Aberropia: A New Refractive Entity

Amar Agarwal, Nilesh Kanjiani, Soosan Jacob, Athiya Agarwal, Sunita Agarwal, Tahira Agarwal, Ashok Garg (India)

INTRODUCTION

The next evolution to come on to the visual science scene in refractive ocular imaging is the aberrometer, the Orbscan and wave front analysis. This technology is based on astrophysical principles, which astronomers use to perfect the images impinging on their telescopes. Dr Bille, the Director of the Institute of Applied Physics at the University of Heidelberg first began work in this field while developing this specific technology for astronomy applications in the mid-1970s. For perfect imaging, astrophysicists have to be able to measure and correct the imperfect higher-order aberrations or wavefront distortions that enter their telescopic lens system from the galaxy. To achieve this purpose, adaptive optics are used wherein deformable mirrors reform the distorted wavefront to allow clear visualization of celestial objects. Extrapolating these same principles to the human eye, it was thought that removal of the wavefront aberrations of the eye might finally yield the long awaited and much desired ultimate goal of "super vision."

So far, the only parameters that could be modified to obtain the optical correction for a given patients refractive error were the sphere, cylinder and axis even though this does not give the ideal optical correction many a times. This is because the current modes for correcting the optical aberrations of the eye do not reduce the higher order aberrations. The ideal optical system should be able to correct the optical aberrations in such a way that the spatial resolving ability of the eye is limited only by the limits imposed by the neural retina i.e. receptor diameter and receptor packing.

Thus, there may be a large group of patients whose best corrected visual acuity (BCVA) may actually improve significantly on removal of the optical aberrations. These optical aberrations are contributed to by the eye's entire optical system, i.e. the cornea, the lens, the vitreous and the retina. This study was conducted to determine the existence of a hitherto unidentified entity which we label as "aberropia" wherein patients with best corrected visual acuity of $\leq$ 6/9 (0.63), corneal topography not accounting for the lack of improvement in BCVA and with no other known cause for decreased vision improved by $\geq$ two Snellen lines after refractive correction of their wavefront aberration.

MATERIALS AND METHODS

16 eyes of 10 patients were included in this retrospective study carried out at the Dr Agarwal's Eye Institute, India between May to December 2002. Only patients who had visual acuity less than 6/9 (0.63) prior to the procedure and whose visual acuity improved by more than or equal to two lines after the procedure were included in the study. None of these patients had any other known cause for decreased vision and their corneal topography did not account for the lack of improvement in BCVA. The routine patient evaluation including uncorrected (UCVA) and best corrected (BCVA), slit lamp examination, applanation tonometry, manifest and cycloplegic refractions, Orbscan, aberrometry, corneal pachymetry, corneal diameter, Schirmer test and indirect ophthalmoscopy had been performed for all the patients. Patients wearing contact lenses had been asked to discontinue soft lenses for a minimum of 1 week and rigid gas permeable lenses for a minimum of 2 weeks before the preoperative examination and surgery. Informed consent was obtained form all patients after a thorough explanation of the procedure and its potential benefits and risks.

The Zyoptix procedure was then performed using the Bausch and Lomb Technolas 217 Z machine. The parameters used were: wavelength 193 nm, fluence 130 mJ/cm^2 and ablation zone diameters between 4.8 mm and 6 mm. The Hansatome (Bausch and Lomb) was used in all the eyes. Either the 180 µm or the 160 µm plate was used in all the eyes. The aberrometer and the Orbscan, which checks the corneal topography, are linked and a zylink created. An appropriate software file is created which is then used to generate the laser treatment file.

Postoperatively, the patients underwent complete examination including UCVA, BCVA, slit lamp examination, Orbscan and aberrometry. The mean follow up was 37.5 days.

For statistical analysis, the Snellen acuity was converted to the decimal notation. Continuous variables were described with mean, standard deviation, minimum and maximum values.

RESULTS

16 eyes of 10 patients satisfied the inclusion criteria. The mean age of the patients was 29.43 years (range 22 to 35 years). 6 patients were females and 4 were males. The mean preoperative pupil diameter measured on aberrometer was 4.69 mm and mean postoperative pupil diameter measured on aberrometer was 4.53 mm.

The mean pre-operative spherical equivalent was –4.94 D (range –12.50 to –1.5 D). The mean spherical equivalent at 1 month post-operative period was –0.16 ± 0.68 D (range –1.0 to 1.5) . Mean preoperative sphere was –4.95 D (range-12.50 to –0.75 D) and the mean postoperative sphere was –0.13 ± 0.68 D (range-1 to 1.5) at 1 month. The mean preoperative cylinder was –1.34 D (range 0 to –3.50). The mean postoperative cylinder was –0.08 ± 0.24 D (range 0 to –0.75 D) at one month. Postoperatively, at the end of first month, 70 percent of the patients were within ± 0.5D and 90 percent were within ± 1D of emmetropia (Figure 15.1). Preoperatively mean RMS (Root Mean square) values (Figure 15.2) were: Z 200 Defocus –9.22, Z 221 Astigmatism 0.12, Z 220 Astigmatism 1.02, Z 311 Coma –0.041, Z 310 Coma –0.04, Z 331 Trefoil 0.23, Z 330 Trefoil 0.016, Z 400 Spherical aberration –0.054, Z 420 Secondary astigmatism 0.103, Z 421 Secondary astigmatism 0.029, Z 440 Quadrafoil –0.103, Z 441 Quadrafoil –0.021, Z 510 Secondary coma 0.025, Z 511 Secondary coma –0.015, Z 530 Secondary trefoil 0.0049, Z 531 Secondary trefoil -0.00219, Z 550 Pentafoil 0.023, Z 551 Pentafoil 0.046. Postoperative mean RMS values were: Z 200 Defocus –0.429, Z 221 Astigmatism 0.07, Z 220 Astigmatism –0.07, Z 311 Coma 0.149, Z 310 Coma –0.079, Z 331 Trefoil –0.102, Z 330 Trefoil –0.004, Z 400 Spherical aberration -0.179, Z 420 Secondary astigmatism 0.015, Z 421 Secondary astigmatism 0.031, Z 440 Quadrafoil 0.019, Z 441 Quadrafoil –0.069, Z 510 Secondary coma –0.008, Z

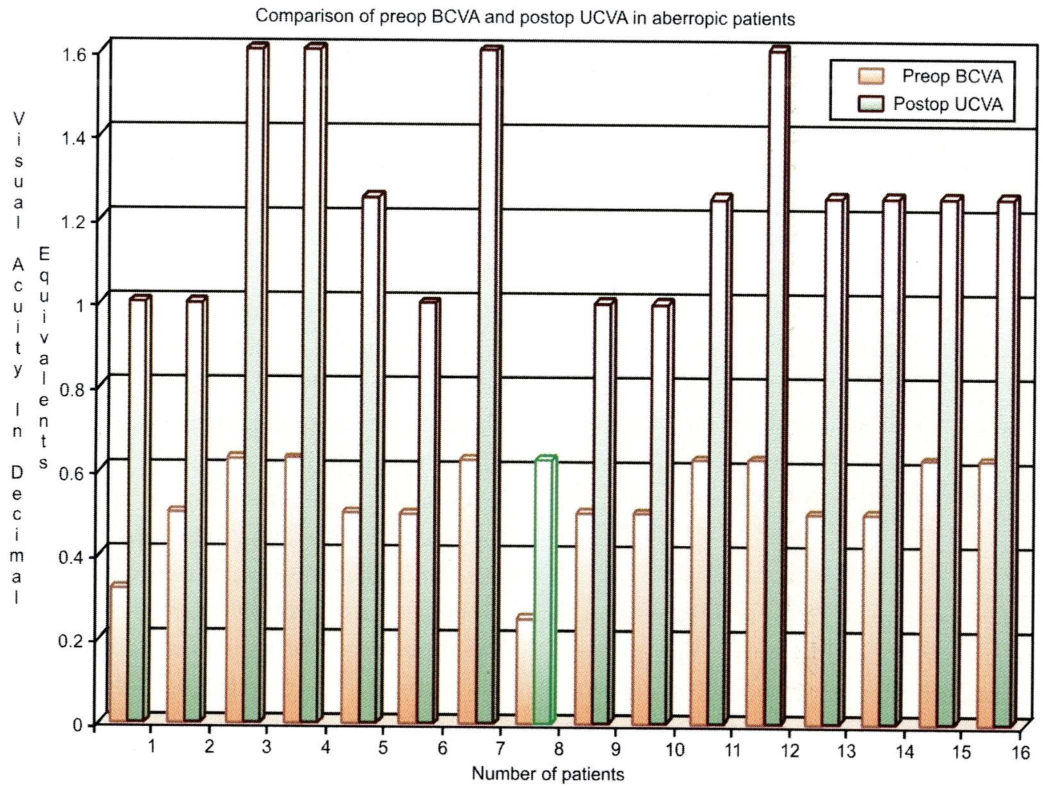

Figure 15.1: Preoperative BCVA versus postoperative UCVA

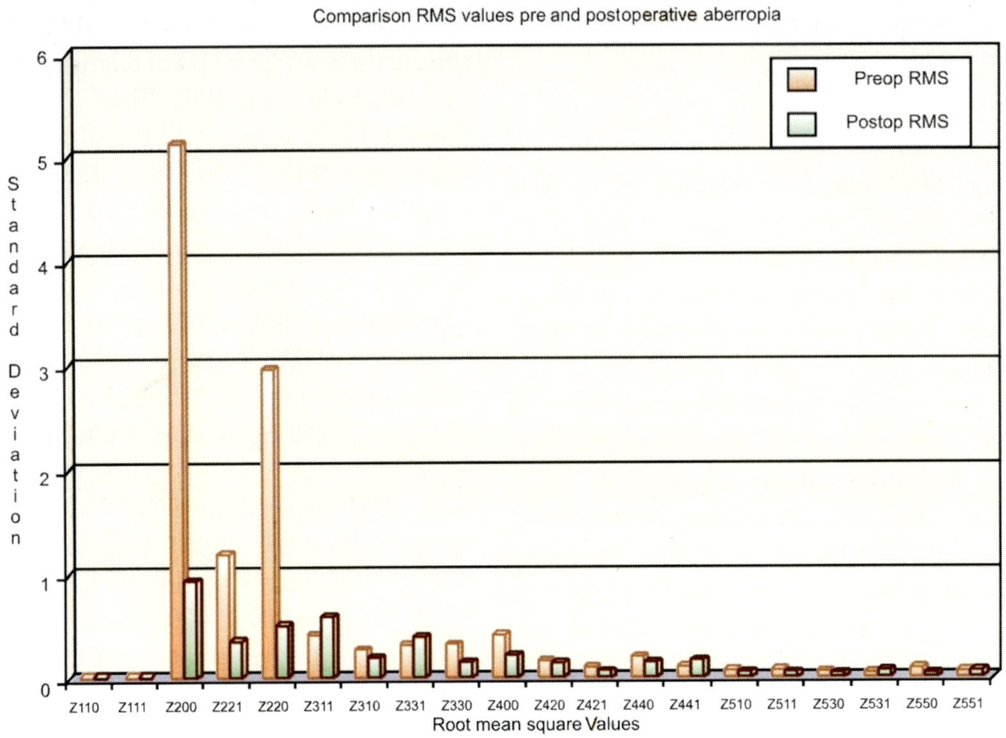

Figure 15.2: RMS values pre- and postoperative

511 Secondary coma 0.008, Z 530 Secondary Trefoil -0.002, Z 531 Secondary Trefoil –0.014, Z 550 Pentafoil 0.006, Z 551 Pentafoil 0.026.

RMS pre- and post-laser showed a reduction in the higher order aberrations (Tables 15.1 and 15.2). 6.25 percent patients achieved 6/9, 31.25 percent patients achieved ≥ 6/6 (1.00), 37.50 percent achieved a BCVA of 6/5 (1.25) and 25 percent achieved a BCVA of 6/4 (1.6) (Figure 15.3). Figure 15.4 shows the pre-op Orbscan picture of a patient showing no abnormality. Figures 15.5 and 15.6 show the aberrometer maps of the right eye and left eye of a patient in which we can see the aberrations reduced post-laser.

DISCUSSION

Zyoptix is the new generation of excimer laser used for the treatment of refractive disorders. Until recently, refractive disorders were treated with standard techniques, which took into consideration only the subjective refraction. Zyoptix technique on the other hand, takes into account the patient's subjective refraction, ocular optical aberrations and corneal topography, with the latter not only for the diagnosis, but also for the therapeutic treatment, in order to design a personalized treatment based on the total structure of the eye. The wavefront technology in Zyoptix uses the Hartmann Shack aberrometer based on the Hartmann-Shack principle[1] demonstrated by Liang et al[2] to measure the eye's wave aberration. This wavefront sensor has been improved by increasing the density of samples taken of the wave-front slope in the pupil[3]. All Hartmann-Shack devices are outgoing testing devices in that they evaluate the light being bounced back out through the optical system. A narrow laser beam is focused onto the retina to generate a point source. The out coming light rays which experience all the aberrations of the eye pass through an array of lenses which detects their deviation. The wavefront deformation is calculated by analyzing the direction of the light rays using this lenslet array. Parallel light beams indicate a good wavefront and non-parallel light beams indicate a wavefront with aberrations, which does not give

Table 15.1: RMS values pre laser

Pat. No	Z 110	Z 111	Z 200	Z 221	Z 220	Z 311	Z 310	Z 331	Z 330	Z 400	Z 420	Z 421	Z 440	Z 441	Z 510	Z 511	Z 530	Z 531	Z 550	Z 551	Z 6
1	0	0	-5.77	4.055.	-6.131	0.299	-0.113	0.725	-0.44	0.009	-0.03	0.102	-0.233	0.109	0.131	0.027	-0.048	-0.041	0.052	0.039	-9999
2	0	0	-4.323	-1.719	6.005	-0.273	0.022	-0.353	0.275	0.092	0.092	-0.145	0.199	-0.013	-0.006	0.011	0.034	-0.039	0.042	0.042	-9999
3	0	0	-11.8	-0.088	0.116	0.435	-0.658	-0.444	-0.567	-0.779	-0.089	0.043	-0.202	-0.053	-0.052	-0.057	-0.04	-0.001	0.13	0.111	-9999
4	0	0	-12.46	0.514	-0.155	0.29	-0.006	0.016	0.529	-0.91	0.124	0.124	-0.431	-0.222	0.074	-0.04	0.001	-0.063	-0.141	0.119	-9999
5	0	0	-6.535	-0.123	-0.886	0.156	-0.09	0.094	-0.128	-0.084	-0.072	0.035	-0.009	-0.044	0.001	-0.031	0.01	-0.005	0.001	-0.041	-9999
6	0	0	-7.867	0.185	1.704	-0.02	0.414	0.441	0.197	0.365	0.197	0.107	-0.155	-0.002	0.123	0.026	-0.001	0.049	0.048	0.032	-9999
7	0	0	-4.28	0.167	2.571	0.007	-0.089	0.356	0.125	0.585	0.101	-0.002	-0.17	-0.062	-0.077	0.198	0.001	-0.104	-0.022	0.029	-9999
8	0	0	-10.4	0.502	-0.587	-0.007	-0.331	0.165	-0.126	-0.054	-0.071	0.036	-0.118	-0.128	0.009	0.017	-0.007	-0.026	0.063	-0.052	-9999
9	0	0	-17.15	-0.414	-1.217	0.093	-0.106	0.343	-0.18	-0.254	0.009	0.002	0.001	-0.025	0.007	-0.022	-0.007	-0.042	0.037	0.04	-9999
10	0	0	-16.78	-0.162	-0.637	0.122	-0.159	0.279	0.2	-0.181	0.115	0.007	-0.002	0.042	-0.034	-0.028	0.021	-0.043	-0.006	-0.017	-9999
11	0	0	-4.513	2.916	4.661	-0.634	-0.205	0.477	0.44	0.094	0.377	0.058	-0.201	0.101	0.133	-0.147	0.009	0.011	-0.055	0.118	-9999
12	0	0	-5.736	-1.501	5.195	-1.126	0.32	0.665	-0.254	0.218	0.479	0.122	-0.253	-0.045	0.099	-0.025	0.012	-0.006	-0.05	0.11	-9999
13	0	0	-15.46	1.605	2.754	0.378	0.443	0.208	0.458	0.643	-0.083	0.09	0.407	-0.006	-0.021	0.09	0.033	0.032	0.239	0.149	-9999
14	0	0	-15.26	-0.557	2.865	-0.26	-0.059	0.107	0.122	0.168	0.025	-0.256	-0.003	0.257	0.007	0.051	0.136	-0.061	-0.114	0.124	-9999
15	0	0	-4.955	0.735	0.383	-0.401	0.003	0.62	-0.494	-0.676	0.391	0.163	-0.421	-0.264	0.039	-0.261	-0.079	0.241	0.103	-0.067	-9999
16	0	0	-4.367	-0.195	-0.238	0.28	-0.04	0.021	0.11	-0.112	0.084	-0.022	-0.061	0.013	-0.018	-0.063	0.004	0.063	0.044	0	-9999

Table 15.2: RMS values post laser

Pat. No	Z 110	Z 111	Z 200	Z 221	Z 220	Z 311	Z 310	Z 331	Z 330	Z 400	Z 420	Z 421	Z 440	Z 441	Z 510	Z 511	Z 530	Z 531	Z 550	Z 551	Z 6
1	0	0	-0.022	0.74	-1.294	0.117	-0.067	0.141	0.052	-0.063	-0.076	0.1	0.054	-0.037	-0.028	0.001	0.008	0.007	0.013	0.006	-9999
2	0	0	-0.508	0.12	0.194	-0.085	0.039	-0.12	-0.018	-9999	-9999	-9999	-9999	-9999	-9999	-9999	-9999	-9999	-9999	-9999	-9999
3	0	0	-1.398	-0.606	0.697	-0.558	-0.351	0.841	0.345	-0.39	0.392	0.038	-0.303	-0.038	-0.001	0.103	-0.066	-0.105	-0.021	0.137	-9999
4	0	0	-2.05	-0.499	-0.375	-0.027	-0.269	-0.534	-0.289	-0.58	0.114	0.058	0.236	-0.161	0.034	-0.083	0.004	0.039	0.01	-0.077	-9999
5	0	0	0.229	0.1	-0.123	-9999	-9999	-9999	-9999	-9999	-9999	-9999	-9999	-9999	-9999	-9999	-9999	-9999	-9999	-9999	-9999
6	0	0	-0.036	-0.17	0.425	-0.002	0.069	-0.045	-0.042	-0.342	-0.032	0.094	0.075	-0.05	0.068	0.03	0.064	-0.014	0.012	0.002	-9999
7	0	0	0.687	0.128	-0.028	-0.117	-0.043	0.062	0.088	-0.178	0.179	0.024	-0.045	0.055	0.013	0.016	-0.034	-0.013	-0.013	0.059	-9999
8	0	0	-2.164	0.279	-0.696	-0.25	-0.398	-0.147	-0.128	-0.581	-0.238	0.02	0.032	-0.088	-0.129	0.028	-0.029	0.007	0.089	0.059	-9999
9	0	0	-0.298	0.002	-0.311	0.158	-0.206	0.129	-0.116	-0.105	-0.045	-0.043	-0.1	-0.1	-9999	-9999	-9999	-9999	-9999	-9999	-9999
10	0	0	0.109	0.241	-0.503	0.233	-0.119	-0.16	-0.204	-9999	-9999	-9999	-9999	-9999	-9999	-9999	-9999	-9999	-9999	-9999	-9999
11	0	0	0.034	-0.092	0.076	0.013	-0.03	-0.067	0.003	-9999	-9999	-9999	-9999	-9999	-9999	-9999	-9999	-9999	-9999	-9999	-9999
12	0	0	0.187	0.061	0.004	-0.097	0.015	0.067	0.035	-9999	-9999	-9999	-9999	-9999	-9999	-9999	-9999	-9999	-9999	-9999	-9999
13	0	0	-0.701	0.291	0.598	2.161	0.349	-1.062	-0.201	-0.428	-0.013	0.204	0.258	-0.636	-0.082	0.113	0.069	-0.239	0.062	-9999	-9999
14	0	0	-0.638	0.094	0.391	0.517	-0.328	-0.336	0.188	-0.118	-0.077	0.003	0.157	0.034	-0.006	-0.025	0.004	0.018	-0.066	-9999	-9999
15	0	0	-0.148	0.493	0.017	0.261	0.017	-0.354	0.302	-0.111	0.053	0.07	-0.019	-0.084	-0.007	-0.051	-0.052	0.063	0.011	-9999	-9999
16	0	0	-0.161	-0.038	-0.331	0.072	0.049	-0.05	-0.086	0.025	-0.008	-0.059	-0.028	-9999	-9999	-9999	-9999	-9999	-9999	-9999	-9999

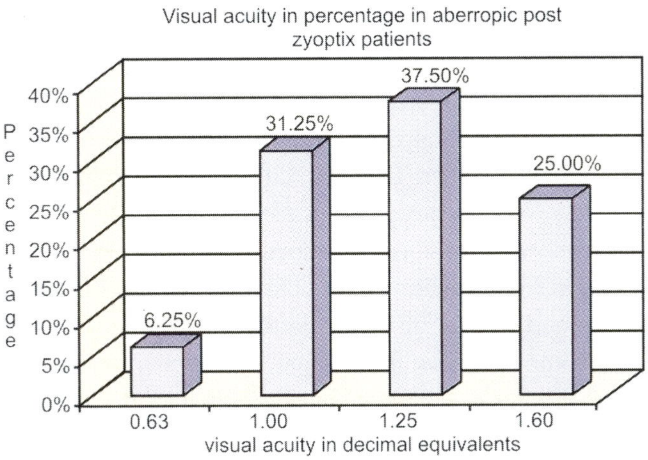

Figure 15.3: Percentage values of visual acuity

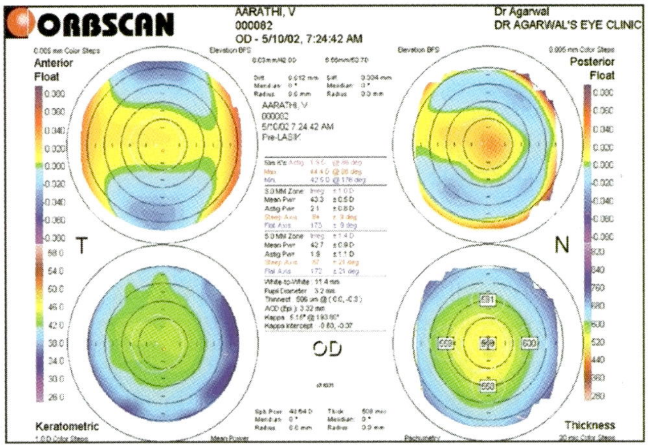

Figure 15.4: Preoperative orbscan

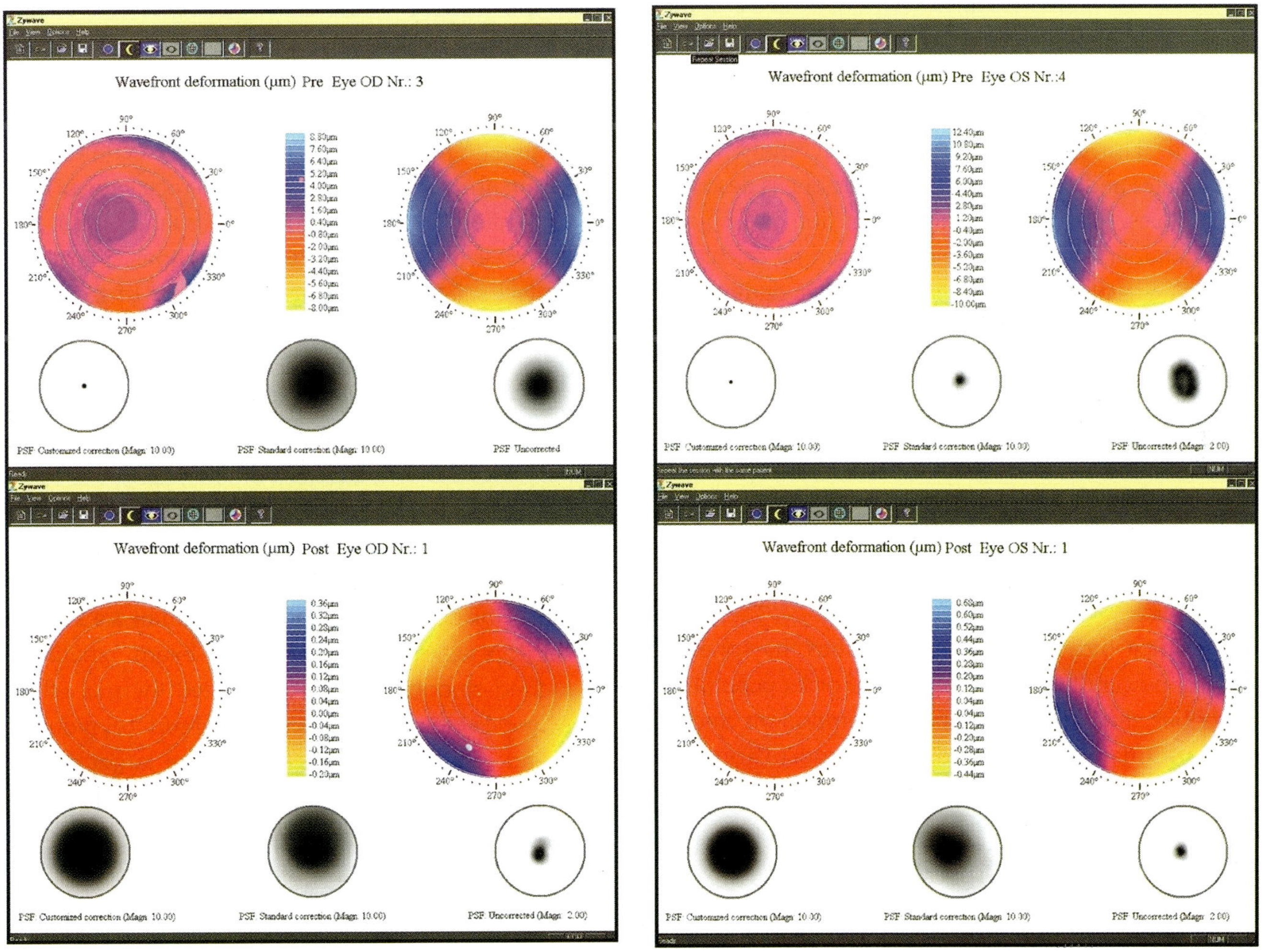

Figures 15.5 and 15.6: Pre- and postoperative aberrometry of the right and left eye of the same patient showing removal of higher order aberrations

equidistant focal points. This image is then captured onto a ccd camera and the wavefront is reconstructed. The data is explained mathematically in three dimensions with polynomial functions. Most investigators have chosen the Zernike method for this analysis although Taylor series can also be used for the same purpose.[4] Data from the wavefront map is presented as a sum of Zernike polynomials each describing a certain deformation. At any point in the pupil, the wavefront aberration is the optical path difference between the actual image wavefront and the ideal spherical wavefront centered at the image point.[5]

Any refractive error which cannot be corrected by sphero-cylindrical lens combinations is referred to by physicists as higher order aberrations, i.e. comma, spherical aberration, chromatic aberration. The Zernike Polynomials, which describe ray points, are used to obtain a best fit toric to correct for the refractive error of the eye. The points are described in the x and y coordinates and the third dimension, height, is described in the z-axis. The local refractive correction of each area of the entrance pupil can be determined by calculating from the wavefront polynomial the corresponding local radii of curvature and hence the required sphero-cylindrical correction.[6] Thus each small region of the entrance pupil has its own three parameters that characterize the local refractive correction: sphere, cylinder and axis.[6] The global aberrations of the entire optical system including the cornea, lens, vitreous and the retina are thus measured. The great advantage of wavefront analysis is that it can describe these other aberrations.

The first order polynomial describes the spherical error or power of the eye. The second order polynomial describes the regular astigmatic component and its orientation or axis. Third order aberrations are considered to be coma and fourth order aberrations are considered to be spherical aberration. Zernike polynomial descriptions for wavefront analysis typically go up to the tenth order of expression. The first and second orders describe the morphology of a normal straight curve. More local maximum and minimum points require higher orders of the polynomial series to describe the surface. Normal eyes exhibit spherical[7,8] and coma[9,10] aberrations in addition to exhibiting defocus and astigmatism.

Ideally, the difference in the magnitude of the local refractive correction of each area of the entrance pupil should not exceed 0.25 D. Lower spherocylindrical corrections are generally associated with lower wavefront aberrations.[6] These observations regarding variation in local ocular refraction along different meridians are also confirmed by Ivanoff[11] and Jenkins.[12] van den Brink[13] also commented on the change in refraction across the pupil. Clinically significant changes of at least 0.25 D in one or both components of the spherocylindrical correction might normally be expected for decentrations of about 1 mm. Rayleigh's quarter wavelength rule states that if the wavefront aberration exceeds a quarter of a wavelength, the quality of the retinal image will be impaired significantly.[14] Thus the aberration in eyes starts to become significant when the pupil diameter exceeds 1 to 2 mm.[6] Thus it is not possible to correct the entire wavefront aberration with a single spherocylindrical lens. As conventional refractive procedures such as Lasik also reduce only the second order aberrations, the visual acuity will still be limited by aberrations of third and higher order aberrations. These patients are likely to undergo tremendous improvement in their BCVA after correction of their aberrations by Zyoptix.

In the Zyoptix system, the aberrometer and the orbscan, which checks the corneal topography, are linked and a zylink created. An appropriate software file is created which is then used to generate the laser treatment file. The truncated gaussian beam shape used in Zyoptix combines the advantages of the common beam shapes, i.e. flat top beam and the gaussian beam, creating a maximized smoothness and minimized thermal effect. Thus Zyoptix gives a smoother corneal surface, reducing glare and increasing visual acuity. The larger optical zones reduce haloes. Zyoptix also causes a reduction of the ablation depth by 15 to 20 percent and a reduced enhancement rate

In a patient with higher order aberrations, lasik does not remove the higher order aberrations and the point-spread function is a large blur. Zyoptix on the other hand, performs customized ablation and removes the higher order aberrations thus minimizing the wavefront deformation. The point-spread function is therefore a small spot of light.

In our study, the mean preoperative spherical equivalent improved from –4.78 D to –0.16 D ± 0.68 and the mean preoperative cylinder improved from –1.34 D to –0.08 D ± 0.24. The aberrations were reduced drastically in all the eyes and the BCVA improved in all cases by ≥ two lines. Reduction of the aberrations of the eye can thus result in an improved BCVA post-operatively.

Improving the optics of the eye by removing aberrations increases the contrast and spatial detail of the retinal image. Reduction of higher order aberrations may not improve high contrast acuity much more in eyes where spherocylindrical lenses alone improve the BCVA to 6/3 (2.00) or better. In contrast, in otherwise normal eyes where the BCVA is limited to 6/9 (0.50) or 6/6 (1.00) due to optical aberrations, reduction of higher order aberrations should improve visual acuity.

Realization of the best possible unaided visual acuity may be limited at the cortical, retinal and the spectacle, corneal, or implant level. All maculae may not be able to support 6/3 (2.00) vision. Insufficient cone density or sub-optimal orientation of cone receptors or a sub-optimal Stiles-Crawford profile of the macula may make 6/3 (2.00) vision impossible. Clinical or subclinical amblyopia may make achievement of super vision impossible. But, in spite of this, there may be a certain patient population who have the potential for an improved BCVA on removal of their wavefront aberrations. The corneal topography does not account for the decreased preoperative visual acuity in these patients, neither do they have any other identifiable cause for the decrease in acuity except for an abnormal wavefront. It is important that this subgroup of patients are identified and their optical aberrations neutralized so that they are not deprived of the opportunity to gain in their BCVA.

Wavefront sensing technology, at present, does not in most cases define the exact locale of the pathology causing the aberration. Hence, clinical examination and other refractive tools, such as corneal topographic mapping, along with sound clinical judgment is required for proper understanding of the eye and its individual refractive status. Also, wavefront aberrations may not remain static. Numerous authors[15-18] have shown that ocular optical aberrations probably remain constant between 20 and 40 years of age but increase after that. Aberrations also change during accommodation[19,20] and may be affected by mydriatics.[21] Thus, the patient should be informed about these possibilities while taking the consent for the procedure. Long term studies are required to determine the stability of the postoperative refraction, residual aberrations and changes in BCVA if any.

The question of magnification factor improving visual acuity does not arise as these patients preoperatively did not improve with contact lenses. Further the refractive error in some of these patients was not very large.

CONCLUSION

In conclusion, removal of the wavefront aberration may extend the benefit of an improved BCVA to patients with an abnormal wavefront. The subgroup of patients with higher order aberrations, normal corneal topography and no other known cause for decreased vision may thus benefit immensely with wavefront guided refractive surgery. Customized refractive surgery tailor-made for these individual patients, aimed at neutralizing the wavefront aberrations of the eye is safer, more predictable, provides better visual acuities and reduces the incidence of unsatisfactory outcomes. Further studies are required to assess the long-term outcomes.

Till now, when we discuss refractive errors we discuss about spherical and a cylindrical correction. But in todays world we have to think of a third parameter which is the aberrations present in the eye which can be anywhere in the optical media. These can be corrected in the corneal level by the laser treatment.

REFERENCES

1. Platt B, Shack RV. Lenticular Hartmann screen, Opt Sci Center News (University of Arizona) 1971;5:15-6.
2. Liang J, Grimm B, Goelz S, Bille J. Objective measurement of the wave aberrations of the human eye with the use of a Hartmann-Shack wavefront sensor. J Opt Soc Am 1994;11: 1949-57.
3. Liang J, Williams DR, et al. Aberrations and retinal image quality of the normal human eye. J Opt Soc Am A 1997; 14(11):2873-83.

4. Oshika T, Klyce SD, Applegate RA, et al. Comparison of corneal wavefront aberrations after photorefractive keratectomy and laser *in situ* keratomileusis. Am J Ophthalmol 1999;127:1-7.
5. Fincham WHA, Freeman MH. Optics. In: Born M, Wolf E (Eds): Principles of Optics. (2nd edn. and 9th edn). London: Butterworths, 1980. New York: Macmillan, 1964:203-32.
6. Charman WN, Walsh G. Variations in the local refractive correction of the eye across its entrance pupil. Optometry and Vision Science 1989;66(1):34-40.
7. Rosenblum WM, Christensen JL. Objective and subjective spherical aberration measurement of the human eye. In Wolf E (Ed): Progress in Optics, (North-Holland, Amsterdam), 1976;13:69-91.
8. Campbell MC, Harrison EM, Simonet P. Psychophysical measurement of the blur on the retina due to optical aberrations of the eye. Vision Res 1990;30:1587-1602.
9. Howland HC, Howland B. A subjective method for the measurement of monochromatic aberrations of the eye. J Opt Soc Am 1977;67:1508-18.
10. Walsh G, Charman WN, Howland HC. Objective technique for the determination of monochromatic aberrations of the human eye. J Opt Soc Am 1984;A1:987-92.
11. Ivanoff A. About the spherical aberration of the eye. J Opt Soc Am 1956;46:901-3.
12. Jenkins TCA. Aberrations of the eye and their effects on vision. Part 1. Br J Physiol Opt 1963;20:59-91.
13. Van den Brink G. Measurements of the geometric aberrations of the eye. Vision Res 1962;2:233-44.
14. Born M, Wolf E. Principles of Optics. 2nd ed. New York: Macmillan 1964;203-32
15. Kaemmerer M, Mrochen M, Mierdel P, et al. Optical aberrations of the human eye. Nature Medicine (in press).
16. Oshika T, Klyce SD, Applegate RA, et al. Changes in corneal wavefront aberration with aging. Invest Ophthalmol Vis Sci 1999;40:1351-5.
17. Calver RI, Cox MJ, Elliot DB. Effect of aging on the monochromatic aberrations of the human eye. J Opt Soc Am A 1999;16:2069-78.
18. Guirao A, Gonzalez C, Redondo M, et al. Average optical performance of the human eye as a function of age in a normal population. Invest Ophthalmol Vis Sci 1999;40:203-13.
19. Krueger R, Kaemerrer M, Mrochen M, et al. Understanding refraction and accommodation through "ingoing optics" aberrometry: a case report. Ophthalmology (in press).
20. He JC, Burns SA, Marcos S. Monochromatic aberrations in the accommodated human eye. Vis Res 2000;40:41-48
21. Fankhauser F, Kaemerrer M, Mrochen M, et al. The effect of accommodation, mydriasis, and cycloplegia on aberrometry. ARVO abstract 2248. Invest Ophthalmol Vis Sci 2000;41:S461.

16

Intacs

- THE TECHNIQUE
- INTACS FOR LOW MYOPIA
- INTACS FOR KERATOCONUS-PELLUCID MARGINAL DEGENERATION
- INTACS FOR POST-LASIK CORNEAL ECTASIA

George D Kymionis, Charalambos Siganos, Ioannis G Pallikaris (Greece)

INTRODUCTION

Barraquer made the first attempts for biocompatible material implantation intrastromally to the cornea in 1949.[1] Since then, a remarkable improvement has been made. In April 1999, the US Food and Drug Administration (FDA) approved Intacs (Intacs; Addition Technology Inc., Fremont, California, USA) for sale in the United States for the correction of low myopia[2,3] (Table 16.1). The potential advantage of Intacs implantation over the current existed refractive techniques such as reversibility (reverse treatment effects), maintaning the natural prolate corneal shape and the preservation of cornea stroma are the main reasons for the expand of Intacs' treatments indications.

THE TECHNIQUE

The procedure is performed under topical anesthesia (anesthetic drops). The surgeon marks the geometric center of the cornea (11 mm zone marker-Sinskey's hook) and measures corneal thickness at the site of the planned incision. An incision, 1.2 mm in length is made with a diamond blade at the 12 o'clock position, approximately 2.0 mm from the limbus. Using a diamond knife set at 70 percent of the corneal thickness at the incision site (calibrated diamond knife with 15° angled-pivot knife) and 2 intrastromal corneal pockets are created using a pocketing hook, stromal spreader, and clockwise and anticlockwise dissection glides, under suction created by a vacuum centering guide (step 1:400 mBar-step 2: 600 mBar). The 2 polymethylmethacrylate segments (150° crescent-shaped inserts) are implanted in the clockwise and counterclockwise tunnels, maintaining a space of 2.0 mm between their ends and 1.5 mm between the opposite edge of each segment and the edge of the incision. After the stromal pocket is carefully washed with balanced salt solution, the incision is being closed with a single interrupted 10-0 nylon suture. Postoperatively, all eyes receive antibiotic/steroid combination eye drops 4 times per day for 1 week. In addition, all patients are instructed to use preservative-free artificial tears frequently. The sutures are removed 2 weeks after surgery.

Table 16.1: Ring segment description

- Made of PMMA
- Outer diameter: 8.1 mm
- Inner diameter: 6.77 mm
- Arc length: 150°
- Positioning holes diameter: 0.28 mm
- Ring cross-section: hexagonal
- Each package contains two segments: Right and left

Table 16.2: Intacs nomogram for myopia

Thickness	*Average correction*
0.25	–1.3 D (1-1.6)
0.30	–2.0 D (1.7-2.3)
0.35	–2.7 D (2.4-3.0)
0.40	–3.4 D (3.1-3.7)
0.45	–4.1 D (3.8-4.4)

The thickness of the Intacs is based on the attempted correction according to the nomogram (five different thickness inserts, 0.25, 0.30, 0.35, 0.40 and 0.45 mm, are currently available). The nomogram for Intacs inserts selection is described in Table 16.2.

INTACS FOR LOW MYOPIA

Indications for Intacs implantation are: patients older than 21 years old and stability of refraction for at least 12 months prior to the preoperative examination. Intacs inserts are contraindicated in patients with collagen vacular, autoimmune or immunodeficiency diseases, in pregnant or nursing women, presence of ocular conditions, such as keratoconus, recurrent corneal erosion syndrome or corneal dystrophy, that may predispose the patient to future complications, in patients who are taking at least one of the following medications: isotretinoin, amiodarone, sumatriptan (Figure 16.1).

The results from phase II and phase III[4] clinical protocols showed that at 1 year, 97 percent of patients who completed follow-up had 20/40 or better uncorrected visual acuity (UCVA). Seventy-four percent of patients had 20/20 or better UCVA. Ninety-two percent of eyes were within ±1 D of intended refractive correction, and 69 percent were within 0.5 D of intended refractive correction. At 3 months, 90 percent of patients had less than 1.0 D of change from the previous examination performed at 1 month. The ocular complication

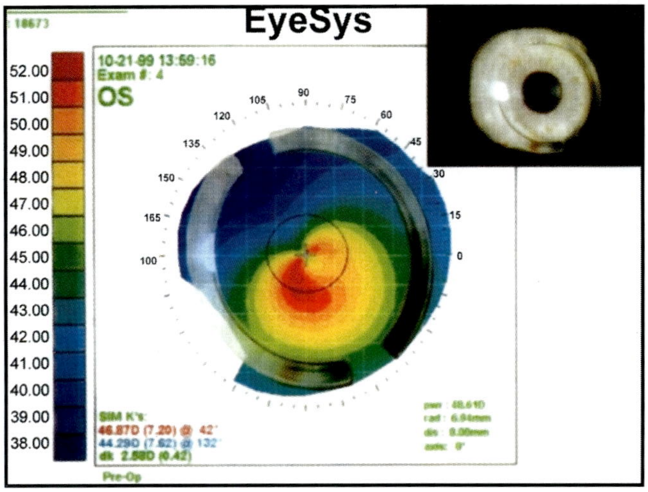

Figure 16.1: Preoperative topography and Intacs position of insertion (top right) of a keratoconic patient

rate was 11 percent at 12 months. Nearly 9 percent of patients requested to have their inserts removed and a total of 3.8 percent of patients required a secondary surgical intervention (Table 16.3).

Recently, a bioptics procedure[5] (combined LASIK and ICRS implantation) reported engouraging results for patients with low pachymetric values or high myopia. Post-Intacs implantation complications are: under- or over- correction, migration of segments toward the wound, neovascularization, extrusion and visual side effects (glare or haloes).

INTACS FOR KERATOCONUS-PELLUCID MARGINAL DEGENETATION

Intacs were designed to achieve a refractive adjustment by flattening the central corneal curvature while maintaining clarity in the central optical zone. Patients must have clear central corneas. Exclusion criteria are: previous intraocular or corneal surgery; history of herpes keratitis; diagnosed autoimmune disease; and systemic connective tissue disease.

Several studies have demonstrated the efficacy of Intacs in correcting low myopia, while several studies reported encouraging results in keratoconic eyes and post-LASIK corneal ectasia. In the year 2000, Colin and associates[6] first published an article about their preliminary results regarding the management of keratoconus with Intacs. One year later, the same authors published a series of 10 keratoconic patients 1-year after Intacs implantation where they support that Intacs reduced the corneal steepening and astigmatism, while visual acuity was improved in almost all eyes.[7] Recently, Siganos et al,[8] reported similar results in keratoconic patients. The surgical procedure is almost the same as myopia correction except the thickness of segments (0.45 mm) and the position of Intacs implantation. Two Intacs segments of thickness are inserted according to the topographic image, aiming at embracing the keratoconus area to try to achieve maximal flattening. With mean follow-up of 11.3 months, intracorneal ring segments implantation improved UCVA and BCVA in the majority of the keratoconus patients. In conclusion, Intacs seem to offer a minimally invasive alternative treatment before PKP for keratoconic patients with clear corneas and contact lens intolerance, especially in early stages of the disease with less topographic irregularities.

Table 16.3: Potential complications during Intacs implantation

Complications	*Cause-precautions*
Abnormal lamellar dissection	Improper stromal channel
Rings on significant different levels	Improper stromal channel
Decentered channel	Slipping of vacuum
Decentered ring placement	Incision placement maker
Corneal perforation (anterior surface)	Slipping of vacuum
Corneal perforation (posterior surface)	Too deep incision (pachymetry)
Perilimbal hemorrage	Vacuum centering guide
Breakage of the ring	Handle with care
Incision gape	Suture incision
Ring ends overlap	Push with sinskey's hook
Incomplete ring advancement	Push with sinskey's hook
Conjuctival chemosis	Vacuum centering guide

Pellucid marginal degeneration (PMD) is a bilateral, noninflammatory disorder characterized by a peripheral band of thinning of the inferior cornea. The disease is usually asymptomatic except for the progressive deterioration in uncorrected visual acuity and best spectacle-corrected visual acuity caused by the irregular astigmatism induced by the corneal ectasia. Recently, Kymionis et al[9] reported a 42-year-old man that had Intacs implantation for early pellucid marginal degeneration (PMD). Two Intacs segments (0.45 mm thickness) were inserted uneventfully in the fashion typically used for low myopia correction (nasal temporal). Eleven months after the procedure, the uncorrected visual acuity was 20/200, compared with counting fingers preoperatively, while the best spectacle-corrected visual acuity improved to 20/25 from 20/50. Corneal topographic pattern was also improved. Although the results are encouraging, concern still exists regarding the long-term effect of this approach for the management of patients with PMD.

INTACS FOR POST-LASIK CORNEAL ECTASIA

The main advantage of Intacs is that, unlike excimer laser refractive techniques, they preserve corneal tissue while maintaining clarity in the central optical zone. In this way, Intacs may represent an interesting surgical alternative for patients with corneal ectasia after LASIK. The procedure is similar to low myopia or keratoconus. The thickness of the Intacs is based on the attempted correction. Using a diamond knife set at 70 percent of the corneal thickness at the incision site, a 0.9-mm radial incision is created, and 2 intrastromal corneal pockets are created using a pocketing lever, stromal spreader, and clockwise and anticlockwise dissection glides. Two tunnels (right and left) are created using clockwise and anticlockwise dissectors under suction created by a vacuum centering guide. The 2 polymethylmethacrylate segments are implanted in the clockwise and counterclockwise tunnels, maintaining a space of 2.0 mm between their ends and 1.5 mm between the opposite edge of each segment and the edge of the incision. Because of the standard 7 mm optic zone diameter of the ring segments, Intacs segments are inevitably ended up more central and deeper to the LASIK flap edge.

In a recent article, Kymionis et al reported that Intacs implantation in post-LASIK cornea ectasia results in statistically significant reducion in spherical equivalent error (pre-Intacs, mean +/– SD: –4.81 +/– 3.24 Diopters (D) (range, –13.75 to –2.50 D) to –0.96 +/– 2.93 D (range, -8.75 to 2.50 D) (P<.001). Pre-Intacs uncorrected visual acuity was 20/100 or worse in all eyes (range, counting fingers to 20/100) while at the last follow-up examination, 9 (90%) of 10 eyes had uncorrected visual acuity of 20/40 or better (range, counting fingers to 20/20). Three eyes maintained the pre-Intacs best spectacle-corrected visual acuity while the rest of the eyes (7) experienced a gain of 1 to 2 lines. The mean difference between pre-Intacs and last follow-up best spectacle-corrected visual acuity was a gain of 1.00 +/- 0.82 lines. In conclusion, Intacs implantation improved uncorrected visual acuity and best spectacle-corrected visual acuity in patients with post-LASIK ectasia. Even though the results are encouraging, concern still exists regarding the long-term effect of such an approach for the management of post-LASIK ectasia.

REFERENCES

1. Burris TE. Intrastromal corneal ring technology: results and indications. Curr Opin Ophthalmol 1998;9:9-14.
2. Schanzlin DJ, Asbell PA, Burris TE, Durrie DS. The intrastromal corneal ring segments. Phase II results for the correction of myopia. Ophthalmology 1997;104:1067-78.
3. Nose W, Neves RA, Burris TE, et al. Intrastromal corneal ring: 12-month sighted myopic eyes. J Refract Surg 1996;12:20-8.
4. Rapuano CJ, Sugar A, Koch DD, et al. Intrastromal corneal ring segments for low myopia: a report by the American Academy of Ophthalmology. Ophthalmology 2001;108(10): 1922-8.
5. Primack JD, Azar DT. Laser *in situ* keratomileusis and intrastromal corneal ring segments for high myopia. Three-step procedure. J Cataract Refract Surg 2003;29(5):869-74.
6. Colin J, Cochener B, Savary G, Malet F. Correcting keratoconus with intracorneal rings. J Cataract Refract Surg 2000;26:1117-22.
7. Colin J, Cochener B, Savary G, Malet F, Holmes-Higgin D. Intacs inserts for treating keratoconus: one-year results. Ophthalmology 2001;108:1409-14.
8. Siganos CS, Kymionis GD, Kartakis N, et al. Management of keratoconus with Intacs. Am J Ophthalmol 2003;135(1): 64-70.
9. Kymionis GD, Aslanides IM, Siganos CS, Pallikaris IG. Intacs for early pellucid marginal degeneration. J Cataract Refract Surg 2004;30(1):230-3.
10. Kymionis GD, Siganos CS, Kounis G, et al. Management of post-LASIK corneal ectasia with Intacs inserts: one-year results. Arch Ophthalmol 2003;121(3):322-6.

17

Phakic Refractive Lens (PRL^{TM}) for Myopia and Hyperopia Correction

- HISTORY OF PRLS BACKGROUND AND DEVELOPMENT
- PATIENT SELECTION
- PREOPERATIVE PREPARATION
- INSTRUMENTATION
- SURGICAL STEPS
- OPERATIVE COMPLICATIONS
- UNUSUAL SITUATIONS AND POSTOPERATIVE COMPLICATIONS
- RESULTS
- CONCLUSION
- PEDIATRIC USAGE
- FUTURE APPLICATIONS
- PRL IMPLANTATION FOR THE CORRECTION OF HIGH AMETROPIA

Dimitrii D Dementiev, Kukrenkov Vetchiaslav (Italy)

INTRODUCTION

The last years more and more refractive surgeons are looking to use not only the corneal refractive procedures (RK, KM, LASIK, PRK, LASEK) for myopia and hyperopia correction, but also the phakic implants. It was just approved that the quality of vision after the refractive implants is much better that after corneal procedures, especially in high refractive error eyes .The evidence of reversibility, stability (no regression was noticed) and high predictability of the final refractive effect of the implants make this kind of surgery to become more popular among the refractive surgeons all over the globe.

In this chapter we want to describe our experience with Phakic Refractive Lense (PRL Medennium-Ciba Vision) implantation and to show the evolution of the phakic refractive lenses we have worked with, to compare the different models of the lenses we used in the past and we use today, to analyze the follow-up and complications we had, to present the instrumentation we developed for this surgery.

HISTORY OF PRLs: BACKGROUND AND DEVELOPMENT

Pupil-fixated Lens (Mushroom) (Figure 17.1)

In 1986, in Moscow Research Eye Institute Drs. V.Zuev and S.Fyodorov proposed a new phakic silicone IOL, named the *mushroom* lens, which was implanted from 1986 until 1990 in Russia. The lens was fixated in the pupil. The main idea was to avoid contact between the lens and the endothelium. We implanted more than 120 lenses with good refractive results. A new era of phakic correction using a lens in the posterior chamber was started. The diameter of the optic zone of this lens was 3.2 mm and the total length of the PRL was 8.0 mm. The haptic was placed in the PC and the optic part remained in the AC; the lens being fixated by the pupil (Figure 17.2).

Despite of the good refractive results many complications were manifested.

The complications such as iridocyclitis (the material was toxic), night glare, night vision acuity loss, pupillary block, endothelial cell loss, cataracts in several cases, and inflammation reaction in long-term follow-up were the serious reason to stop the study of this implant design.

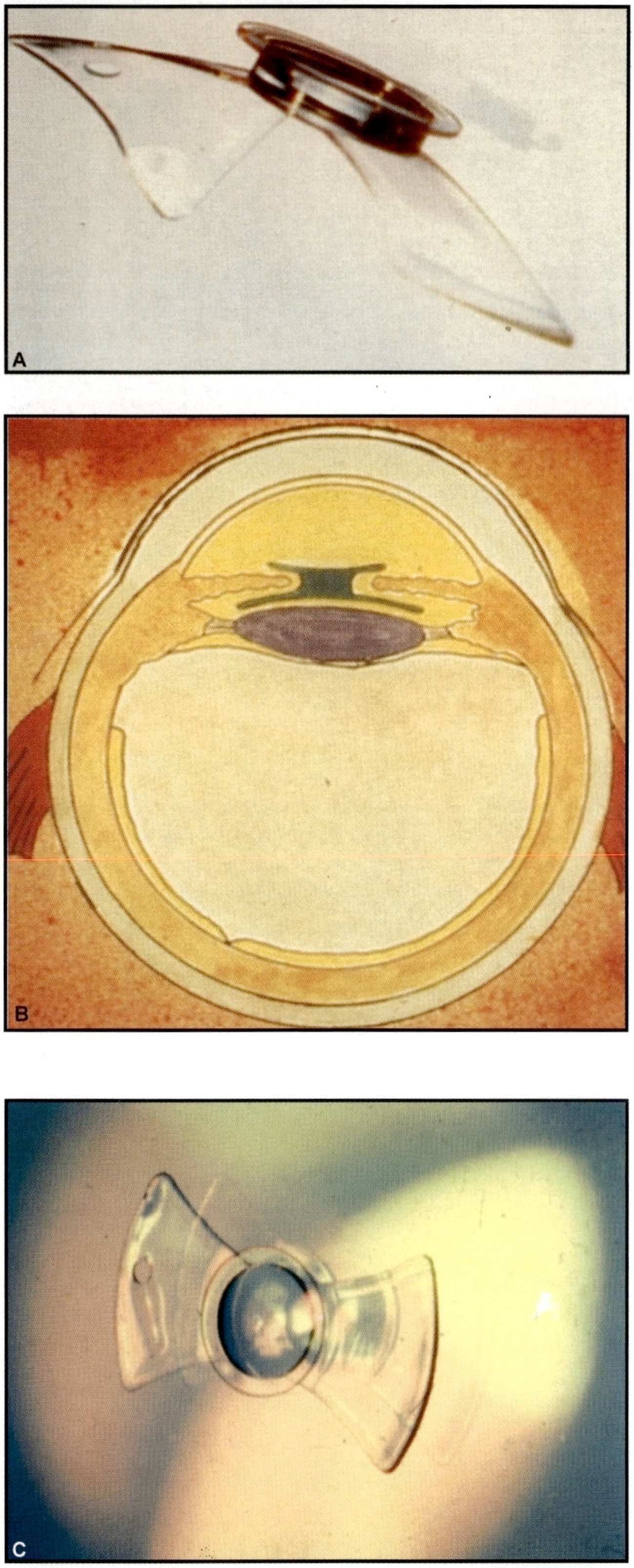

Figure 17.1: Mushroom lens

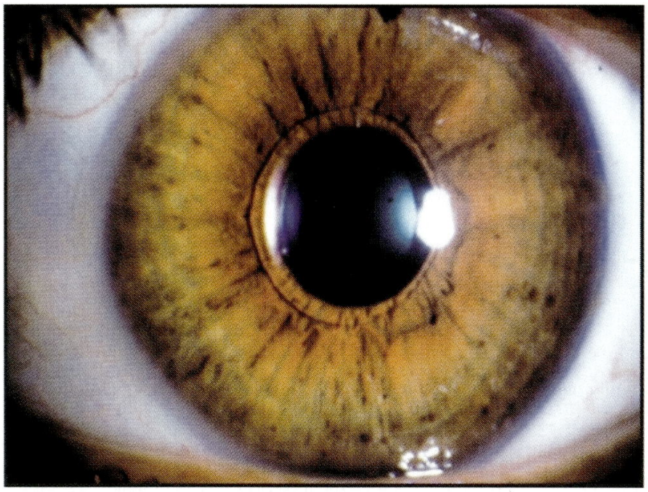

Figure 17.2: Phakic IOL fixated by pupil

Posterior Chamber Phakic Lens made in Russia (Figure 17.3)

Based on the work with the *Mushroom* lens the concept of a purely posterior chamber PRL was proposed at MERI in Russia and was made from a completely new silicone material, which was not toxic but biocompatible and had a higher refractive index than previous silicon.

Its configuration, parameters and the mechanism of fixation of this PRL were completely different from the previous *Mushroom* model. It was intended for implantation entirely in the posterior chamber with fixation on the zonular fibers. The OZ diameter was 4.5 mm and the total length was 10.6 mm. The lens was created for surgical high myopia correction starting from –10.0 D. This lens was the first prototype of all other posterior chamber PRLs available on the market today.

The problems with endothelium cells loss, cataract formation, severe glare were resolved. But a new complication like an implant decentration occurred in many cases (Figure 17.4).

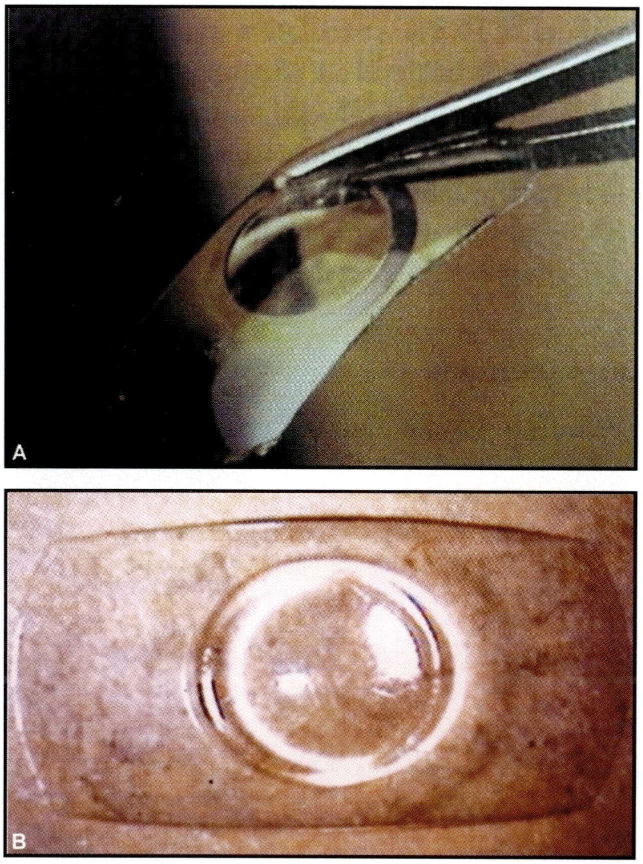

Figures 17.3A and B: Posterior chamber phakic IOL (Russian)

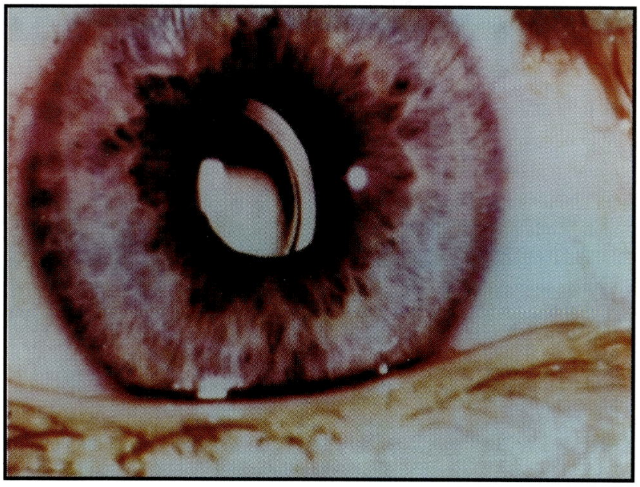

Figure 17.4: Decentration of the PC phakic IOL

Posterior Chamber Phakic Lens (PRL™) by IVI-Medennium (Figure 17.5)

International Vision, Inc

This Company was set up in Cincinnati, Ohio to produce the PC PRL that we have been using for the past 6 years. The idea of PRL design was moved from Russia to USA, modifyeied and improved according to the complications we had in the past. The size and the curvature of the implant were changed, and FDA study started. The

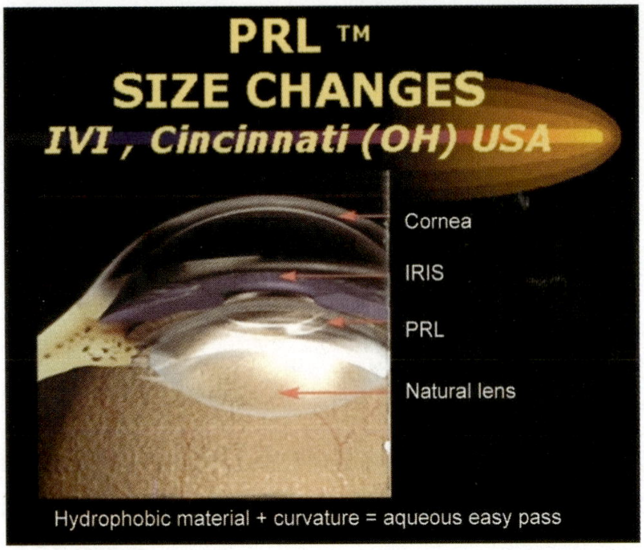

Figure 17.5: The last modifications of phakic refractive lens PRL™

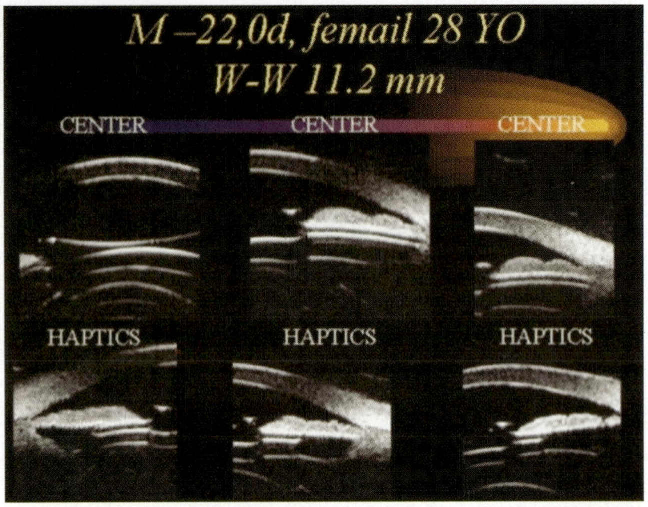

Figure 17.6: UBM picture shows floating of PRL in PC. No contact with the anterior capsule, contact with the iris

Phakic Refractive Lens (PRL) is made from silicone with a 1.46 refractive index. The diameter of the optic zone is from 4.5 to 5.5 mm depending upon the dioptric power of the lens. They produce PRLs for myopia and hyperopia (range from+3.5 to+13.5 and from –5.0 to –20.0), which permits a maximum correction of 27.0 D of myopia and 11.0 D of hyperopia. The material is soft, elastic, and hydrophobic. It is easy to perform the implantation through a 3.0 to 3.5 mm clear cornea incision. The lens doesn't contact the anterior capsule of the crystalline lens. Beeing done from hydrophobic material and having the curvature that repeats the curvature of the crystalline lens the edges of the PRL are lying on the zonulars and all the body floats in the posterior chamber keeping the space between the implant and anterior capsule of the lens. This floating phenomena let the aqueous easy to pass under the PRL keeping the lens metabolism unchanged (Figure 17.6). No synechiae have been noted in long-term follow-up. It is easy to remove if it should become necessary. After changing the size parameters of the PRL, decentration has not been observed. Other possible complications are cataract formation and pigmentary glaucoma.

PRL Medennium/Ciba Vision Surgical (Figure 17.7)

Today the PRL has received the CEE mark and available on the markets of Europe and South America. In the USA it is under the phase III FDA study. Manufactured by IVI/Medennium Inc. Irvine, CA , USA and distributed by Ciba Vision Corp. (Surgical), Dulith, GA USA.

When implanted PRL functions as an optical element to correct refractive error and avoids contact with the natural lens of the eye. PRL does not have the contact with the anterior capsule of the crystalline lens. PRL

Myopic and hyperopic implants are available. PRL is done from high refractive index (1.46) highly purified, optically clear silicone elastomer that has undergone biocompatibility testing in Russia and USA. The specific gravity of the PRL is 0.99. PRL has spherical, thin, flexible and elastic haptic for ease of insertion and conformance to the natural shape and dynamic changes of the eye. The PRL is not fixed in the ciliary sulcus, but floats in the posterior chamber touching the natural lens zonulars with its edge. The implant's width is 6.0 mm. Myopic implant (MI) is 11.3 mm length (one size fits all) and hyperopic implant (HI) is 10.6 mm length (one size fits all).

The optic diameter of MI is varying from 5.0 to 4.5 mm.

HI has 4.5 mm diameter in all the implants.

The Power of MI is from –3.0 D to –20.0 D

The power of HI is from +3.0 D to + 15.0 D

With 0.5 D increment both MI and HI.

From here we shall describe our study of the PRLs and our experience of its implantation.

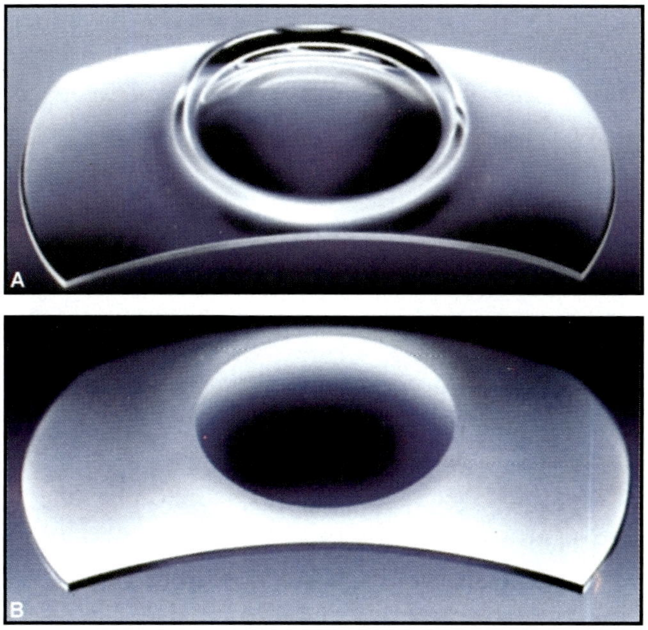

Figure 17.7: A. Myopic PRL B. Hyperopic PRL

Model	*Myopic*	*Hyperopic*
• Optic dia	4.5-5.0 mm	4.5 mm
• Length	11,3 mm	10.6 mm
• Width	6.0 mm	6.o mm
• Power D	–3.0 to –20.0	+3.0 to + 15.0
• Increments	0.5 D	0.5 D

Table 17.1: No. of lenses implanted during three generations

Generation I	97 implants	from 1987 to 1990
Generation II	224 implants	from 1990 to present
Generation III	162 implants	from 1996 to present

Beginning in 1987 we implanted 483 lenses of three generations (Table 17.1).

In this study, we analyze the clinical data of 122 implants in 72 patients. The patients age ranged between 9 and 53 years. The dioptric power of the implanted lenses ranged between +3.5 and +16.0 D (hyperopic implants) and between –5.0 and –18.5 D (myopic implants) performed in our Day-Hospitals in Milano and Bari, Italy from 1992 to the present time. We used the II and III generation implants in this study.

PATIENT SELECTION (TABLE 17.2)

A. Myopic range:
From –3.00 D to –27.00 D

B. Hyperopic range:
From +3.00 to +16.00 D.

Table 17.2: Criteria for patient selection based on previous experience

Myopia (refraction)	*Hyperopia (refraction)*	*Unilateral myopia in children (refraction)*	*Combined astigmatism*	*Keratoconus*	*Error after previous refractive procedures*	*Poor candidates*
From –6.0D To –23.0D	From+3.0 D To +16.0 D.	From –7.0 D. To –14.0 D.	Max. 3.75 D.		From +3.5 D. To + 6.0 D.	Cataract. Glaucoma. Lens sublux. Shallow AC Vitre-retinal problems. Previous eye surgery. Diabetes Age >60
110 cases	12 cases	7 cases (ages 9 to 14)	13 cases	1 case	4 cases (2 PRL exchange of previous models) – dislocation	
Total cases:				**122 cases, Ages 9 to 53**		

A +16.0 D hyperope is the maximum we have corrected.

Because the anterior chamber of the hyperopic patients is usually shallow, it is safer to limit the hyperopic correction for PRL implantation to a maximum of +11.00 D unless there is a deep AC.

C. Unilateral high myopia with amblyopia in children:
So far we have performed seven implantations for correction of unilateral high myopia in children with amblyopia. In cases of progressive myopia, scleral reinforcement surgery is recommended.

D. Combined astigmatism:
In cases with astigmatism greater than 1.0 D we performed PRL implantation with additional AK surgery.

E. Keratoconus correction and correction of the refractive error of the previous surgery
PRL implantations can be performed for keratoconus correction with a high myopia component and for overcorrection of a previous refractive procedure such as RK, PRK, or LASIK.
Exchange of a previous model of PRL

F. Poor candidates:
1. Clouded or non-transparent cornea
2. Cataract
3. Lens subluxation
4. Glaucoma or ocular hypertension
5. Shallow anterior chamber (less then 2.5 mm)
6. Vitreoretinal problems that would preclude good vision or require posterior segment intervention
7. Previous ocular surgery: vitreoretinal surgery, glaucoma filtration, etc.
8. Age limited to age 60.

PREOPERATIVE PREPARATION

PRL Power Calculation

It is important to obtain a precise refraction of the eye (with accurate vertex distance measurement) as well as an accurate axial length and corneal power readings to use the various methods. *Vertex Chart*

The spherical equivalent of the most accurate refraction of the eye is used to interpolate the power of the posterior chamber PRL. These powers are based on a simple vertex correction from 12 mm to the corneal plane. This does not seem to make sense optically, but so far has resulted in excellent accuracy in our experience (Table 17.3).

Clinical Rules

1. Cycloplegic Rx must be less minus than manifest Rx in myopes.
2. Cycloplegic Rx must be more plus than manifest Rx in hyperopes.
3. If cycloplegic Rx is different, see if patient can accept full cycloplegic correction.
4. Best to attempt correction of cycloplegic Rx in hyperopes and manifest Rx in myopes.
5. Hyperopic patients 18 to 35 can accommodate a small undercorrection (up to +1.00).
6. Myopic patients 18 to 35 should not be over-corrected but left emmetropioc or small myopia.
7. All patients 36 to 50 must obtain emmetropia or slight overcorrection (up to –1.00).
8. If cylinder is not to be corrected, using the SE plans for PO mixed astigmatism.
9. If correcting cylinder prior to PRL, use the SE of the resultant healed refraction.
10. If correcting cylinder after the PRL:
    a. If your astigmatic surgical correction will not change the average K, use the SE.
    b. If your astigmatic surgical correction will change the average K (flatten), use the sphere only.

Iridectomy

Surgical

Usually we recommend performing a surgical iridectomy at the time of PRL implantation. We feel it should be a basal iridectomy made at 12:00 and we prefer to perform it after the PRL is inserted. It is of the utmost importance to make sure that it is a complete iridectomy by checking to be sure the pigment layer has been cut through. This must be done carefully so as not to damage the crystalline lens.

Laser

Those surgeons who prefer not to make it surgically must do it by YAG-laser. It is recommended that two YAG

Table 17.3: CIBA-Medennium PRL power table
Based on 12 mm Vertex Formula: PRL=Rx/(1-0.012*Rx)

Each PRL causes what RX?				*Each Rx needs what PRL?*			
Myopia		*Hyperopia*		*Myopia*		*Hyperopia*	
PRL	*RX*	*PRL*	*RX*	*RX*	*PRL*	*RX*	*PRL*
–3,0	–3,11	**3,0**	2,90	**–3,0**	–2,90	**3,0**	3,11
–3,5	–3,65	**3,5**	3,36	**–3,5**	–3,36	**3,5**	3,65
–4,0	–4,20	**4,0**	3,82	**–4,0**	–3,82	**4,0**	4,20
–4,5	–4,76	**4,5**	4,27	**–4,5**	–4,27	**4,5**	4,76
–5,0	–5,32	**5,0**	4,72	**–5,0**	–4,72	**5,0**	5,32
–5,5	–5,89	**5,5**	5,16	**–5,5**	–5,16	**5,5**	5,89
–6,0	–6,50	**6,0**	5,60	**–6,0**	–5,60	**6,0**	6,47
–6,5	–7,00	**6,5**	6,00	**–6,5**	–6,03	**6,5**	7,05
–7,0	–7,64	**7,0**	6,50	**–7,0**	–6,46	**7,0**	7,64
–7,5	–8,24	**7,5**	6,88	**–7,5**	–6,88	**7,5**	8,24
–8,0	–8,85	**8,0**	7,30	**–8,0**	–7,30	**8,0**	8,85
–8,5	–9,50	**8,5**	7,71	**–8,5**	–7,71	**8,5**	9,47
–9,0	–10,09	**9,0**	8,12	**–9,0**	–8,12	**9,0**	10,09
–9,5	–10,72	**9,5**	8,50	**–9,5**	–8,53	**9,5**	10,72
–10,0	–11,36	**10,0**	8,93	**–10,0**	–8,93	**10,0**	11,36
–10,5	–12,00	**10,5**	9,33	**–10,5**	–9,33	**10,5**	12,01
–11,0	–12,67	**11,0**	9,72	**–11,0**	–9,72	**11,0**	12,67
–11,5	–13,34	**11,5**	10,11	**–11,5**	–10,11	**11,5**	13,34
–12,0	–14,00	**12,0**	10,50	**–12,0**	–10,49	**12,0**	14,02
–12,5	–14,71	**12,5**	10,87	**–12,5**	–10,87	**12,5**	14,71
–13,0	–15,40	**13,0**	11,25	**–13,0**	–11,25	**13,0**	15,40
–13,5	–16,11	**13,5**	11,62	**–13,5**	–11,62		
–14,0	–16,83	**14,0**	12,00	**–14,0**	–11,99		
–14,5	–17,50	**14,5**	12,35	**–14,5**	–12,35		
–15,0	–18,29	**15,0**	12,71	**–15,0**	–12,71		
–15,5	–19,00	**15,5**	13,07	**–15,5**	–13,07		
–16,0	–19,80	**16,0**	13,42	**–16,0**	–13,42		
–16,5	–20,50			**–16,5**	–13,77		
–17,0	–21,36			**–17,0**	–14,12		
–17,5	–22,15			**–17,5**	–14,46		
–18,0	–23,00			**–18,0**	–14,80		
–18,5	–23,78			**–18,5**	–15,14		
–19,0	–24,61			**–19,0**	–15,47		
–19,5	–25,50			**–19,5**	–15,80		
–20,0	–26,32			**–20,0**	–16,13		
				–20,5	–16,45		
				–21,0	–16,77		
				–21,5	–17,09		
				–22,0	–17,41		
				–22,5	–17,72		
				–23,0	–18,03		
				–23,5	–18,33		
				–24,0	–18,63		
				–24,5	–18,93		
				–25,0	–19,23		
				–25,5	–19,53		
				–26,0	–19,82		
				–26,5	–20,11		

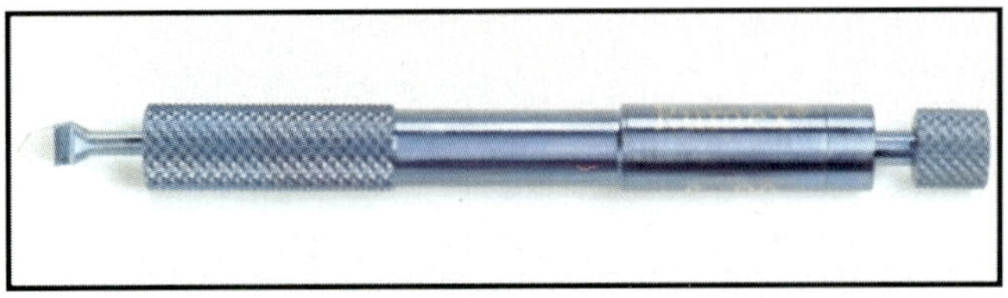

Figure 17.8: Trapezoid diamond Dementiev blade

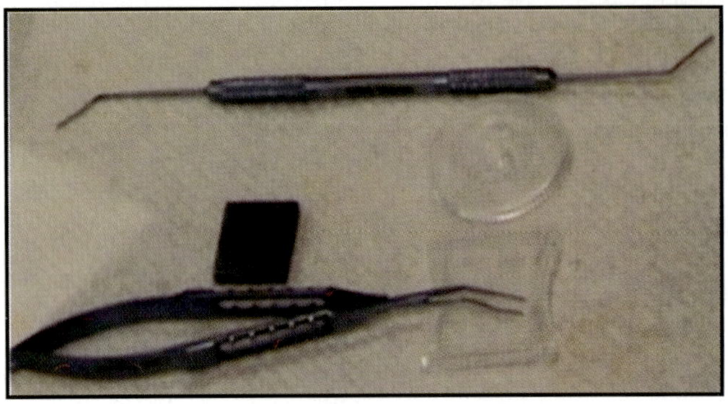

Figure 17.9: Double ended manipulator

iridectomies always be performed at around two weeks before the surgery and that they be made at 10:00 and 2:00. To avoid light and additional images passing through the iridectomies, it is very important not to make them too large and to make them as peripheral as possible. We had one patient with severe complaints of night glare. The iridectomy was found to be too large and located nearer to the pupil. We decided to suture it and after it became smaller, the patient complained much less. We have concluded that the iridectomy's size and placement is very important.

INSTRUMENTATION (Figure 17.10)

A. Incision: Incision trapezoid diamond Dementiev blade for clear cornea incision 3.0-3.2-3.5 mm (Rumex Int., USA) (Figure 17.8).

B. Paracenthesis: Dementiev diamond paracenthesis 1.0 mm blade (Rumex Int.).

C. Implant loading: PRL titanium loading block (DK, UK) (Figure 17.9).

D. Insertion: Titanium Dementiev forceps for PRL implantation (DK, UK)

Titanium diamond dust covered Dementiev PRL forceps (Rumex int, USA) (Figure 17.10)

E. Manipulation: Dementiev PRL titanium double ended haptic spatula (DK,UK).

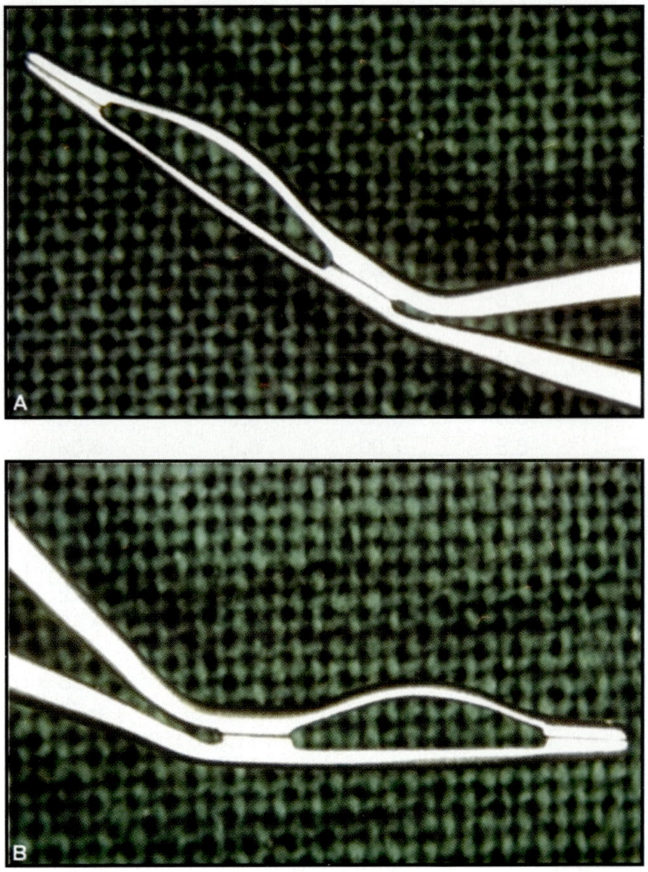

Figures 17.10A and B: Forceps for PRL implantation

Dementiev PRL titanium diamond dust covered manipulator (Rumex Int, USA)

F. Iridectomy: PRL set for manual iridectomy (iris scissors + iris forceps) [Rumex Int, USA].

G. Other: Standard blepharostat and eye fixation forceps (Rumex Int, USA).

Handling the Implant

The PRL implant is supplied in a plastic sterile container. After the container is opened, the implant has to be picked up using PRL Dementiev forceps. It is important to be careful to be sure that the lens does not come into contact with the skin, conjunctiva, lids, lashes or epithelium of the cornea because some microelements can be attracted to and become deposited on the lens surface. It is necessary to be sure that the implant is grasped with the forceps in the correct position. The anterior surface of the lens should be up and posterior surface should be down. This can be seen by observing the fact that the PRL has a similar convexity (curvature) paralleling that of the natural lens. While grasping the lens with the forceps, don't squeeze too hard its optics since it can be easy damaged. Implant is put on the PRL loading block, after that is grasped by the forceps in length.The edge of the implant has to correspond to the end of the forceps. We don't fold the lens; it is self-folding during its insertion. After the implant has been grasped in the correct manner and orientated in the forceps, we irrigate it profusely using BSS from a syringe. It is important to inspect it carefully and with fine forceps gently remove any foreign particulate matter or fibers that may have become attached to its surface. The lens is now ready for insertion (Figures 17.11A and B).

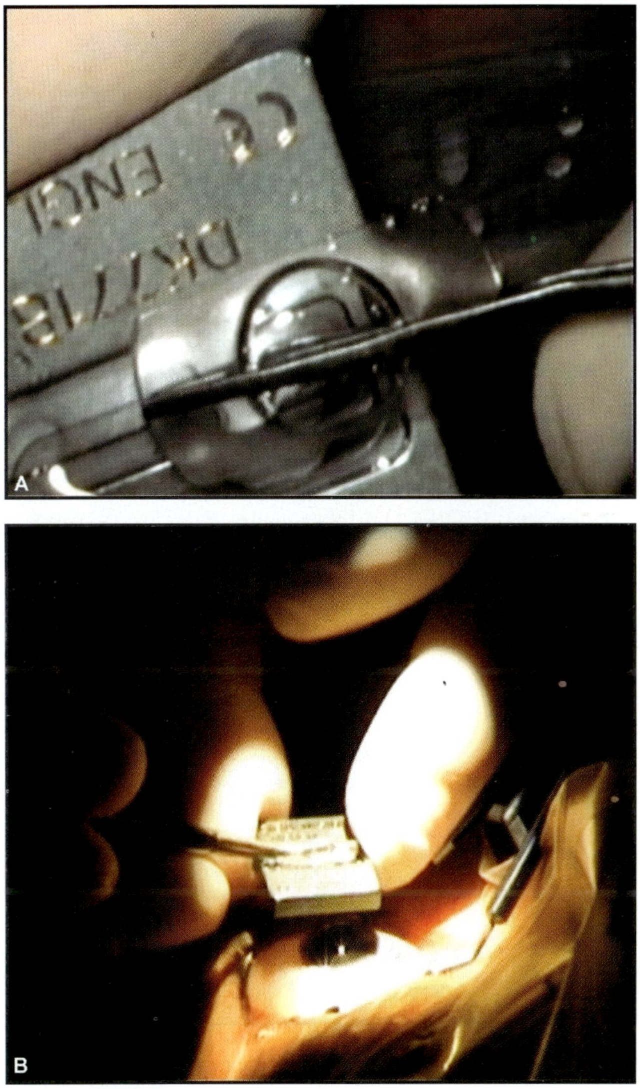

Figures 17.11A and B: Handling the implant

SURGICAL STEPS

Do not start the surgery if the pupil is not wider than 5.0 mm.

Incision

Usually the incision is placed at the temporal cornea. Our experience recommends performing a clear corneal, self-sealing incision of 3.0 to 3.2 mm in width. The incision can be made with either a diamond or stainless steel blade.

Any method of fixation may be used to ensure that there is no possibility of the blade contacting the anterior lens capsule since the pupil is widely dilated. The incision architecture should be one the surgeon is familiar with for self-sealing cataract surgery. Non-suture closure is the intended aim (Figure 17.12A).

Viscoelastic Insertion

Next the anterior chamber should be filled with viscoelastic to achieve a chamber of not less than 3.0 mm in depth. It is also helpful to place some viscoelastic under the iris to make more room to facilitate lens insertion in the posterior chamber (Figure 17.12B).

Paracentesis

This incision is needed to perform the iridectomy and to create an additional entry point for the lens manipulator that will be needed in the next step to position the PRL in the posterior chamber. We make it no larger than 0.5 mm and it should be placed at the 12:00 position. It can be made with a stainless steel or diamond knife. The position of the knife has to be perpendicular to the cornea surface and the cut has to be made at the limbus so that the iridectomy will be more basal (Figure 17.12C). This will avoid:

1. Light passing through the iridectomy and the upper lid will cover it (less halos).
2. The possibility of the iridectomy being blocked by the edge of the PRL (pupillary block).

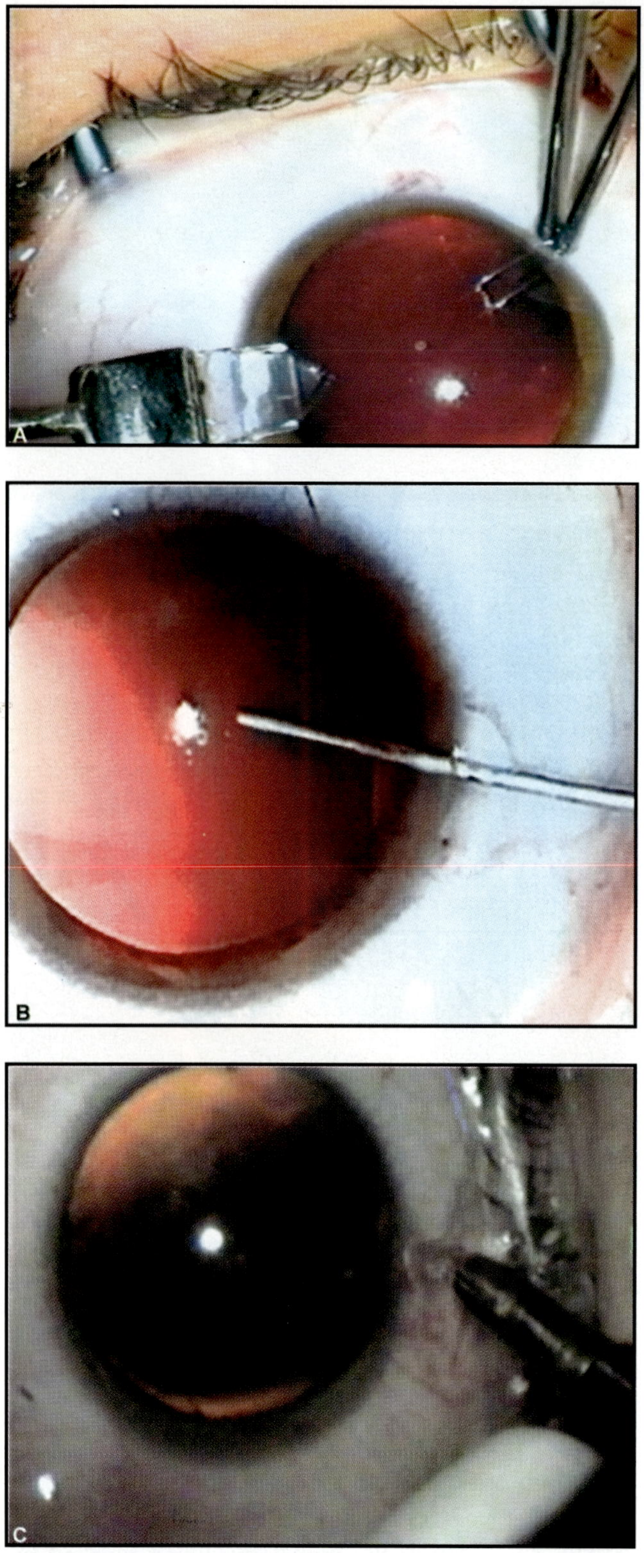

Figures 17.12A to C: PRL is loaded in the forceps A. 3.0 mm clear cornea incision, B. Visco insertion, C. Paracentesis

Lens Insertion

This is the most important and delicate step of the procedure.

The surgeon has to be extremely careful:

1. Not to damage the implant (very soft, thin and rather expensive).
2. Not to damage the anterior capsule with the forceps.
3. Not to touch the endothelium with the implant or the forceps.

The implant is grasped by the special forceps that is designed to prevent damage to the PRL (protection of the optical zone of the PRL). Only the haptic area of the implant is in contact with the forceps. Since the lens is very thin, we can insert it through a 3.0 to 3.2 mm incision without any additional folding. After the implant has been inserted into the anterior chamber, the forceps must be opened gently to allow for the release of the lens. Care must be taken that there are no unexpected sudden movements of the eye during this crucial maneuver.

If, after the lens is inserted, it is discovered that it is upside down it, is necessary to correct this (Figures 17.12D and E).

Retroiris Placement and Centration

Next, we must manipulate the peripheral edges of the implant under the iris. Using the spatula-PRL Manipulator (entered through the paracentesis at 12:00), we move the two lateral edges of the lens under the pupil margin and under the iris. In this step, it is very important to pay maximum attention so as not to put pressure on the crystalline lens capsule. It is important to avoid anterior capsule and cortical damage. It is very important not to push too hard to get it under, but rather try to fold it with the spatula and then release it under the iris to avoid damage to the zonular fibers. When all four "feet" are under the iris satisfactorily, the PRL optic zone is then gently centered using the same manipulator (Figures 17.12F and G).

Iridectomy

I prefer to perform the iridectomy at 12:00 through the paracentesis site. The iridectomy has to be as peripheral

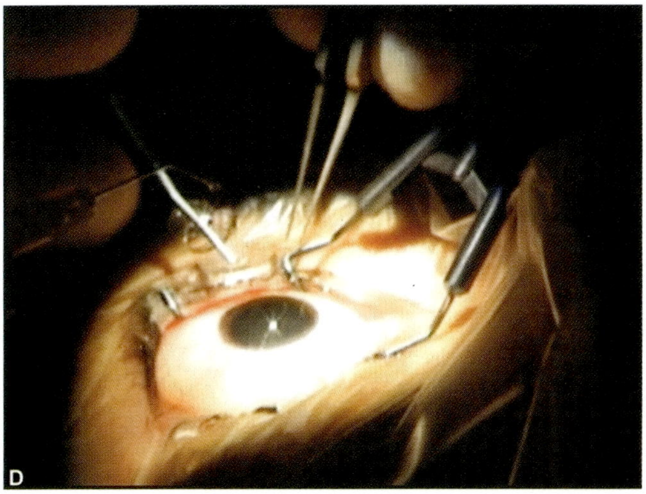

Figure 17.12D

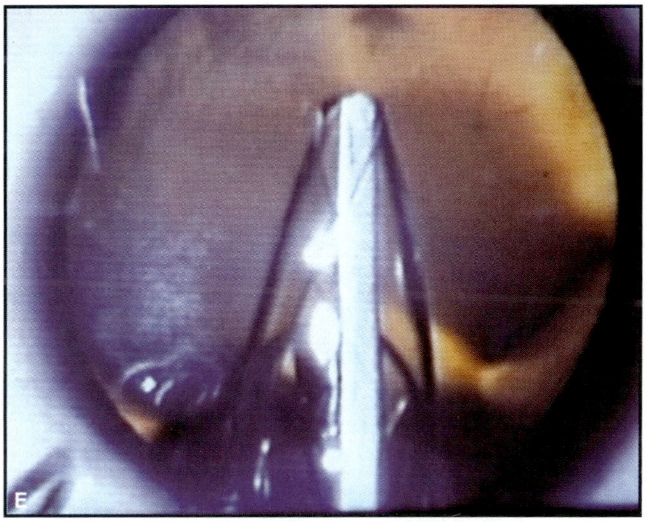

Figure 17.12E: PRL Insertion (self folded)

as possible. This decreases the risk of the PRL blocking it. During this step, bleeding is possible. If this should happen, I prefer to reinject viscoelastic in the area of bleeding to act as a tamponade. After an appropriate waiting period (and clotting has occurred), the viscoelastic must again be removed.

Viscoelastic Removal

We now must try to remove all the viscoelastic by irrigation. It is extremely important to remove as much as possible and not to leave any in the anterior or posterior chamber. If this is not accomplished it may create (Figures 17.12H to K):

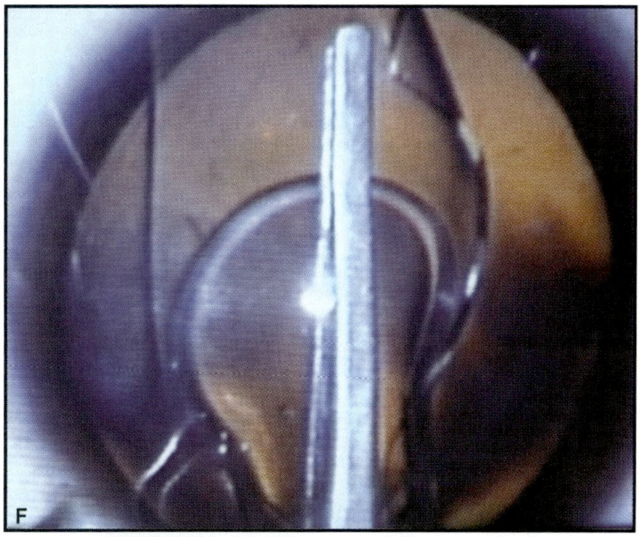

Figure 17.12F: PRL opening in the AC

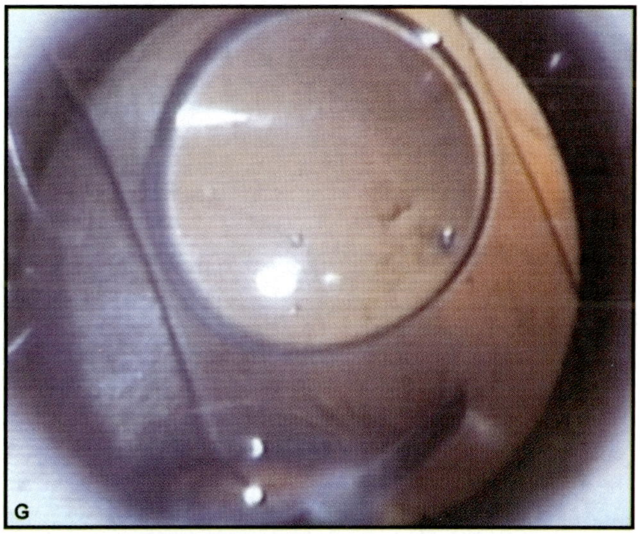

Figure 17.12G: Under iris placement

1. Postoperative IOP increase,
2. Viscoelastic crystallization between the anterior capsule and the posterior surface of the implant.

If it is not possible to remove all the viscoelastic by irrigation, irrigation-aspiration may be used, but be thoughtful of damaging the endothelial cells.

Pupil Constriction

It is important to constrict the pupil as much as possible before the iridectomy is performed. We recommend injecting acetylcholine solution into the AC to accomplish this.

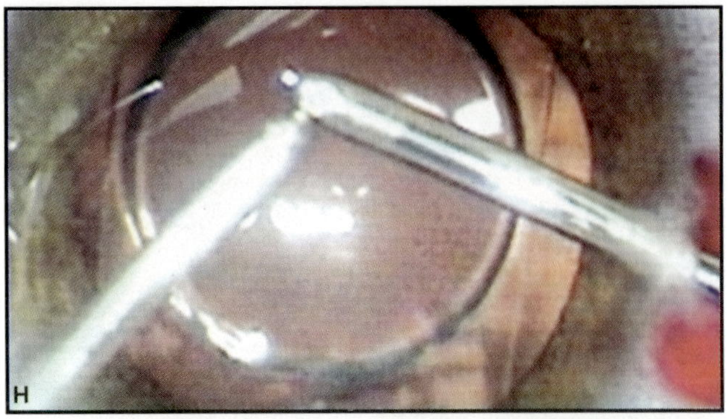

Figure 17.12H: I/A phaco machine

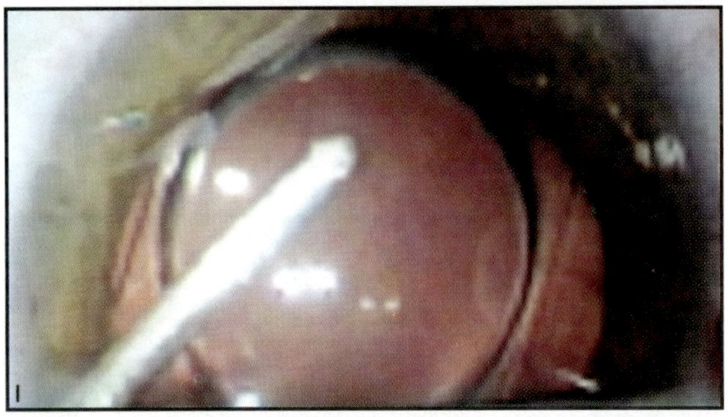

Figure 17.12I: Aspiration

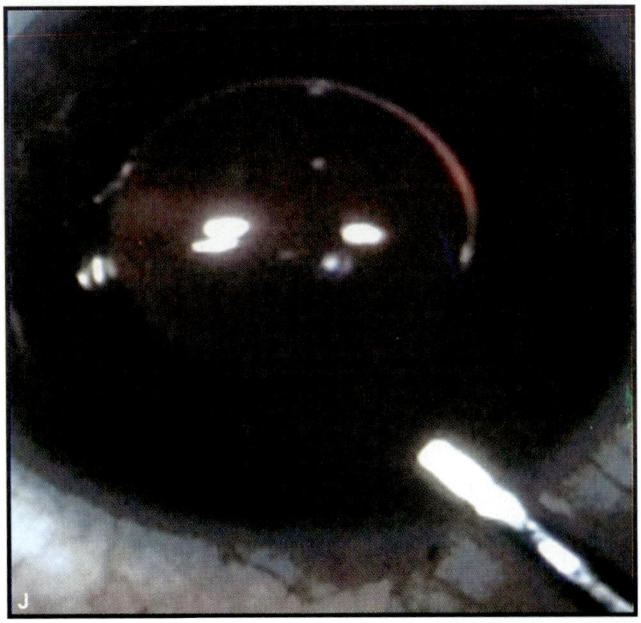

Figure 17.12J: Washing out

Incision Closure

It is not necessary unless security of wound closure is in doubt (Figures 17.12L and M).

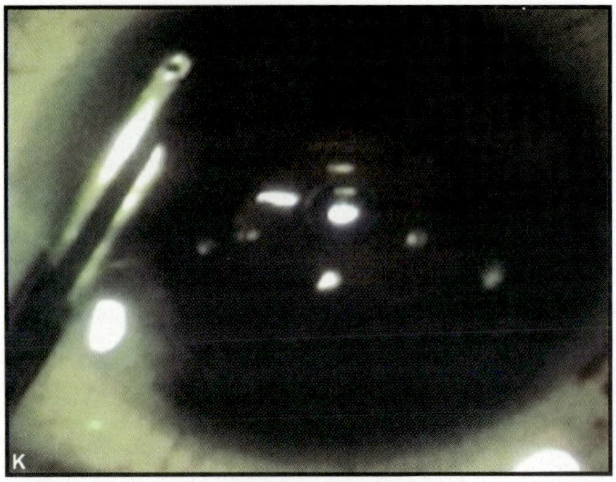

Figure 17.12K: Manual I/A

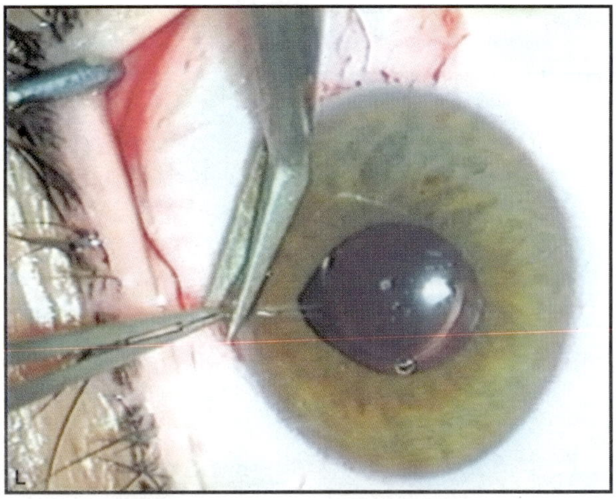

Figure 17.12L: Surgical PI

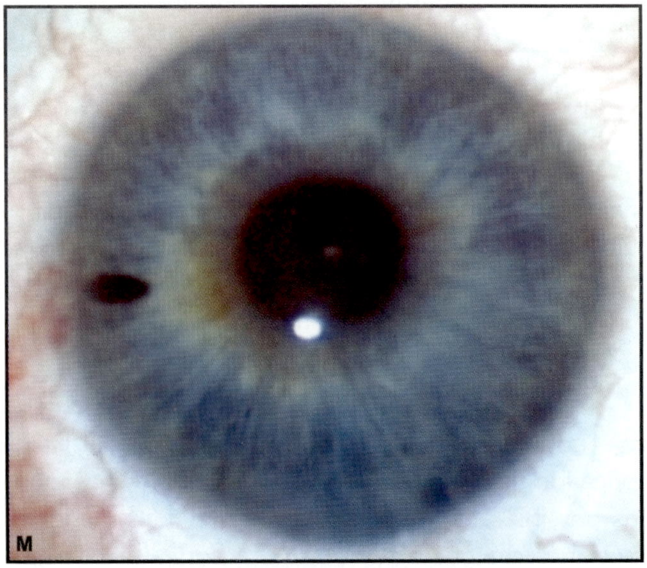

Figure 17.12M: No stitches are needed

Patch

Placing a patch on the eye is not obligatory.

OPERATIVE COMPLICATIONS

Implant Damage

Damage to the implant can occur during its insertion into the AC if the special forceps are not used. It can also happen during its release and manipulation under the iris. Both the surgeon and the technician must be very careful when the lens is taken from the package and inserted into the forceps. Do not forget that the implant is very thin and rather expensive and can be damaged easily.

Hemorrhage

Bleeding can occur during the manual surgical iridectomy. It should not be common. If happens, it is recommended injecting some viscoelastic through the paracentesis and wait several minutes for the bleeding to stop, then remove it.

Iris Damage

It is possible to damage the posterior pigment surface of the iris with the implant, so we recommend injecting viscoelastic under the iris to avoid this complication. The surgeon has to be very careful during the manual iridectomy:

1. Don't pull and tear the iris strenuously through the paracentesis; this can cause iris damage and actual bleeding,
2. But, be sure that the iridectomy is completely open including the pigmentary surface of the iris, to prevent postoperative pupillary block.

Lens Damage

The worst complication that the surgeon can have during the actual procedure is the immediate creation of lens damage and a cataract. One must always be ready to convert the surgery (in case of lens damage) to phacoemulsification with IOL implantation.

The lens can be damaged in the following steps of the surgery:

1. Corneal Incisions: due to sudden knife insertion or eyeball movement.
2. Paracentesis: due to insufficient viscoelastic in the AC, too quick blade movement, or eyeball movement.
3. Implant Insertion: due to contact between the forceps and the anterior capsule of the lens.
4. Implant manipulation: due to pushing the implant on the lens.
5. Viscoelastic removal: due to inadvertent movement of irrigation or aspiration needle, and excessively forceful BSS irrigation.

Endothelial Damage

Inadequate viscoelastic protection may allow endothelial cell damage during the implant insertion. It is necessary to be sure to avoid contact of the forceps with the endothelium. The implant lens is soft, but it is made of silicone and studies have shown that silicone contact can be damaging to endothelial cells. My experience has shown, however that even if the edge of the lens touches the endothelium damage has not been noticed. This may be due to the high endothelial cell density in this age range.

Zonular Fiber Damage

Pushing the implant too strenuously under the iris may cause the edge of the implant to damage the zonular fibers. We have to remember that there are a large number of zonular fibers that stretch across the anterior periphery of the lens capsule. This could lead to implant dislocation and optic zone decentration in the future. That is why we try to fold and then release the implant allowing it to go under the iris never pushing it there with force.

UNUSUAL SITUATIONS AND POSTOPERATIVE COMPLICATIONS

IOP Increase on First or Second Day PO

The patient feels pain in the eye, complains of vision loss, or headache in the temple.

Slit-lamp examination: The chamber may be shallow, pupil doesn't react to light or is sluggish, residual viscoelastic is noted in the AC or PC, the gap between the PRL and the anterior capsule is larger.

Be sure to check the patency of the iridectomy (visual and red reflex).

What to do?

a. Treat the iridectomy: if it is small or closed by making it larger or making an additional one (possible YAG).
b. Residual viscoelastic in the chamber: Diamox up to 1.0 g. a day and keep the pupil dilated to help reabsorb the viscoelastic. Use betablocker drops until the pressure is normalized.

Four cases of increased IOP were observed at the 1 week postoperative visit. The increased IOP ranged from 21 to 27 mm Hg. All four cases were treated topically with timoptol ophthalmic drops and oral acetazolamide (Diamox). At the next (2 weeks) postoperative visit IOP was within normal limits (17 mm Hg or less) for all four cases.

Pupilary block was observed in one eye 3 weeks postoperatively. The iridectomy was surgically enlarged, which relieved the pupilary block. No further recurrence was observed in this case. This case occurred with a II generation lens.

Traumatic Cataract (Lens Damage during Surgery)

What to do?

Be ready to convert the procedure to phaco with IOL implantation, keep an IOL ready in the OR with all IOL power calculations done in advance.

Subcapsular Opacity

So far, we have only one case of a subcapsular opacity 13 month after the surgery.

The patient lost 1 line of the BCVA and has poorer contrast sensitivity. In the future phacoemulsification with IOL may be necessary (Figure 17.13).

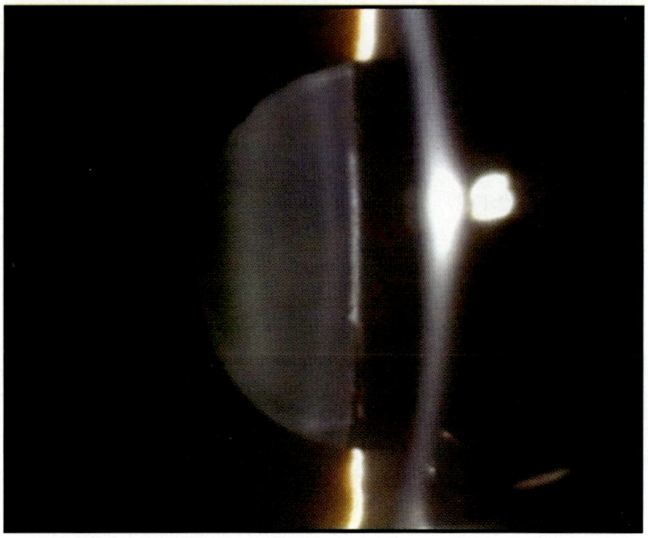

Figure 17.13: Capsular opacification 13 months PO

Iridocyclitis Early Postoperative

This is very rare, but more common in hyperopic eyes (3 cases.)

Patient complains that the vision is decreasing, but no pain.

Slit-lamp exam: Flare and cell in AC, some synechiae noted between the PRL and the pupil, the pupil is small and it is not easy to dilate it.

What to do?

Steroids + atropine + adrenaline subconjunctival injection, systemic steroids, and maximum mydriasis is needed.

We have had 3 such cases, 2 of them occurred in the same patient who had both eyes implanted. Using the above treatment, we achieved a normal result within 2 to 3 days. We do not yet know the reason for this complication, but all of them were hyperopic eyes and occurred approximately one to two months after surgery. So far, we consider this type of reaction as a sterile iridocyclitis with low pigment dispersion (Figure 17.14). Perhaps some implant surface problem was present. An unsmooth surface might have irritated the posterior surface of the iris and started a mechanism of sterile inflammation. We didn't exchange the implants in these 3 cases and there are no further reactions or cataract formations up to now.

Implant decenteration occurred in 4 eyes of 3 patients that had negative power II generation lenses implanted, one patient had implant decenteration of both operated eyes (Figure 17.15). All four decentered lenses were exchanged for the III generation implant. Design changes in the III generations implants were made to improve its centration and avoid decenteration of its OZ (Table 17.4).

Table 17.4: Adverse events and complications

Adverse event	*Number of occurrences*	*% Incidence (n/N) N=122*	*Implant generation*
Corneal edema after one month	0	0.00%	
Hyphema	0	0.00%	
Macular edema	0	0.00%	
Raised IOP requiring treatment in early postop period (≤ 1 month)	4	3.28%	II/III
Raised IOP persistent	0	0.00%	
Pupilary block	1	0.82%	II
Retinal detachment	0	0.00%	
Cataract	1	0.82%	
Non specific inflammatory reaction	3	2.45%	II
Implant decentration	4	3.27%	II
Endoftalmitis	0	0.00%	
Iridocyclitis	3	2.45%	II
Pigment dispertion	1	0.8%	III

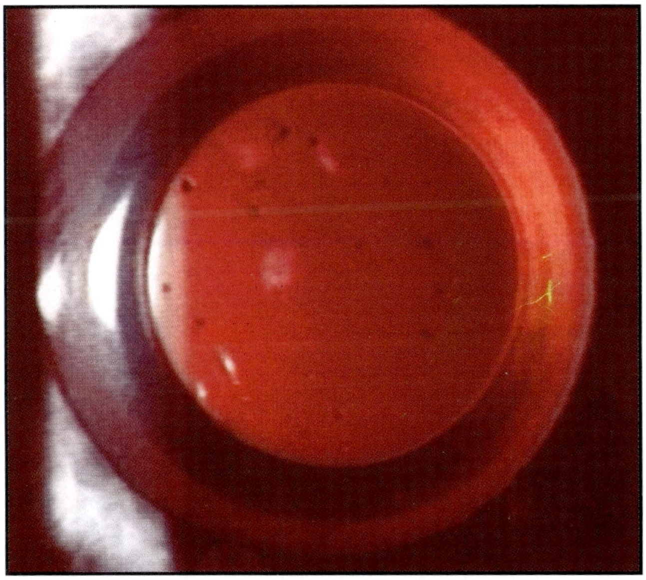

Figure 17.14: Pigment dispertion, (YAG iridectomy performed 1 day before implantation)

RESULTS

The preoperative spherical equivalent refractive error of the patients we have implanted so far were 16 percent from 5 to 7, 37 percent from 7 to 10 D and 47 percent greater than 10 D.

The PO refractive results, of the 122 eyes reported here, were obtained the earliest days after surgery and have not changed substantially to my knowledge. For patients with preoperative astigmatism, AK was performed anywhere from 1 month after the PRL procedure. In 66.1 percent of the cases, we obtained emmetropia. In 26.8 percent we saw a residual under-correction (myopia) of no greater than –1.00 D and 7.1 percent of the eyes needed additional spectacle correction of more than –1.0D and less then –2.5 D (in all 6 eyes the goal was to leave some residual myopia and all of them were presbyopic.). In 46.6 percent of the eyes we achieved no loss of any lines of best corrected visual acuity (BCVA). In 54 percent we noted an increase in lines of vision (increase in BCVA). In 3.3 percent, we lost one line of BCVA. Postoperative UCVA was superior to preoperative BCVA in 55.1 percent (66/122) of the cases. None of the eyes had UCVA worse than 20/200 at the last postoperative visit.

In the 26 eyes that required a PRL exchange due to dislocation, only two are included in this study, but we achieved the same best-corrected vision as before the first surgery in all 26. The average endothelial cell loss (including patients to whom two procedures were performed) is 4.87 percent. This is not different than reported with cataract surgery. All the children with amblyopia improved their best corrected vision after six months postoperatively and occlusion therapy (Tables 17.5 to 17.7).

negative-powered silicon PRLs but some slow dispersion in the positive-powered PRLs. The UBM ultrasound study showed us that the implant does not touch the anterior capsule, but we need to know more about contact between the PRL and the capsule and iris.

The goal of any refractive procedure is emmetropia, and the predictability of the PRL implantation is very promising in providing stable long-term emmetropia.

The most important point concerning PRL implantation is it reversibility. There are no refractive procedures which can be reversed. With the promising results, and more modern materials, surgical and diagnostic equipment, it will be one of the most exciting areas of ocular surgery.

PEDIATRIC USAGE

In cases of high unilateral myopia in children, PRL implantation can be used instead of amblyopia treatment with aniseikonic spectacles or forcing a contact lens.

The youngest patient in which we have implanted a myopic PRL was –14.00 D at the age of seven. Twenty months PO, 20/40 vision without correction was obtained in this amblyopic eye which was 20/100 best corrected preoperatively. There are not many reasonable alternatives today to help these young patients. Spectacle correction is practically impossible and it is not easy to make them wear contact lenses. These eyes are destined to become strabismic with deep amblyopia for life. With PRL implantation, we cannot only correct myopia but treat amblyopia and prevent strabismus. We prefer and recommend performing scleral reinforcing surgery one to two months prior to implantation for the purpose of slowing the growth of the eyeball. Even if the refractive error changes when the child grows to adulthood, the PRL implant can be easy exchanged and the procedure can be repeated.

We are planing to start correcting hyperopia in the near future, but up to now, we don't have any clinical experience in hyperopic correction with PRL implantation in children. The surgical technique is the same that we use for our adult patients. The only difference is that general anesthesia is recommended, and manual iridectomy at the time of surgery is preferable.

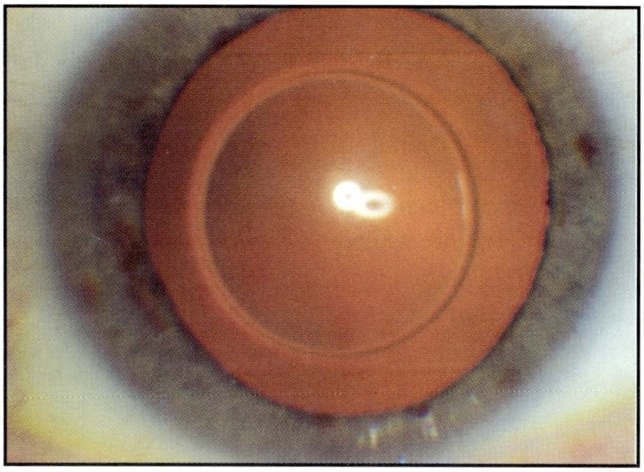

Figure 17.16: Myopic PRL

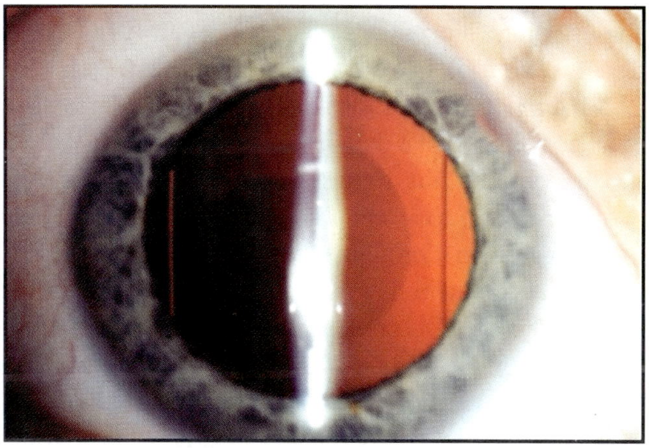

Figure 17.17: Hyperopic PRL

FUTURE APPLICATIONS

Piggy Back Over IOLS

When two IOLs are necessary, it is certainly conceivable that the second lens could be a posterior chamber PRL that could be easily inserted in the capsular bag or in the ciliary sulcus. In such special eyes that require piggyback lenses the calculations of IOL power are often not as accurate and it may be necessary to exchange the more anterior lens. A PRL is much easier to remove and replace than an IOL is (Figures 17.16 and 17.17).

Pseudophakic Ametropia Correction

Every patient who is unhappy with the refractive results of their cataract/IOL surgery could be offered a rather simple procedure of posterior chamber PRL implantation over the top of the IOL. This would open a whole new market for the anterior segment surgeon and replace the dangers inherent in removing and replacing a well-placed IOL in the bag. Patients could be almost assured of obtaining the refractive result they desire.

Those patients who wish to try monovision could have the nondominant eye implanted with an additional appropriate plus power PRL over the emmetropic IOL. If they could not tolerate the monovision, the PRL could be easily and atraumatically slipped out.

Multifocal Correction

The posterior chamber PRL could open two fronts in the use of multifocal IOLs:

1. Any and all patients could try the concept by having an emmetropic IOL implanted with a multifocal PRL placed on top of it during their cataract removal. After the patient has had sufficient time to become accustomed to it, they could decide whether they wish to keep it or have it easily slipped out.
2. All patients who have missed the chance for getting a multifocal IOL could now have a multifocal PRL placed on top of their IOL to try it out. Again, if they didn't like it, it could be easily removed. Perhaps any over or under-correction in the original IOL could also be taken into account in the PRL distance power.

PRL IMPLANTATION FOR THE CORRECTION OF HIGH AMETROPIA

Informed Consent

All visual errors can be corrected by refractive surgery. The most advantageous application of surgery, apart from the simple esthetic-practical aspects of being able to abandon the use of spectacles and contact lenses, are the ocular and environmental conditions that prevent the optimal use of visual capacity. This understanding is critical for the high dioptric values of the visual error that tie the patient tightly to the vision-aid, in the marked differences in refraction between one eye and an other, limit binocular vision and the visual field, particularly where there is intolerance to comfortable contact lenses wearing and in some types of activity where the traditional optical aids are unquestionably contraindicated.

According to the specialist who has been treating you, you may benefit from the implantation **of a so-called Phakic Refractive Lens**, a soft, flexible implant inserted surgically inside the eye, between iris and the crystalline.

This technique, when performed correctly, has the following **advantages:**

1. The operation is rapid. It lasts 10 to 15 minutes. It is performed in day-hospital on outpatient basis, under topical anesthesia, more specifically with the sole instillation of anesthetic eyedrops and peri-ocular infiltration of anesthetic. The PRL is implanted through a small self-sealing incision measuring about 3.0 mm that normally does not require sutures. The lens is inserted with a special forceps, if it is necessary the PRL can be removed through the same incision, restoring the clinical situation and the refraction as before.
2. It is reversible technique: contrary to what happens with the corneal refractive surgery (incisional or laser), the natural structures of the eye are not modified in a unidirectional manner.
3. Visual rehabilitation is rapid. The patient can normally appreciate the visual result the next day of the surgery and the result is stable in time. We didn't see the cases of vision fluctuation, it is no regression of the obtained result in follow-up.
4. The predictability of the results is high.

The Risks and Possible Problems

1. Some patients, with particularly large pupils under low light conditions complain of haloes with night vision, similar to those reported by contact lens wearers, but the brain usually adapts to this problem during the first 2 to 6 months after the surgery.
2. In order to avoid pupilary block and intaocular pressure increase after the PRL implantation ,the periphery iridectomy will be performed (small hole in the iris) or during the surgery or by YAG laser 1 week before the procedure.
3. As we are dealing with a surgical operation that requires the eyeglobe to be opened, and even through very small incisions, the risk of infection persists. In order to avoid this potentially complication

pre and postoperative prophylaxis is necessary. (Drops installation, oral medications or I/M injections in some cases).The slight inflammation is possible in immediate postoperative period.

4. The implantation of PRL runs the risk of developing opacities in the crystalline lens (cataract) in time. It should be remembered that in subjects with serious errors, especially myopic ,the risk of developing a natural cataract is much higher and more precocious than in the 'normal' population. Moreover, the surgical replacement of the cataractous lens is now considered to be a routine technique, it is well-known, safe and simple, and in the vast majority of cases produces excellent results, with simultaneous correction of the myopia and the removal of the cataract.
5. There is also possible that the PRL may provoke intraocular pressure increase. In the more serious cases, the patient may feel severe pain along the trigeminal nerve irradiating from the eye to the forehead, accompanied by nausea and vomiting. This situation should be treated immediately with the oral medicamentations and drops.

Issued by Dr Dimitrii Dementiev.

The undersigned, expressing his/her full, free, unconditioned will,

First Name and Family name of patient

....

Date and Place of birth

....

Place of residence

....

Consent of the surgery of the PRL implantation. He/she declares that the information provided regarding the implications of the operation has been full and thorough. He/she declares that he/she has carefully evaluated the possible benefits and potential risks inherent to this type of surgery.

Signature of patient ....

Date..

BIBLIOGRAPHY

1. Alberti M. PRK and Lasik Versus Intraocular Contact Lenses for High Myopia Correction ASCRS Annual Meeting, Boston, USA 1998.
2. Apple DJ. Complications of Phakic IOL,s AAO annual meet New Orleans 1998.
3. Asseto, Benedetti, Pesando. Collamer intraocular contact lens to correct high myopia. J Cataract Refract Surg 1996;22.
4. Avalos G. Comparison Between LASIK and Phakic Posterior Chamber Intraocular Lenses in High Myopia and High Hyperopia ASCRS annual meet, San Diego, USA 1998.
5. Avalos G. Silicone Posterior Chamber Intraocular Lens (P-PCIOL) in the management of LASIK complications ASCRS Annual Meet, San Diego, USA 1998.
6. Baikoff G, Colin J. Intraocular lenses in phakic patients Ophtalmol Clin North Am 1992;5.
7. Baikoff G, et al. Angle fixated Anterior Chamber Lens for Myopia of –7.0 to –19.0 Diopters. Jornal of Refractive Surgery 1998;14:(3).
8. Baikoff G, Joly P. Comparison of minus power anterior chamber intraocular lenses and myopic epikeratoplasty in phakic eyes. Refract Corneal Surgery 1990;6:252-60.
9. Baikoff G. 5 years follow-up on anterior chamber phakic IOLs Chiron's ZB5-XXVIII International Congress of Opathalmology, Amsterdam, 1998.
10. Baikoff G. Antrior Chamber Phakic IOLs AAO Annual Meeting, New Orleans,USA 1998.
11. Baikoff G. Contrast sensitivity in patients with PRK in one eye and refractive implant in the fellow eye, Last evaluation of the Phakic Myopic Baikoff lens ASCRS Annual Meeting, Boston, USA 1997.
12. Brauweiler P, Busin M, Wehler T. High incidence of cataract formation after implantation of a silicon Posterior Chamber Lens in Phakic, highly myopic eyes AAO Annual Meeting, New Orleans, USA 1998.
13. Brown D. Use of the STAAR Surgical Implantable Contact Lens for High Myopia ASCRS Annual Meeting, Boston USA 1997.
14. Chatitterjee A, Shah S. Predictability of spherical PRK based on initial refraction. Jornal of Refractive Surgery 1998;14:(2 suppl).
15. Davidorf JM, Zaldivar R, Oscherow S. Posterior Chamber Phakic Intraocular Lenses for Hyperopia of +4 to +11 Diopters and Posterior Chamber Phakic Intraocular lenses for Myopia of –8.0 to –19.0 Diopters. J Refract Surg 1998;14:3.
16. Dementiev D, Rozakis G, Hatsis A, Hoffer K, Sborgia G, Marucchi P. The 5 Years Experience in the Phakic Refractive Posterior Chamber IOL Implantation for the correction of High Ametropia Binkhorst Symposium during XXVIII International Congress of Ophtalmology, Amsterdam, Holland 1998.
17. Dementiev D. Comparison of tree generations of Posterior Chamber Phakic Lenses for the Correction of high myopia and hypropia, ASCRS, Boston, USA 1997.

18. Dementiev D. Silicone Phakic Posterior Chamber Intraocular Lens (P-PCIOL) and the management of pediatric Anisometropia. ASCRS annual meeting, San Diego, USA 1998.
19. Fechner PU. Intraocular lenses for the correction of myopia in phakic eyes: Short long success and long-term caution. Refract Corneal Surgery 1990;6:242-4.
20. Fechner PU. Phakic IOLs is promising for high myopia by Schonfeld AR. Ocular Surgery News 1993,4:12.
21. Fyodorov, Zuev Tumanian, Suheil. Clinical and functional follow up of minus IOL implantation in high-grade myopia. Ophtalmosurgery 1993;2:12-7.
22. Fyodorov, Zuev, Aznabaev. Intraocular correction of high myopia with negative posterior chamber lens. Ophtalmosurgery 1991;3:57-8.
23. Gelender H. Corneal endothelial cell loss, cystoid Macular Edema, and iris- suported intraocular lenses. Ophtalmology 1984;91:841-6.
24. Grabby, Deitz, Fyodorov. Staar implantable contact lens (ICL). In: Martin RG, Dills JP, Sanders DR (Eds): Foldable Intraocular Lenses. Slack, INC, Thorafare, 1993;251-5.
25. Guell JL. Cataract formation after phakic IOL Implantation, World Refractive Surgery Symposium,Orlando in Eurotimes 1998;15.
26. Hatsis A. Phakic Posterior IOLs for the correction of high Hyperopia and high Myopia, ASCRS, Boston,USA 1997.
27. Hatsis A. Silicone posterior chamber intraocular lens (P-PCIOL), American Blind Eye Study. ASCRS Annual Meet, San Diego, USA 1998.
28. Hodkin M, Lemos MM, McDonald MB, Holladay J, Shhidi SH. Near vision sensitivity after photorefractive keratectomy. J Cataract Refractive Surgery 1997;23:2.
29. Hoffer KJ. Predicting silicone phakic posterior chamber IOL power in the management of high hyperopia ASCRS Ann. Meet, San Diego, USA 1998.
30. Holladay JT. Refractive power calculation for intraocular lenses in the phakic eye. Amer J Ophthalmol 1993;116 (2A):63-6.
31. Izak M. Worst Myopia Iris Claw IOL implantation ASCRS Annual Meeting, Boston, USA 1997.
32. Kanski J. Clinical Ophthalmology. Butterworth Ltd, 1989; 360. In: Woo GC, Wilson MA (Eds): Current methods of treating and preventing myopia. Optometry and Vision Science 1990;67(9):719-27.
33. Kariger U. Refractive Baikoff anterior chamber lenses implantation, ASCRS 1997.
34. Landesz M, Worst JGF, Siertsema JV, Van Rij G. Correction of high myopia with the worst myopia claw intraocular lens" XXVIII International Congress Ophtalmology, Amsterdam, Holland 1998.
35. Lavery F. Laser *in situ* keratomilesusis for myopia. Journal of Refractive Surgery 1998;14:2.
36. Luger MHA. The Staar Collamer phakic posterior chamber IOL to correct myopia and hyperopia, XXVIIIth ICO, Amsterdam 1998.
37. Marinho A, et al. Phakic IOLs: The state of the art. ASCRS annual meeting, Saqn Diego, USA 1998.
38. Marinho A, Neves MC, Pinto MC, Fernando Vaz. Posterior chamber silicone phakic intraocular lens. Jorn Refrac Surg 1997;13:3.
39. Pallicaris I. Barraquer lecture AAO Annual Meeting, San Francisco, USA 1997.
40. Rozakis G, Dementiev D, Avalos G, Hatsis A. Complications of Silicone Phakic Posterior Chamber Intraocular Lens (P-PCIOL) for the Correction of High Ametropia. ASCRS annual meet, San Diego, USA 1998.
41. Rozakis G, Dementiev D, Hatsis A, Avalos G. Complications of Silicon Phakic Posterior Chamber Lenses for the Correction of high ammetropia. ASCRS, San Diego, USA 1998.
42. Saragoussi JJ, et al. Damage to the Corneal Endothelium by minus Power Anterior Chamber Intraocular Lenses Refract Corneal Surg 1991;7.
43. Saragoussi JJ, Puech M, Assouline M, Reard G, Pouliquen Y. Ultrasound biomicroscopy of Baikoff Anterior Chamber Phakic Intraocular Lenses Jornal of Refractive Surgery, 1997;13:2.
44. Sosnier Z. Evaluation of the effect of Synder-Thompson scleroplasty based on the behavior of the axial dimension of the eye ball. Klin Oczna 1989;91:19-20.
45. Strampelli B. Supportalita di lenti acriliche in camera anteriore nella afachia e nai vizi di r refrazione Ann Ottalmol Clin Oculist 1954;80:70-82.
46. Tarutta E, Saksanova E. Peripheral segments of the fundus oculi in highly myopic patients after scleroplasty. Vestn Opht 1991;107(4):19-23.
47. Tereschenko A. Complications of minus silicone Posterior Chamber Phakic Lenses ASCRS Annual Meet, Boston, USA 1997.
48. Tratta E, Shamlokova E. An analysis of the late results of scleroplasty in progressive myopia. Ophthal Zh 1989; (4):204-7.
49. Tumanian E, Zuev VK, Koslova TV. Hydrodynamics Before and After Implantation of Negative IOL in Highly Myopic Phakic Eye. Ophtalmosurgery 1997;4:50-6.
50. Tumanian E. Surgical correction of high myopia by the method of implantation of negative phakic IOL. In Russian, Diss Kand Medic 1989;158-64.
51. Vorotnikova K, Kurenkov VV, Polunin GS. Retreatment of Regression after photorefractive keratectomy for myopia. Jornal of Refractive Surgery, 1998;14:(2 suppl).
52. Wang Y, Zhao K, Wang H. Histopatoplgy of corneal wound healing after PRK in rabbit eyes. Jornal of Refractive Surgery 1998;14:2.
53. Werblin T. Barraquer lecture AAO Annual Meeting, New Orleans, USA 1998.
54. Worst J. Phakic high myopia correction. ASCRS Meet, Boston 1997.
55. Worst JGF. Iris Anatomy and its Surgical Implications XXVIII International Congress of Ophtalmology, Amsterdam, Holland 1998.

56. Worst JGF. Recent improvements in phakic refrative correction with Iris Claw Lens ASCRS Annual Meeting, San Diego, USA 1998.
57. Zaikova M, Molokova N. Scleroplasty results in progressive myopia with use of allogenic. Vestn Opht 1990;106(3):16-9.
58. Zaldivar R, Davidorf J, Osheraw S. Intarocular contact lens in Lasik 2000. In: Buratto L, Ferrari M, Fabiano (Eds): Belbo (CN), 1998;359-75.

18

Phakic Intraocular Surgery in Hyperopia

- CHALLENGES IN HYPEROPES
- LASIK VS. PHAKIC IOLs IN HYPEROPIA
- CONTRAINDICATIONS TO PIOL
- PROPER SELECTION AND ASSESSMENT OF PATIENTS
- CHOICE OF LENSES
- SPECIFIC COMPLICATIONS IN HYPEROPIC ARTISAN LENS IMPLANTATION

Jorge L Alio (Spain), Hany S Elsaftawy (Egypt)

INTRODUCTION

The surgical correction of hyperopia, especially for medium to high hyperopic errors, has been a continuous challenge in refractive surgery . A safe, efficient, and predictable refractive surgical technique has been sought as a solution for patients with high hyperopia or induced hyperopia from previously unsuccessful refractive corneal surgery.[1]

Years ago, different techniques were described to steepen the central cornea, as with electro coagulation to shrink peripheral corneal collagen or with para-central hexagonal keratotomy,[2] to decouple the central cornea biomechanically from the periphery, had limited applicability because of its reduced predictability, induction of astigmatism, loss of spectacles-corrected visual acuity and high complication rate.[2-4]

Other surgical techniques such as keratoplasty, keratomileusis, and epikeratoplasty were quickly abandoned due to technical difficulties or complications.[3]

Laser thermal keratoplasty (LTK) with the holmium laser, is not suitable in high hyperopia due to regression, especially in young patients.[3,4] Fyodorov proposed radial thermal keratoplasty, but had unpredictable results.[7,8] The use of thermal keratoplasty either with Holmium laser (LTK), diode laser, or conductive keratoplasty needle are not suitable for hyperopia of more than +3.00 D, and usually are not effective in young patients as they are affected by regression.[4,5,19] In addition, laser in situ keratomileusis (LASIK) results are good only in eyes with low to medium hyperopia.[10,17]

Refractive lensectomy mutilates the natural lens and does not preserve accommodation.[11] Hence, high hyperopia, more than +5.00 dioptres (D) of cycloplegic refraction, remains a consistent unsolved problem in refractive surgery.

For high hyperopia correction, the surgeon can increase the refractive power of the eye in four ways: increase the axial length of the eye, modify the curves of corneal surface, modify the intraocular refraction index, or add a new optical system to the eye. The latter seems to be the only successful alternative.[4]

Improvements in instrumentation, surgical technique, and quality of the optical design of phakic intraocular lenses (PIOLs) have improved expectations in the use of intraocular lenses for the correction of high refractive errors The development of new intraocular surgical techniques including corneal incisions, new biomaterials, and sutures, has resulted in new and better intraocular lenses that have favorably changed expectations for intraocular lenses in the correction of high refractive errors.[4]

The implantation of anterior or posterior chamber intraocular lenses in phakic eyes is now an alternative that has good results in high errors , and a low complication rate.[12,13]

Worst and Fechner introduced the iris claw anterior chamber lens for the correction of high myopia in 1990, with initial satisfactory results.[14]

CHALLENGES IN HYPEROPES

The decision to perform intraocular phakic lens surgery for hyperopia should satisfy certain medical requirements, such as patient desire not to use spectacles or contact lenses, and adequate comprehension of the medical implications of phakic IOLs, evidenced by signing a written informed consent.[15]

The best patients are usually young individuals able to fully exploit their crystalline lens powers to accommodate. In patients aged 50 and over, with severe accommodation loss , the cost/benefit ratio (possible extra-risk of angle closure glaucoma, early lens opacities, and benefits of implanting an accommodative or multifocal IOL after clear lens extraction) is fully explained to the patient.[16]

Due to the lack of technologies able to accurately measure the sulcus-to-sulcus (S-to-S) distance and the posterior chamber volume, there is no perfect anatomic correspondence between external linear measurements and internal distances and spaces, therefore, the crucial role of a proper sizing must be stressed in hyperopic eyes, with particular attention must be paid to the biometric evaluation of the anterior segment to identify flat corneas, shallow chambers and narrow irido-corneal angles.[17]

Pupillometry must be performed as it can predict the potential for visual symptoms in dim light conditions. In our experience, the diameter of the optic(5.5-mm) matched well the mesopic pupil diameter (on average:

5.7 ± 0.5 mm) and the percentage of patients complaining of halos, star bursting, disks, and glare is significantly lower than in the myopic population, in a perfectly centred lens.[18]

Anterior chamber depth (ACD) and axial length measurements can be measured by resorting to optical (IOL Master, Zeiss; Depth Measuring Device II, Haag-Streit; EAS 1000, Nidek; Orbscan II, Bausch and Lomb) or ultrasound A-scan techniques where as for ACD, we like the precision provided by Orbscan´s tomographic analysis of anterior segment structures,[19,20] allowing for point-to-point 3-D scanning measurements to create anterior chamber geometry maps. Peripheral data of the chamber volume, the corneal thickness, and the endothelium-to-iris and endothelium-to-anterior lens surface distances are particularly appreciated.

For those surgeons lacking access to high-frequency ultrasound or the newest optical equipment we provide a sizing special nomogram based on the regression analysis of two variables: W-to-W and anterior chamber depth (Table 18.1). It is valid for hyperopic implantations only.[15]

Table 18.1: Sizing nomogram for hyperopic ICLs

ACD (mm) (Central endothelium to anterior crystalline lens distance)	Overall Length (mm)
2.8–2.9	W-to-W- 0.6
3.0–3.1	W-to-W- 0.4
3.2	W-to-W- 0.2
≥ 3.2	W-to-W

According to Staar guidelines (Table 18.2), the external horizontal white-to-white (W-to-W) distance is the crucial element in the choice of the overall lens length by applying the " golden rule": W-to-W minus 0.5 mm = Overall Diameter.

Since ICHs are available in 0.5-mm steps, with intermediate values (for example, W-to-W = 12.35 and ACD = 2.9 mm, overall length = 11.75 mm), the space of the irido-corneal angle is taken into consideration. If its opening is wider than 0.6-mm, the 12.0-mm overall length is chosen; if it is narrower than 0.6-mm, the 11.50-mm length is preferred.[15]

Table 18.2: Guidelines by the manufacturer for ICH implantations (Staar Inc.)

- Age = 18 and = 55
- Hyperopia >+ 4.50 D or other LASIK contraindications.
- Anterior Chamber depth (ACD) = 2.8 mm
- Endothelial cell count (ECC) = 2500 cells/mm^2
- No crystalline opacity
- No relevant eye disease as glaucoma (even borderline cases) and uveitis

As regarding the endothelial cell count, the qualitative-quantitative analysis of the endothelial cell population is a basic standard to evaluate the quality of intraocular surgery, including ICL implantation.[18] Taking the physiological cell deprivation observed over time into consideration, we refer to age-adjusted personal criteria for establishing the minimum endothelial cell count:

- 20 years of age: = 2500 cells/mm^2.
- 30 years of age: = 2200 cells/mm^2.
- 40 years of age: = 2000 cells/mm^2.

The anterior chamber angle examination in our opinion, becomes now a prospective prerequisite for phakic IOL implantation surgery in hyperopes. An angle of grade GII or less (according to Scheie's classification) is considered a contraindication for ICH implantation since the main risk seems to be an acute or subacute angle closure glaucoma in the postoperative periods. The Urrets.Zavalia Syndrome,[21] the ischemic paresis of the iris sphincter muscle occurring at night without pain or other symptoms, has been observed after ICH implantation (0.9% in our series). Intermittent or subacute, prolonged angle closure episodes with IOP rise cause a " blown" pupil of 7 to 7.5-mm in diameter with direct an indirect areflesia. Problems are both cosmetic an functional (mainly halos), given the "edge" effect of the 5.5-mm ICH optical zone.

However, the peculiar anatomic shape and size of the hyperopic anterior segment, combined with the continuous growth of the crystalline lens and the modified relationship among anterior segment structures over time probably limit phakic IOL technology and are almost impossible to overcome.[55]

The preoperative assessment of the planned lens vaulting is critical to avoiding concerns, such as endothelial cell loss, cataract, and glaucoma from significant aqueous flow disruption, anterior and posterior synechiae, iris ischemia and pigment dispersion. The choice of overall length, central and peripheral thickness of the optic geometry (front and base curve) and elasticity of the material will be the crucial factors.[22] The higher anterior vaulting provided by the last version(V4) of the ICL permits the physiological turnover of the nutrients through the aqueous flow, and does not disturb the metabolism of the subcapsular epithelium.[15]

Given the lack of statistical correlation between the external W-to-W or other empirical "golden rules" or nomograms. The ideal situation would be to measure angle-to-angle and/or S-to-S directly and enable a predictable clearance between phakic IOL and inner structures (corneal endothelium, central iris, crystalline lens anterior surface) by using sophisticated technologies (high frequency ultrasonographers, like the I^3 ABD™ by innovative, or the Artemis 2™ by Ultralink, the computerized Scheimpflug camera, the EAS 1000™ by Nidek, and the optical coherence tomography, the OCT™.[23]

LASIK VS. PHAKIC IOLs IN HYPEROPIA

LASIK is now the standard of care in corneal refractive surgery, and in some centres is the only refractive procedure performed. But is LASIK a possible option for almost all the refractive errors? . As with PRK, LASIK has been suggested to treat an important range of myopia (–1.00 to –20.00 D) and of hyperopia (+1.00 to +6.00 D).[24,25] However, important complications have led most surgeons to lower dramatically the limits of LASIK.

LASIK became the most popular form of refractive surgery until now, both for ophthalmologists and the general public mostly for the following reasons:

a. Easy surgery
b. Associated with few complications during surgery and immediate postoperatively
c. Almost no pain
d. Extremely rapid recovery of vision.

In hyperopia, the laser ablates tissue in an annular form, leaving the center undisturbed, inducing the following changes:

a. The central cornea becomes steeper (increases curvature)
b. No change in thickness in the central cornea.

Laser ablation, not only changes corneal thickness, but also changes corneal shape. It flattens the cornea in myopia and steepens it in hyperopia. Moreover, it changes the normal aspheric form of the cornea, creating new edges (transition zones of the present day lasers minimize this effect, but do not annul it). The normal cornea has a curvature between 39 and 46 D. A cornea with a curvature of more than 47 D is considered a keratoconus suspect and should not be ablated . The physical properties of the cornea allows us to flatten it to a maximum of 34D and to steepen it to a maximum of 48 D. Exceeding this range leads to important regression (due to "biological memory" of the corneal tissue) and important visual aberrations (due to dramatic change in corneal shape.[26]

If LASIK is the state of the art for corneal refractive surgery, the surgical possibilities to change the refractive status of the eye are not confined to the cornea. The lens, the other important refracting surface of the eye, has been manipulated for the correction of myopia for more than 50 years, and more recently for hyperopia. Despite the possibility of easily correcting any spherical ametropia by clear lens exchange with an appropriate posterior chamber IOL, the loss of accommodation and some retinal risks (mainly in myopia) make this type of surgery inadvisable in young patients. On the other hand, clear lens exchange is the procedure of choice in refractive surgery outside the LASIK range in patients 50 or older and in all cases where some form of lens opacity is present.[27]

There is, however, a third option in refractive surgery that does not interfere with the cornea or the lens. It is the placement of an IOL inside the phakic eye. This is called the phakic IOL. However, despite differences between them, phakic IOLs have common characteristics that are important when comparing their performance with LASIK in high ametropias:[28]

a. Phakic IOLs have the potential to correct any ametropia, including astigmatism.
b. The power of a phakic IOL does not depend on tissue healing (no regression).
c. The surgery is reversible.

Table 18.3: Qualitative comparison of LASIK and phakic IOLs

Refractive error treated	–1.00 to –10.00 D	–10.00 to –23.00 D
Myopia	+1.00 to +5.00 D	+5.00 to +12.00 D
Hyperopia	1.0 to 6.00 D	up to 7.00 D (some models)
Astigmatism	Good	Excellent
Stability of refraction	Good to excellent	Good to excellent
Predictability	Under correction, good	Good
Adjustability	No	Yes
Quality of vision	Good	Excellent
Patient satisfaction	High	Very High
Surgical complexity	High	Moderate
Location for surgery	Clean room	Surgical Room
Corneal contour	Abnormal	Normal
Optical aberrations	Moderate	Mild
Cost for surgeon and facility	Very High	Low

To respect the limits of LASIK, almost all eyes with myopias exceeding –12.00 D and hyperopias exceeding +4.00 D are, in one way or another, out of LASIK range[29] (Table 18.3).

Advantages of Phakic IOLs

Phakic IOL implantation has the following advantages:

a. Accuracy and predictability
b. Stability
c. No loss of lines of BCVA
d. Glare and halos are present in some cases (if disabling, explantation is feasible).

CONTRAINDICATIONS TO PIOL

Refractive surgery aims to alter the refractive condition of the eye to eliminate or reduce spherical an cylindrical refraction errors and thus to eliminate or reduce the patient's dependence on optic correction. Thus, refractive surgery usually has no medical indication, but is justified by the patient's desire to eliminate glasses or contact lenses. The ophthalmologist's role should be to perform the necessary medical examinations to verify the correct status of the eye and the absence of contraindications, as well as to indicate the best surgical technique for each case. The ophthalmologist should give a detailed explanation of the advantages and

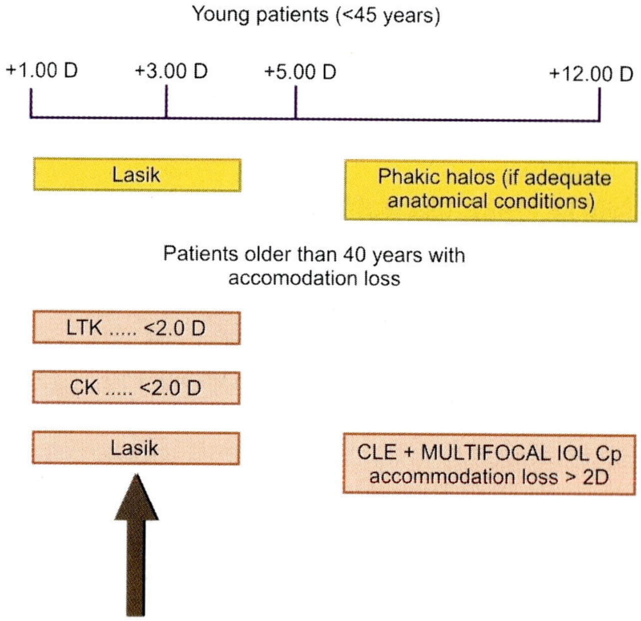

Figure 18.1: Algorithm for the surgical correction of hyperopia: LTK-Laser thermokeratoplasty; CK- Conductive keratoplasty; CLE-Clear lens extraction

disadvantages of surgery and the possible risks and complications, and should make sure that the patient not only understands and assumes them but that he/she has realistic expectations.[30]

In hyperopia, phakic implants are indicated for over +5 D since efficacy, predictability and safety of corneal surgical techniques (LASIK and collagen shrinkage procedures) decrease considerably with hyperopia above 5 D.[16]

We consider phakic IOL implantation to be contraindicated when any of the following conditions are present:

1. Previous intraocular surgery.
2. Evidence of any lens opacity or developing cataract.
3. Glaucoma or ocular hypertension.
4. Personal history of uveitis, intraocular inflammation, pseudoexfoliation or pigmentary dispersion.
5. Personal history of retinal detachment or macular pathology.
6. Chronic infection of the ocular adnexa.
7. Corneal disorders, such as corneal scars, keratoconus or degenerative diseases, and previous corneal or kerato-refractive surgery are only relative contraindications.
8. Endothelial disorders and any infectious or inflammatory corneal conditions that can be reactivated are also a surgical contraindication.
9. One-eyed patients are always a contraindication for this type of surgery, and this includes the fellow eyes of patients with a deep amblyopia.
10. Systemic disorders as pregnancy, diabetes mellitus, autoimmune diseases, immune suppression and severe systemic pathology.[30]

PROPER SELECTION AND ASSESSMENT OF PATIENTS

As in any other refractive procedure, phakic lens implantation should not be performed when the patient is under 21 years of age since the ametropia is generally not stable and the eyeball has not fully developed. However, there are exceptions, such as anisometropic amblyopia, that can justify this type of surgery earlier.[31,32]

In 2002 Alio et al considered as contraindications for hyperopic IOL implantation previous history of iridocyclitis, glaucoma or intraocular pressure higher than 20 mm Hg, cataracts, anterior or posterior synechiae, corneal dystrophy, central endothelial cell count lower than 2250 cells/mm^2, and anterior central chamber depth less than 2.8 mm, associated with normal anterior chamber angle configuration at gonioscopy (at least Grade 3 of Shaffer's classification).[33] Patients with corneal astigmatism > 2.00 D or values between K1 and K2 > 2.00 D were excluded. Eyes that had myopic pupil measurements larger that 6 mm were also excluded.

Preoperative Assessment

All patients should remove contact lenses before preoperative examination to assure that corneal moulding does not affect final refraction and Keratometric measurements.[30]

Every candidate for correction of refractive errors by phakic lens implantation should undergo a general ophthalmic examination to verify the indication and to guarantee that ocular contraindications are not present. The general ophthalmic study should include the following examinations:

- **Uncorrected and best-corrected visual acuity** (UCVA, BCVA), measured by the Snellen's chart.
- **Manifest and cycloplegic refrac**tion, measured on the spectacles plane.
- **Calculation of phakic lens power** is based on the patient's refraction, in contrast with the calculation for a lens used in cataract surgery, for which we only need the keratometry and the axial length. The predictability of the measurement of the corneal curvature by manual keratometry. Automated keratometer, corneal topography, or with the Orbscan anterior segment analysis system, or by the tangential map of the EyeSyes Technologies, Houston, TX, measured at 33 mm-diameter zone.
- **Anterior segment examination** by slit-lamp. Biomicroscopy should be performed with both undilated pupil and in mydriasis. In the preoperative examination, special attention should be given to the condition of the cornea and crystalline lens, eliminating all ocular conditions that could contraindicate the surgery.
- **Gonioscopy** with Goldman's three-mirror lens. Implantation of angle-supported and posterior chamber phakic lenses are only indicated when the anterior chamber angle is open enough, with grade 0 to 1 according to the Scheie's classification, or 3 to 4 according to Shaffer's grading. Generally,

patients with high myopia have an anterior chamber angle with these characteristics, while it is not rare to find hyperopic patients with lower angular openings. The gonioscopy, besides studying the angular opening degree, allows us to verify the normality of the angular structures and the absence of alterations.

- **Intraocular pressure (IOP) measurement** by means of applanation tonometry (Perkins or Goldman). An IOP > 21 mm Hg contraindicates the implantation of any type of phakic lens.
- **Fundus examination** by means of indirect ophthalmoscopy to evaluate the peripheral retina and posterior pole. Prophylactic laser retinal treatment, if needed, should be performed and controlled before any refractive surgery.
- **Pupillary size** and diameter should be measured under photopic, mesopic and scotopic conditions to avoid night aberrations at night when dilatation occurs. Several technologies are introduced in this field as the Colvard's pupillometer and the Orbscan who are likely to be the most accurate up to this date.[34]
- **Measurement of the horizontal corneal diameter (White to White measurement):** Calculation of the lens length for anterior chamber (angle-fixated) and posterior chamber (sulcus-supported) phakic lenses depends on the horizontal corneal diameter (white-to-white distance). This measurement is not necessary for iris claw (iris-fixated) lenses, where one size fits all eyes.
- White-to-White limbal measurement can be performed with a surgical calliper under direct visualization through the operating microscope, under topical anaesthesia. The Holladay-Godwin corneal gauge, a small hexagonal instrument with a series of black half-moons marks varying in diameter from 9.0 to 14.0 mm in 0.5 mm steps, can be used in a similar way. The horizontal white-to-white distance can also be obtained with photographic techniques by the Orbscan anterior segment analysis system, or even with conventional computerized videokeratoscopy.

Based on general studies,[35] a minimum preoperative endothelial density is about 2.250 cells/mm^2 in all patients who are candidates for phakic lens implantation so that the cellular loss due to all the factors mentioned do not lead to corneal decompensation over time.

- **Ultrasound pachymetry**, which has replaced optical pachymetry because of its ease of use, portability, accuracy, and reproducibility, is an additional diagnostic tool in the study of the normal and pathological corneal. Corneal thickness can also be obtained with the Orbscan anterior segment analysis system, which, in addition to the numeric values, provides a pachymetric map of almost the entire cornea on a colored scale that is similar to that used in the conventional corneal topography .
- **Biometry and IOL power calculations**

The power of the lens is accurately calculated by proprietary software based on the Vander Heyde formula (Ophtec BV).

The parameters used for calculation are anterior central chamber depth, angle Keratometric power, and cycloplegic refraction. Anterior chamber depth was measured with an ultrasonic biometer (Ocuscan, Alcon, Ft. Worth, TX). Keratometric power was estimated from the tangential map of corneal topography (EyeSys Technologies, Houston, TX), measured at the 3-mm-diameter zone.

- **Anterior Chamber Depth:** The ACD necessary to implant a phakic lens varies according to the type and model chosen, and this value is provided by the manufacturer. In general, the minimum space between the corneal endothelium and anterior crystalloids necessary to implant a phakic lens is about 2.8 mm (3.2 mm from the corneal surface), with slight variations from one lens to another.[36]

The anterior chamber depth can also be obtained with the Orbscan anterior segment analysis system, a three-dimensional analysis system for the surfaces and structures of the anterior segment. By the Orbscan it is possible to obtain not only the topographic map of the anterior and posterior surfaces of the cornea and the White-to-White distance, but also the corneal thickness and the endothelial-lens surface distance, which converts it into an examination method that is especially suited to the preoperative study of potential phakic implant patients.[37]

- **Ultrasound Biomicroscopy.** UBM is a high resolution technique that allows examination of the anterior segment and peripheral retina.[37,38] It is an ideal method for produce . Its resolution and produce images of the anterior and posterior chamber provide a unique method to test the exact phakic IOL location and its relationship with the adjacent intraocular structures including the cornea, anterior chamber angle, iris, lens, zonules, and ciliary body.[38] UBM also provides reproducible measurements, so it can also be used to measure distances between phakic IOLs and these structures.[39] Therefore, UBM constitutes an important exploratory technique for evaluating aspects related to safety of phakic IOLs.

CHOICE OF LENSES

Currently, phakic IOLs are mainly useful in treating high hyperopia from +5.00 to +12.00 D in young patients while low hyperopia (up to +3.00 D) can be corrected by LTK, CK, or LASIK in patients older than 40 years or by LASIK in young patients. The lower limit for phakic IOLs is the upper limit for LASIK, as previously discussed, and the upper limit is determined by the availability of phakic lenses.

Moderate hyperopia (up to +5.00 D) can also be corrected by LASIK, and high hyperopia in patients older than 45 years can be corrected by clear lens extraction and posterior chamber IOL implantation. Astigmatism correction is also possible with some phakic IOLs (toric phakic IOLs) in addition to high myopia/hyperopia correction.[40]

There are currently three sites of fixation for phakic IOLs: anterior chamber angle, iris surface, and posterior chamber. Phakic IOLs are usually classified according to these sites of fixation:

a. **Angle-supported anterior chamber phakic IOLs.** This group includes phakic anterior chamber IOLs with 4- or 3-point fixation in the anterior chamber angle.
b. **Iris-fixated phakic IOLs.** These lenses are based on the lobster claw design proposed originally by Worst in 1977 and modified for phakic refractive purposes. Iris-fixated lenses have two diametrically opposed claw haptics that fixate the lens on the iris by enclavation of midperipheral iris stroma.
c. **Posterior chamber phakic IOLs.** This group of lenses are implanted in the posterior chamber, occupying the slit-like potential space between the posterior surface of the iris and the anterior surface of the crystalline lens.

Angle-Supported Anterior Chamber Phakic IOLs

Baikoff Angle-supported Phakic IOLs (ZB, ZB5M, Nuvita)

In 1987 Joly , Baikoff and Bonnet[41] modified the Kelman four-point fixation multiflex implant into a negative biconcave lens for the correction of high myopia. The first generation lens, the ZB lens, was a polymethyl-methacrylate (PMMA) biconcave lens with a 4.5 mm optic, and it was associated with a high endothelial cell loss.[42, 43] Because of these endothelial problems, Baikoff modified the lens design to reduce the possibility of contact with the corneal endothelium. The new design, called ZB5M lens, has a 4-mm biconcave effective optic and is fluorine-treated. Recent clinical studies [44,13] have shown a reduced long-term endothelial cell loss with the ZB5M lens, although night-vision problems and pupil ovalization remained as complications without a clear answer. In order to avoid these complications, a third generation lens was designed, the Nuvita MA20 lens. This is a PMMA lens with a 4.5 mm effective meniscus optic, no optic shoulder, anti-glare edge treatment and larger curved footplates.

The major advantage of such a lens is ease of insertion. A 6-mm incision is made either at the temporal or superior limbus, and viscoelastic is placed in the anterior chamber. The lens is inserted into the inflated anterior chamber with a constricted pupil. A lens glide may be used so that the distal haptics find the proper place in the angle, or the distal haptics can be directly inserted against the peripheral cornea. When this is done, the proximal haptics should be compressed with a smooth forceps so that the distal haptics, once placed in the angle, and a very tiny peripheral iridectomy can be done between the haptics. Alternatively, a peripheral iridectomy can be done with a laser before the surgery.[45]

The ZSAL4/Plus

The ZSAL4/Plus lens, the fifth generation of the ZS series,[46] is a plano-concave lens made of one-piece PMMA. This lens has an effective optical diameter enlarged from 5.0 to 5.3 mm (total optical zone 5.8 mm), keeping the transitional edge of the optic to reduce night halos. The haptic geometry has been improved to increase haptic flexibility and disperse compression forces against angle structures. With this lens night-vision problems and pupil ovalization are rare. This lens is available in 12.0, 12.5 and 13.0 mm overall length, and the lens power also ranges from –6.0 D to –20.0 D, in 0.5 dioptre steps.

Phakic 6, 6H and 6H2 Lens

The Phakic 6 and 6H IOLs (Ophthalmic Innovations International, Ontario, CA, USA) are made of PMMA. The Phakic 6 and 6H (H for heparin coating) have a 1.0 mm vault, optic of 6.0 mm up to –10 dioptres and then 5.5 mm up to –25 dioptres. The haptic sizes range from 11.5 mm to 14.0 mm in increments of 0.5 mm. In addition, the IOL heparin coating is believed to have anti-inflammatory and antibacterial properties. A more recent modification of the footplates and a reduction of the optic edge from 0.77 mm to 0.56 mm in the higher dioptric powers is designated as Phakic 6H2. This lens is available for hyperopic corrections, with lens power ranging from +2.0 D to + 10.0 D.[46]

The hyperopic intraocular contact lens (ICH) optical geometry (thicker in the center, thinner at the periphery) should prevent the central starvation from aqueous pooling frequently seen after myopic implantation with previous ICL models (V2 and V3), thus allowing for an adequate metabolic turnover of the lens subcapsular epithelial cells. For such a reason we plan lower vaulting values (250 to 350 μm) with respect to the corresponding myopic ones.[3]

Posterior Chamber Phakic IOLs

Two different models of posterior chamber phakic IOLs are now commercially-available for hypermetropes, the Implantable Contact Lens (ICL) and the Phakic Refractive Lens (PRL).

Implantable Contact Lens (ICL)

The ICL (Staar Surgical Co., Monrovia, CA, USA) is a single-piece plano-concave plate lens made of Collamer, which is a collagen-polymer constituted by 62.9 percent poly-HEMA (hydrosyethylmethacrylate), 33.4 percent water, 3.4 percent benzophenone and 0.2 and porcine collagen. This " collagen-copolymer" is a soft and elastic material with high light transmittance. Its refractive index is 1.452 at 35°C. The Collamer is highly biocompatible and permeable to gas and metabolites.[60]

The ICL V4, the fourth version available on the market today, has a range of powers from –3.00 to –20.0 D for myopia , and from +3.00 to +17.0 to 13.0 mm, in 0.5 mm steps.[47]

Phakic Refractive Lens (PRL)

The PRL was developed by Medennium Inc. (Irvine, CA, USA) in 1987 based on previous models of posterior chamber phakic Halos introduced by Fyodorov. At present, it is distributed internationally by CIBA Vision (Duluth, GA, USA). The PRL is a single-piece plate lens, made of pure silicone with a refractive index of 1.46. It is soft, elastic and hydrophobic. The optic is biconcave (myopia) or concave-convex (Hyperopia).

The hyperopic implant (PRL-200) has an optic diameter of 4.5 mm, the length of the lens is 10.6 mm, and the lens power ranges from +3.00 to +15.00 D, in 0.5 D steps (maximum hyperopic correction +11.0 D).[60]

Iris Fixated Phakic IOLs

Artisan Iris-fixated Lens

History of iris claw lenses in hyperopia surgery In 1978 Worst developed the iris claw lens in Pakistan to be implanted after intracapsular cataract extraction.[48] This anterior chamber lens is fixated on the iris, leaving the chamber angle free. The diametrically opposed haptics can be "pinched" on the midstromal iris tissue as "claws."

In this way the lens stays fixated on the immobile part of the iris. Many of these lenses have been implanted in Europe and India following cataract surgery with good results.[9]

Artisan TM aphakia IOLs this fixation principle can be applied in many different situations, including: intracapsular cataract extraction for mature lenses, extracapsular cataract extraction for mature lenses, extracapsular cataract extraction, primary and secondary implantation, capsule rupture (backup IOL), triple procedure (Keratoplasty, cataract extraction, and lens implantation), reconstruction of complex anterior chamber damage (custom design with colored haptics), pupil occlusion in case of diplopia (black material), and secondary implant in children (proportionally reduced size IOL).[53]

In 1997 a plus-powered convex-concave lens was introduced to correct phakic hyperopia, the ArtisanTM Hyperopia PIOL. This lens has the same convex-concave configuration. In our opinion the iris claw lens has the highest popularity among all the other types of hyperopic lenses due to the following facts;

- It has no angular support which reduces the possibility of peripheral contact with the corneal endothelium.[52] The anterior chamber angle becomes narrower by age in hyperopes in whom natural lenses are growing in a narrow anterior chamber.
- This PIOL should perform well in patients who have a shallow anterior chamber and a narrow angle such as in high hyperopia in which implantation becomes impossible.[55]
- The iris claw lens has a high rate of efficiency , predictability and safety in correction of hyperopia.[54]
- The lens respects the angle issue which becomes narrower by age ,avoiding angle supported lens complications.
- There is no stress exerted on the Zonules as in posterior chamber IOLs.

The ArtisanTM Toric PIOL for the correction of astigmatism in hyperopes was added in 1999.

In 1980 a modified iris claw lens with an occluding optic was implanted for the first time in an aphakic eye of a patient suffering from untreatable diplopia after cerebral trauma. This lens is still in situ today and the patient has a clear cornea and no lens opacification.[10] The ArtisanTM phakic IOL is a typical spin-off of the fixation principle of the claw lenses

The one-piece convex-concave ArtisanTM PIOL is made of Perspex CQ (clinical quality UV absorbing PMMA). The lenses are manufactured by Ophtec Bv in Groningen, The Netherlands using a special compression moulding technology to obtain "claws" with a high tensile strength and superb flexibility of the haptics[56] The overall diameter of the lenses is 8.5 mm with an optic of 5 or 6 mm. The height of the lenses (regardless of power) does not exceed 0.96 mm. The two diametrically opposed haptics attach the lens to the mid-peripheral, virtually immobile, iris stroma, allowing relatively unrestricted dilation and constriction of the pupil.[53]

The power of the ArtisanTM Myopia PIOL with 5 mm optic ranges from –3.0 to –23.0 D. The ArtisanTM Myopia PIOL with 6 mm optic ranges from –3.0 to –15.5 D while the ArtisanTM Hyperopia PIOLs range from +1 to +12 D).[54] The ArtisanTM Toric PIOLs correct cylinders from 2 to 7 D. All lenses are manufactured in 0.5 D increments. The ArtisanTM Phakic IOLs can correct:

- Myopia, hyperopia, astigmatism (Toric PIOL)
- Presbyopia (monocular low plus power IOL)
- Incorrect power of posterior chamber (PC) IOLs (Piggyback IOL).

Designs In 1990 Worst and Fechner modified the Worst-Fechner biconcave lens in order to reduce postoperative complications.[57] The new design, called Artisan iris fixated lens (Ophthec BV. Groningen, The Netherlands), is a one-piece all-PMMA lens with a convex-concave optic of 5 or 6 mm in diameter (Figures 18.2 and 18.3). The vault height of the lens does not exceed 0.96 mm in myopic lenses, regardless of their power, and 1.0 mm in hyperopic lenses.[60] The Artisan Hyperopia lens (model 203) has a power range from +1.0 D to +12.0 D, and optic diameter of 5 mm. All the lenses are manufactured in 0.5 D steps. The two diametrically opposed haptics fixate the lens on the iris by enclavation of midperipheral iris stroma. The distance from the edge of the optic to the corneal endothelium is 1.5 to 2.0 mm depending on the eye anatomy and lens power.[60]

The Artisan lens is also available for hyperopic astigmatism correction since 1999. The Artisan Toric lens corrects astigmatism from 2 to 7 D, and it is a biconcave lens. The fixation is versatile, as the lens may be fixed

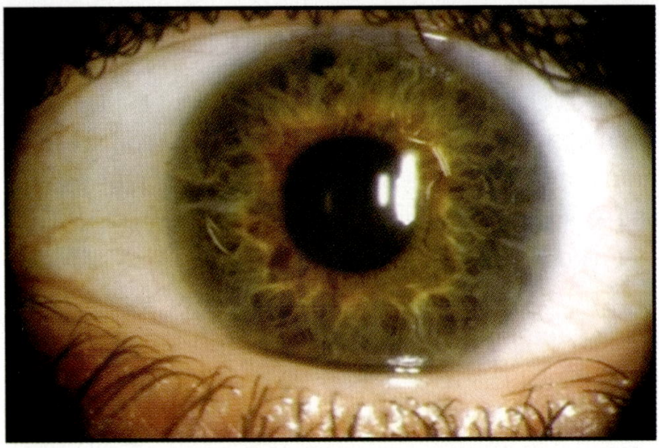

Figure 18.2: Artisan (Ophtec, Netherlands)

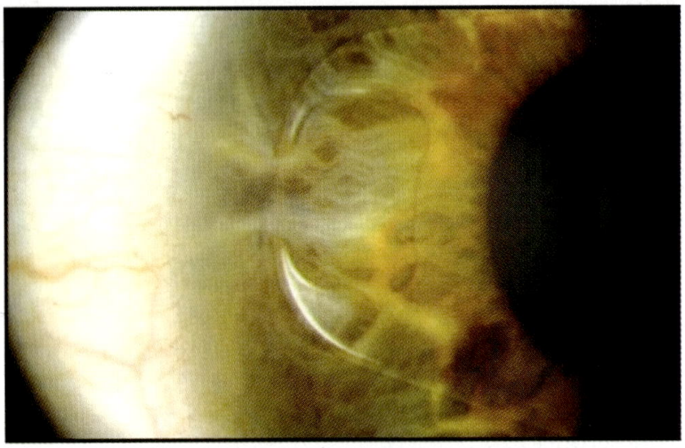

Figure 18.3: Artisan lens, details of the iris claw

with the necessary angle to correct any astigmatism. There are two different models of this lens depending on the axis location:

a. **Model "A":** The cylinder axis runs on the axis that runs through the claws.
b. **Model "B":** The cylinder axis is perpendicular to the axis that runs through the claws.

Techniques of Artisan Lens Implantation: Personal Experience and Technique

Local anesthesia is preferred. Topical anesthesia is not advisable for Artisan lens implantation.

If local anesthesia is given, the para-bulbar injection of 8 ml of bupivacaine 0.75 percent and lidocain 2 percent with 1 cc of hyaluronidase. This technique is preferred. and should result in total immobility of the globe and the eyelids. Perform orbital compression with a Honan Balloon (Lebanon Corporation, Lebanon, IN) and /or massage for 20 minutes until low preoperative pressure is obtained. This will improve the accessibility to and operative space in the anterior chamber. Pupillary miosis , using one drop of pilocarpine 2 percent (Alcon–Cusi, Barcelona , Spain), 30 minutes before surgery.[15]

Cover all eye lashes since they are potential sources of infection. Do not allow fluid-filled reservoirs between the plastic drapes and the skin and eyelashes during surgery.

Because the white-to-white distance is shorter vertically than horizontally, we recommend a horizontal enclavation and also a superior approach for the Artisan™ hyperopia lens.[53]

With an astigmatic marker (Katena, Denville, NJ) the horizontal 180° corneal axis is identified and two 1.5 mm stab incisions ,2 mm away from the limbus and directed toward the peripheral iris are done at the 3 and 9 o'clock position using a 1.4 mm MVR blade (Sharpoint, Surgical Specialities Corporation Reading, PS).[3]

Inject a miotic solution through the lateral incision, followed by regular cohesive viscoelastic material (Healon). Be careful with dispersive viscoelastics because their removal is difficult and there is a postoperative pressure risk. Dispersive and cohesive viscoelastic have different effects on lens epithelial cells. Dispersive viscoelastics could cause the lens to float in the viscoelastic material and have no contact with the iris during the implantation. The enclavation would also be more difficult.[5] High viscosity cohesives such as Healon GV are not advised due to rise in intraocular pressure.

A 6 mm incision is made at the superior clear cornea just in front of the vascular arcades .This incision size was selected after finding difficulties in lenses with power higher than +5 through 5.5 mm.[3]

Cover the conjunctiva with the viscoelastic material to avoid any contact between it and the PIOL during the implantation. Then the implant is inserted using a specially designed implantation forceps (Artsan lens forceps, Ophtec) and then rotated to a horizontal position in the center of the anterior chamber with a Lester hook (Catena, Denville, NG). It is then held in this position at the 12 o'clock position of the optic with Artizan lens forceps and the optic was centered on the pupil.[3]

There are, two techniques of enclavation available: the hook technique and the forceps. With the hook technique, hold the lens in the center of the optic with the implantation forceps, push a fold of mid-peripheral iris tissue forward with the blunt enclavation Needle (snow-ploughing) and place the fold between the claws. The handle provided carries a right and a left needle.[5]

If using the enclavation forceps, through the stab incision take a fold of mid-peripheral iris tissue into the specially designed iris forceps (Alio iris forceps, ASICO, Westmont, IL) and engage into the claw of the lens. During these maneuvers, hold the lens in the center over the pupil with the implantation forceps and depress the lens slightly.

For both instruments it is important not to pull on the iris, but bringing the iris fold gently betweer the claws. Never pull on the iris. The pupil is used as a reference for centering the lens.

Make a peripheral iridotomy using a specially designed iris forceps (Alio iris scissors , ASICO) as an additional precaution to prevent pupillary block, glaucoma, and iris prolapse during surgery. An iridotomy is cosmetically more attractive and prevents ghost images.[3]

The incision is then sutured with a three –bite running nylon 10/0 suture (ALCON).

Before closing the knot ,the cohesive viscoelastic should be removed by careful washing with a 27 –gauge cannula using a total of 10 cc of balanced saline solution (BSS , Alcon –Cusi , Barcelona Spain). It was found that automated irrigation is not a safe maneuver when performed after the fixation of the implant.[3]

The big advantage of this lens is that it can be centred over the pupil. The disadvantage is that more surgical skill is required for its insertion than for insertion of other kinds of lenses.

Although these lenses are more difficult to insert, the clinical results are usually spectacular. The quality of vision after insertion of the iris claw and the anterior chamber lenses appears to be significantly better than the quality of vision after LASIK, and usually these patients see well either the next day or shortly thereafter with improvements that are dramatic.

The future challenging phakic IOL for implantation should be designed to:

- Not put a pressure on the angle ,
- Not move in the anterior chamber
- Not flex against the peripheral endothelium
- Not rub against the iris
- Not cause damage to the endothelium on insertion
- Not cause damage to the lens on insertion
- Not require an incision of more than 1.5 to 2mm
- Not be difficult to insert
- Not be difficult to remove
- Not be difficult to exchange.[4]

Long-term follow-up shows that the Artisan is a lens made to stay for life in the eyes of hyperopes. The lower incidence of complication , the high BCVA, and the minimal effect on the total endothelial count is on its behalf in front of the other PIOLs.

In 2002 we carried on a study on the Artisan PIOL,[3] for high hyperopic patients, which is a modified model of the iris claw Fechner Worst phakic lens for the correction of myopia. Its lack of angular support reduces the possibility of peripheral contact with the corneal endothelium. This PIOL works well in patients who have an anterior chamber less than 3.4 mm or a narrow angle, as it is placed at the central anterior chamber without interfering with the anterior chamber angle, allowing an intact accommodation mechanism. This is especially important when we consider previous reports that hyperopia greater than + 6.00 D shows a shallower anterior chamber when compared with the emmetrope or low myope, a tendency that becomes even more evident with increase in age. This fact makes it even more compelling to have a PIOL placed at the central area of the anterior chamber, where this space will be better maintained over time.

The hyperopic Artisan PIOL seems to be an adequate lens to correct high hyperopia; further improvement in predictability and implantation technique, using a foldable model, will enhance its application for correction of hyperopia. Alió, advocated its use in hyperopia higher than +5.00 to +6.00 D, or in eyes in which central corneal steepening induced by corneal surgery will be higher than 50 D, a limit frequently associated with night vision disability and loss BSCVA.

A three years follow up study carried by Sexana et al, 2003, recorded that implantation of the Artisan

Table 18.4: Recent FDA study data: Artisan lens. mean endothelial cell change pre-pp vs. 6 months, 1 year, 2 years

	Pre-op	6 Months	1 Year	2 Year
Mean (SD)	2628(474)	2628 (474)	2599 (482)	2572 (469)
Cummulative % Change		0%	-1.10%	-1.06 %
Net Change @ 2 year				-2.15%

hypermetropic lens leads to accurate and stable refractive results with no significant loss of vision. More attention should be paid to convex irides and shallow anterior chamber during the preoperative screening to avoid unnecessary complications.[61]

SPECIFIC COMPLICATIONS IN HYPEROPIC ARTISAN LENS IMPLANTATION

How to Avoid Complications

Any kind of complication is surgery dependent and not due to the implant itself. Therefore, learning the exact technique is essential. It is very important for the surgeon to receive training before operating in vivo (Table 18.4).

For beginners, general anesthesia is more comfortable for both the patient and the surgeon. If, a local anesthetic is chosen, a peribulbar is less dangerous than a retro bulbar. A scleral perforation can always arise, especially in myopic eyes (= –17 D). A purely topical anesthetic appears dangerous, in our opinion. Any uncoordinated movement may cause contact between the implant, the anterior capsule, or the endothelium. Patient sedation never protects the surgeon from a sudden, brusque movement and the subsequent consequences.

When the pupil is insufficiently constricted , viscoelastic material may be trapped in the pupillary area under the implant and is the difficult to remove. Insufficient miosis might also lead to touch of the natural lens during implantation. Under these circumstances centring of the PIOL is more difficult. Manipulation of the PIOL in the anterior chamber can cause endothelial touch or touch of the crystalline lens. This contact could happen when the anterior chamber has collapsed due to external loss of viscoelastic material. That is why the use of a high viscosity viscoelastic material such as Artivisc™ or HealonGV™ is mandatory. It should be entirely washed out. Other viscoelastic materials with lower viscosity fail to maintain the anterior chamber and cannot be washed out completely.

Due to the typical hydrostatic and hydrodynamic conditions present during insertion of a high myopia implant, iris prolapse tends to occur more easily than in normal cataract surgery. Once incarcerated in the incision, reposition is more difficult and the incarceration tends to recur. Iris prolapse tends to occur more often in corneoscleral incisions than in tunnel incisions.

The most difficult step of this surgical technique is encountered when the surgeon enclavates the iris fold in the slit of the haptics. This could make perfect centring of the PIOL difficult. Proper centring needs a lot of attention because of the possible postoperative problems of glare and halos. One should also pay attention to creating a fold that is not too small; otherwise the PIOL can luxate into the anterior chamber and cause damage to the corneal endothelium . Another potential complication that can occur during enclavation is the traumatizing effect on the iris or endothelium, especially when instruments are used that are not made for this type of surgery. Iris damage can easily occur when "home-made" enclavation needles are used, which have sharp tips. The special "Ophtec Enclavation Needles" have soft polished tips.[56]

Intraoperative Complications

Implant Damage

Damage to the implant can occur during its insertion into the anterior chamber if the special forceps are not used. It can also occur during its release and manipulation under the iris . Both the surgeon and the technician must be very careful when the lens is taken from the

Table 18.5: Recent FDA study data: complications with the Artisan lens			
Complication	*6 Months N = 549*	*1 Year N = 378*	*2 Year N = 108*
Glare/Halos 5 mm Optic	7.8 %	2.5%	11.7%
Six mm Optic	2.9%	2.7%	3.2%
Non-pigmented Precipitates	0.5%[2]	0%	0%
Iris-pigmented Precipitates	2.9%[2]	1.3%[2]	8.3%[2]
Anterior Capsule Vacuoles	1.0%[2]	0.8%[2.3]	2.8%[2.3]
Irregular Pupil	2.9%[2]	1.0%[2]	2.8%[2]
Synechia	0.4%[1.3]	0.3%[3]	0%

1 Resolved by 9th month postop

2 Clinically insignificant, no treatment

3 No change since 6 months postop

Data submitted in 2004 by Ophtec USA to Food and Drug Administration. Reprinted by permission of Ophtec USA

package and inserted into the forceps. Do not forget the implant is very tin and rather expensive and can be damaged easily[57] (Table 18.5).

Hemorrhage

Bleeding can occur during the manual surgical iridectomy, but should not be common. If it occurs , inject some viscoelastic through the paracentesis, wait several minutes for the bleeding to stop, then remove it.

Iris Damage

It is possible to damage the posterior pigment surface of the iris with the implant , and we recommend injecting viscoelastic under the iris to avoid this complication. The surgeon has to be very careful during the manual iridectomy not to pull and tear the iris strenuously through the paracentesis because this can cause iris damage and actual bleeding.

Lens Damage

The worst complication during the actual procedure is the immediate creation of lens damage and cataract. The surgeon must always be ready to convert the surgery to phaco-emulsification with IOL implantation. The lens can be damaged in the following steps during surgery.

Corneal incisions due to sudden knife insertion or eye ball movement

- Paracentesis due to insufficient viscoelastic in the anterior chamber, too quick blade movement , or eye ball movement.
- Implant insertion due to contact between the forceps and the anterior capsule of the lens.
- Implant manipulation due to pushing the implant on the lens.
- Viscoelastic removal due to inadvertent movement of irrigation or aspiration needle, and excessively forceful BSS irrigation.

Endothelial Damage

Inadequate viscoelastic protection may allow endothelial cell damage during implant insertion. Postoperative endothelial cell loss was found by Alió to be similar to that reported in previous studies with anterior chamber PIOLs[58] although other reports on the Artizan lens in myopic eyes have shown larger losses and a trend to chronic cell loss[58,52,60] (Table 18.5).

Zonular Fiber Damage

Pushing the implant too strenuously under the iris may cause the edge of the implant to damage the Zonular fibres. We have to remember that a large number of Zonular fibers stretch across the anterior periphery of the lens capsule. This could lead to implant dislocation and optic zone decentration if the future. That is why we try to fold and the release the implant allowing it to go under the iris, never pushing it there with force.[57]

Postoperative Complications

Corneal Edema

A persistent corneal edema, especially at 12 o'clock, is due to implant endothelium contact at the time of the implantation. This edema usually disappears.

Iris Damage

At the time of enclavation , the surgeon may damage the iris, which will result in a localized iris atrophy that is not progressive.

Implant Decentration

This implies that if the implant is not well centered at the end of procedure it will remain that way and this will cause halos and glare that the patient will complain about. Therefore, it must be re-centered, preferably during the primary surgery.

Pupil deformation was present in small degrees in three eyes (5.26%). Two eyes (3.51%) showed minor degrees of decentration of the PIOL optic of less than 1 mm from the pupillary center. None of these eyes were symptomatic.[2]

Early Rise of IOP

Pupillary blocks occurs if an iridectomy or an iridotomy is not well checked. This can be performed with an Nd:Yag laser preoperatively. Make sure that both layers of iris are perforated and that the anterior capsule of the crystalline or the zonular fibers is visible. Preferably it should be performed at 12 o'clock to avoid any diplopia.

Another cause of high pressure in the immediate postoperative period is the persistence of viscoelastics in the anterior chamber. Therefore, cohesive viscoelastic material is recommended because it can be removed more easily than a dispersive one.

Retinal Detachment

It was reported in 0.8 percent of eyes in the same publication. No relationship with the implant has been shown.[53]

Implant Induced Astigmatism

If the implant has induced astigmatism of more than 1.25 D to 1.50 D, remove the stitches five weeks after the operation.

Cataract

An age-related cataract may develop in some patients. Since postoperative keratometry readings are practically unchanged and because a preoperative biometry will always be carried out, the implant is removed and cataract surgery is proceeded as usual.

Postoperative Inflammation

Most of the cases develop mild uveitis grade 1+/- 2. rarely grade 3 iridocyclitis is seen with membranes and small sterile hypopyon and absence of ciliary injection. or pain. This anterior iridocyclitis is controlled with an intensive steroid therapy and cycloplegics

Endothelial Cell Density Changes

The endothelial cell loss in the first six months was 6.8 percent of the baseline endothelial count ,while after one year the losses accounts for 9.4 percent of baseline records.[3]

Halos and Glare

The problem of halos and glare is secondary to the relationship between the pupillary diameter and the diameter of the Artisan lens (Table 18.5)

Haloes and night glare usually occurs if pupillary diameter in scotopic or mesopic conditions exceeds the lens optical diameter. Decentration and tilting of the implant may cause in addition diplopia and astigmatism. If necessary, a 5 mm Artisan lens can be replaced by a 6 mm one.

REFERENCES

1. Alió JL, Ismail MM, Artola A, Pérez-Santonja JJ. Correction of PRK induced hyperopia by holmium laser 12 months follow-up. J Refract Surg 1997;13:13-16.
2. Werblin TP. Hexagonal Keratotomy: should we still by trying? Jrefract surgery 1996;12:613-20.

3. Jorge L. Alió, Emilia Mulet M, Ahmad MM, Shalaby. Artisan Phakic Iris Claw Intraocular Lens for High Primary and Secondary Hyperopia. Journal of Refractive Surgery 2002;18.
4. Ismail MM, Alio JL, Perez-Santonja JJ. Non-contact thermokeratoplasty to correct hyperopia induced by laser in situ keratomileusis .J Cataract Refractive Surgery 1998; 24:1-4.
5. Alio JL, Ismail MM, Artola A. Correction of hyperopia induced by photorefractive keratotomy using non contact HO Yag laserthermal keratoplasty. J Cataract Refractive Surgery 1997;13:17-22.
6. Pietila J, Makinan P, Pajari S, Uusitalo H. Eximer laser photorefractive keratectomy for hyperopia . J Refract Surg 1997;13:504-10.
7. Fyodorov SN, Durnev VV. Anterior keratotomy method application with the purpose of surgical correction of myopia. In: Pressing Problems of Ophthalmosurgery. Moscow, 1997.
8. Koch DD, Abarca A, Villarreal K. Hyperopia correctic n by non-contact holmium laser thermokeratoplasty. Clinical study with two years follow up. Ophthalmology 1996; 103:731-40.
9. Suarez E, Tones F, Duplessie M. LASIK for correction of hyperopia and hyperopia with astigmatism. Intl Ophthalmol clin 1996;36:65-71.
10. Pérez-Santonja JJ, Sakla HF, Ayala MJ, Alió JL. Queratomileusis in situ con láser excimer (LASIK) para hipermetropía. Resultados preliminares. Arch Soc Esp Ophthalmol 1999;74:89-96.
11. Fink AM,Gore C, Rosen ES. Refractive lensectomy for hyperopia. Ophthalmology 2000;107:1540-48.
12. Alió JL, De la Hoz F, Ismail MM. Subclinical inflammatory reaction induced by phakic anterior chamber lenses for correction of high myopia. Ocular Immunology and Inflammation 1993;1:219-23.
13. Alió JL, De la Hoz F, Pérez-Santonja JJ, Ruiz-Moreno JM, Quesada JA. Phakic anterior chamber lenses for the correction of miopía. A 7-year cumulative analysis of complications in 263 cases. Ophthalmology 1999;3:458-66.
14. Worst JGF, Van Der Veen G, Loss LI. Refractive surgery for high myopia. The Worst-Fechner biconcave iris claw lens. Documenta Ophthalmologica 1990;75:335-41.
15. Jorge L Alió, Carlo F Lovisolo, Enrico Giacomotti. Phakic Intraocular Lenses for Hyperopia . Refractive Surgery with phakic IOLs Fundamentals and Clinical Practice 2004.
16. Glasser A, Campbell MC. Presbyopia and the optical changes in the human crystalline lens with age. Vison Res 1998;38:209-29.
17. Lowe RF. Anterior lens displacement with age. Br J Ophthalmol 1970;54:117.
18. Campbell MC, Harrison EM, Simonet P. Psychophysical measurement of the blur on the retina due to optical aberrations of the eye. Vision Res 1990;30:1587-1602.
19. Auffarth GU, Tetz MR, Biazid Y, Volcker HE. Measuring anterior chamber depth with the Orbscan Topography System. J Cataract Refract Surg 1997;23:1351-55.
20. Yaylali V, Kaufman SC, Thompson HW. Corneal thickness measurements with the Orbscan Topography System and ultrasonic pachymetry. J Cataract Refract Surg 1997; 23:1345-50.
21. Flament J, Schraub M, Guimaraes R, Bronner A. Urretz-zavalia syndrome and glaucomatous cataract. Etiopathogenetic and nosologic discussion. Ophthalmologica 1984; 189:186-94.
22. Strampelli B. Anterior chamber plastic lenses:present technique. Arch Ophthalmol 1961;66:12-17.
23. Zaldivar R, Davidorf J, Oscherow S, et al. Combined posterior chamber phakic intraocular lens and laser in situ keratomileusis ; Bioptics for high extreme myopia. J Refract Surg 1999;15:139-46.
24. Knors M, Weisienger B, et al. Laser in situ keratomileusis for moderate and high myopia and myopic astigmatism. Ophthalmology 1998;105:932-40.
25. Hans H, Song J, Kim H. Long term results of laser in situ keratomileusis for high myopia . Korean J Ophthalmol 2000;14:1-6.
26. Pérez-Santonja J, Bellot J, Claramonte P, et al. Laser in situ keratomileusis to correct high myopia. J Cataract Refract Surg 1997;23:372-85.
27. Colin J, Robinet A. Clear lensectomy and implantation of low power posterior chamber intraocular lenses for the correction of high myopia. Ophthalmology 1994;101:107-12.
28. Antonio A Marinho, Maria Ceu Pinto, Fernando Vaz. The Limits of LASIK. Comparative Analysis between Corneal and Phakic IOL Refractive Surgery. Refractive Surgery with phakic IOLs 2004.
29. Malecaze FJ, Hulin H, Bierer P, et al. A randomized paired eye comparison of two techniques for treating moderately high myopia. LASIK and Artisan phakic lens. Ophthalmology 2002;109:1622-30.
30. Alberto Artola, Ignacio Jiménez-Alfaro, José M, Ruíz-Moreno, Carlo F Lovisolo, Dan Z Reinstein. Proper Patient Assessment, Selection and Preparation. Refractive Surgery with phakic IOLs 2004.
31. Lesueur LC, Arne JL. Phakic posterior chamber lens implantation in children with high myopia .J Cataract Refract Surg 1999;25:1571-75.
32. BenEzra D, Cohen E, Karshai I. Phakic posterior chamber intraocular lens for the correction of anisometropia and treatment of amblyopia. Am J Opthalmol 2000;130:292-96.
33. Chan RY, Smith JA, Richardson KT. Anterior segment configuration correlated with Shaffer's grading of anterior chamber angle. Arch Ophthalmol 1981;99:104-07.
34. Colvard M. Preoperative measurement of scotopic pupil dilation using an office pupillometer. J Cataract Refract Surg 1998;24:1594-97.

35. Werblin TP. Long-term endothelial cell loss following phacoemulsification: Model for evaluating endothelial damage after intraocular surgery. Refract Corneal Surg 1993;9:29-35.
36. Fontana ST, Brubaker RF. Volume and depth of the anterior chamber in the normal aging human eye. Arch Ophthalmol 1980;98:1803.
37. Auffarth GU, Tetz MR, Biazid Y, Volcker HE. Measuring anterior chambert depth with the Orbscan Topography System. J Cataract Refract Surg 1997;23:1351-55.
38. Saragoussi JJ, Puech M, Assouline M, et al. ultrasound biomicroscopy of Baikoff anterior chamber pkakic intraocular lens. J Refracr Surg 1997;13:135-41.
39. Kim DY, Reinstein DZ, Silverman RH, et al. Very high frequency ultrasound analysis of a new phakic posterior chamber intraocular lens *in situ*. Am J Ophthalmol 1998; 125:725-29.
40. Dick HB, Alió JL, Bianchetti M, et al. Toric phakic intraocular lens: European multicenter study. Ophthalmology 2003; 110;150-62.
41. Joly P, Baikoff G, Bonnet P. Mise en place d'un implant négatif de chambre antérieure chez des sujets phakes. Bull Soc Ophthalmol Fr 1989;5:727-33.
42. Saragoussi JJ, Cotinat J, Renard G, et al. Damage to the corneal endothelium by minus power anterior chamber intraocular lenses. Refract Corneal Surg 1991;7:282-85.
43. Mimouni F, Colin J, Koffi V, Bonnet P. Damage to the corneal endothelium from anterior chamber intraocular lenses in phakic myopic eyes. Refract Corneal Surg 1991;7:277-81.
44. Baikofff G, Arne JL, Bokobza Y, et al. Angle-fixated anterior chamber phakic intraocular lens for myopia of –7 to –19 diopters. J Refract Surg 1998;14:282-93.
45. Charles D Kelman. The Kelman DUET Angle-Supported Phakic IOL. In: Alio JL, Pérez-Santonja JL (Eds). Refractive Surgery with phakic IOLs. Highlights of Ophthalmology International 2004.
46. Pérez-Santonja JJ, Alió JL, Jiménez-Alfaro I, Zato MA. Surgical correction of severe myopia with an angle-supported phakic intraocular lens. J Cataract Refract Surg 2000;26:1288-1302.
47. Bechmann M, Ullrich S, Thiel MJ, et al. Imaging of posterior chamber phakic intraocular lens by optical coherence tomography. J Cataract Refract Surg 2002;28:360-63.
48. Worst JGF. Iris claw lens. Am Intra-ocular Implant Soc 1980;6:166-67.
49. Alpar JJ, Fechner PU. History of modern lens implantation. In: Fechner PU, (Ed). Fechner's intraocular lenses. New York: Thiem Inc, 1986:6-23.
50. Drews RC. Risk benifit análisis of anterior chamber intraocular lenses for the correction of myopia in phakic patients. Eur J Implant Refracr Surg 1991;3:171-94.
51. Landesz M, Worst JGF, van Rij G, Houtman WA. Opaque iris claw lens in a phakic eye to correct acquired diplopia. J Cataract Refract Surg 1997;23:137-38.
52. Budo C, Hessloehl JC, Izak M, et al. Multicenter study of the Artisan™ phakic intraocular lens. Cataract Refract Surg 2000;26:1163-71.
53. Camille JR Budo, Monika Landesz, Jan GF Worst. Iris-Fixated Phakic IOLs. The Artisan Lens. Refractive Surgery with phakic IOLs 2004.
54. Rao GN, Stevens RE, Harris JK, Aquavella JV. Long-term changes in corneal endothelium following intraocular lens implantation. Ophthalmology 1981;88:386-97.
55. Hosni M, Alió JL, Claramonte P, Attia WH, Pérez-Santonja JJ. Relationship between anterior chamber depth, refractive state, corneal diameter and axial length. J Refract Surg 2000;16:336-40.
56. Herbert E Kaufmann, Stephen C Kaufman. Phakic Intraocular Lenses – Where Are We Now? Refractive Surgery with Phakic IOLs 2004.
57. Dimitrii D Dementiev, Kenneth J Hoffer, Aleksandra Sonecka. PRL-Medennium Posterior Chamber Phakic Intraocular Lens .Refractive Surgery with phakic IOLs 2004.
58. Alpar JJ, Fechner PU. History of modern lens implantation. In: Fechner PU, (Ed). Fechner's intraocular lenses. New York: Thiem Inc, 1986:6-23.
59. Landez M, Worst JG, Van Rij G. Long-term results of correction of high myopia with an iris claw phakic intraocular lens. J Cataract Refract Surg 2000;16.3:310-16.
60. Juan J Pérez-Santonja, Luca Antico, Jorge L Alió. Refractive Surgery with Phakic IOLs 2004.
61. Saxana R, Landesz M, Noordzij B, Luyten GP. Three –years follow-up of the Artisan phakic intraocular lens for hypermetropia. Ophthalmology 2003;110(7):1391-95.

19

"Newlife" Multifocal Phakic Implant for the Correction of Presbyopia

- NEWLIFE BIFOCAL PHAKIC IMPLANT
- ANTERIOR CHAMBER DIMENSION
- SURGICAL TECHNIQUES
- RESULTS
- ANATOMICAL RESULTS—INCIDENTS AND COMPLICATIONS

Georges Baikoff (France)

INTRODUCTION

Correcting presbyopia is an essential challenge for refractive surgery. This particular type of surgery is not so much to do with restoring accommodation, but more a question of giving patients an opportunity of living without spectacles for distant and near vision. This opens the door to a number of compromises or alternatives to real accommodation surgery.

Presbyopia affects most people over the age of 45 years and if we consider that in the United States 50 percent of the population is presbyopic,[1] through extrapolation, this represents several billion individuals throughout the world.

Considering the degree of ametropia (high/low myopia, high/low hyperopia, emmetropia) several options are available. Unilateral myopization (monovision) of the dominant eye or multifocal correction of either the cornea or crystalline lens, either by adding a new lens or exchanging the crystalline lens if it is still transparent.

A choice is therefore available to both surgeons and patients as not one of all these techniques provides the perfect solution and in the years to come, it is quite probable that several different but complementary solutions will be available. We decided to work on three possible options: the cornea, the crystalline lens and the sclera and will give the results we obtained following implantation of a bifocal lens for correcting both slight ametropia and an average presbyopia of + 2.50 D

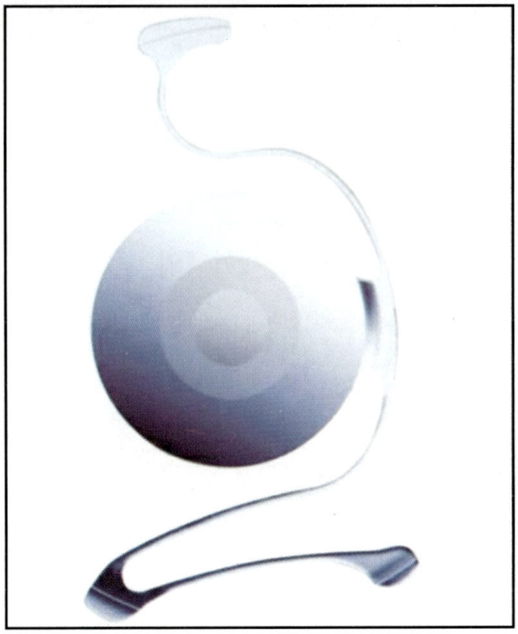

Figure 19.1: Drawing of presbyopic anterior chamber implant

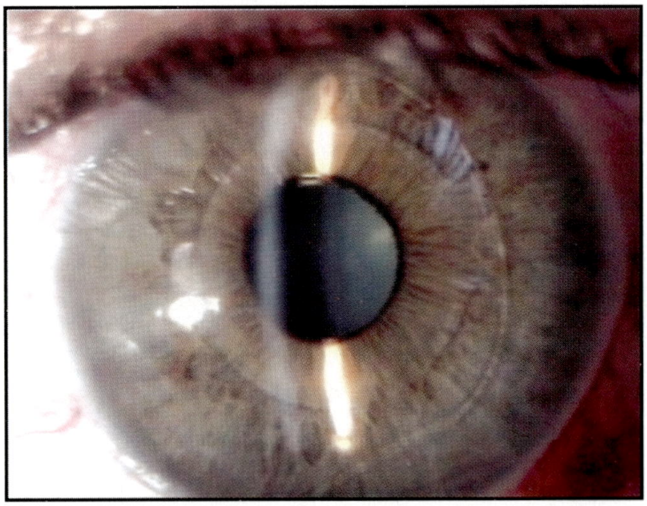

Figure 19.2: Postoperative aspect

NEWLIFE BIFOCAL PHAKIC IMPLANT

The bifocal refractive phakic IOL is an anterior chamber angle-supported lens marketed under the trade name of NEWLIFE (**Ioltech**,)*. The optic is of soft 28 percent hydrophilic acrylic, the haptic is of poly (methyl methacrylate) (PMMA), and the footplates at the extremities are of hydrophilic acrylic. The 5.5 mm diameter optic is divided into 3 zones: the center, which is for distance vision, the medium periphery which is for near vision; and the periphery which is for distance vision. The central zone diameter is 1.50 mm, and the near intermediate zone is 1.1 mm wide (Figures 19.1 and 19.2). The haptic is shaped-like the number 2 and is available in overall diameters of 12.0, 12.5 and 13.0 mm.

The IOL comes in powers between –5,00 D and +5,00 D for distant vision with a single addition of +2,50 D for near vision. This addition is a compromise,

* **Ioltech**, Avenue Paul Langevin, BP 5, 17053 La Rochelle, France, Tel + 33 5 4644 8550 ; Fax + 33 54 644 8560

allowing a slight over correction for 50 years old subjects and a slight under correction for 60 years old subjects; these slight refractive inaccuracies will prove to be generally well accepted

ANTERIOR CHAMBER DIMENSION

Internal Diameter

For all angle-supported implants, it is essential to carry out a precise evaluation of the internal diameter of the anterior chamber. We began by using the white-to-white method, then we used a PMMA graduated sizer which was inserted into the anterior chamber during surgery. In fact, all these measurements are relatively approximate and for an implant to remain stable in the anterior chamber, it must not only be adapted to the eye's largest diameter in order to avoid rotation but also as near as possible in size to this diameter so that there is no pressure on the iris which in the long run gives rise to pupil ovalization.

These problems can not be solved with the actual ultrasound A and B Scan techniques. However, modern imaging techniques such as the Artemis, ultra-high frequency ultrasound equipment and the anterior segment OCT give more precise measurements of the anterior chamber's internal diameter. We were able to demonstrate in-vivo, and this was confirmed by Liliana Werner on cadaver eyes, that in 75 percent of cases, the anterior chamber's internal vertical diameter was bigger than the horizontal one. In daily practice, we, therefore, systematically preoperatively measure the anterior segment helping us in the choice of implant (Figure 19.3).

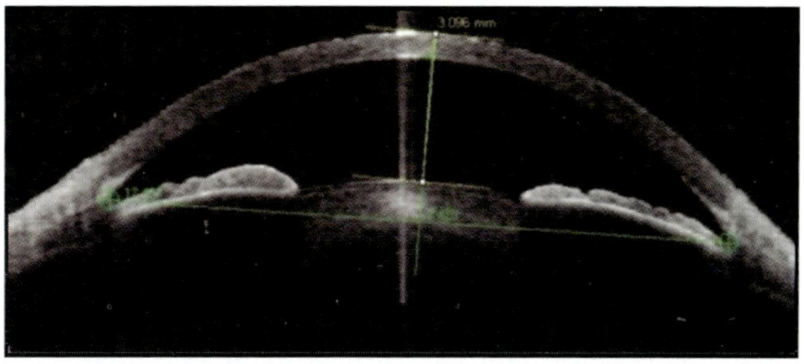

Figure 19.3: AC measurements with the Visante™ OCT prototype

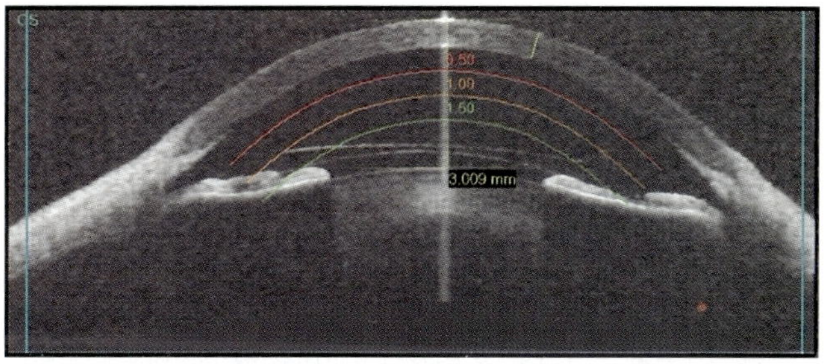

Figure 19.4: Endothelial safety distances

Anterior Chamber Depth

Minimum anterior chamber depth must be equal to or above 3,1mm (measured from the corneal epithelium to the anterior surface of the crystalline lens). This is of course a safety notion but does not in fact take into account the implant's vault (Figure 19.4).

SURGICAL TECHNIQUES

Topical, local regional or general anesthesia was used based on the surgeon's or patient's choice. Surgery

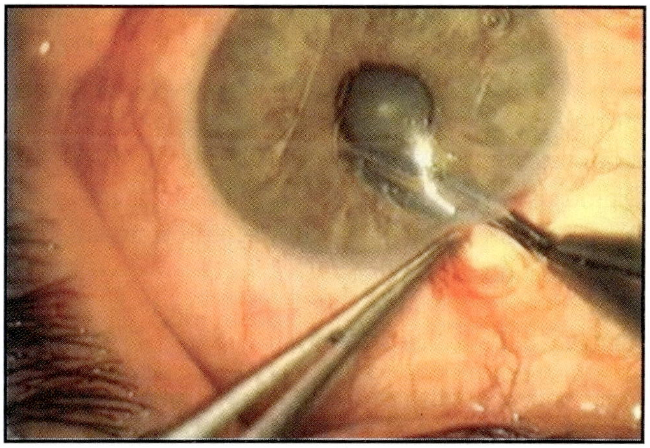

Figure 19.5: Insertion of the implant with optic folded in three

(Figure 19.5) is relatively simple and consists in placing the lens, which is folded at the time of surgery, into the anterior segment of the eye in front of the iris.

A preoperative myosis is essential (preoperative installation of 2 percent pilocarpine drops). A corneal or corneo-scleral incision is carried out with a 2.8 mm calibrated knife. Viscous substance was injected into the anterior chamber, two paracenteses were made at 3 and 9 o'clock to allow subsequent maneuvers in the anterior chamber.

The lens is folded into three with a special folder before being inserted . First the two leading footplates are introduced into the anterior chamber followed by the optic and trailing haptic. Once the lens is in the anterior chamber, pressure on the forceps is gently released and the optic unfolds. When the lens is open in the anterior chamber and depending on the largest axis, the implant will be rotated to fit this axis. It is essential that all the viscous substance is removed at the end of surgery to avoid postoperative hypertonia with Urrets Zavalla syndrome (fixed dilated pupil). The viscous substance is replaced with BSS. No sutures are required with the self-sealing incision. An iridectomy is not routinely suggested because the optic is soft and the optic/haptic junction can act as a gentle hinge. If mechanical blockage of the pupil in the anterior chamber occured, the iris was pushed forward and the optic, which is soft, would in turn be pushed forward letting the aqueous humour escape through the pupil. In the event of an inflammatory pupil blockage, mydriatic therapy would be proposed first and if that failed, an iridectomy with the YAG laser was done. At the end of surgery, *500 mg of Diamox®* is systematically administered intravenously and a tablet of 250 mg Diamox is also prescribed on the first night after surgery. A one-month antibiotic steroid eye-drop treatment is prescribed postoperatively.

Anatomical Exclusion Criteria

Only patients with normal anterior segments, normal endothelium cell counts, without ocular hypertonia or associated pathologies are considered. It is essential to have a clear crystalline lens and a normal macula.

Choice of Implant

To avoid rotation, the implant is placed along the axis of the anterior chamber's biggest diameter, which, in general is the vertical diameter. If for instance, the vertical diameter is the bigger diameter and the implant is placed on the horizontal diameter, this will lead to instability and a risk of the implant rotating. If the implant is well placed on the largest axis, there is no longer any risk of rotation.

Power of the Implant

Choice of the IOL optical power was based on distant refraction according to the Holladay's formula.[2] The IOL comes in powers between – 5.00 D and + 5.00 D. A single addition is available with this model (+ 2.50D). All hyperopes between the age of 50 and 60 years can be corrected in this way, knowing that the younger subjects will be slightly over corrected and the older subjects slightly under corrected. This under or over correction has no incidence on everyday life.

Any corneal astigmatism, (which alters the quality of the IOL), must be corrected beforehand either with laser or lasik in order to make the most of this multifocal implant.

RESULTS

Our initial study concerned 55 eyes of 33 patients: 21 women, 12 men, 29 right eyes, 26 left eyes. Preoperative refraction was between –5.00 D and +5.00 D.. There were 9 myopic eyes and 46 emmetropic or hyperopic eyes. The anterior chamber was over 3.1 mm in almost all of the cases and the endothelial cell density equal to or above 2000 C/mm^2. Average age of patients was 54 ± 5.4 years (ranges between 45 and 70 years). The average follow-up was 42.6 weeks (ranges between 83 and 2 weeks).

Refraction

Mean preoperative refraction is + 1.8 D ± 1.3 D (ranges –2.75 D to + 5.00 D). Postoperative mean refraction is – 0.12 D. ± 0.51 D. (ranges –1.5 D to 1.25 D). There is, therefore, a very satisfactory precise refractive effect. Without going into detail, the first series of patients (Baikoff[3]) for whom we used the Van der Heijde formula,[4] showed a higher rate of myopisation than the patients subsequently operated on using the more precise Holladay's refractive formula.[2]

On the diagrams showing the evolution of the results after one-year follow-up, refraction remains stable (Figure 19.6).

Distant Visual Acuity

Uncorrected preoperative visual acuity was 0.41 ± 0.29 (decimal scale), and postoperative uncorrected visual

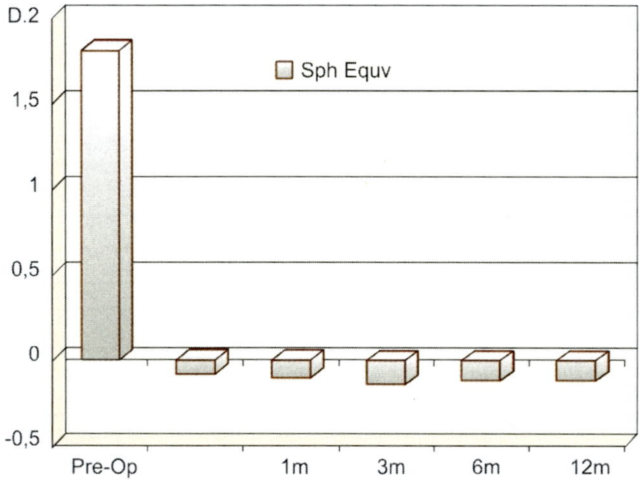

Figure 19.6: Evolution of postoperative refraction. Stability at 12 months

acuity (UCVA) was 0.78 ± 0.20 (decimal scale). This uncorrected visual acuity (UCVA) result is equivalent to the other refractive surgery techniques where the mean result is around 0.8.[5-7] Preoperative best corrected visual acuity is 0.98 ± 0.02 and postoperatively best corrected visual acuity drops to 0.92 ± 0.09. This loss of visual acuity is the result of a drop in contrast sensitivity due to the multifocal lens. It is a well known fact that multifocal lenses reduce image lighting, decreasing contrast sensitivity and BCVA. This has been observed in pseudophakic IOLS.[8]

Near Visual Acuity

Before surgery, near BCVA is PARINAUD 2.03* ± 0.1. Postoperative UCVA is PARINAUD 2.3 ± 0.6 (ranges 2 to 3).

Efficacy and Safety Ratio

The optical and refractive target was obtained, as distant UCVA was satisfactory with an 94 percent safety ratio (Postoperative BCVA / preoperative BCVA) and an 80 percent efficacy ratio. (Postoperative UCVA/ Preoperative BCVA). These results were slightly below those that we normally observe with refractive implants where the two factors are respectively between 120 percent and 140 percent and around 100 percent.[9-12] Finally, UCVA was satisfactory in most cases as 84 percent of eyes operated on obtained 0.6 or better for distant vision and Parinaud 3 or better for near vision both without correction. These figures correspond to a normally demanding population leading normal everyday lives.

ANATOMICAL RESULTS – INCIDENTS AND COMPLICATIONS

Loss of Visual Acuity

One patient showed a 3-line loss of BCVA three months after surgery of both eyes. Residual myopia existed but despite the correction of this myopia, the patient's visual acuity did not improve. The posterior pole was explored (angiography, OCT, Visual field, color vision) and was normal. Three or four months after surgery visual acuity returned to 1.0. This patient had PRK at a later date to correct her residual myopia with an excellent optical result.

A second patient found her visual acuity reduced to 0.5 and it was impossible to improve after surgery whereas preoperatively she had 0.8. In fact, this 70 year old patient presented a moderate cataract.

The addition of a multifocal lens in front of a slightly opalescent crystalline lens leads to a very severe drop in visual acuity for two reasons: decrease in light transmission due to the incipient cataract, and a decrease in the lighting of the focused image. Infact, crystalline lens opalescence can reduce retinal illumination by 30 percent and the added effect of a multifocal lens is, therefore, particularly harmful. The implant was removed at the same time as cataract surgery was performed by phakoemulsification using the same 3.2 mm incision. A monofocal implant was inserted into the bag with excellent visual results and a postoperative corrected visual acuity of 1.0.

Loss of Contrast Sensitivity:

Loss of contrast sensitivity was not studied objectively, and patients maybe sensitive to it after surgery of the first eye as they can compare with the other non operated eye. A slight grayish sensation is perceived. Once the second eye has been operated on, there is no

* Parinaud 2 / 3 is very similar to JAEGER 1 / 2

element of comparison and the discomfort is better accepted. In mesopic vision, that is to say reading at night in dim light conditions, some patients occasionally wear additional glasses.

Reduction of Retinal Illumination

We have seen that the problem with multifocal lenses was a reduction of retinal illumination. One patient suffered from this problem because of an pre-existing crystalline lens pathology (c f. supra).

The problems we are faced with concern anatomical predispositions such as senile myosis. A study should be carried out to define the acceptable minimum pupil diameter for this type of implant.

Therefore, multifocal lenses must be contraindicated for patients with slight macular pathologies such as Drüsens or epithelium pigment disorders because they are particularly sensitive to reductions in retinal illumination.

Halos

One of the problems of multifocal lenses is the possibility of parasite optical side effects. We have mentioned before that multifocal lenses reduce contrast sensitivity, however, they also produce halos that are particularly disturbing in night vision. About 18 percent of eyes and 24 percent of patients complained of halos, but these had no incidence on night driving except in two patients out of 33 (6%).

This high percentage of complaints concerning halos disappears in time because the brain adapts to this inconvenience. In the end, very few patients complained of this discomfort and in time none of them requested change or removal of the implant for this particular reason. Thanks to the Visante™ OCT pupil ovalizations have almost disappeared as the size of the implant is now correctly adapted to the largest axis which is generally the vertical one.

Pupil Ovalization

Ten percent of slight pupil ovalizations showed up under the slit lamp's intensive light. There were fewer under normal lighting. Generally, pupil ovalizations are the result of over sizing the implant.

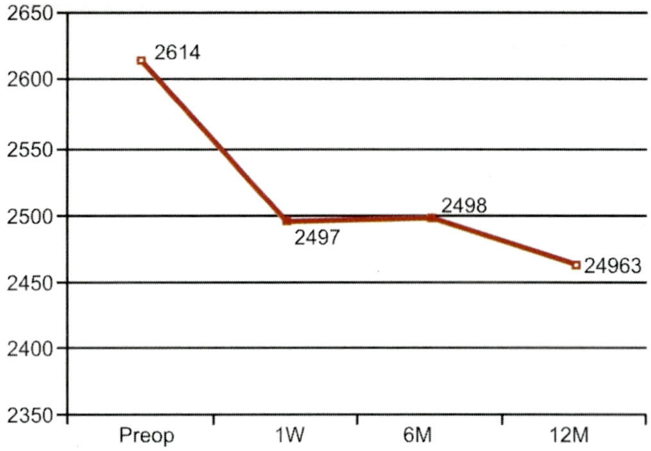

Figure 19.7: Evolution of corneal endothelium at 1 year

Cataract

No implant-induced cataracts have been observed in this study to date.

Ocular Hypertonia

No ocular hypertonia induced by the implant has been observed in this series to date.

Endothelium

After a year, mean endothelial cell loss is below 5 percent. The results meet the FDA's guidelines (Figure 19.7).

Explantations

Four explantations were carried out on patients who were disappointed with the results. One patient had excellent near and distant vision, 1.0 (decimal scale) and Parinaud 2 but was not satisfied with the intermediate vision. He therefore requested that the implant be removed.

Two explantations were suggested because of insufficient visual results. (c f. supra patient with cataract). One was due to unsolvable postoperative diplopia. In both cases, they recuperated their initial visual status. Optical defects are inevitable with multifocal lenses, therefore patient selection must be very strict. Patients too demanding and who think that they will recuperate the vision they had at the age of 20 must be excluded and before surgery, it is essential to provide precise information concerning the risks and drawbacks of this procedure.

SUMMARY

Since this preliminary study, we have continued to use this technique and to continue rigorous patient selection. The results are confirmed and more than 80 percent of the patients have an distant UCVA over 0.6D and Parinaud 3 or better for near vision also uncorrected. This means all the patients lead normal lives without glasses in diurnal conditions; only a few (less than 10%) need them in mesopic conditions, for instance to read at home in the evenings. In this series, everyday acts are done without glasses. Halos are generally well tolerated and the loss of contrast sensitivity is unavoidable. This technique can therefore be proposed but very strict inclusion criteria must be taken into account with regards to anatomy and psychology. This procedure can only be offered to patients with an anterior chamber depth equal to or above 3.0 mm, with an open angle, with a healthy endothelium and without anterior segment or retinal disorders (Figure 19.8). Any astigmatism must be corrected either before or after implantation. Patients that are too demanding must be excluded as well as patients who, for professional reasons, have to drive at night. The interest of phakic implants is their reversibility, in our series we had no persistent pupillary ovalization after explantation. In certain cases, a mono correction is possible on an emmetropic subject by placing an implant in the dominated eye only. If the result is satisfactory, surgery can be limited to just one eye, and surgery of the other eye proposed only if the patient wishes it. Experience has shown us that patients who had postoperative slightly hypermetropic refraction were more satisfied than patients slightly myopic. This had already been proved with multifocal pseudophakic implants (Steinert[13]). However, to obtain a satisfied patient, it is important to explain that the correction of presbyopia with this multifocal implant for phakic eyes is a compromise between an excellent preoperative vision with glasses and a good postoperative vision without glasses.

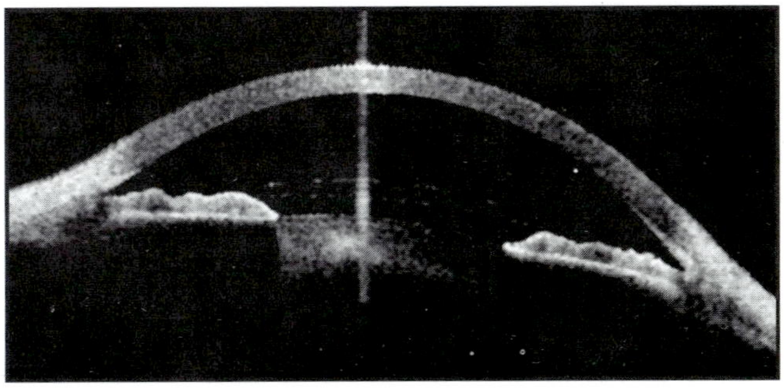

Figure 19.8: Aspect of a NEWLIFE presbyopic IOL with the AC OCT

Newlife Multifocal phakic implant for the correction of presbyopia, G. Baikoff.[3]

NB: An important part of this article (text and illustrations) has already been published in the Journal of Cataract and Refractive Surgery 2004;30:1454-1460 courtesy of Elsevier, Philadelphia USA.

REFERENCES

1. Lindström R. Correction of presbyopia with intraocular and intracorneal lenses Binkhorst Lecture. American Society of Refractive and Cataract meeting. San Francisco California 2003;12.
2. Holladay JT. Refractive power calculations for intraocular lenses in the phakic eye. Am J Ophthalmol 1993;116(1):63-66.
3. Baïkoff G. Presbyopic phakic intraocular lenses. In: Agarwal A (Ed). Presbyopia A Surgical Textbook: Thorofare NJ-Slack Inc 2002;225-28.
4. Fechner PU, Van Der Heijde GL, Worst JGF. The correction of myopia by lens implantation into phakic eyes. Am J Ophthalmol 1989;107:659-63.
5. Sawelson H, Marks RG. Ten years refractive and visual results of radial keratotomy. Ophthalmology 1995;102:1892-1901.
6. Hersh PS, Stulting RD, Steinert RF, et al. Results of phase III Excimer laser photorefractive keratectomy for myopia The Summit PRK study group. Ophthalmology 1997;104:1535-53.
7. Davidorf JM, Zaldivar R, Oscherow S. Results and complications of laser in situ keratomileusis by experienced surgeons. J Refract Surg 1998;14:114-22.
8. Monte –Mico R, Alio J. Distance and near contrast sensitivity function after multifocal intraocular lens implantation. J Cataract Refract Surg 2003;29(4):703-11.
9. Perez-Santoja JJ, Alio Jl, Jimenez–Alfaro I, Zato MA. Surgical correction of severe myopia with an angle supported phakic intraocular lens. J Cataract Refrat Surg 2000;26(9):1288-302.

10. Baïkoff G, Arne JL, Bokobza Y, et al. Angle fixated anterior chamber phakic intraocular lens for myopia of -7 to-9 diopters. J Refract Surg 1998;14:282-93.
11. Menezo JL, Avino JA, Cisneros A, et al. Iris claw phakic intraocular lens for high myopia. J Refract Surg 1997;13: 545-55.
12. Zaldivar R, Oscherow S, Ricur G. Implantable contact lens. In Clear corneal lens surgery. Thorofare, NJ: SlackInc, 1999;287-324.
13. Steinert RF, Aker BL, Trentacost DJ, et al. A prospective study of the AMO-Array zonal progressive multifocal silicone intraocular lens and a monofocal intraocular lens. Ophthalmology 199;106:1243-45.

20

Epi-LASIK: An Advanced Surface Ablation Procedure

- EPI-LASIK: AN EVOLVING TECHNIQUE
- HISTOLOGICAL FINDINGS OF MECHANICALLY SEPARATED EPITHELIAL SHEETS
- EPI-LASIK: THE SURGICAL PROCEDURE
- POSTOPERATIVE TREATMENT
- CLINICAL RESULTS

Vikentia J Katsanevaki, Maria I Kalyvianaki, Ioannis G Pallikaris (Greece)

INTRODUCTION

Since the introduction of excimer lasers for photorefractive corrections the surgical trends are continuously changing in order to achieve the best possible clinical results with minimal complications. Photorefractive Keratectomy (PRK) initially introduced in the beginning of 90s[1,2] was the first technique to be used for photo refractive corrections. Despite its encouraging results for low and moderate myopia, during the evolvement of refractive surgery PRK was partially abandoned mostly due to the postoperative pain of the treated patients as well as the risk of corneal postoperative haze. Laser in situ keratomileusis (LASIK),[3,4] which involves the ablation deeper in the stroma after the creation of a corneal flap, soon became popular among refractive surgeons. Providing fast visual rehabilitation as well as the ability to correct higher degrees of ametropias LASIK is currently the undisputable leader within photorefractive treatments. However, LASIK is not without complications. Complications unique to LASIK such as those related to the use of the microkeratome,[5,6] LASIK induced diffuse lamellar keratitis[7] and the increasing reports of LASIK patients that developed corneal ectasia;[8] have set the stage for the revival of surface treatments.

Laser assisted subepithelial keratectomy[9] (LASEK) was the first attempt to modify surface treatments in order to control the major drawbacks of PRK, i.e. the postoperative pain and the risk of haze formation. The modification of the surgical technique as compared to the conventional PRK, was the separation of corneal epithelium as a sheet rather than its scrapping prior to the photo ablation. This epithelial sheet which is separated en toto and is replaced onto the ablated cornea, is thought to act as a natural contact lens on the operative eye[10] is expected to control the epithelial healing and thus provide better postoperative results as compared to PRK.

EPI-LASIK: AN EVOLVING TECHNIQUE

The separation of the epithelial sheet in LASEK as described by Camellin, requires the preparation of the cornea with a short-term exposure to a diluted (18%-20%) alcohol solution. In order to avoid the probable toxic effect of alcohol on the epithelium and the underlying stroma[13,14] Pallikaris described Epi- LASIK.[11,12] With this modality, the epithelial sheet is separated mechanically with the use of a customized device (Centurion Epiedge Epikeratome, Ciba Vision Surgical, GA) without the need of prior corneal preparation with alcohol. This device has recently granted CE mark and 510K aproval for clinical use and is commercially available. Epi-LASIK,[11,12] is currently the treatment of choice for low myopia in the University of Crete and up to now has been performed in more than 400 eyes worldwide (Figure 20.1). Its name is derived from the Greek word "epipolis" that means superficial and LASIK.

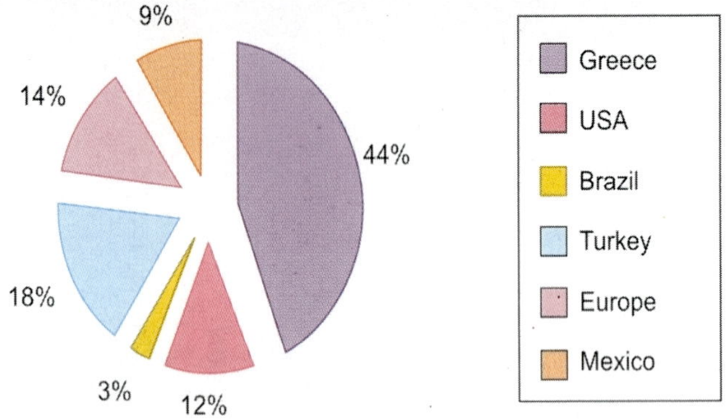

Figure 20.1: Epi-LASIK: experience around the globe (N = 402)

HISTOLOGICAL FINDINGS OF MECHANICALLY SEPARATED EPITHELIAL SHEETS

Transmission electron microscopy of harvested epithelial sheets in eyes that the treatments were reversed to PRK demonstrated that the cleavage plane of mechanical separation was located under the level of the basement membrane.[11] Basal epithelial cells had normal morphology with minimal evidence of trauma and edema and rested upon the prominent basal lamina, which consisted of an apparently structure less lamina lucida and an electron-dense lamina densa. Under the basal lamina an upper part on Bowman's layer was evident in the epithelial sheets (Figure 20.2). Intracellular organelles and intercellular desmosomal connections, as well as hemidesmosomal connections with the basement membrane appeared close to normal with only focal disruptions.

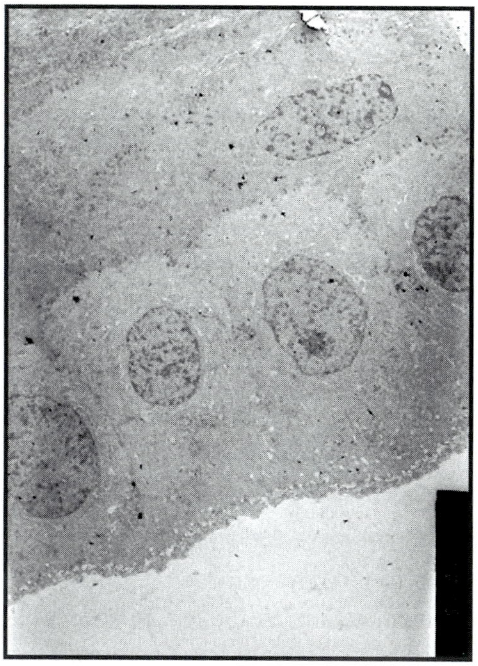

Figure 20.2: Transmit ion electron microscopy of a mechanically assisted separated sheet harvested from the operative eye immediately after the separation

Alcohol assisted epithelial separations are reported to take place within the basement membrane thus affecting its integrity.[11,15,16] The presence of an intact basement membrane has been shown to be important in the control of epithelial wound healing[17] minimizing the fibrotic activation of keratocytes. Even though alcohol solutions are not reported toxic in the specific concentrations and exposure times that are advocated for epithelial separations in LASEK,[18,19] mechanical separation appears to have the advantage of a deeper cleavage plane over alcohol assisted separations thus being expected to provide better control of corneal healing within the first postoperative days.

EPI-LASIK: THE SURGICAL PROCEDURE

The operative eye is prepared with three drops of topical tetracaine hydrochloride 0.5 percent (applied every 5 minutes before the procedure) and povidone-iodine and is covered with a sterile drape. Before the epithelial separation the cornea is marked with a customized Epi-LASIK marker (Epi-LASIK marker, Duckworth and Kent,

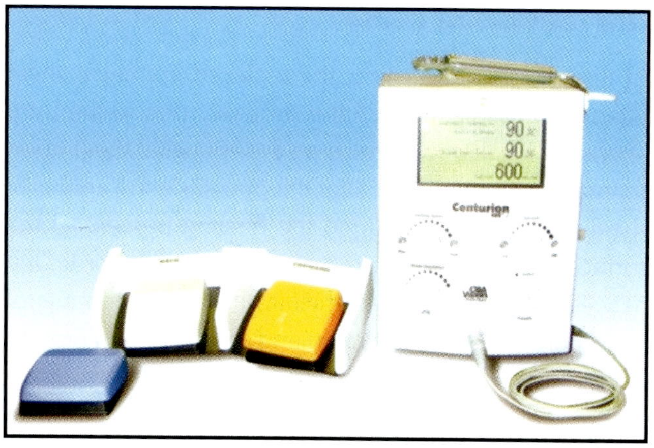

Figure 20.3: The Centurion sub epithelial epikeratome

Baldock, UK). This marker features two concentric circles crossed by 8 radial arms. Upon the replacement of the epithelial sheet, any deformity of the preoperative marks dictates its proper repositioning.

The Centurion EpiEdge Epikeratome is an electrically powered device (Figure 20.3) that operates under low suction similarly to a conventional microkeratome. Instead of a blade it features a disposable, oscillating polymethylmethacrylate (PMMA) separator with an advance speed of 3.5 mm/sec. The resulting separated epithelial sheet has a nasal hinge and a diameter of 9.5 to 10 mm. Any manipulations of the epithelial sheet both for its reflection and replacement, are performed with the use of a moistened sponge. The replacement of the separated epithelial sheet is often achieved with a single movement. Any inward or outward folds of its edges can be restored with the use of an anterior chamber irrigation canula under constant irrigation. Once the epithelial sheet is stuck to the underlying stroma, a therapeutic contact lens is applied onto the operative eye.

POSTOPERATIVE TREATMENT

Postoperative treatment includes eye drops of diclofenac sodium 0.1 percent qid for two days and combined eye drops of tobramycin-dexamethasone qid until the removal of the therapeutic lens. After the removal of the lens all treated eyes receive fluorometholone eye drops qid for five weeks in a tapered dose. Artificial tears are prescribed to be used at the patients' discretion.

Early Postoperative Course

At the end of the surgery, the replaced epithelial sheet often overlays its initial gutter probably due to the intra operative mechanical stretch on the epithelial sheet upon separation. Immediately after the operation the epithelial sheet is transparent. During the healing process of the surface, slit-lamp biomicroscopy reveals the borderline between the migrating epithelium and the remnants of the separated sheet. The migrating cells gradually replace the separated epithelial sheet, which is subsequently constricted in the central area. Starting from its peripheral part around the edges on the first postoperative day the sheet becomes hazy in its total area until about the third day after the treatment. At that time the hazy area measures about the central 1 to 2 mm whereas a front of newly synthesized, transparent epithelium migrates from the corneal periphery toward the center of the corneal surface. After that stage, the transparency of the corneal epithelium is restored within 24 to 48 hours and the therapeutic contact lens is removed. The time of epithelial healing ranges from 3 to 5 days between the treated eyes.

CLINICAL RESULTS

Up to date we have performed 183 mechanically assisted epithelial separations in the University of Crete. Seventy six eyes were left to heal as epi-LASIK whereas the rest of the separated sheets underwent histological evaluation and the treatments were reversed to PRK. The preoperative spherical equivalent of the treated eyes was up to –7.75 D, with cylinder up to –2.25 D.

Postoperative pain of the treated patients was assessed subjectively with a use of a questionnaire that graded pain in a scale from 0 to 4. The patients graded postoperative pain in two-hour intervals on the operative day and once daily in the following days. No patient reported pain after the operative day.On the operative day, the mean scores remained below the threshold of pain in the reported series of eyes (Figure 20.4). Similarly as after LASEK,[25, 26] epi-LASIK was not proved a totally pain –free procedure. We observed that discomfort or pain was mainly reported within the first postoperative hours. In order to deal with this finding we included intra

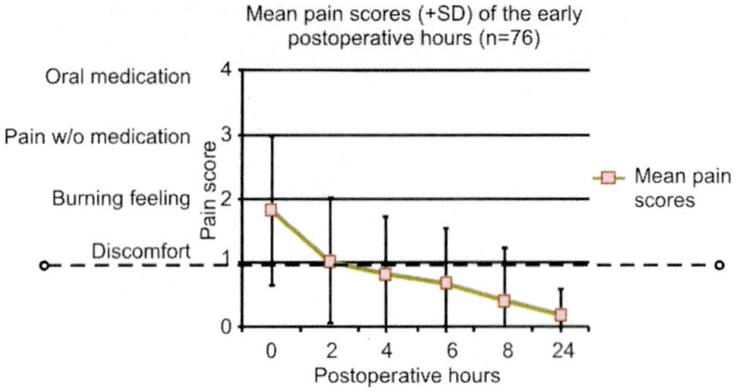

Figure 20.4: The mean pain scores remained below the threshold of burning feeling in the reported series of eyes

operative corneal cooling in the standard treatment of the last 20 eyes. We cooled the cornea immediately before the separation and after the ablation with the instillation of pre freezed balanced salt solution. After this alteration of the technique, the reported discomfort was below the threshold of pain in all patients even in the first postoperative hours.

During the early postoperative course, the mean uncorrected visual acuity (UCVA) of the treated eyes corresponded well with the progress of the epithelial healing and the transparency of the replaced epithelial sheet. More particularly, UCVA was better on the first postoperative day, when the epithelial sheet was transparent, to decrease around the third postoperative day, as the epithelial sheet became hazy, and, finally rise again, when the epithelial healing was complete (Figure 20.5). On the sixth month interval 94 percent of eyes had visual acuity of 20/25 or better whereas 48 percent of eyes have gained one or two (8%) Snellen's lines of best-corrected visual acuity.

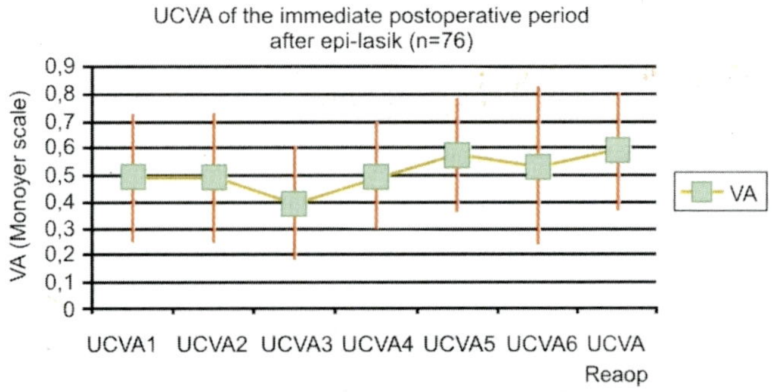

Figure 20.5: Early postoperative course

The vast majority of epi-LASIK eyes had clear corneas or trace haze at three (96%) and six month's (100%) postoperative intervals.

CONCLUSIONS

Histological findings of mechanically separated epithelial sheets have shown that mechanical separation preserves the epithelial cell viability, the stratification of the sheet and the integrity of the epithelial basement membrane. In contrast to the varying solution dilutions and exposure times required for alcohol assisted separations[20-22] the epikeratome can achieve mechanically assisted separations in a repetitive and fully automated way with a short learning curve for experienced LASIK surgeons. Preliminary clinical results are comparable to that of LASEK[15, 21,23,24] and suggest epi-LASIK as an efficient and safe alternative surgical modality for low myopia. Given the preliminary encouraging results for low myopia the next goal will be to apply this technique for higher myopic corrections. Intraoperative corneal cooling has an additive effect to the retained epithelial sheet minimizing discomfort below the threshold of pain in all the treated eyes. Future randomized comparative studies between epi-LASIK and PRK are expected to prove the advantages of the retained epithelial sheet in surface treatments.

REFERENCES

1. Seiler T, Wollensak J. Myopic photorefractive keratectomy with excimer laser; one-year follow up. Opthalmology 1991; 98:1156-63.
2. Epstein D, Fagerholm P, Hamberg-Nystroem H, Tengroth B. Twenty four-month follow up of excimer laser photorefractive keratectomy for myopia; Refractive and visual outcome results. Opthalmology 1994;101:1558-63.
3. Pallikaris IG, Papatzanaki ME, Siganos DS, Tsilimbaris MK. A corneal flap technique for laser in situ keratomileusis. Human studies. Arch Ophthalmol 1991;109(12):1699-702.
4. Hersh PS, Brint SF, Maloney RK, et al. Photorefractive keratectomy versus laser in situ keratomileusis for moderate to high myopia; A randomized prospective study. Opthalmology 1998;105:1512-22.
5. Pallikaris IG, Katsanevaki VJ, Panagopoulou SI. Laser in situ keratomileusis intraoperative complications using one type of microkeratome. Ophthalmology 2002;109(1):57-63.
6. Melki SA, Azar DT. LASIK complications: Etiology, management, and prevention. Surv Ophthalmol 2001(2); 46:95-116.
7. Smith RJ, Maloney RK. Diffuse lamellar keratitis. A new syndrome in lamellar refractive surgery. Ophthalmology. 1998;105(9):1721-26.
8. Pallikaris IG, Kymionis GD, Astyrakakis NI. Corneal ectasia induced by laser in situ keratomileusis. J Cataract Refract Surg. 2001;27(11):1796-802.
9. Camellin M, Cimberle M. LASEK technique promising after 1 year of experience. Ocular Surg News 2000;18(1):14-17.
10. Lee JB, Seong GJ, Lee JH, Seo KY, Lee YG, Kim EK. Comparison of laser epithelial keratomileusis and photorefractive keratectomy for low to moderate myopia. J Cataract Refract Surg 2001;27(4):565-70.
11. Pallikaris IG, Naoumidi II, Kalyvianaki MI, Katsanevaki VJ. Epi-LASIK: Comparative histological evaluation of mechanical and alcohol - assisted epithelial separation. J Cataract Refract Surg 2003;29(8):1496-501.
12. Pallikaris IG, Katsanevaki VJ, Kalyvianaki MI, Naoumidi II. Advances in subepithelial excimer refractive surgery techniques: Epi-LASIK. Curr Opin Ophthalmol 2003;14(4): 207-12.
13. Kamm O. The relation between structure and physiological action of the alcohols. J of the American Pharmaceutical Association 1921;10:87-92.
14. Kim SY, Sah WJ, Lim YW, Hahn TW. Twenty percent alcohol toxicity on rabbit corneal epithelial cells: Electron microscopic study. Cornea 2002;21(4): 388-92.
15. Azar DT, Ang RT, Lee JB, Kato T, Chen CC, Jain S, Gabison E, Abad JC. Laser subepithelial keratomileusis: electron microscopy and visual outcomes of photorefractive keratectomy. Curr Opin Ophthalmol 2001;12(4):323-28.
16. Espana EM, Gruetereich M, Mateo A, Romano AC, Yee SB, Yee RW, Tseng SCG. Cleavage plane of corneal basement membrane components by ethanol exposure in laser-assisted subepithelial keratectomy. J Cataract Refract Surg 2003;29: 1192-97.
17. Stramer BM, Zieske JD, Jung JC, Austin JS, Fini ME. Molecular mechanisms controlling the fibrotic repair phenotype in cornea: implications for surgical outcomes. Invest Ophthalmol Vis Sci 2003;44(10):4237-46.
18. Chen CC, Chang JH, Lee JB, Javier J, Azar DT. Human corneal epithelial cell viability and morphology after dilute alcohol exposure. Invest Ophthalmol Vis Sci 2002;43(8): 2593-2602.
19. Gabler B, Winkler von Mohrenfelds C, Dreiss AK, Marshall J, Lohmann CP. Vitality of epithelial cells after alcohol exposure during laser-assisted subepithelial keratectomy flap preparation. J Cataract Refract Surg 2002;28:1841-46.
20. Camellin M. Laser epithelial keratomileusis for myopia. J Refract Surg 2003;19:666-70.
21. Chalita MR, Tekwani NH, Krueger RR. Laser epithelial keratomileusis: Outcome of initial cases performed by an experienced surgeon. J Refract Surg 2003;19:412-15.
22. Litwak S, Zadok D, Garcia-de Quevedo V, Robledo N, Chayet AS. Laser-assisted subepithelial keratectomy versus photorefractive keratectomy for the correction of myopia. A prospective comparative study. J Cataract Refract Surg 2002;28:1330-33.

23. Anderson NJ, Beran RF, Schneider TL. Epi-LASEK for the correction of myopia and myopic astigmatism. J Cataract Refract Surg 2002;28:1343-47.
24. Claringbold VT. Laser-assisted subepithelial keratectomy for the correction of myopia. J Cataract Refract Surg 2002; 28:18-22.
25. Shahinian L. Laser-assisted subepithelial keratectomy for low to high myopia and astigmatism. J Cataract Refract Surg 2002;28:1334-42.
26. Rouweyha RM, Chuang AZ, Mitra S, Phillips CB,Yee RW. Laser Epithelial Keratomileusis for myopia with the Autonomous Laser. J Refract Surg 2002;18:217-24.

21

Presbyopic Multifocal LASIK (PML): A New Approach in Corneal Refractive Surgery

- APPROACHES TO THE SURGICAL CORRECTION OF PRESBYOPIA
- THE PML™ PROCEDURE
- RESULTS
- PEARLS AND LESSONS LEARNED

Roberto Pinelli (Italy)

INTRODUCTION

In all refractive surgery, our goal has been to surgically correct the visual defects, i.e. myopia, hyperopia, astigmatism, and presbyopia. Correction of these defects is possible through corneal surgical procedures or lenticular surgery.

Of all the visual defects, presbyopia has been the most challenging to correct, partly because the mechanisms of accommodation and the causes of presbyopia are complex and not fully understood. Thus far, it has largely been managed through the use of progressively stronger spectacles, which gradually take over the near focus work of the crystalline lens. Presbyopia is also unique in that it is the only refractive error that is considered to be progressive in nature. Although our management and most of our experience seems to point to the progressive nature of presbyopia, in truth, we don't know for sure that it truly progresses. It maybe that in our "prosthetic culture" we have merely become unnecessarily dependent on our glasses and contacts.

In any case, a surgical alternative to the correction of presbyopia is appealing because of the enormous pool of presbyopic patients with a desire for good uncorrected vision. Mild hyperopes and emmetropes who have never worn glasses are particularly uncomfortable with presbyopia and its associated inconveniences.

APPROACHES TO THE SURGICAL CORRECTION OF PRESBYOPIA

The mission of presbyopic surgery—as with all other refractive surgeries—should be to eliminate the symptoms of the refractive error, rather than to correct the anatomical defect itself. For this reason, I think an approach that provides pseudoaccommodation is natural and appropriate. If we can provide patients with good functional vision at multiple distances, it is not necessary to restore true accommodative function in the form of a dynamically adjusting optical power of the eye.

There are several potential sites for correction of presbyopia. The cornea is probably the most common target, as it is the area refractive surgeons are most comfortable operating on. Theoretically, the anterior chamber provides another site for the correction of presbyopia, but this is as yet theoretical and would likely prove extremely difficult in reality. The human crystalline lens can be replaced with a multifocal or accommodative intraocular lens, of which many different styles are now under development and coming to market. Finally, a number of scleral implant or ciliary muscle surgical procedures have been developed. This approach, however, is complicated, largely untested, and seems "more surgical" than is necessary.

As a familiar corneal procedure, LASIK has been the most popular and easiest surgical approach. In addition to the surgeon comfort level with the procedure, patients in the presbyopic baby boomer generation are also familiar with and accepting of the procedure. In addition, LASIK can be performed bilaterally on the same day, is relatively quick and painless, and has proven to be quite safe.

Even with LASIK, we have several options for addressing presbyopia. Most conventionally, we have taken a monofocal approach with surgically-induced monovision, but bifocal and multifocal approaches are increasing. LASIK is ideal for presbyopia because of the absence of haze and its associated refractive complications, the absence of regression, and the presence of a regular and, hopefully, thin flap that can protect the multifocality created in the stroma.

In designing a multifocal LASIK procedure, we must take advantage of some of the lessons learned from current and past procedures. Some myopes treated with radial keratotomy have retained good near and distance vision well into the presbyopic age range. Why is that? Similarly, some hyperopic LASIK patients also have retained their pseudoaccommodative function well into their older years. Again, why would that be? The secret lies in the asphericity of the cornea. A prolate cornea seems to have the capability to focus both far and near better than an oblate cornea. We have seen that again recently with conductive keratoplasty, which author performs and have been involved in studying in Italy. CK is an excellent technique for correcting hyperopia and restoring near vision. It appears to provide some degree of multifocality because eyes corrected for near visual acuity with CK typically have much better distance visual acuity than would be expected. This may be due to the prolateness of the post-CK cornea. In any case, the "blended vision" of CK permits the presbyopic patient to read by treating just the non-dominant eye.

In the past three years, my purpose has been to create a truly multifocal corneal procedure that can be performed bilaterally if necessary, and that will work for any eye, regardless of preoperative refractive error. Intuitively, we know that many zones should do a better job of mimicking natural vision than just two zones, but obtaining a gradual but effective multifocality is nonetheless challenging. The ultimate presbyopic LASIK procedure must also be easy to perform, with standardized nomograms that any surgeon can use as a basis for successful surgery.

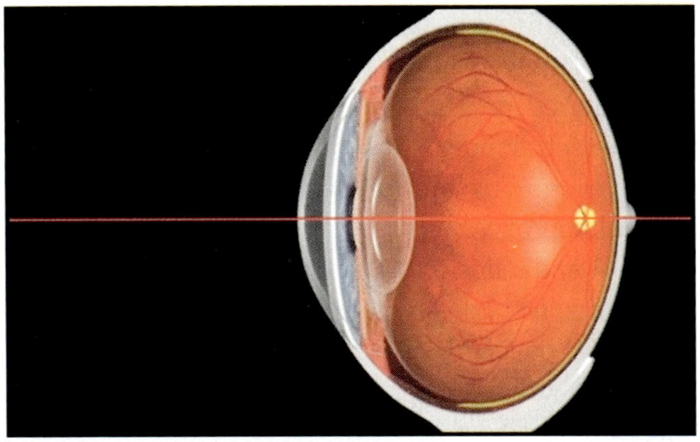

Figure 21.1: Central area of the cornea: Focus on the retina

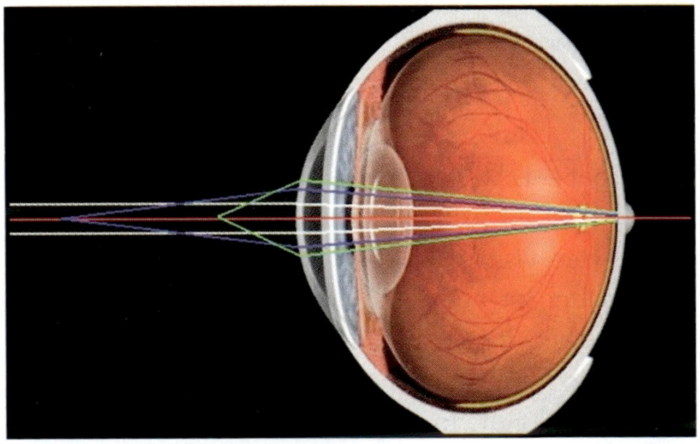

Figure 21.2: Multifocality permits to focus both far and near objects on macula (pseudo-accommodation)

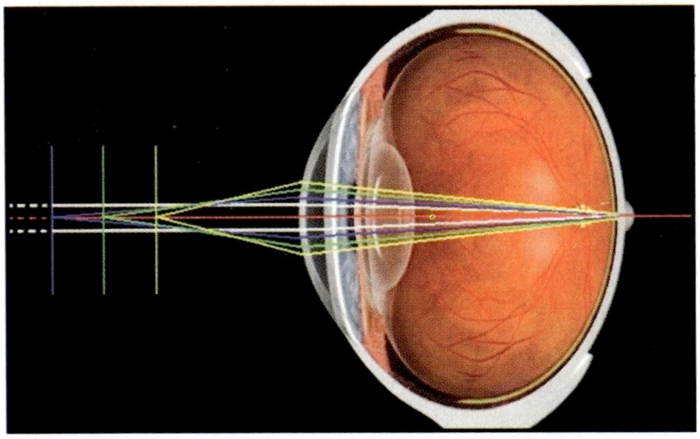

Figure 21.3: Effects of a completely multifocal cornea

THE PML™ PROCEDURE

With the above goals in mind, the author developed and have been investigating at ILMO a patented procedure which we call PML™ (Presbyopic Multifocal LASIK). This procedure can be performed on presbyopic myopes, hyperopes, astigmats, and emmetropes. Multifocality on the cornea is created using a multi-step treatment in which several independently calculated ablations are performed at various optical zones. Depending on the patient's refractive error, there may be anywhere from three to eight different concentric zones. In all cases, the goal is to treat the central cornea for distance vision, with a multifocal peripheral cornea that is able to provide functional near vision. Some other multifocal LASIK procedures take the opposite approach, with the near correction in the center. However, the central cornea provides an excellent site for distance vision because it is relatively aberration-free, while peripheral aberrations may actually be useful for near focusing (Figures 21.1 to 21.3).

In this multi-step process, we first treat astigmatism in the classic manner, as if we were doing a purely astigmatic laser correction. Next we treat the distance defect in a zone on the central cornea. Then, we treat the near defect in a larger optical zone. Finally, other zones maybe created to ensure that the overall power of the cornea is emmetropic, even though there are varying powers in the different optical zones. It is a procedure that is highly customizable for each patient's optical needs.

The author began doing this procedure in 2002, starting cautiously by treating 10 patients in only their non-dominant eyes. One year postoperatively, five of these patients were happy with their outcomes; the other five required retreatment. These unilateral patients experienced some of the benefits and problems of monovision. The author became convinced that a bilateral approach would be more effective, and began to adjust and refine the nomograms toward this end.

For our first bilateral study cohort, we treated 100 eyes of 50 patients with. Our studies so far have been performed with the Technolas 217 Z (Bausch and Lomb) and the Lasitome microkeratome (Gebauer). However, the procedure is technology-independent and was designed to work with any keratome and laser combination.

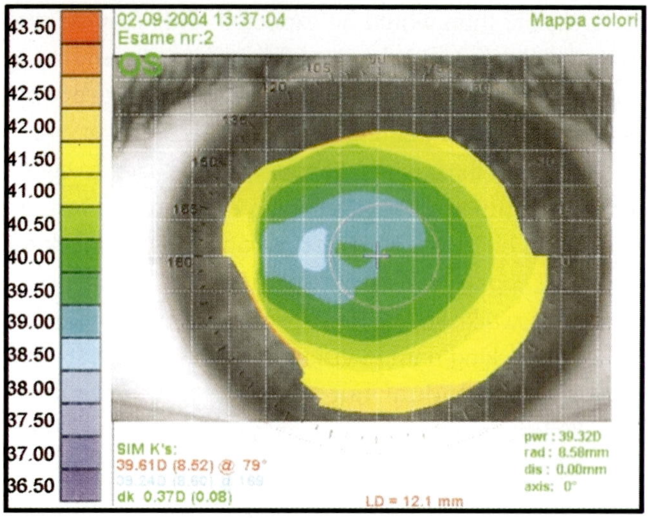

Figure 21.5: A prolate cornea after PML™ case # 1

RESULTS

All 50 patients were seeing at least 20/25 for distance and at least J3 for near. Eighty percent had bilateral uncorrected vision of 20/20 or better for distance *and* J2 or better for near. Another 10 percent were 20/25 and J2, while the remaining 10 percent were 20/25 and J3. Patient satisfaction levels have been very high, and there have been no retreatments thus far. Typically, patients experience a myopic shift during the first month postoperatively, then stabilize at plano (Figure 21.4).

A few cases illustrate well the potential of this procedure. The first example is a 50-year-old female who was a –6.0 D myope with a +1.5 D add for reading. We treated the cornea in six different zones: a –1.5 D correction in each of the following optical zones: 4.8, 5.2, 5.4, 5.6, and 6.0 mm; and a +2.00 D correction at the 6.5-mm optical zone. Six months postop, her uncorrected vision is 20/20 and J2 in both eyes (Figure 21.5).

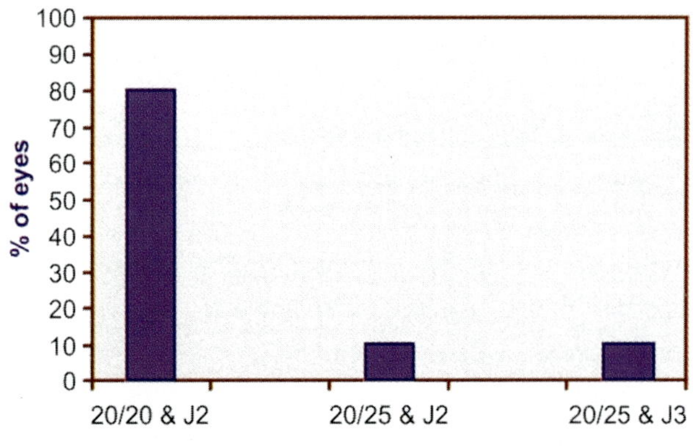

Figure 21.4: 50 patients' eyes post-op results

The second case is a 54-year-old patient who was plano in both eyes preoperatively but using a +1.5 D add for near vision. We performed two treatment rings for near vision, each +0.75 D, at the 6.0 and 6.5-mm optical zones. In addition, author did three treatment rings for distance vision, ablating a –0.50 D spherical correction at the 5.0, 5.2, and 5.4-mm optical zones. After a myopic reaction initially, the eyes are now emmetropic, and six months postop, this patient's uncorrected visual acuity is 20/20 and J2 in both eyes. Ultimately, my goal is to be able to correct emmetropes like this as soon as they start experiencing presbyopic symptoms at age 45 or 50 (Figure 21.6).

PEARLS AND LESSONS LEARNED

We have found that it is better to overcorrect hyperopia and to undercorrect myopia, and that astigmatism must be fully corrected for a satisfactory outcome. In some cases (hyperopes and emmetropes), the cornea becomes more prolate; in other cases (primarily myopes) it actually becomes more oblate. Pupil size is not an important factor in determining outcomes from this procedure. We have not had to manage patients with especially large pupils any differently than we would with a monofocal LASIK procedure.

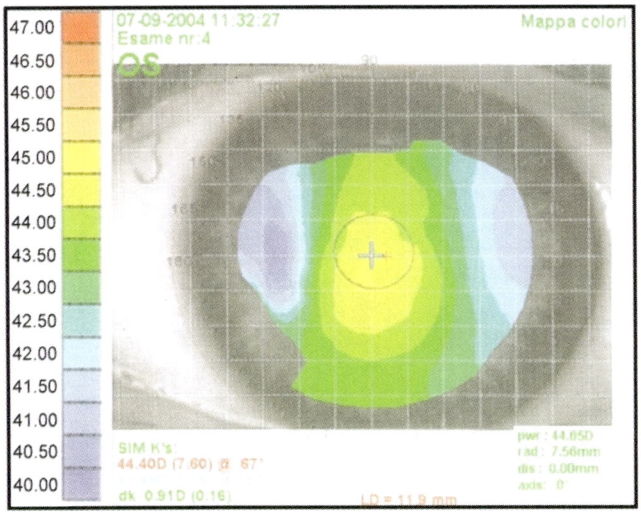

Figure 21.6: An oblate cornea after PML™ case # 2

The PML™ technique uses the same or less tissue as other laser vision correction procedures, so although pachymetry is important, it is no more a factor than in monofocal LASIK. Keratometry is very important, as it is essential to keep the pre- and post-operative K values constant.

Patients must be willing to participate in training their eyes to learn how to see at near with the multifocal correction. Our patients are instructed not to use reading glasses after the procedure at all and to do visual exercises (for which we provide instruction) in order to maintain the eye's focusing power with age.

In our experience so far, is a very successful procedure that has been well-accepted by patients and is in high demand at our center. Currently, about 30 percent of our patients are PML™ candidates. The procedure and the excellent results experienced by patients have enhanced the reputation of our center and generated many referrals. Ongoing research is required to determine whether and when regression might occur.

22

Aberrometric Correction of Presbyopia: Theory and Results

- PRESBYOPIA AND ACCOMMODATION
- HELMHOLTZ'S THEORY
- SPHERICAL ABERRATION

Franco Bartoli (Italy)

PRESBYOPIA AND ACCOMMODATION

The word presbyopia (which comes from Greek πρεσβυς οψ = old eye), identifies the age-related reduced ability in near vision.

In spite of last century's technical progress, the mechanisms of accommodation and the reason for which its decrease causes presbyopia remain a partly solved problem. Recently measurements with two different units (VISANTE OCT and UBM) confirm probably the Helmholtz's theory (Marchini).

There are two opposite theories:

Helmholtz's Theory

Helmholtz's theory (1855) and subsequent modifications derive the accommodation from a decrease in zonular tension, with a relative curving of the crystalline lens front surface (greater refractive power) and an increase in its front-rear diameter. Presbyopia is due to a crystalline lens sclerosis (lack of elasticity) and to an atrophy of ciliary muscle with consequent impossibility to obtain such a curving (Figure 22.1).

Schachar's Theory

Schachar's theory (1994) assumes that zonula fibers can be divided into three groups: front, equatorial and rear fibers. Accommodation only involves the equatorial ones, while front and rear fibers have almost solely a support function. During the accommodation process there would be an increase in equatorial fibers tension and a decrease in that of front and rear ones; therefore, there is an increase in central curvature and a decrease in the peripheral one, related to an increase in front-rear diameter (thickness) of crystalline lens (Figure 22.2). The loss of accommodation is bounded to the increase of crystalline lens equatorial volume (about 20 mm, per year) and to the consequent decrease in distance between the ciliary muscle body and the crystalline lens equator, with relative loss of efficiency of tractional activity by the equatorial fibers.

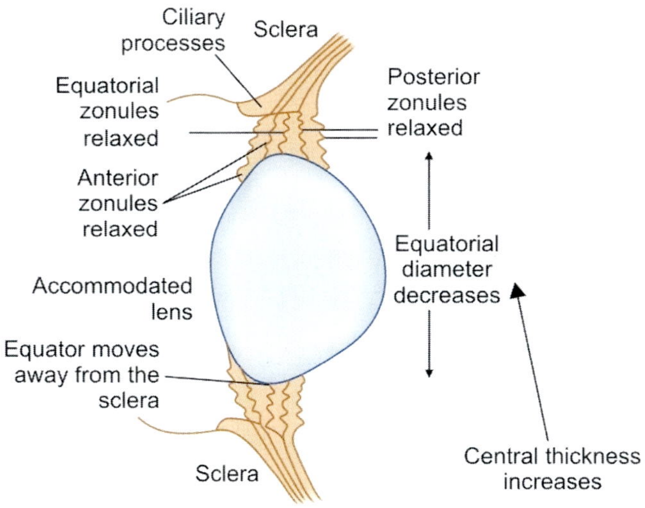

Figure 22.1: Helmholtz's model of accommodation

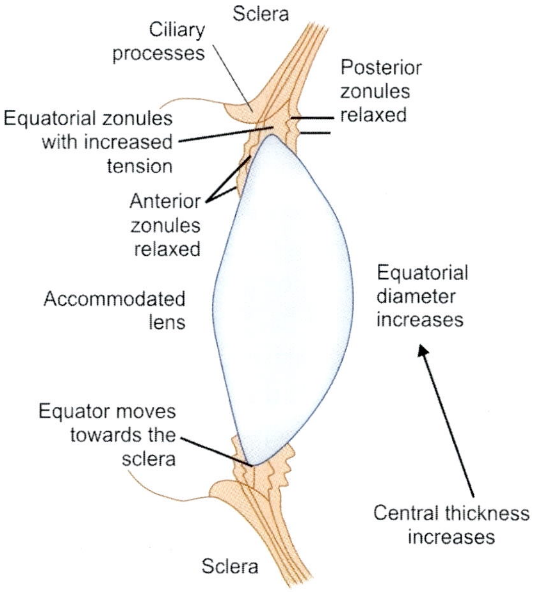

Figure 22.2: Schachar's model of accommodation

According to the above theories, during the accommodation process the increased crystalline lens refractive power (accommodation) is caused by the increased curvature of the entire front surface (Helmholtz) or by an increase of the central one with a decrease in the peripheral one (Schachar). Theories apart, presbyopia correction has always been realized with positive lenses (either monofocal, bifocal, or multifocal) which guaranteed focus at about 30 to 40 cm.

After finding solutions for myopia, hypermetropy and astigmatism, in the last few years refractive surgery has been fighting for a new goal: correct presbyopia. Schachar's hypothesis, based on practical experimentation (SEB), has started a race between all people involved in refractive surgery (manufacturers, ophthalmologists, etc.) toward a possible practical solution. Scleral expansion bands (Schachar) have been proposed to move the ciliary muscle away from the crystalline lens equator.

Excimer laser ablation assumes that the cornea, interpreted a glass lens, is transformed into a bifocal or multifocal lens. Another possible solution is monovision, and so on. For the last three years Bartoli have been proposing a slight different solution with excimer laser. Taking advantage of the newest aberrometric acquisitions, it offers a possible solution in this field.

SPHERICAL ABERRATION

When an optical system has an axis of revolution, the light rays emitted from a point *P* remain on the plane of incidence containing the axis and hit it again at a point P_1 (Figure 22.3).

If the rays converge at *1*, the plane of the pupil of entrance, which is perpendicular to the axis at *C*, the length *C-I* is defined as the height of incidence *h*. All rays of equal *h* that arrive from *P* reach a certain point P_1 (Figure 22.4), but the position of this point is a function of *h*.

$$X^1 = a_o + a_1 h + a_2 h_2 + \dots \dots = a_o + \delta x^1$$

The coefficients *a* are functions of the abscissa *x*, the sources and the wavelength λ.

The term a_o is the abscissa of the paraxial image or image according to Gauss's approximation, and corresponds to the value x^1 when *h* is infinitely small.

In the above formulation, the quantity δx^1, which unites all terms other than a_o, is called spherical

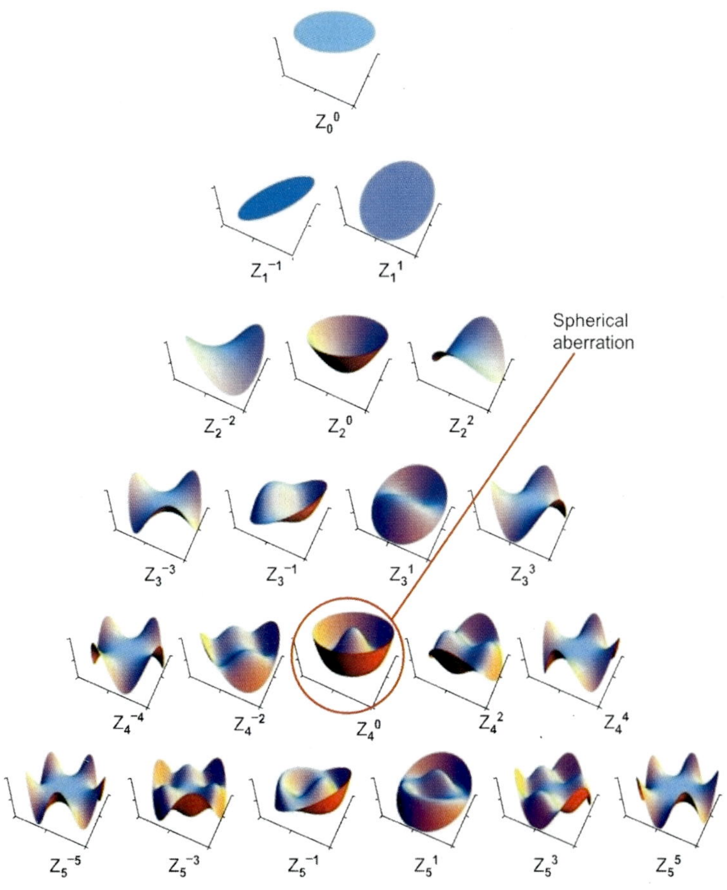

Figure 22.3: Spherical aberration

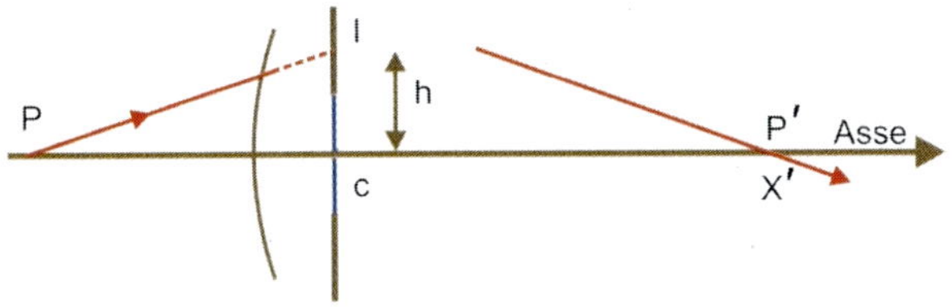

Figure 22.4: Schematic diagram showing spherical aberration

aberration and expresses the divergence between the paraxial image and the point where the rays actually focus on the axis; it is a function of h, x and λ.

An optical system is called "correct" when spherical aberration is zero for a certain value of x and λ; this system is called stigmatic for the point object and the set λ. In most cases, the spherical diopter is not a correct system.

Spherical aberration is due to the fact that the peripheral regions of a lens have a refractive power different from that of the central areas. For example, in a biconvex lens the rays that hit a central area are focused at a greater distance and those that hit the peripheral area focus at a shorter distance from the lens (Figure 22.5).

There are two focus, one for the central rays and another for the peripheral rays. The distance between the two focus determines a triangular area called the caustic.

In an incorrect system, the spherical aberration (δx^1) can be positive or negative. As h increases, P^1 moves towards or away from the light source, and the system is called overcorrect or undercorrect. The caustic defined as the surface fashioned from an outer envelope of light rays has its point P^1 in either one sense or the other, depending on whether there is overcorrection or undercorrection.

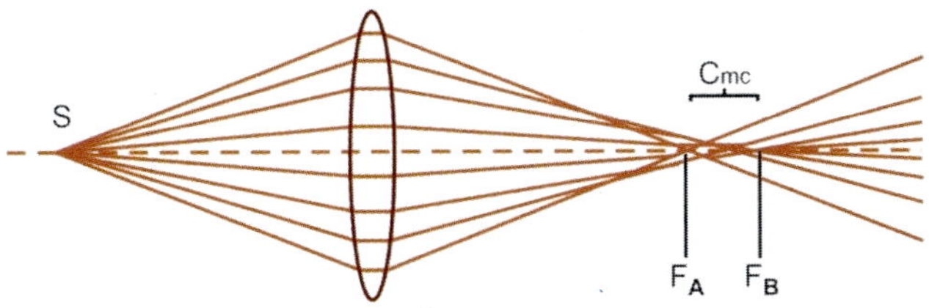

Figure 22.5: Spherical aberration: Peripheral regions of lens have different refractive power than that of central areas

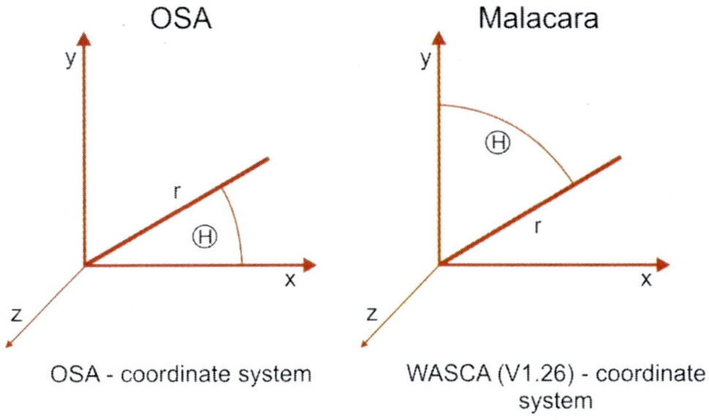

$$\sqrt{5}(6R^4 - 6R^2 + 1)$$

Figures 22.6A and B: Calculation system to determine spherical aberration: A OSA system; B. WASCA system

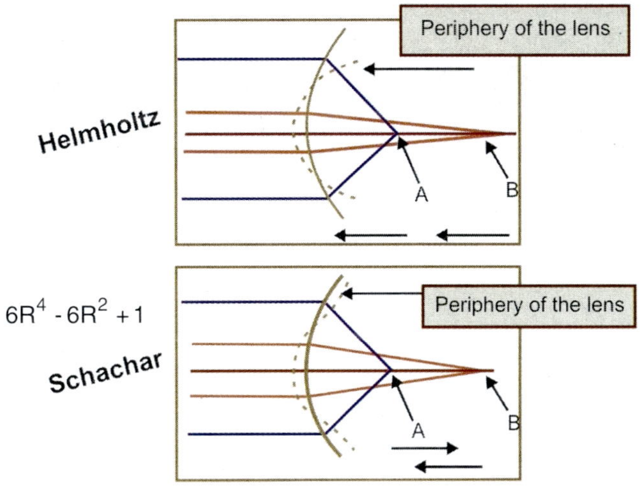

Figure 22.7: Helmholtz's and Schachar's theory of accommodation determining a positive spherical induction

In the last few years, depending on the calculation systems (WASCA or OSA) and thus on the aberrometer, front wave being equal, the same spherical aberration could be defined as positive or negative and even change its numeric value, inducing confusion. That is the reason why a conversion system has been prepared. It is always necessary to specify which one notation is used (Figures 22.6 to 22.11).

In our description results we always use the MALACARA notation:

1. When marginal rays focus is closer to the crystalline lens than paraxial rays, a positive spherical aberration is present.

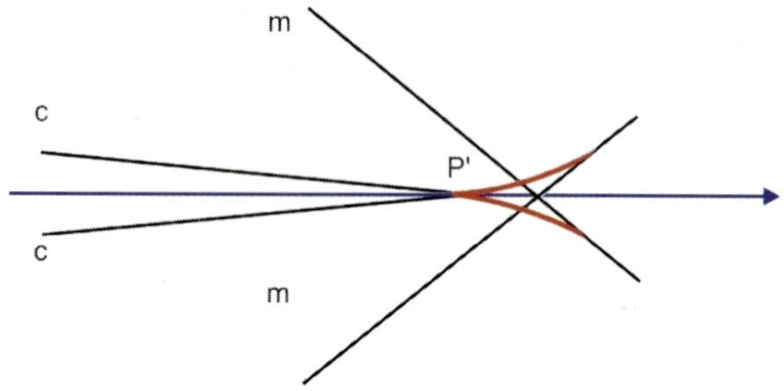

Figure 22.8: Positive spherical aberration

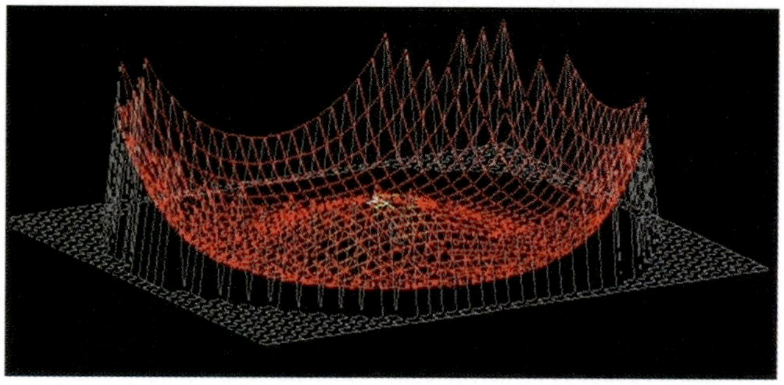

Figure 22.9: 3D image of positive spherical aberration

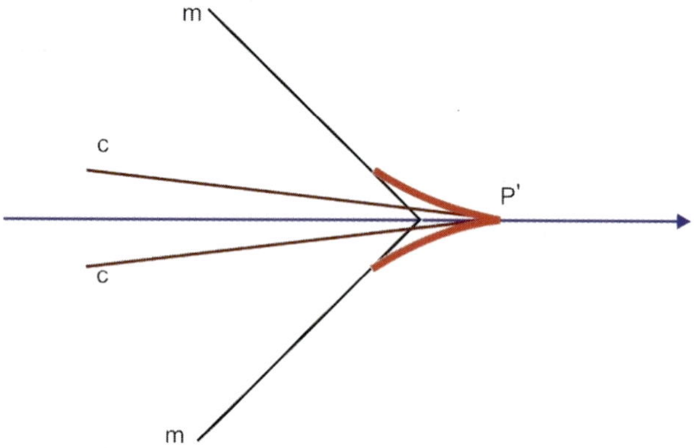

Figure 22.10: Negative spherical aberration

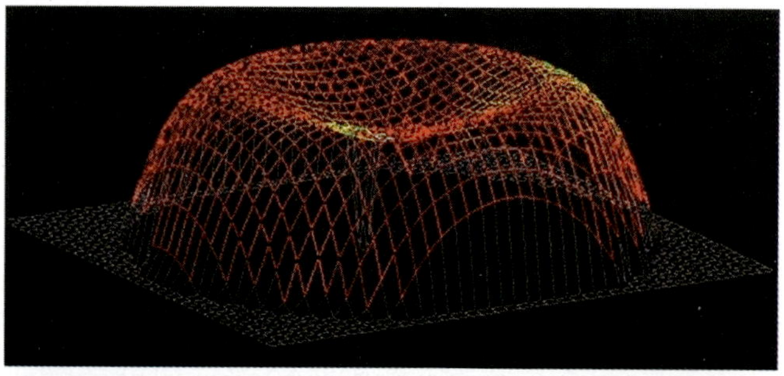

Figure 22.11: 3D image of negative spherical aberration

2. When marginal rays focus is farther from the crystalline lens than that of paraxial rays, a negative spherical aberration is present.

Out of Helmholtz's and Schachar's theory, during accommodation, there is always positive spherical aberration induction, with two focus A and B identifying a caustic defined as the surface fashioned from an outer envelope of light rays (Figure 22.7).

Since the cornea of the eye is aspherical (correct optical system), spherical aberration is due to the lens. In accommodation at rest, spherical aberration is almost zero or slightly negative; during accommodation it increases and becomes positive. Hence, the eye's optical system is undercorrect in accommodation at rest and overcorrect during accommodation.

The Eye and the Spherical Aberration

In a study of the human eye in 1500 patients conducted with a WASCA aberrometer, spherical aberration was found to be zero or slightly negative in accommodation at rest (Pallicaris).

The cornea is a practically aspherical lens, as is the lens in the absence of accommodation. During accommodation, both for near vision or compensation of a hypermetropic defect for far vision, the central anterior surface of the lens curves, inducing positive spherical aberration.

With dynamic wavefront analysis using a WASCA aberrometer it was possible to quantify both accommodation (Figure 22.12A) and induced positive spherical aberration (Figures 22.12B and 22.13); or impossibility of accommodation and apherical aberration induction in presbiopic eye (Figure 22.14).

At this point, a direct correlation can be assumed between spherical aberration and accommodation. In confirmation of what was stated above, it can be shown that in presbyopes over 60 years of age there is no increase in spherical aberration since they try to accommodate. Briefly:

1. In presbyopia there is a lack of accommodation with increasing age
2. During accommodation there is a shift in spherical aberration from zero or negative to positive or only positivation of spherical aberration

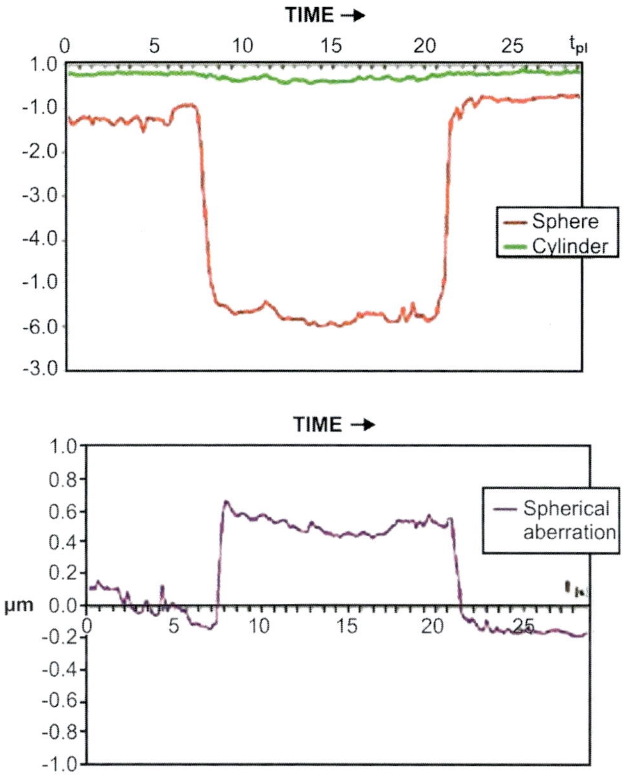

Figures 22.12A and B: Variation of spherical aberration during accommodation

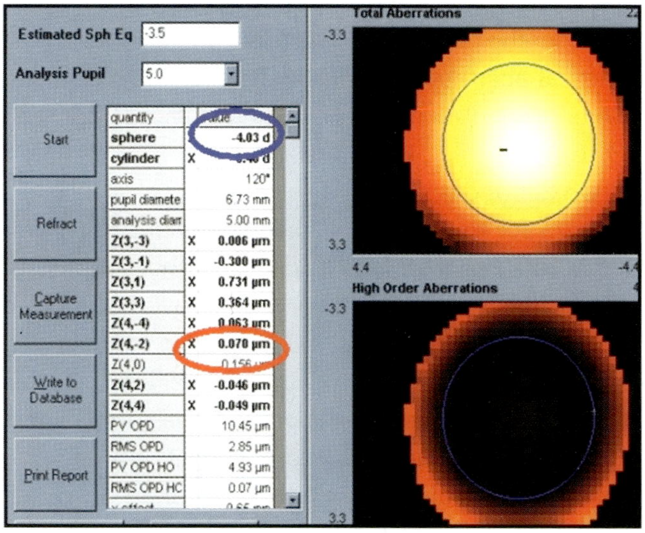

Figure 22.13: Positive spherical aberration during accommodation (–4.03D)

3. A close correlation exists between accommodation and spherical aberration

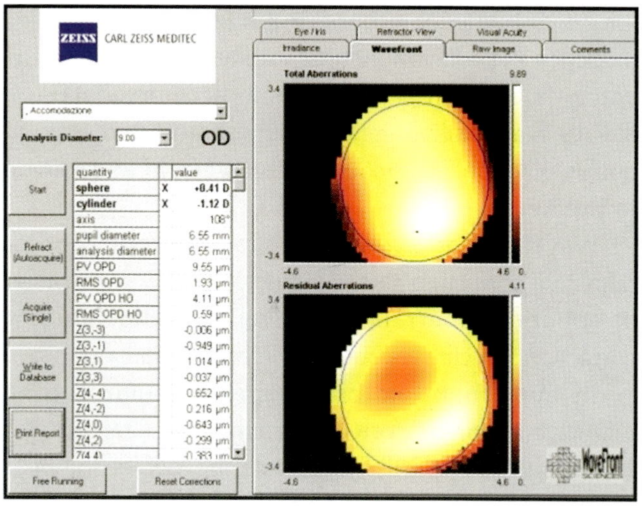

Figure 22.14: In presbyop there is not accommodation and spherical aberration induction

4. In presbyopes, the loss of accommodation is accompanied by a loss of the ability to induce spherical aberration
5. Inducing an increase in positive spherical aberration can compensate for the loss of accommodation in the presbyope.

To confirm what previously stated, the following experiment can be performed, on the basis that placing in front of the eye a neutral lens, the optical system is not modified (Peyman).

- Using an excimer laser, spherical aberration is induced on a neutral lens
- The lens is applied on a emmetrope, presbyopic patient
- The patient will have a normal distance vision and will acquire a good near vision.

Dynamic wavefront analysis allows accommodation to be objectively assessed and changes in the wavefront it induces, i.e. there is an increase of spherical aberration from almost zero or slightly negative to positive. In moderately hypermetropic patients in non-presbyopic age with good farsightedness and near-sightedness without corrective lenses, the correlation between the change of accommodation and the change of spherical aberration is particularly significant.

A young, moderately hypermetropic eye focuses far and near objects thanks to the increased curvature of the central anterior surface of the lens, with a relative induction of positive spherical aberration. The eye of the young hypermetrope is always in accommodation; it always has positive spherical aberration and a good quality of vision. It is evident that: **spherical aberration is the key**.

Wavefront analysis after hypermetropic photorefractive correction shows an increase and positivation of spherical aberration; conversely, after myopic correction it increases but still remains negative.

In hypermetropic presbyopes, circular corona refractive treatment corrects the refractive defect for far vision and also partially corrects the defect for near vision. If associated with aberrometric treatment, which corrects spherical aberration and raises it from negative to zero, a further increase is obtained with positivation of spherical aberration, thus fully correcting near vision. In addition, coma aberration is improved, with a subsequent enhancement of quality of vision. Hence, there is an evident correlation between hypermetropic treatment, positive spherical aberration and accommodation.

In the optical system of the eye, the first diopter (cornea) remains aspherical, the second (lens) does not; despite the induction of spherical aberration, the quality of the image does not deteriorate but improves instead, nor is there any alteration in contrast perception. The objective, therefore, is to make the presbyopic eye resemble a hypermetropic eye in constant accommodation by inducing a certain amount of spherical aberration on the cornea.

Research on spherical aberration and its measurement in the human eye has always been hampered by the fact that the optical system could only be studied from one side, unlike the examination of telescopic lenses or a photographic objective.

The first observations on spherical aberration in the human eye were made by Juren (1738) and the first measurements by Young (1801), and later studies by Tscherning and Gullstrand. But it was not until 1950 that an effective method was found to objectify measurements, wherein the image of a light source was formed on the retina and then used as a source of light to study aberrations of the eye as done with any objective. It was discovered that the light diffused by the retina suppresses the distribution of optical phase caused by the first passage of light through the eye, so that the results were referable only to the reverse/return trajectory.

During the early 1950s, Francon and Ivanoff (1951-1953) demonstrated that, contrary to previous thought, an increase of spherical aberration did not deteriorate the quality of the image. In fact, except for a small central area, the emerging wave was in concordant phase for the entire pupillary area, so that only when the pupils were very constricted could spherical aberration play a certain role. From this evidence it was clear that spherical aberration did not affect vision and that the quality of the image was not distorted (Y Le Grand).

In recent years, however, wavefront analysis using new aberrometers has confirmed the theoretical bases and experimental measurements of 50 years earlier.

RESULTS

On 2002, we treated mostly hyperopic patients, with PRK and a MEL 70 excimer laser. Results were encouraging, and continue to be so. The higher the hyperopia (3-4 diopters), with a highly hyperprolate final cornea, the better the near vision. The reach a good near vision, spherical aberration had to be made positive of 0.6 to 0.7 μm, regardless of initial curvature (Figures 22.15 and 22.16).

On 2003, despite modification of the photoablative program for myopic eyes, treatment with PRK/LASIK and MEL 70 excimer laser lead to better but still unsatisfactory results. As on February, 2004, we had treated 142 eyes—120 hyperopic, 20 myopic, 2 emmetropes. On 2004 we adopted the MEL 80 excimer laser, capable of reaching a certain degrees of prolateness for low and medium myopia, and reached the target. It is easier to make hyperprolate a refracted cornea than an oblate cornea. This means making positive a spherical aberration not excessively negative. At the same time the mathematical calculations for refractive compensation, for unit of positivization of spherical aberration, became more precise, allowing a standardization of the technique.

PREOP		S.G.	POSTOP 2 YEARS	
BCVA	Near BCVA	56 y.	UCVA	Near UCVA
+2.75sph 10/10	+4.75sph IJ	Left Eye	10/10	IJ
High order aberrations	Zernike polynomials			High order aberrations
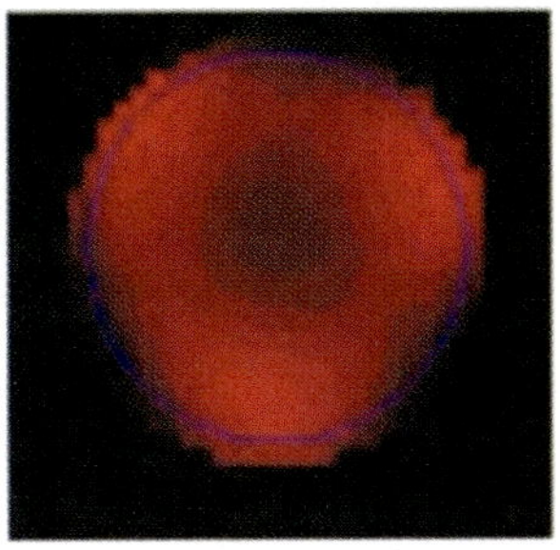	Value	Zernike term	Value	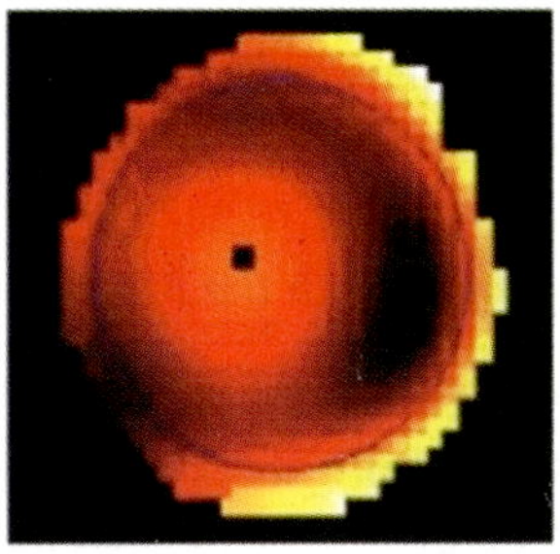
	-0.337 µm	Z(4,0)	0.650 µm	

Figure 22.15: Full correction of refractive defect for farsightedness. A major increase in spherical aberration Z (4.0) which changes from negative to positive. Pseudoaccommodation with near-sightedness *IJ* without lenses

PREOP		M.A.	POSTOP	
BCVA	Near BCVA	60 y.	UCVA	Near UCVA
+2.50sph 10/10	+4.75sph IJ	Left Eye	11/10	IJ
High order aberrations	Zernike polynomials			High order aberrations
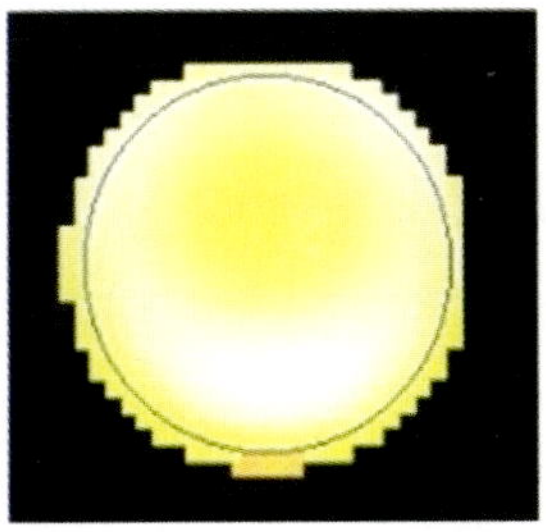	Value	Zernike term	Value	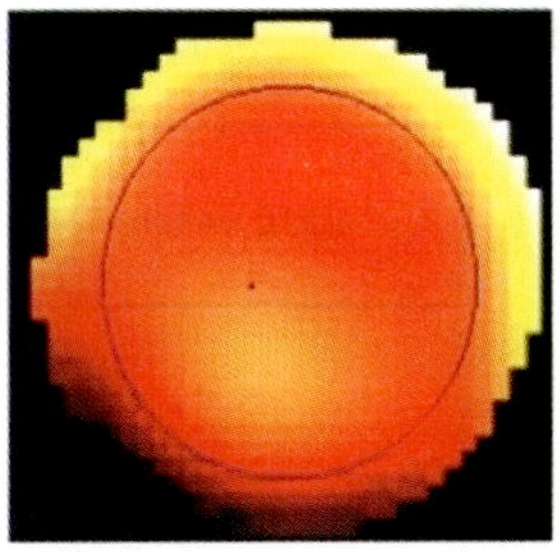
	-0.483 µm	Z(4,0)	0.277 µm	

Figure 22.16: Full correction of refractive defect for farsightedness with an increase of 1/10 in vision. A major increase in spherical aberration *Z* (4.0) which changes from negative to positive. Pseudoaccommodation with near-sightedness *IJ* without lenses

In hyperopic eyes, positivization of spherical aberration had to be of 0.8 to 1.0 µm, with a refractive hypercorrection for compensation of 0.5 to 0.75 diopters. In presbyopic myopic eyes positivization of spherical aberration had to be of 1.1 to 1.2 µm, with a refractive hypocorrection of 2 to 2.5 diopters. This always considering the positivization (hyperops) or negativization (myops) induced by standard treatment.

From all these calculations, derived clearly the correction for the emmetrope: positivization of spherical aberration and refractive treatment for compensation. Single or compound astigmatism could be treated with the same rules defined for spherical defects, according to their sign.

From March 2004 to today, April 2005, we have treated a total of 128 eyes – 86 hyperops, 32 myops, 10 emmetropes. During the last year-and –half, Carl Zeiss Meditech in Germany started new experiments with MEL and CRS Master (Dieter Dausch, Eckard Schroder), with similar results. Furthermore, they could highlight safety of treatment, without loss in contrast sensitivity at distant and close vision, no halos, etc.

A Few Examples with the MEL 80 Excimer Laser

Hyperopic patient of forty-eight-year-old, + 4.00 spherical (Figures 22.17 and 22.18A and B). All refractive and aberrometric data reported, final refraction was satisfactory, and inversion of spherical aberration, turning from negative to positive. Topographical examination shows how the cornea becomes hyperprolate after the treatment.

Fifty-year-old myopic and astigmatic patient (Figures 22.19 and 22.20). Pre- and postoperative refractive and aberrometric data are presented, as well as the power difference map. Besides the good refractive result, both for distance and near vision, it is interesting to note how pre- and postoperative spherical aberration is quite similar and always negative. It is important to remember, however, that without the positivization treatment (presbyopic correction), the simple refractive treatment would have induced a 2.5 times negative spherical aberration. This is very important in order to understand the results. Thus, when we talk about positivization, this does not mean only to achieve a positive spherical aberration, but even a substantially less negative one. Another interesting data: on topography, instantaneous algorithm, no sign of presbyopic correction can be perceived, meaning that no central island is observed.

Fifty-seven-year Old Emmetropic Patient (Figures 22.21 and 22.22)

As it almost always happens, emmetropia is a virtual reality. Usually, a small positive or seldom negative component is present, as in the case shown below. Refractive results for distance and near have been

Preop		B.P.	Postop	
BCVA	Near BCVA	49 y.	UCVA	Near UCVA
10/10 +4sph	+6,50sph IJ	OS	10/10	I-II J

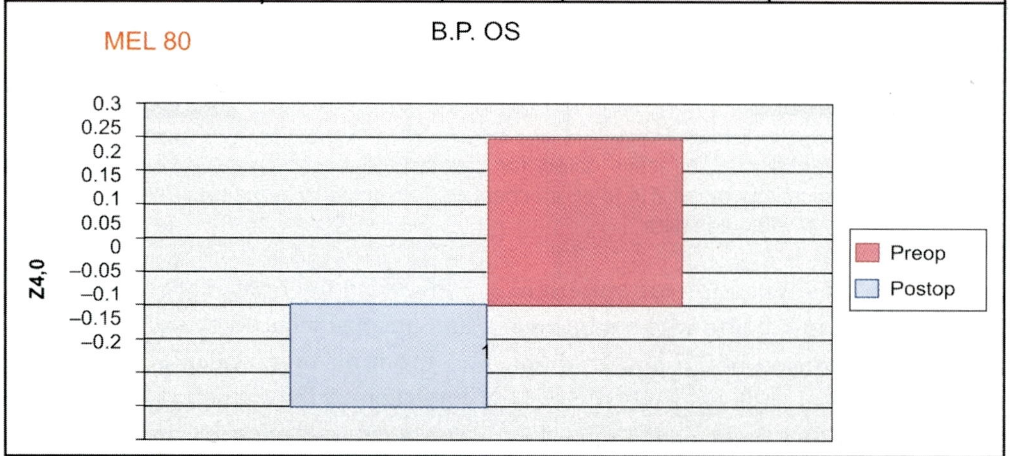

Figure 22.17: Pre- and postoperative state of hyperopic patient. Treatment made by MEL 80 LASER

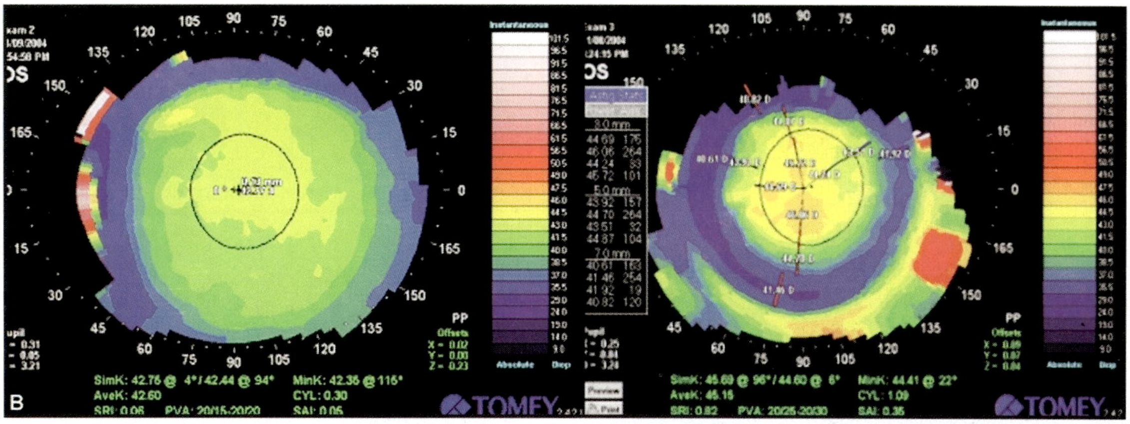

Figures 22.18A and B: Topographic examination shows prolateness of cornea

Preop		N.F.	Postop 6 months	
BCVA	Near BCVA	50 y.	UCVA	Near UCVA
8-9/10 -6,00sph; -3,00 cyl 180°	I Aw -4,50 sph; -3,00 cyl 180°	OS	8-9/10	I Aw

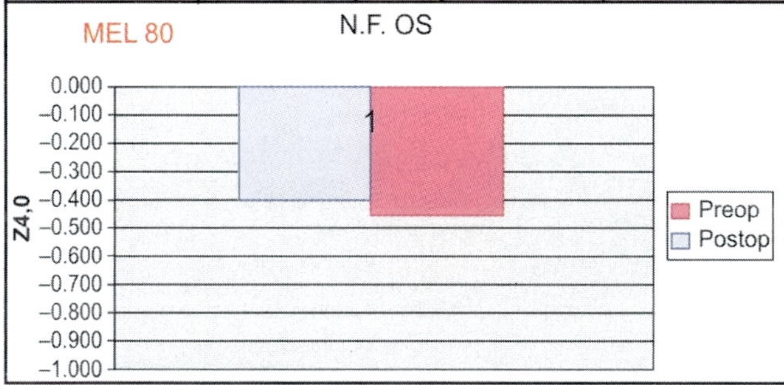

Figure 22.19: Pre- and postoperative states of a myopic and stigmatic patient treated by MEL 80 LASER

Preop pseudofachico		S.A.	Postop 6 months	
BCVA	Near BCVA	57 y.	UCVA	Near UCVA
10/10 -0.25 sph	I Aw -1,50 sph	OD	10/10	I Aw

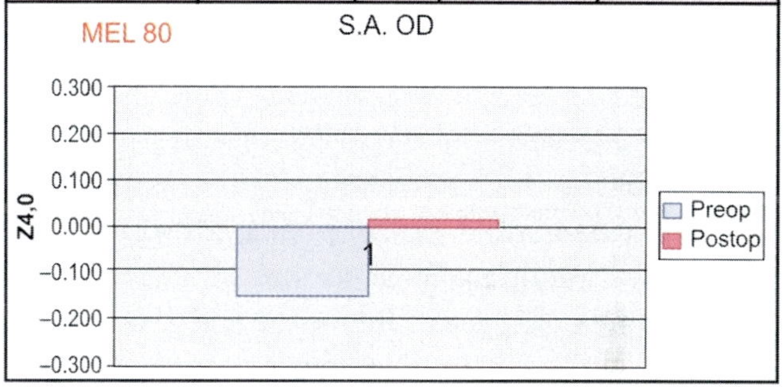

Figure 22.21: Pre- and postoperative state of a emmetropic patient, treated by MEL 80 laser

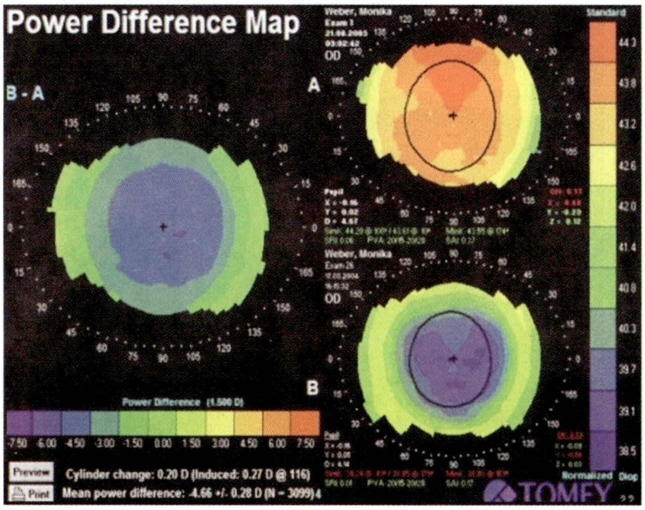

Figure 22.20: Power difference maps

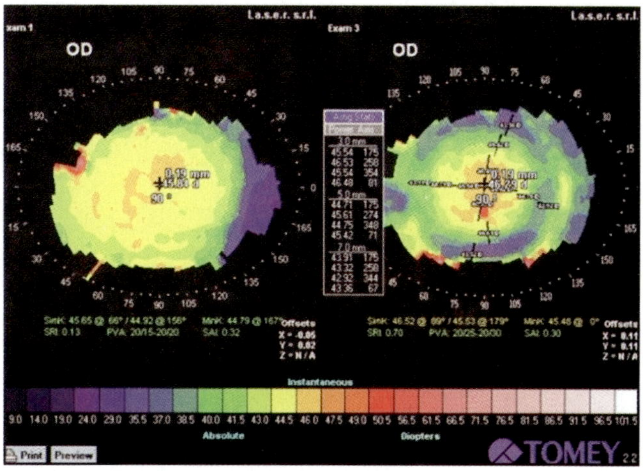

Figure 22.22: Topographic image of the same patient of Figure 22.21

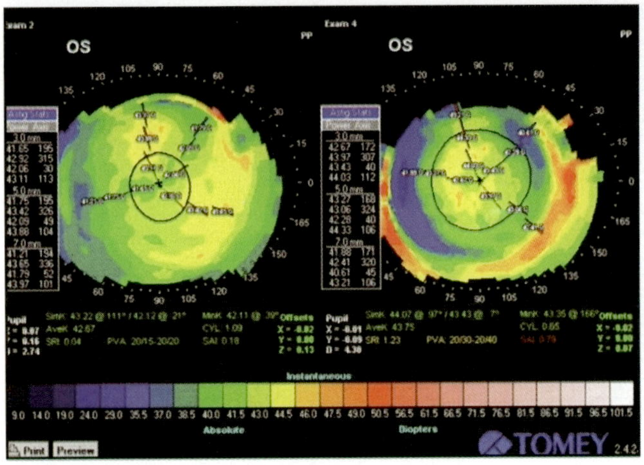

Figure 22.23: Topographic image of pseudophakic patient

satisfactory, spherical aberration changed from negative to slightly positive. Postoperative corneal map shows the features of a hyperopic treatment, as always when treating emmetropic eyes.

During the last months, we started the treatment of pseudophakic eyes. Presently we have treated 8 of them, with refractive defects related to IOL miscalculation, and other problems.

Sixty-two-year-old pseudophakic patient (Figure 22.23). Treatment is similar to that of a presbyopic, phakic, hyperopic patient. Refractive and aberrometric results are similar, as well as topographic views.

The main interest in this technique is related to its possible alternative to pseudoaccommodative or diffractive IOLs for the correction of presbyopia. For the correction of IOL calculation error-derived refractive

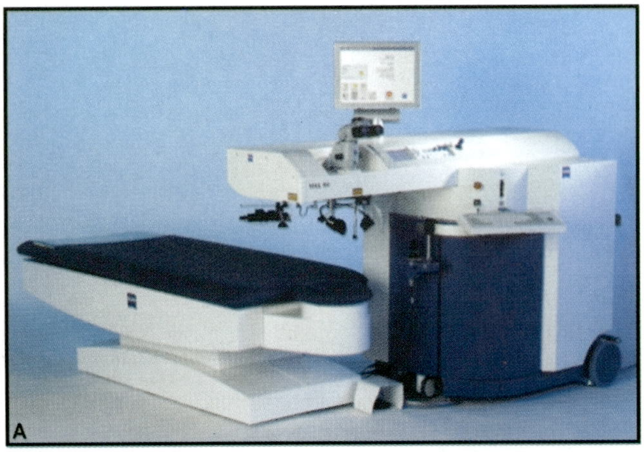

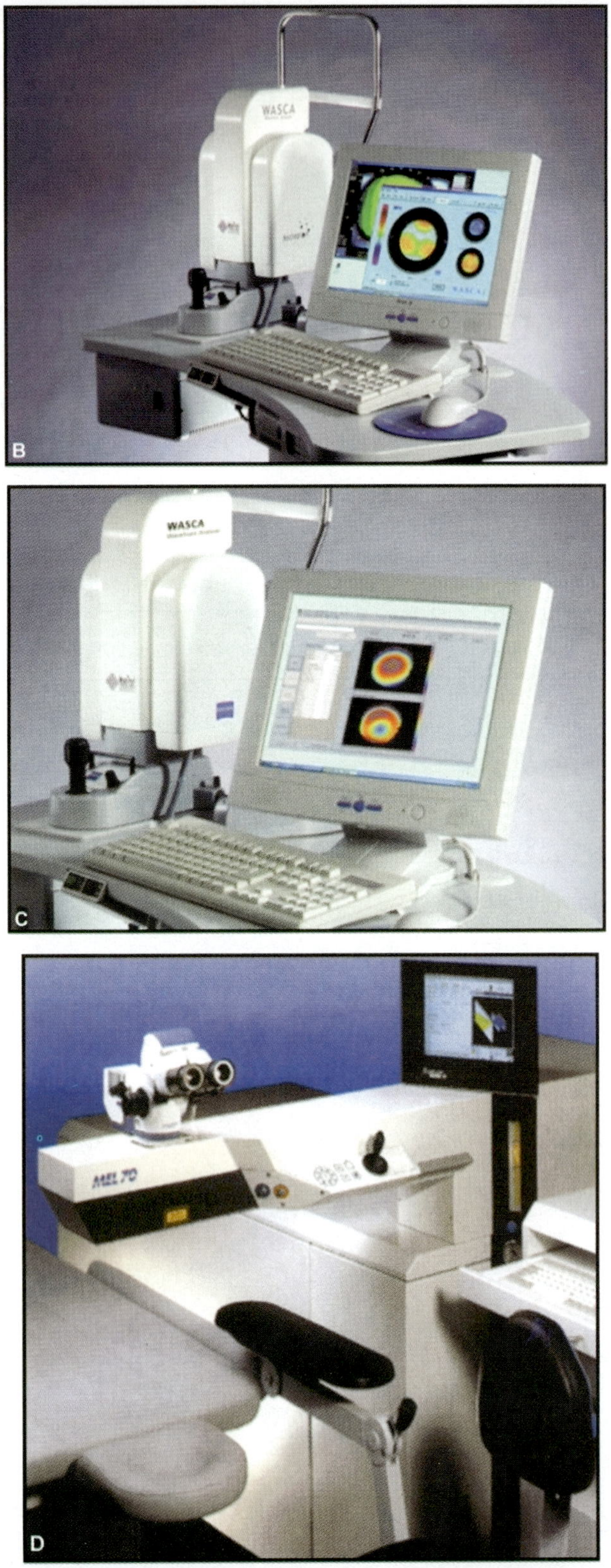

Figures 22.24A to D: Machines for aberrometric corrections

defects, the advantages are two-fold: the error is eliminated and the patient acquires near vision correction. After cataract surgery it can be utilized to restore near vision capabilities.

The latest development, still undergoing the experimental phase, concerns the making of corneal contact lenses for the correction of presbyopia, with the same scheme and analysis used for corneal treatment. Similar studies have been conducted in the past, without substantial results. Difficulties are manifold – i.e. ablation rate, different hydration if the contact lens is of the soft type, leons motion on the cornea, etc. We are persuaded that presently most of these difficulties are solved, and the refractive results in the correction of presbyopia are really encouraging.

If these preliminary results would be confirmed, through the use of custom-made trial lenses, we could have the patient try the actual result of his possible refractive treatment (see Figures 22.24A to D machines for aberrometric corrections).

BIBLIOGRAPHY

1. Agarwal A. Presbyopia, Slack Inc 2002.
2. Applegate RA, Thibos LN, Hilmantel G. "Optics of aberroscopy and super vision", J Cataract Refrac Surg 2001.
3. Artal P, Hoffer H, Williams DR, Aragon JL. Dynamic of ocularaberration during accomodation, Optical Society of America Annual Meeting 1999.
4. Bartoli F, Ipotesi di correzione aberrometrica della presbiopia, SOI 2002.
5. Bartoli F. Aberrometric correction of presbyopia, Refr@active on-line 2004.
6. Bartoli F. Aberrometro ad alta definizione WASCA, link aberrometrico con Mel 70 G-Scan, The aberrometers, Fabiano 2002.
7. Bennett Arthur G, Rabbetts, Ronald B. Clinical Visual Optics 3e, Butterworth-Heinemann, 1998.
8. Born M, Wolf E. Principles of Optics 7e, Cambridge University Press, 1999.
9. Buratto L, Cantera E, Dal Fiume C, Genisi C, Merlin U, Topografia corneale, CAMO editore 1995.
10. Buratto L, Picardo V. Focal points in chirurgia rifrattiva, Fabiano 2001.
11. Burkhard Dick H, Werner T, Kaiser S, Wrede J. Dynamic wavefront measurements of eyes with accommodative IOL, 3rd Internationan congress of wavefront sensing and aberration-free refractive correction 2002.
12. Caimi F, La correzione laser dell'ipermetropia, Fabiano 2001.
13. Dausch D, Klein RJ, Schroeder E, Laserb ad eccimeri in oftalmologia,Medical Books 1992.
14. Dausch D, Lee S, Schroeder E, Wottke M. Wavefront Guided Correction of Presbyopia, 8th ESCRS Winter Meeting 2004.
15. Dick B, Goes F, Grabner G. The importance of resolution in aberrometry, ASCSRS-ASOA 2002.
16. Dossi F, Dossi R, Suppo E. Tecniche chirurgiche per la correzione dei difetti rifrattivi, Chirurgia rifrattiva, Fabiano 2000.
17. Geary, Joseph M. Introduction to wavefront sensing, SPIE Press, 1995.
18. Goodman, Joseph W. Fourier Optics 2e, McGraw-Hill, 1996.
19. Hecht, Eugene: Optics 3e, Addsion Wesley, 1997.
20. Le Grand Y. Optique physiologique,Revue d'optique, Paris 1956.
21. Liang J, Brimm B, Goelz S, Bille JF. Objective measurement of wave aberrations of the human eye with the use of Hartmann-Shack wave-front sensor. J Opt Soc Am Acad 1994;11:1949-57.
22. Liuzzi L, Bartoli F, Manuale di Oftalmologia, ed. Minerva Medica 2002.
23. Machat JJ. Excimer laser refractive surgery, Slack Incorporated 1996.
24. Mahajan Virendra N. Optical Imaging and Aberrations, SPIE Press, 1998.
25. Mastropasqua L, Nubile M. Lo studio delle aberrazioni oculari L'oculista italiano n°131 2001.
26. Miller Donald T. Retinal imaging and vision at the frontiers of adaptive optics. Physics Today, 2000;531,31.
27. Neal D, Copland J, Topa D, Vogelsang H, Bergt M. Wave Front Sciences/Asclepion Meditec WASCA: The technology, calibration, dynamic range, resolution, pecision and accuracy. The Aberrometers, Fabiano 2002.
28. Neal Daniel R, et al. Complete light analysis system user's manual, wavefront. sciences, May 1999.
29. Neal Daniel R, Hedlund E, Lederer M, Collier A, Spring C, Yanta W. Shack-Hartmann wavefront sensor testing of aero-optic phenomena, 20th AIAA Measurement and Ground Testing Technology Conference, June 1998.
30. Neal DR, Alford WJ, Gruetzner JK, "Amplitude and phase beam characterization using a two-dimensional wavefront sensor," SPIE 2870, 1996;72–82.
31. Neal DR, Armstrong DJ, Turner WT. "Wavefront sensors for control and process monitoring in optics manufacture," SPIE 2993 1997.
32. Pallikaris IG, Panagopoulu SI. Dynamic wavefront refractomy with asclepion aberrometer in the accommodation process, ASCSRS-ASOA 2002.
33. Piovella M, Camesasca FI, Kusa B. LASIK custom ablation based on WASCA aberrometry, Refr@active on-line 2002.
34. Salmon T, West R, Kenmore T, Gasser W. "Evaluation of the COAS Shack-Hartmann Aberrometer as an Autorefractor," Optometry and Vision Science 2001;78(12):94.
35. Salz JJ. Chirurgia laser della cornea,Medical books 1996.
36. Schachar RA. Retinal imaging aberrometry, Ophtalmology 2002.

37. Smith, George, Atchison, David A. The Eye and Visual Optical Instruments, Cambridge University Press 1997.
38. Spadea L, Sabetti L, Bianco G, Santacroce B, Balestrazzi E. Standard vs wavefront-driven corneal ablation: Results of an intraindividual comparison, ASCRS 2002.
39. Thibos L, Hong X. Clinical applications of the Shack–Hartmann aberometer. Optom Vis Sci 1999;76,817-25.
40. Vinciguerra P, Atlante di topografia corneale, Fogliazza Editore 1995.

23

Conductive Keratoplasty for the Treatment of Hyperopia and Presbyopia

- TREATMENT EFFECTS
- PERFORMING CONDUCTIVE KERATOPLASTY
- CLINICAL STUDY RESULTS

Marguerite B McDonald (USA)

INTRODUCTION

The variety of approaches that have been used to correct hyperopia and increase near vision in presbyopia testifies to the challenges inherent in surgical steepening of the central cornea. Hot wire thermokeratoplasty used in the 1980s showed lack of predictability and stability and further development was abandoned.[1-4] Similarly, non-contact Ho:YAG laser thermal keratoplasty (LTK, Sunrise Technologies, Fremont, Calif.) ultimately failed to achieve commercial acceptance for lack of predictability and stability.[5-9]

Non-thermal, excimer laser based techniques for correcting hyperopia have included photorefractive keratectomy (PRK)[10-14] and laser-assisted subepithelial keratectomy (LASEK).[15] Because of postoperative pain and corneal haze, PRK has been mostly replaced by hyperopic laser in-situ keratomileusis (H-LASIK).[16-23] However, LASIK also has a number of potential complications, mostly related to the flap, such as striae, displacements, button-hole flaps, and diffuse lamellar keratitis that can limit postoperative visual results.[24-28] These risks do not seem warranted when a low to moderate amount of hyperopia is being corrected or a small amount of overcorrection is being induced to improve vision in a presbyopic eye.

Conductive keratoplasty® (CK®) (Refractecâ, Inc., Irvine, Calif.), is an entirely different approach to corneal steepening.[29-33] With CK, the cornea is reshaped through a non-ablative, non-incisional, collagen-shrinkage procedure that works through radiofrequency energy that the cornea converts to heat in a controlled fashion. Treatment is applied through a fine tip inserted into the peripheral corneal stroma in a ring pattern outside of the visual axis (Figures 23.1 and 23.2). A full circle of treatment spots acts like a belt tightening the cornea in the periphery so that the central cornea steepens. When a series of treatment spots are placed in up to three rings in the corneal periphery (6, 7, and 8 mm optical zones), striae form between the spots and create a band of tightening. This causes a steepening of the central cornea and corrects hyperopic refractive error.

In April 2002, the United States Food and Drug Administration granted approval of the ViewPoint CK System for the treatment of mild to moderate (+0.75 D to +3.00 D) spherical hyperopia in patients 40 years old or older. In March 2004, CK was approved for improvement of near vision in emmetropic and hyperopic presbyopes by inducing 1.00 to 2.00 D of myopia in the non-dominant eye. This chapter describes the technique and presents results of studies conducted on the treatment of hyperopia and presbyopia.

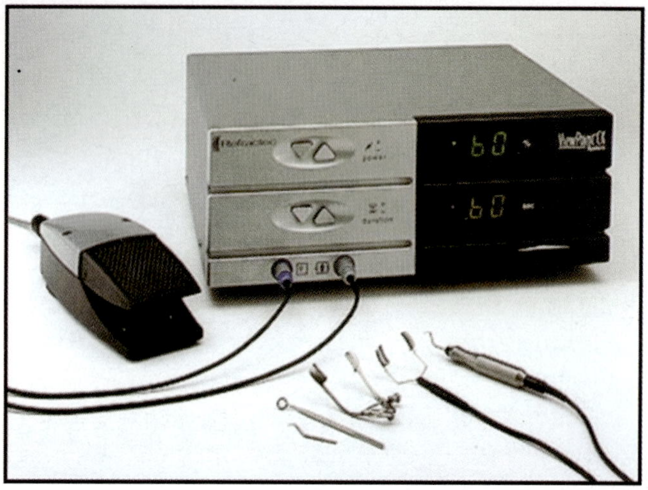

Figure 23.1: The ViewPoint™ CK System consists of a 14 pound portable console, a handpiece that holds the 450 μm long and 90 μm wide Keratoplast tip™, a corneal marker, a speculum, and a foot pedal. The speculum is a return path for the radiofrequency energy. *[[color]]*

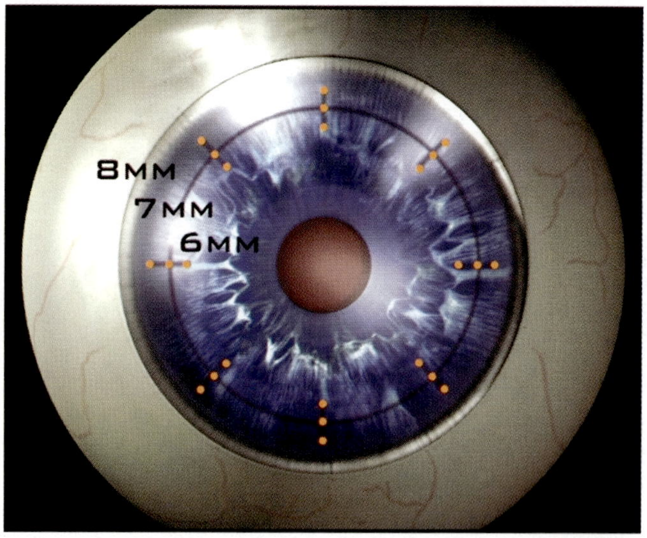

Figure 23.2: Radiofrequency energy is delivered to the stroma by means of a fine tip inserted into the peripheral cornea in a ring pattern outside of the visual axis. *[[probe in cornea – color]]*

TREATMENT EFFECTS

Although corneal collagen has great tensile strength and thermal stability, exposure to elevated temperatures for specific time periods transforms its native helical structure into a randomly coiled structure during the denaturation process. This is accompanied by contraction (shrinkage) of the collagen and changes in the mechanical behavior of the tissue.[34-36] In hyperopia treatment procedures, the desired mechanical change is peripheral corneal flattening and the resulting central corneal steepening.

Conductive keratoplasty uses the optimal combination of radiofrequency energy characteristics, including current, waveform, frequency, and duration of exposure, to raise the temperature of corneal collagen long enough to cause localized shrinkage of collagen fibers. The default CK treatment parameters are 0.6 W for 0.6 seconds at 350 kHz. Treatment application at these default parameters causes the surrounding tissue to undergo a temperature increase. As the heated tissue dehydrates, its resistance to radiofrequency current increases. Since current seeks the path of least resistance, the current path moves up the shaft of the Keratoplast tip (Figure 23.3).

Tissue heating progresses from bottom (deep in the stroma) to top (corneal surface), and creates a thermal lesion that is uniformly cylindrical. The Keratoplast tip only *delivers* radiofrequency energy and heats up only in response to the increase in tissue temperature. The tip acts as a heat sink (takes heat away) rather than as a heat source (supplies heat). Histology studies on a pig cornea show that the cylindrical thermal lesion (footprint) formed as a result of CK treatment extends to approximately 80 percent of the depth of the stroma (Figure 23.4).

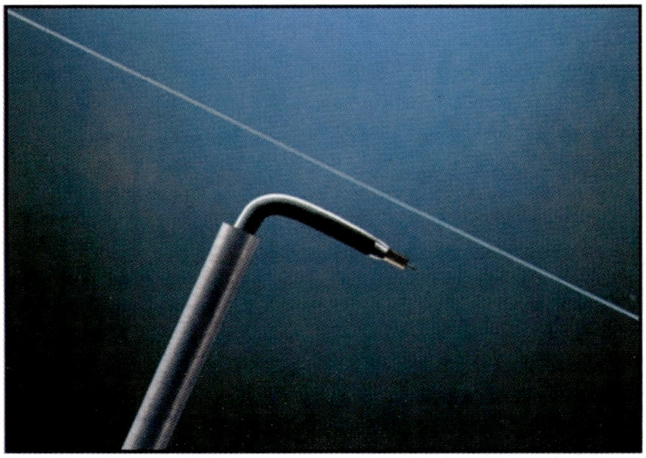

Figure 23.3: Conductive keratoplasty handpiece with Keratoplast tip (90 μm wide, 450 μm long) and insulated stop at the distal end. Shown next to a 7-0 suture

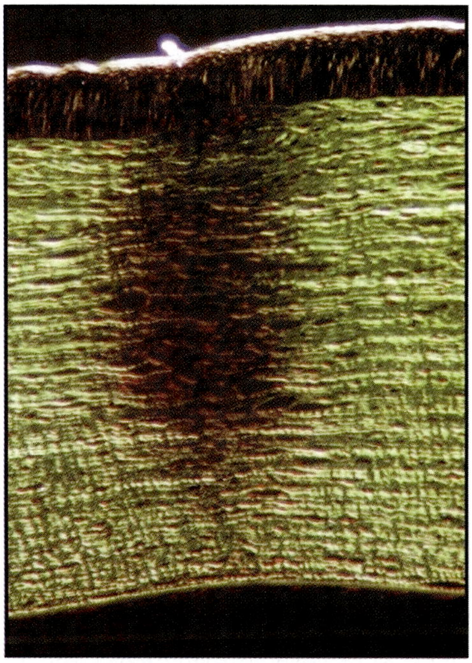

Figure 23.4: A polarized light micrograph of a histological section from a pig cornea, approximately 650 μm thick, seven days after CK treatment. The CK-treated spot (dark region) shows a cylindrical footprint, approximately 80 percent deep

PERFORMING CONDUCTIVE KERATOPLASTY

Patients suitable for the CK procedure should have visual acuity correctable to at least 20/40 in both eyes, and pachymetry readings of 560 mm or more at the 6 mm optical zone. Contact lens wearers should have a stable refraction. Hard lens wearers should discontinue lens use three weeks and soft contact lens wearers two weeks before the procedure.

Assessment of preoperative topography is important to outcome. Avoid atypical or unusual corneas, such as those with keratoconus or pellucid marginal degeneration and be aware of potential sources of induced cylinder. These include corneas with a decentered apex or peripheral, asymmetric, or non-orthogonal astigmatism. Also avoid surgery on eyes with significant dryness or tear-function compromise.

To perform the procedure, the surgeon inserts the Keratoplast tip into the stroma at defined spots in a ring pattern around the peripheral cornea according to the supplied nomogram. (Different nomograms are supplied for treatment of hyperopia and for emmetropic and hyperopic presbyopes.) The number and location of spots determines the amount of refractive change, with an increasing number of spots and rings used for higher amounts of correction. The CK procedure is performed under topical anesthesia and takes a few minutes to complete.

For the improvement of near vision in presbyopic emmetropes and hyperopes, the goal is to overcorrect the non-dominant eye by inducing slight to moderate myopia, –1.0 to –2.0 D for near vision tasks. If the dominant eye is significantly hyperopic, it can be treated as well. Treated patients display a reduction of symptoms of presbyopia without compromising binocular functional distance vision. Most well-selected patients will initially only need one eye corrected with the application of 16 to 24 spots. Patients with high target anisometropia or strong ocular dominance should be avoided.

CLINICAL STUDY RESULTS

Hyperopia Treatment

A total of 400 eyes were treated for low to moderate spherical hyperopia (0.75 D to 3.00 D) in the two-year, FDA phase III multicenter, prospective clinical trial of the CK system. Emmetropia was intended for all eyes. No retreatments were performed and all data are the result of one treatment. Cohort follow-up data was 98 percent (391/401) at one year and 94 percent (378/401) at 2 years. The mean baseline cycloplegic spherical equivalent (SE) refraction of these eyes was +1.86 ± 0.63 D.

The procedure demonstrated good stability. Manifest refractive spherical equivalent (MRSE) changed a mean of 0.03 D per month during the 6 to 9 month postoperative interval, 0.05 D per month during the 9 to 12 months interval and 0.03 D per month for the 12 to 24 months interval. Figure 23.5 shows the percentage of eyes with

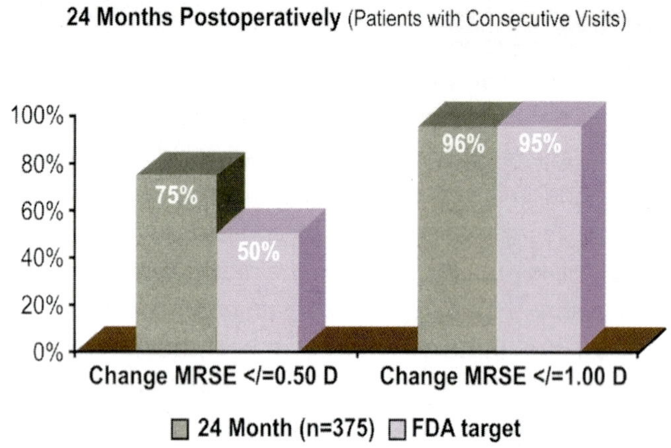

Figure 23.5: Hyperopia Study: Stability of Manifest Refraction

change of manifest refractive spherical equivalent of equal to or less than 0.50 D and 1.00 D 2 years postoperatively.

CK safety results were remarkably good (Table 23.1). Three percent of the eyes showed loss of two lines of BSCVA at 12 months and 1 percent at 24 months. However, all of these eyes with 2-line losses had at least 20/25 vision after the 2-line loss. No eye lost more than 2 lines of BSCVA at 12 months and 1 eye (0.29%) lost 2 lines at 24 months.

Only one of 351 eyes (0.25%) had >2 diopters of cylinder induced at 12 months, but the percentage was zero at 24 months. (Any cylinder induced by CK usually disappears with time).

Thus there was no effect of induced cylinder on BSCVA, and the effect of induced cylinder was reflected largely in the UCVA 20/20 or better data.

Confocal microscopy and histology showed a deep, cylindrical footprint, which is compatible with a more effective and longer-lasting result. Corneal topography showed central corneal steepening with mid-peripheral

Table 23.1: Hyperopia study safety results

	12 Months N = 351	*24 Months N = 349*
>2 Lines Lost BSCVA	0%	0.29%
BSCVA Worse than 20/40	0%	0%
Increase > 2.00 D Cylinder	0.25%	0%
Patients preop = 20/20 who had = 20/25 postop	0%	0.29%

flattening. The incidence of adverse events was very low and all resolved without sequelae. Patients showed a high degree of satisfaction with the results of the procedure. At 24 months, 76 percent were satisfied or very satisfied with results of CK procedure, and 95 percent noted improvement in quality of vision.

Presbyopia Treatment

A multicenter study was also conducted to determine the safety and efficacy of CK for the treatment of presbyopic symptoms in emmetropic and hyperopic eyes. Eligible patients were treated to correct up to 2.0 D of presbyopia. To be eligible for the study, patients had to have a preoperative spherical equivalent (SE) from plano (considered as +0.5 to –0.5 D) to +2.0 D and less than or equal to 0.75 D of refractive astigmatism, as determined by cycloplegic refraction. Screening for eligibility included a history of monovision contact lens wear or success with a contact lens trial of monovision.

In addition, preoperative assessment using loose lenses was performed to demonstrate the effects of CK to the candidate. Based on nominal corrections with CK, lenses of three different dioptric powers were used: 1) a +0.75 D lens for 1 ring of CK treatment, 2) a +1.25 D lens for 2 rings of CK treatment, and 3) a +1.75D lens for 3 rings of CK treatment. If a patient could not find a satisfactory endpoint, we did not proceed with the surgery.

The target refraction was up to –2.0 D (myopic endpoint) in the non-dominant eye. Emmetropic patients were treated unilaterally in the non-dominant eye with an intended correction of up to 2.0 D (target of –1.0 to –2.25 D) to attain near vision in that eye. Hyperopic patients were treated bilaterally: the non-dominant eye was treated up to 3.0 D (target of –1.0 to –2.0 D) to provide near vision, and the dominant eye was treated with a correction of up to 2.0 D (target of plano) to improve distance vision.

A total of 188 eyes (150 patients) at five centers in the United States who met eligibility requirements were enrolled consecutively into the study and signed informed consent forms. Of these, 150 eyes were

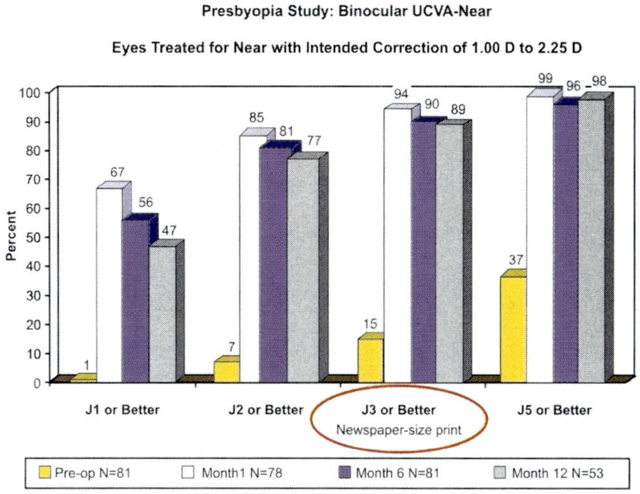

Figure 23.6: Binocular UCVA-near following CK presbyopia treatment

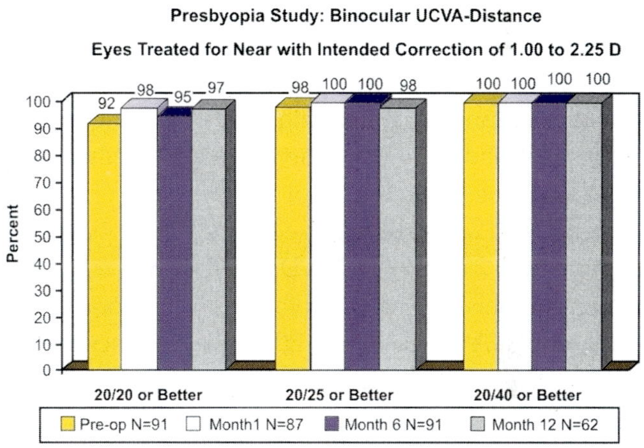

Figure 23.7: Binocular UCVA-distance following CK presbyopia treatment

emmetropic or hyperopic presbyopes and were treated to improve near vision. The patients' mean age was 53 ± 4.7 years, and the intended refraction was 2.03 D ± 0.625. All eyes were treated once (no retreatments).

At 12 months post-op, 89 percent of the eyes treated for near with the full correction (1.00 to 2.25 D) had binocular uncorrected near visual acuity (UCVA-Near) of J3 or better (newspaper-size print) (Figure 23.6). A total of 97 percent had UCVA-Distance of 20/20 or better and 100 percent had 20/40 or better (Figure 23.7). For binocular combined UCVA Distance and Near, only 15 percent of eyes had 20/32 or better distance together with J3 or better near preoperatively, At 12 months,

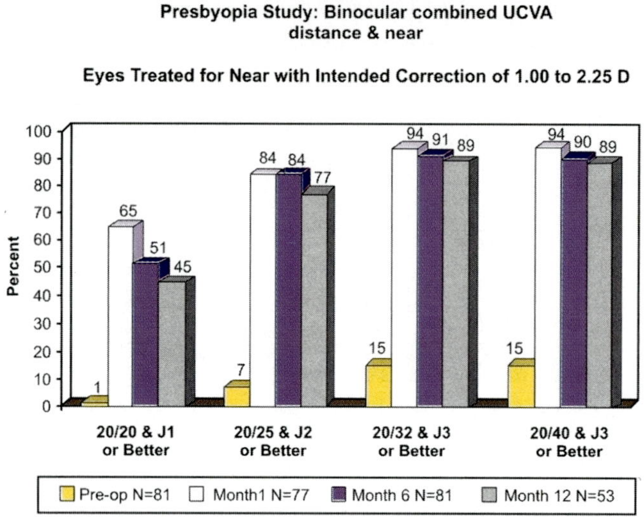

Figure 23.8: Binocular combined UCVA-distance and near following CK presbyopia treatment

however, 77 percent had 20/25 or better distance together with J2 or better near, 89 percent had 20/32 or better distance together with J3 or better near, and 89 percent had 20/40 or better distance together with J3 or better near (Figure 23.8).

Safety at 12 months was exceptional. A transient loss of more than 2 lines of BCVA-D was seen in 2 eyes at 1 month, but this resolved in both eyes by 3 months. No eye had BCVA-D worse than 20/40, had an increase of >2.00 D cylinder, or had BCVA-D of 20/20 or better preop that became 20/25 or worse postop (Table 23.2). Mesopic contrast sensitivity was unchanged from pre-op through month 12. Extreme/marked/ or moderate improvement in quality of vision was noted by 89 percent to 95 percent of the patients over the course of the study. A range of 79 percent to 86 percent reported being satisfied or very satisfied with the results. Patient

Table 23.2: Presbyopia study safety results

	Month 1 N = 90	*Month 6 N = 93*	*Month 12 N=63*
Loss of >2 Lines BCVA-D	2%	0%	0%
BCVA-D Worse than 20/40	0%	0%	0%
Increase >2.00 D Cylinder	0%	0%	0%
Patients preop ≤ 20/20 who had ≥ 20/25 postop	0%	0%	0%
BCVA-N Worse than J3	0%	0%	0%

satisfaction with the procedure is similar to that of monovision LASIK. Quality of depth perception was rated excellent, very good, or good in 91 percent to 93 percent over the study course.

CONCLUSIONS

Treatment of hyperopia with CK produces safe and effective results in a large majority of patients. As a non-ablative, non-incisional procedure, CK does not invade the central cornea, cause flap-related complications, compromise the integrity or structure of the cornea, cause dry eye, or central haze. In addition, CK can be performed in the office setting with only topical anesthesia, is technically easier to perform than other hyperopic procedures, and involves use of a portable unit that is much less expensive than most other refractive surgery platform.

When performed in one eye to improve near vision, CK improved binocular vision so that 89 percent saw 20/32 uncorrected distance as well as J3 near. CK causes minimal to no compromise to distance vision binocularly and does not reduce contrast sensitivity or depth perception (which are reduced after monovision LASIK). CK appears to be very safe and effective in producing functional visual acuity in presbyopic eyes. Patients report a high rate of patient satisfaction.

REFERENCES

1. Neumann AC, Sanders D, Raanan M, DeLuca M. Hyperopic thermokeratoplasty: Clinical evaluation. J Cataract Refract Surg 1991;17:830-38.
2. Feldman S, Ellis W, Frucht-Pery J, et al. Regression of effect following radial thermokeratoplasty in humans. Refract Corneal Surg 1989;5:288-91.
3. Charpentier DY, Nguyen-Khoa JL, Duplessix M, et al. Intrastromal thermokeratoplasty for correction of spherical hyperopia: A one-year prospective study. J Fr Ophthalmol 1995;18:200-06.
4. McDonnell PJ. Radial thermokeratoplasty for hyperopia. I. The need for prompt prospective investigation. Refract Corneal Surg 1989; 5:50-52.
5. Koch DD, Kohnen T, McDonnell PJ, et al. Hyperopia correction by non-contact holmium:YAG laser thermal keratoplasty. United States phase IIA clinical study with a 1-year follow-up. Ophthalmology 1996;103:1525-36.
6. Koch DD, Abarca A, Villareal R, et al. Hyperopia correction by non-contact holmium:YAG laser thermal keratoplasty.

Clinical study with two-year follow-up. Ophthalmology 1996;103:731-40.
7. Koch DD, Kohnen T, McDonnell PJ, et al. Hyperopia correction by non-contact holmium:YAG laser thermal keratoplasty. US phase IIA clinical study with 2-year follow-up. Ophthalmology 1997; 104:1938-47.
8. Alio JL, Ismail MM, Sanchez Pego JL. Correction of hyperopia with non-contact Ho:YAG laser thermal keratoplasty. J Refract Surg 1997;13:17-22.
9. Durrie DS, Schumer JD, Cavanaugh TB. Holmium:YAG laser thermokeratoplasty for hyperopia. J Refract Corneal Surg 1994;10(suppl):S277-80.
10. Jackson WB, Mintsioulis G, Agapitos PJ, Casson EJ. Excimer laser photorefractive keratectomy for low hyperopia: safety and efficacy. J Cataract Refract Surg 1997;23:480-87.
11. Daya SM, Tappouni FR, Habib NE. Photorefractive keratectomy for hyperopia. Six months results in 45 eyes. Ophthalmology 1997;104:1952-58.
12. Vinciguerra P, Epstein D, Radice P, Azzolini M. Long-term results of photorefractive keratectomy for hyperopia and hyperopic astigmatism. J Refract Surg 1998;14:S183-85.
13. Pietila J, Makinen P, Pajari S, Uusitalo H. Excimer laser photorefractive keratectomy for hyperopia. J Refract Surg 1997;13:504-10.
14. Dausch D, Smecka Z, Klein R, et al. Excimer laser photorefractive keratectomy for hyperopia. J Refract Surg 1997;23:169-76.
15. Autrata R, Rehurek J. Laser-assisted subepithelial keratectomy and photorefractive keratectomy for the correction of hyperopia. Results of a 2-year follow-up. J Cataract Refract Surg 2003;29:2105-14.
16. Argento CJ, Cosentino MJ. Laser *in situ* keratomileusis for hyperopia. J Cataract Refract Surg 1998;24:1050-58.
17. Ditzen K, Huschka H, Pieger S. Laser *in situ* keratomileusis for hyperopia. J Cataract Refract Surg 1998;24: 42-47.
18. Rashad KM. Laser *in situ* keratomileusis for the correction of hyperopia from +1.25 to 5.00 diopters with the Technolas Keracor 117C laser. J Refract Surg 2001;17: 113-22.
19. Tabbara KF. El-Sheikh HF, Islam SM. Laser *in situ* keratomileusis for the correction of hyperopia from +0.50 to 11.50 diopters with the Technolas Keracor 117C laser. J Refract Surg 2001;17:123-28.
20. Esquenazi S, Mendoza A. Two-year follow-up of laser *in situ* keratomileusis for hyperopia. J Refract Surg 1999; 15:648-52.
21. Goker S, Er H, Kahvecioglu C. Laser *in situ* keratomileusis to correct hyperopia from +4.25 to +8.0 diopters. J Refract Surg 1998;14:26-30.
22. Carones F, Vigo L, Scandola E. Laser *in situ* keratomileusis for hyperopia and hyperopic and mixed astigmatism with LADARVision using 7 to 10-mm ablation diameters. J Refract Surg 2003;19:548-54.
23. Salz JJ, Stevens CA; LADARVision LASIK Hyperopia Study Group. LASIK correction of spherical hyperopia, hyperopic astigmatism, and mixed astigmatism with the LADARVision excimer laser system. Ophthalmology 2002;109:1647-56.
24. Lin RT, Maloney RK. Flap complications associated with lamellar refractive surgery. Am J Ophthalmol 1999;127: 129-36.
25. Ambrosio R Jr, Wilson SE. Complications of laser *in situ* keratomileusis: Etiology, prevention, and treatment. J Refract Surg 2001;17: 350-79.
26. Doughman DJ, Hardten DR. Loss of vision after laser *in situ* keratomileusis. Eye Contact Lens 2003;29(1 Suppl): S135-38.
27. Sciscio A, Hull CC, Stephenson CG, Baldwin H, O'Brart D, Marshall J. Fourier analysis of induced irregular astigmatism. Photorefractive keratectomy versus laser *in situ* keratomileusis in a bilateral cohort of hyperopic patients. J Cataract Refract Surg 2003;29:1709-17.
28. Stulting RD, Carr JD, Thompson KP, Waring GO 3rd, Wiley WM, Walker JG. Complications of laser *in situ* keratomileusis for the correction of myopia. Ophthalmology 1999;106:13-20.
29. McDonald, MB, Durrie DS, Asbell PA, Maloney R, Nichamin L. Treatment of presbyopia with conductive keratoplasty: Six-month results of the United States FDA clinical trial. In press, Cornea. 2004.
30. Haw WW, Manche EE. Conductive keratoplasty and laser thermal keratoplasty. Int Ophthalmol Clin 2002 Fall;42: 99-106.
31. McDonald MB, Hersh PS, Manche EE, Maloney RK, Davidorf J, Sabry M. Conductive keratoplasty for the correction of low to moderate hyperopia: US clinical trial 1-year results on 355 eyes. Ophthalmology 2002; 109: 1978-89.
32. Asbell PA, Maloney RK, Davidorf J, Hersh P, McDonald M, Manche E. Conductive Keratoplasty Study Group. Conductive keratoplasty for the correction of hyperopia. Trans Am Ophthalmol Soc 2001;99:79-84.
33. Lin DY, Manche EE. Two-year results of conductive keratoplasty for the correction of low to moderate hyperopia. J Cataract Refract Surg 2003;29:2339-50.
34. Pearce J, Thomsen S. Rate process analysis of thermal damage. In: Welch AJ, van Gemert MJC, eds. Optical-Thermal Response of Laser-Irradiated Tissue. New York: Plenum Press: 1995; 561-605.
35. Chen SS, Humphrey JD. Heat-induced changes in the mechanics of a collagenous tissue: Pseudoelastic behavior at 37° C. Journal Biomechanics 1998;31:211-16.
36. Chang J, Soderberg PG, Denham D, et al. Temperature induced corneal shrinkage. In: Parel JM (ed) Ophthalmic Technologies VI. Proc SPIE. 1996;2673:70-76.

24

A New System (DTK-Plus) for Thermal Keratoplasty Using IR Lasers

- **HYPEROPIA CORRECTION**
- **PENETRATION DEPTH**
- **TEMPERATURE PROFILE**
- **SAFETY AND EFFICACY**

JT Lin (USA), Vivek Kadambi (India)

INTRODUCTION

Corneal reshaping procedures, such as photorefractive keratectomy (PRK) and laser assisted in situ keratomileusis (LASIK) have been performed by lasers in the ultraviolet (UV) wavelength of (193 - 213) nm. The commercial UV refractive lasers include ArF excimer laser (at 193 nm) in US Pat. 4,773,414 of L'Esperance, et al. and other non-excimer, solid-state lasers such as those proposed by Lin in 1992 (US pat. no. 5,144,630) and in 1996 (US pat. No. 5,520,679). The above-described systems using lasers to reshape the corneal surface curvature, however, are limited to the corrections of myopia, hyperopia and astigmatism. They do not significantly contribute to the treatments of presbyopia or glaucoma.

Refractive surgery using a scanning device and iasers in the mid-infrared (mid-IR) wavelength was first proposed by Lin in US Pat. No. 5,144,630 and 5,520,679 and later proposed by Telfair et al. in US Pat. No. 5,782,822. These inventions disclosed the generation of mid-IR wavelength of 2.5 to 3.2 microns, by various methods including, but not limited to, the Er:YAG laser (at 2.94 microns), the Raman-shifted solid-state lasers (at 2.7-3.2 microns) and the optical parametric oscillation (OPO) lasers (at 2.7-3.2 microns).

Hyperopia may be surgically corrected by LASIK which involves corneal tissue removal. Alternatively, minimally invasive techniques may be employed using Ho:YAG laser (at 2070 to 2120 nm) or the diode laser (at 1885 nm), through thermal keratoplasty procedures known as Holmium Laser Thermokeratoplasty (Ho:LTK) and Diode Laser Thermokeratoplasty (DTK), respectively. Radio frequency (RF) wave can also be used to create the same effect by a procedure known as conductive keratoplasty (CK).[1-4] Procedures of LASIK, Ho:LTK, DTK and CK have also been recently used for the correction of presbyopia which is limited to monovision treatment by inducing myopia in the non-dominant eye. This is in contrast to the laser scleral ablation (LASA) procedure which normally treats both eyes and does not result in any Myopic shift[5,6] (Figure 24.1 and Table 24.1).

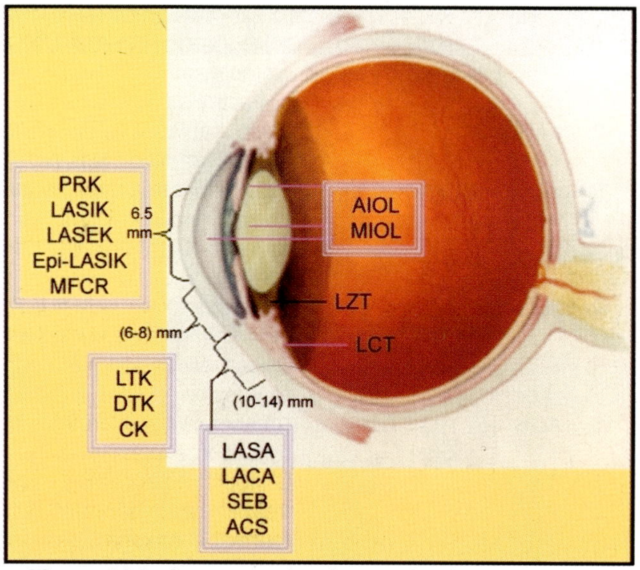

Figure 24.1: Summary of various technologies for vision correction (referred to Table 24.1 for notations)

HYPEROPIA CORRECTION

The recent paper of Rehany and Landa[3] reported results of DTK using a diode laser having a focusing optics for contact mode with deeper penetration of the laser thermal energy in the corneal stroma. However, their data still showed significant six-month postoperative regression of about 0.7 diopter. Papadopauls et al[2] using non-contact Ho:LTK in 50 hyperopic eyes showed that 32 cases reached refraction stability within 1 to 3 months follow-up, 5 cases within 3-6 months and 3 cases within 12 months. Their data also showed a similar regression as that of DTK. The major factor responsible for postoperative regression with Ho:LTK and DTK, is the *cone-shaped* laser power profile (or temperature profile) within the corneal stroma, where the penetration depth (d) is limited by the strong tissue absorption of the laser energy. While the existing DTK system with a tightly focused beam within the stroma may have successfully improved the penetration depth, it did not improve the effective tissue volume (ETV) for collagen shrinkage. The non-focused Ho:LTK has its majority of laser energy absorbed by superficial stromal layer of about 0.15 mm. To overcome the limitation of penetration depth and maximize the ETV for thermal shrinkage, we propose a new concept based on an *optimized focusing beam*

Table 24.1: Summary of technologies for vision corrections (laser and non-laser methods)

No.	Technology	Description
1.	PRK, LASEK, EPI-LASIK	Corneal surface ablation with laser (epithelium removed or preserved); suitable for low diopter corrections (<3.5 D) or high diopter with thin cornea; simple procedure.
2.	LASIK	Stroma ablation by laser after a "flap" is prepared by microkeratome; (less pain, fast recovery, epithelium intact, less haze); potential keratome failure, thin cornea, flap complication.
3.	LASA, LACA	Presbyopia treatment by laser scleral ablation (LASA) to increase accommodation via ciliary body contraction; combining effects of change in scleral elasticity,lens curvature change and anterior chamber shift. Efficiency may be improved by deeper laser ciliary-body ablation (LACA)
4.	LZT, LCT	Laser zonules thermal (LZT) stimulation for presbyopia: non-invasive method using gona lens and focused laser. Laser ciliary-body thermal shrinkage (LCT) for presbyopia
5.	SEB	Scleral expansion band implanted in scleral layer to cause near vision improvement; major regression
6.	ACS	Anterior ciliary sclerotomy by diamond knife incision; major regression which may be reduced by silicon expansion plug.
7.	CK	Conductive keratoplasty using radio frequency wave for hyperopia and monovision correction; treated eye to see near but losing its far vision; non-surgical, corneal curvature changed via thermal shrinkage
8.	LTK and DTK	Laser thermal keratoplasty (LTK) using Ho:YAG (at 2.1 um) or diode laser (1.45 to 2.1 micron) (DTK)
9.	MFCR	Multi-focal corneal reshaping by excimer LASIK
10.	AIOL	Accommodative IOL implanted to lens capsule; forward movement for accommodation; good for post-cataract eyes; loop, thin plates, human optics
11.	MIOL	Multi-focal IOL implanted for patient with high refraction errors
12.	Super Vision	Customized LASIK combined with wave-front technology; flying-spot scanning laser with eye tracking is required for customized and irregular corneal reshaping

*Major technologies (inventors): Broad beam Excimer (L'Esperance, Blum, Taboada); LTK (Sand); SEB (Schachar); Flying-spot LASIK (Lin); LAPR and LACA (Lin), LZT (Lin, Martinez); Eye-tracking (Lai); Solid-state UV Laser for LASIK (Lin, Lai); MFCR (Ruitz). Most of the above technologies have been patented (1988-2004) and greater details may be found in their patents by online searching of "US Patent" files or by the following US pat. No: 4718418, 5484432, 5520679, 5144630, 6263879, 6258082, 5533997, 5354331.

which was used in a system called DTK-plus by New Vision, Inc. (patent pending) (Figure 24.1 and Table 24.2).

PENETRATION DEPTH

The laser power density profile (or irradiance/transmittance profile) of a focused laser inside an absorbing medium, in this case, ocular tissue, may be calculated by a revised Beer's law:

$$P = B\exp(-dA) \quad \text{.......... (Eq. 1)}$$

$$B = [f / (f-d)]^2 \quad \text{........... (Eq. 2)}$$

where A is the absorption coefficient of the cornea tissue at a given laser spectrum; B is a focusing factor which is inversely proportional to the focused beam spot size(derived from simple geometry); f is the focal length of the optics and d is the penetration depth or position away from the corneal surface,which in case of contact mode equals zero. It should be noted that when d approaches f, B is calculated by the square of the ratio between the initial beam spot size (at d=0) and the beam waist (a diffraction-limited finite size at d=f) to avoid the singularity of formula (2). From above formula, one may readily see that the laser irradiance has a fast exponential decrease due to its absorption in ocular tissue, which is competing with the increasing factor B in a focused beam. The net result of power absorption and beam spot decrease (or increase of power density) produces a peak value (P*) of the laser irradiance profile located at the focal point or position of minimal beam spot. For example, given a laser spot size (diameter) of 1.0 mm on the corneal surface (or d=0) which is focused to a

Table 24.2: Comparison of technologies for hyperopia correction

Method	Features
LASIK	ArF excimer laser corneal surface ablation
Ho:LTK	Ho:YAG laser (at 2.1 micron) non-focused beam, shallow penetration
DTK	Diode-laser (at 1.88 micron), focused CW beam
DTK-Plus	Diode-laser (at 1.4 to 1.9 micron), optimal focused beam
CK	Penetration depth controlled by electrode length

minimal spot of 0.25 mm (at d=f), one may easily calculate, from Eq. 2, B=(1, 4, 16, 4, 1) at d/f= (0, 0.5, 1.0, 1.5, 2.0).

Using the published transmittance data (Atchi:ıson and Smith, "Optics of human eye, p. 108) to calculate the absorption coefficient (A) to be about 20 to 70 cm^{-1} for laser wavelength at about 1.4 to 2.1 micron, the absorption term exp(-dA) may be calculated at various penetration depth (d).

Several important features may be addressed based on the above calculated profiles. The peak irradiance (P*) of a focused laser is inversely proportional to the absorption coefficient (A), i.e. a laser having a larger A value has a lower P* than that having a smaller A value. However, this peak power effect from focusing factor (B) may be totally suppressed by the exponentially decreasing term by an appropriate choice of the focal length (f). Mathematically, a perfect flat-top (PFT) profile would be possible under the condition of B=exp (+dA) for all depth (d). For A=55 cm^{-1} as an example, the PFT condition is given by B= (1.0, 3.96, 7.9, 15.7) at depth position of d= (0, 0.25, 0.375, 0.5) mm. This PFT condition is fundamentally impossible to meet under a typical lens design having B= (1, 4, 7.1, 16) for spot size of (1, 0.5, 0.37, 0.25) R, R being the spot size on the corneal surface which produces an almost flat-top (AFT) oscillating function. These AFT profiles require a deeper focal point (f) at 1.0 mm (or two times of the corneal thickness) for the case of A=30 cm^{-1}. In general, the condition for AFT profile is given by B*=exp (f*A), therefore, f*= (0.92, 0.7, 0.62, 0.55, 0.46) mm, for A= (30, 40, 45, 55, 60) cm^{-1}.

The laser irradiance profile is almost flat in the vertical (depth), the laser footprint (spot size) is conical in shape in a focused beam. Therefore, no homogeneous laser irradiance profile exists in both vertical and horizontal directions. The most one may achieve is an *approximate* flat-top (AFT) profile in the depth direction and under the condition defined above. To achieve maximal thermal shrinkage tissue volume (MTTV), the preferred focal length includes f=f*+/-0.2 mm for small A= (20 to 35) cm^{-1}, and f=f*+/-0.05 mm for large A= (40 to 70) cm^{-1}.

TEMPERATURE PROFILE

For RF devices, the penetration depth is controlled by the configuration of the electrode tip. For IR laser of 1.4 to 2.2 microns, the absorption (0.5 mm path) in cornea, sclera or conjunctival tissue is about 60 percent (at 1.4 micron), 75 percent (at 1.45, 1.87 and 2.1 micron), 50 percent (at 1.8 micron), 95 percent (at about 1.89 micron) and over 99 percent (at about 1.92 microns) for non-focused beam.[7] These are the criteria for the selected IR lasers in addition to the focusing factor (B) discussed earlier. The absorption depth at various laser spectra for various ocular tissues is one of the critical elements in defining system parameters of this invention. Given value of "A" with respect to the treated tissue, we may predict the penetration depth (d) by the revised Beer's law, Bexp (-A x d) discussed earlier. However, the penetration depth is also an increasing function of the power of the thermal energy beam.

As shown earlier, higher "A" values tend to move the temperature peak profile forward towards the corneal epithelium. Therefore, to avoid cornea epithelial damage while achieving significant deep thermal penetration, the laser wavelength and the focal length must be carefully specified.

Figure 24.2 schematically shows the temperature profile of the treated tissue relative to the surface temperature "Ts" based on the calculated laser power density profiles. Figure 24.2A to D, respectively represents temperature profiles for non-focused, short-focused (f<f*), optimally focused (with f=f*) and long focused (f>f*) cases, where f* is defined by B*=exp (f*A), or f*= (ln B*/A), and where B*= (7-16) is the value at focal point.

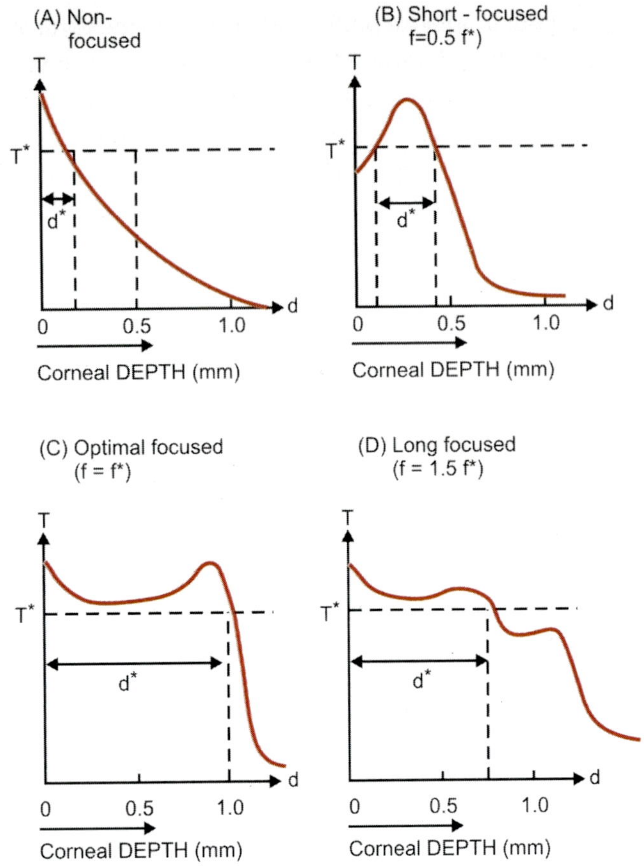

Figure 24.2: Temperature profiles for non-focused and focused laser, where the threshold temperature (T*=58°C) defines the penetration depth (d*)

It was known (Stringer HPT, Nature, vol. 204, p.1307, 1964) that stroma collagen shrinkage temperature is 58°C (defined as the threshold temperature "T*") to 75°C. Given the T*, we may evaluate the effective penetration depth (d*), the depth where tissue thermal shrinkage starts to effectively occur. As shown by Figures 24.2A to D), d* increases with f up to about f=f*, then it starts to decrease after f* and approaches to the non-focused value.

The significance of Figure 24.2 may be summarized as follows:

a. Non-focused laser has the shortest effective penetration, d*=(0.1-0.2) mm depending on A and T*.
b. Short focused case with f<f* has lower temperature on the treated surface, and therefore less risk of surface damage. However, this scenario results in a higher temperature in the vicinity of the endothelial (about 0.5 mm for the case of cornea) and hence the concern of endothelial damage increases.
c. At the optimal focusing case (f=f*), the temperature profile is almost flat-top, similar to that of laser power profile shown in Figure 24.2, therefore it has the maximal d* whereas the risk of epithelial or endothelial layers may be reduced under controlled laser power and treatment time, typically about 1 to 5 seconds.
d. For long focused beam (f>f*), the value of d* decreases. To keep d* at least 80 percent of the corneal stroma thickness (0.5 mm), as an example, the preferred parameters of this invention includes f is about (0.8-1.5) and most preferable (0.9-1.1) times of f*, where f* is about 0.4 to 1.4 mm, for B*=16. The preferred range selection of focal length also significantly reduces the risk of overheating on the epithelial or endothelial tissue of the cornea.

SAFETY AND EFFICACY

Non-focused LTK used in Ho:YAG laser (by Sunrise Technologies, Inc.) suffers the disadvantages of shallow penetration, typically less than 1/3 of the cornea stroma thickness. In order to increase the effective penetration depth (d*), defined by the region where stroma temperature is higher than the shrinkage threshold (T*), one needs to use a higher laser power which causes excessive injury to the epithelial layer. Using a focused laser will improve d* and reduce the risk of epithelial damage. However, for short focal length case, used in the conventional DTK system (ProLaser), as shown in Figure 24.2B, with the focal point inside the stroma increases the risk of endothelial layer damage because of the peak-power profile may be too close to the layer. DTK-Plus system (New Vision, Inc.) using an optimal focal length (f*) about 0.8 to 1.2 mm, longer than the corneal thickness, has a minimal risk of epithelial or endothelial damage, while offering a much deeper d*, in the range of about 0.4 to 0.6 mm.

Conductive keratoplasty (CK) using RF wave electrode may offer a rather deep thermal penetration, controlled by the length of the conductor tip, however, it has been shown to cause scaring and postoperative regression. Regression and poor predictability are the two major drawbacks of existing systems of the CK device, Ho:YAG LTK and conventional DTK. These problems are mainly caused by epithelial or stroma tissue healing and poor control over the temperature profile produced by the thermal energy beam, which may be laser induced or RF wave generated. The conventional-DTK (ProLaser) uses a diode laser at about 1885 nm and having a tolerance of 5 nm which causes the absorption coefficient (A) to change from 40 to 55 cm^{-1}. This uncertainty in A value and the rather long exposure time (about 4 seconds in each treated spot) may result in the change of d* and temperature profile which leads to poor predictability. The new DTK-Plus system (New Vision, Inc.) uses a lower and narrower "A" value at a proprietary wavelength. This not only offers a deeper d*, which is controlled by the optimal local length given by f*= (ln B*)/A, with B* about 16, but also repeatable temperature profiles from spot to spot at a shorter exposure time of about 2 to 3 seconds. Therefore, it offers better predictability of refractive outcomes with less regression due to less damage to epithelial or endothelial layer. In addition, a smaller spot size of about 200 micron in DTK-Plus versus about 50 micron in conventional DTK system, reduces the stromal overheating caused by the hot-spot of small laser spot size at the focal point.

Both conventional-DTK and DTK-Plus produce a conical temperature profile, however, DTK-Plus, by virtue of its energy focal length, has a horizontal profile about two times wider than that of conventional DTK. It is important to note that the hyperopic refractive change at a given laser power exposed to the treated spot is proportional to d*W, which is equal to (effective penetration depth) x (mean width of the conical profile). Therefore deeper "d*" and wider width "W" will result in higher diopter hyperopia correction, even when a lower laser power is used. In the CK device, a cylindered temperature profile and deep d* are achievable by the length of conductor tip (about 450 micron). However, a typical tip diameter is only about 90 micron which limits the width (W) of the temperature profile to about 200 micron or less, in comparison to about 200 – 600 micron width in DTK-Plus, and about 50 – 150 micron width in conventional DTK.

The currently used Ho:LTK, DTK devices still suffer instability and postoperative regression which may be significantly reduced by choosing an optimal focusing depth associated to the absorption coefficient (A) at a given laser spectrum.

The threshold temperature (T*) for permanent thermal shrinkage (PTT) of the treated tissue is about 58 degree C. It is important to note that PTT occurs near the surface layer of the treated area in a collimated beam, whereas it penetrates deeply into the area defined by the focal point (or focal length f) in a focused beam. Deep penetration is one of the critical elements for efficacy and postoperative stability presented in this new system. The Ho:LTK system of Sand suffers major regression due to its non-contact, non-focused superficial laser heating. The new system of DTK-Plus in focused mode overcomes the drawback of prior systems and also provides other advantages including less damage to the corneal epithelial and endothelial layers. It creates sufficient coagulation in almost the entire stroma versus only less than 30 percent in non-focused cases. The prior system of Sunrise Technologies using a non-focused short pulsed Ho: YAG laser results in epithelial damage since the laser power peaks on the surface and causes insufficient coagulation in deep stroma. The currently used conventional DTK using tightly focused CW diode laser (with f about 0.3 to 0.5 mm) improves the penetration depth, however, it still has a narrow peak profile which results in postoperative regression and a low initial efficacy, of less than 2.0 diopter of correction. The broader laser profile under the AFT condition introduced in this chapter not only provides better efficacy for higher hyperopic correction of up to +4 diopter, but also reduces the postoperative regression.

CONCLUSION

Thermal keratoplasty using either CK, non-focused, pulsed Ho:YAG laser (Ho:LTK) or focused CW diode lasers (conventional DTK and DTK-Plus) offer the advantages of being minimally invasive with reduced risk of complication in comparision with LASIK for hyperopia or mono-vision presbyopia treatment. CK, Ho:LTK and DTK also have the advantage of low system cost. However, the refractive predictability and postoperative regression are the major drawbacks when compared to LASIK. The new DTK-Plus system, with better predictability and higher refractive correction capability than the conventional-DTK and CK, therefore, may be a better alternative for hyperopia correction. Furthermore, a combined procedure (JT Lin, unpublished, pending patent) for thermal shrinkage of corneal stroma and ocular tissues located outside the limbus would have futuristic applications in the treatment of presbyopia.

REFERENCES

1. Alio JL, Ismail MM, Sanchez-Pego JL. Correctional of hyperopia with non-contact Ho:YAG laser thermal keratoplasty. J. Refract Surg 1997;13:17-22.
2. Papadopauls NT, Balidis M, Brajitikos PD, et al. Non-contact Ho:YAG laser thermal keratoplasty for hyperopia: Two-year follow-up. J Refract Surg 2005;21:82-86.
3. Rehany U, Landa F. Diode laser thermal keratoplasty to correct hyperopia. J Refract Surg 2004;20:53-61.
4. Pallikaris IG, Nroumidi TL, Pangopoulou SI, Alegakis AK, Astyrakakis NI. Conductive keratoplasty for low moderate hyperopia: 1-year results. J Refract Surg 2003;19:496-506.
5. Lin JT, Mallo O. Treatment of presbyopia by infrared laser radial sclerotomy. J Refract Surg 2003;19:465-67.
6. Lin, JT, Kadambi V. The new mechanism for laser presbyopia reversal and accommodation: Presbyopia, A Surgical Textbook. Thorofare, NJ: SLACK Inc; 2002;63-70.
7. Atchison, Smith. Optics of the human eye, Butterworth-Heinemann, 2000;110.

25

Solid-State Lasers for Refractive Surgery

- KATANA, SOLID-STATE UV LASER FOR REFRACTIVE SURGERY SINCE 2003
- CLINICAL EXPERIENCE
- SOLID-STATE LASERS VS. EXCIMER LASERS

Matteo Piovella, Fabrizio I Camesasca, Barbara Kusa (Italy)

INTRODUCTION

Laser technology for refractive surgery advanced with unrelentless pace during the past 20 years. The introduction of concepts such as wavefront analysis and customized ablation required manifold developments dealing with an increased, outmost precision of treatment.

Solid-state lasers in ophthalmic surgery have meant increased energy efficiency, as well as reduced size and costs. Presently, a new generation of UV generating solid-state lasers is becoming available even for refractive surgery, including lasers such as the LaserSoft and the CustomVis.[1, 2]

KATANA, SOLID-STATE UV LASER FOR REFRACTIVE SURGERY SINCE 2003

A good example of solid-state laser for refractive surgery, LaserSoft, is a continuous wave diode-pumped all-solid-state UV laser for refractive surgery recently introduced by Katana Technologies GmbH. A solid-state is not an excimer laser, since the UV laser ablation radiation is generated by nonlinear frequency conversion of infrared laser light in a laser crystal. A sequential frequency conversion with nonlinear crystals shifts the wavelength of the laser radiation into the range of 208 to 210 nm. The resonator structure and the beam delivery ensure an emission of the laser radiation with a TEM_{00} transversal mode, as well as an emission of laser radiation with a true Gaussian beam. The continuous wave-diode pumping provides a very stable shot-to-shot UV output with impressive long-term stability.

A Gaussian beam means excellent UV light spot distribution on the cornea. In fact, differently from the usual excimer laser, the solid-state laser does not need beam-forming elements – i.e. mirrors - in the beam path. Thus, energy at the corneal surface – fluency – is very stable. The laser beam is highly collimated, providing an increased beam precision and the technical features adequate to a fast scanning. Furthermore, the ablation pattern utilized in LaserSoft ensures an extremely homogenous cornea surface due to the accurate overlap made possible by true Gaussian spots.

Differently from an excimer laser, in a solid-state laser there is no gas exchange and gas discharge involved, with the related instabilities in output radiation, due to the physical nature of the discharge process. The solid-state approach reduces the requirements for maintenance and costs, providing high stability and long lifetime.

This device generates a flying spot of 0.2 mm in diameter, operating at repetition rate of 1 kHz. Thanks to this high repetition rate, the energy per pulse is lower then in standard excimer treatments. Ablation has strongly reduced shock waves, and to no audible sound due to ablation or laser firing. The whole procedure takes place in a silent environment, much reassuring to the patient, without the risk of noise-induced abrupt motion.

To fully exploit the opportunities provided by custom ablation, a very fast laser like LaserSoft requires a fast eye-tracker. The LaserSoft eye-tracker has a latency of 1 ms and controls ablation centration at very high repetition rates. This very fast eye-tracker ensures a reliable, high repetition centration of ablation on the x-y axes as well as well as the ocular rotation.

All these features makes the solid-state laser an ideal device for accurate custom ablation (Figures 25.1 and 25.2).

The ablation profiles currently adopted by this laser are designed to preserve the strongly aspherical physiological corneal curvature, as well as to minimize the induced spherical aberration.

Different reflection losses and fluence values for different angles of incidence of the ablating laser radiation during surgery are also taken into account in the ablation algorithm.

CLINICAL EXPERIENCE

We hereafter illustrate our clinical experience with a solid-state laser. Patients were treated at two different centers: Messina (PRK) and Campobasso (LASIK), Italy. The results were gathered after one year and were analyzed with the software Datagraph, using graphs recommended by GO Waring III.[3, 4] After signing a specific informed consent, 37 eyes, were treated with LASIK and PRK procedures with LaserSoft ablation. Preoperative

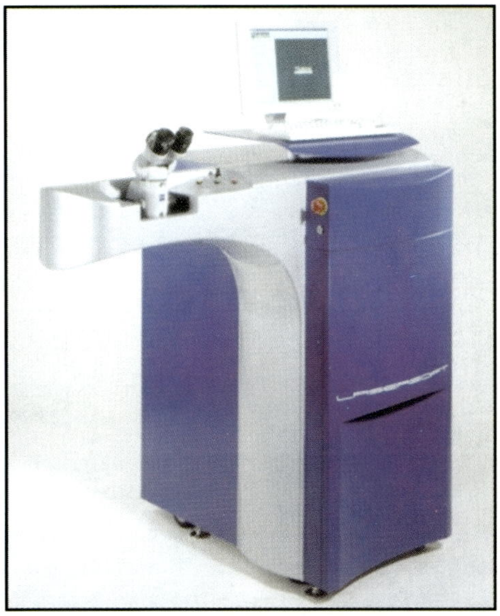

Figure 25.1: LaserSoft solid-state laser

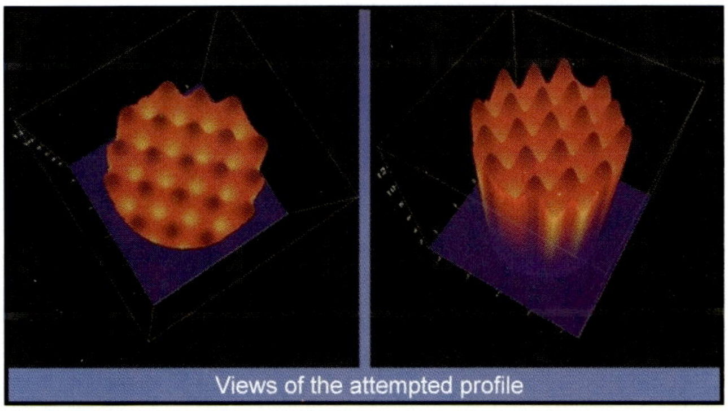

Figure 25.2: Experimental model, possibilities for custom ablation offered by small spot size. Views of the attempted profile

refractive data are reported in Table 25.1. Preoperative BSCVA of all eyes was between 0.3 and 1.0. LASIK was performed with the Hansatome microkeratome, choosing a flap thickness of 180 micrometer. Treatment diameters ranged between 6 and 7 mm, and transition zones between 8 and 9 mm.

One-year results were well within the current standards provided by normal excimer lasers (Table 25.1). Figure 25.3 shows the scattergram of the attempted versus the achieved refractive change for each eye. Figure 25.4 shows the spherical equivalent refractive outcome with the corresponding numbers. At one year, 100 percent of the eyes were in the so called happiness zone of ± 1D, 94 percent were within ± 0.5 D, and 87 percent were within ± 0.25 D. Figure 25.5 shows stability of refraction. The mean achieved change of spherical equivalent with time is also given. Table 25.2 provides the refractive and BSCVA results at one year.

Efficacy consists of two components: component 1 is the spectacle corrected visual acuity at baseline (BSCVA); component 2 is the cumulative graph of uncorrected visual acuities after refractive surgery (UCVA). In our study, 45 percent of the eyes show a postoperative UCVA better then 20/20 from a cohort with 41 percent being preoperatively at 20/20 with best correction. The preoperative BSCVA of all eyes was between 1.0 and 0.3.

SOLID-STATE LASERS VS EXCIMER LASERS

Table 25.3 presents the differences between common excimer lasers and solid-state laser. Presently, solid-state laser presents several significant examples of technical evolution in refractive surgery lasers. The solid-state laser features a tiny flying spot with a diameter of 0.2 mm and it operates at repetition rate of 1 kHz. Its very small spot size fits the present requirements for effective custom ablation.

The vast majority of excimer lasers commonly available on the market features a 1 mm flying spot, and they never have spots smaller than 0.65 mm, thus with a much wider spot ablation area than a solid-state laser

Table 25.1: Preoperative vs one-month data, 37 eyes

	SE refractive defect (mean ± SD)	*Sphere (mean ± SD)*	*Cylinder (mean ± SD)*	*SE refractive defect, range*	*BSCVA*
Preoperative	–1.71 D ± 3.71 D	–1.46 D ± 3.32 D	–0.51 D ± 1.97 D	–8.00 D to +6.75 D	0.80 ± 0.23
One year	–0.03 D ± 0.13 D	–0.03 D ± 0.19 D	–0.01 D ± 0.19 D	–0.50 D to +0.25 D	0.83 ± 0.23

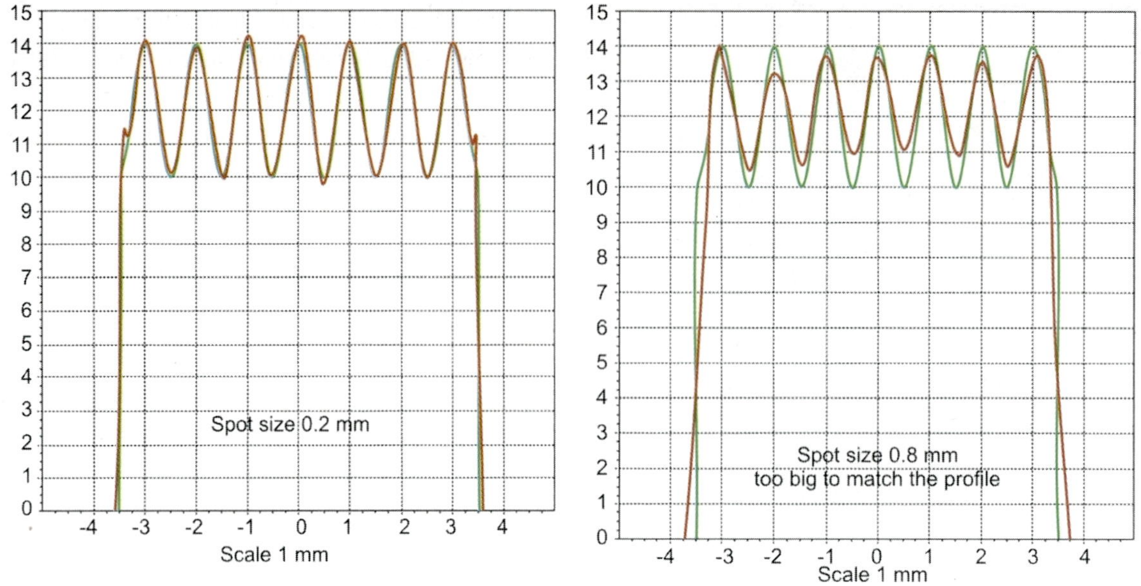

Figure 25.3: Experimental model, small spot size and custom ablation. Views of the attempted profile with a 0.2 mm spot size solid-state laser vs. that of a 0.8 mm spot size

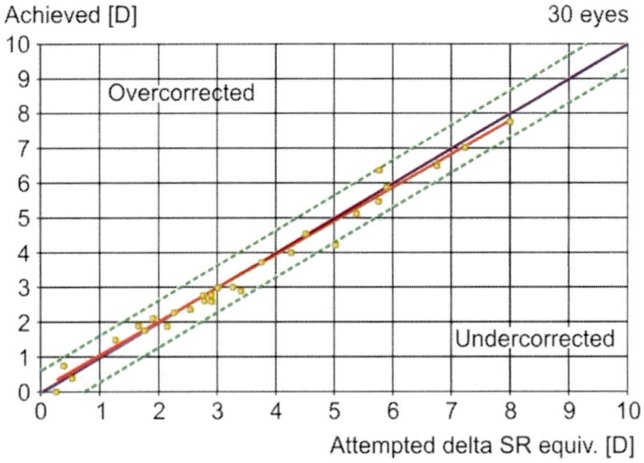

Figure 25.4: Show the scattergram and therefore an impression of the spread of cases of the attempted versus the achieved refractive change for each eye for LASIK

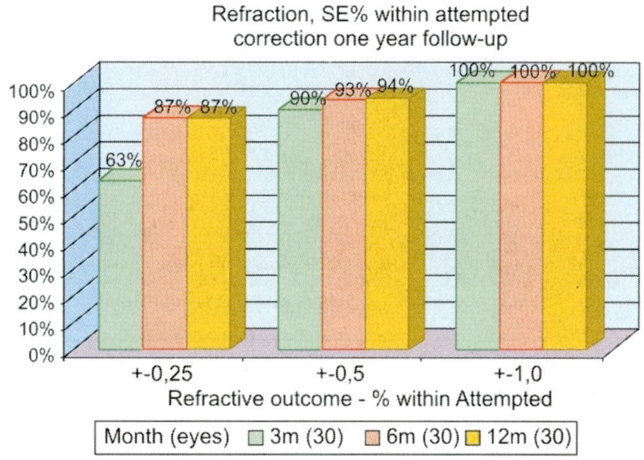

Figure 25.5: Spherical equivalent refractive outcome at one year. Of all eyes, 100 percent are in the so-called happiness zone of ± 1D, 94 percent are within ± 0.5 D, and 87 percent are within ± 0.25 D

Table 25.2: Refractive and BSCVA results at one-year follow-up, 37 eyes

SE refractive defect, Attempted vs Obtained	*BSCVA Preoperative vs One-year*
–0.03 D ± 0.20 D	0.0 ± 0.2

(Figure 25.6). There is a technical limit in decreasing the spot size of an excimer laser, as smaller spots would have a less homogeneous beam. Utilizing the usual excimer laser repetition rates, a 0.2 spot size would mean a very long treatment time, with the entire precision problem related to eye motion. To maintain ablation time within acceptable limits, and thanks to its technical features, the repetition rate of a solid-state laser is much higher in the solid-state than in excimer lasers (Figure 25.7).

The mirrors in a solid-state laser transmit the UV light without further elaborating it, unlike an excimer laser. This thanks to the true Gaussian profile of the beam.

Solid-state lasers appear to be easier to use lasers for refractive surgery, requiring less maintenance.

Table 25.3: Excimer vs solid-state lasers for refractive surgery

	Common excimer laser	*LaserSoft solid-state laser*
Spot size (mm)	0.8–1.0	0.2
Beam quality	Multimode (additional optics for clearing the excimer beam)	Single mode (Gaussian)
Repetition rate	50-500 Hz	1 kHz
Eye-tracker speed	Approximately 150 Hz	More than 1 kHz

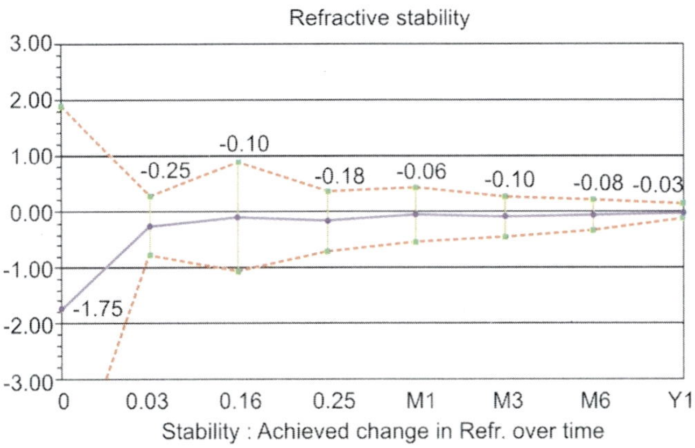

Figure 25.6: Refractive stability of the study group, at one year

The fast eye tracking ensures a reliable centration of ablation for x-y directions as well as the rotation of the eye at high repetition rates.

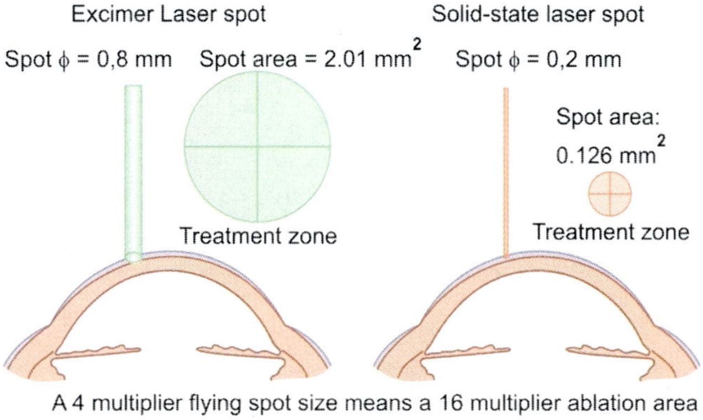

Figure 25.7: Solid-state vs. excimer laser spot size

CONCLUSION

Solid-state lasers appear to be a promising solution for a refractive surgery, applying less energy to the cornea and using a small flying spot of 0.2 mm, thus with the theoretical potential of inducing less scarring.

LaserSoft and solid-state UV lasers in general appear as a safe, reliable, stable, more compact as well as less costly alternative to gas-operating excimer lasers for refractive surgery.

REFERENCES

1. Personal Communications, 2003 Meeting of the ISRS/AAO, November 14-15, 2003, Anaheim, CA. Syllabus 289.
2. Personal Communication, 2004 Meeting of the ISRS/AAO, October 22-23, 2004, New Orleans, LA. Syllabus 10.
3. Datagraph med (Medical Data Analysis Software) Ingenieurbüro Pieger, Germany.
4. Waring G. Standard Graphs for Reporting Refractive Surgery. J Refract Surg 2000;16:459.

26

VisioDynamics Theory: A Biomechanical Application for the Aging Eye and LaserACE™ Natural Vision Restoration

- **BIOMECHANICAL IMPACT OF AGE-RELATED CHANGES IN OCULAR TISSUE**
- **BIOMECHANICAL SOLUTIONS FOR THE AGING OCULAR ORGAN**
- **LASERACE™ NATURAL VISION RESTORATION SURGICAL SOLUTIONS**

AnnMarie Hipsley (USA), Dimitrii Dementiev (Italy)

INTRODUCTION

VisioDynamics: Biomechanical Model for the Aging Ocular Organ

The defining concept of VisioDynamic Theory is that *presbyopia is not a refractive error or simply the loss in the ability to focus on near objects, rather it is an Aging Disease* whereas the age-related consequences on connective tissue as they occur throughout the body produce significant but reversible impact on biomechanical efficiency of ocular function which includes visual function, ocular biotransport, and ocular metabolic efficiency among other ocular organ functions.[1] The limiting factors for eye function throughout development and during aging can be broken down into *three* basic categories:

- Structural/mechanical
- Physiological
- Extracellular and intracellular.

Connective tissues (CT) can change their strength depending on the forces applied to them. Without force acting on them, the chemical structures and property of the tissues change, and therefore the fibers and mechanical properties of the tissue change. In muscle tissue this is called atrophy; in other supporting CT this is called hysteresis.[2] The SAID (Specific Adaptation to Imposed Demands) principle applies here, whereas the internal design of CT works as a feedback loop which is responsive to force, mass and gravity.[3] The opposite can happen if a CT begins to receive a persistent stress. If you do something to stress the CT, it will gradually add new CT at the point of stress, this is called hypertrophy.

The *internal design of* CT also responds to organismal experience such as environmental stress, biological stress, chemical stress which can manifest itself into various disease processes or traumas if the cycle is not broken. CT remodels itself in order to accommodate the new stress.[4] Chronic stress which exceeds the threshold of tissue healing can produce a low-grade chronic inflammatory process which triggers a cycle of cell damage ultimately resulting in cell death and or irreversible tissue changes which affect homeostatic equilibrium—this is 'aging'.[5] Despite the normal loss of elastin, collagen and dehydration of tissue, tissue morphology is limited by genetic predisposition, cultural (race) and environmental (altitude/sunlight) impact and inherent structural characteristics of health.[6] In the VisioDynamic Theory, the loss of accommodation in presbyopia is due to age-related changes of the eye which affect its normal biomechanical and therefore physiological function.[7] Biomechanical dysfunction leads to increased mechanical load, shear stress and consequential tissue strain. Tissue strain and deformation has effects on micro tissue layer interactions, collagenous integral structure/remodeling and ultimately extracellular matrix chemical and nutrient balance and efficiency.[8] Tissue properties and architecture are critical considerations when determining the impact of the pathophysiology of age-related changes (Figure 26.1).[9] The cornea is responsible for two-thirds of the eye's total focusing power, while the crystalline lens accounts for the remaining one-third. The focusing power of the cornea is fixed, whereas focusing power of lens complex is not fixed and depends largely on the mechanical efficiency of accommodation mechanism which is dependent upon the biomechanical relationships of the structures of the eye. Therefore, any surgical solution implemented for an aging ocular organ would be enhanced by restoring biomechanical balance in the structures included in the *Kinematic chain* of the *Oculociliary complex*.

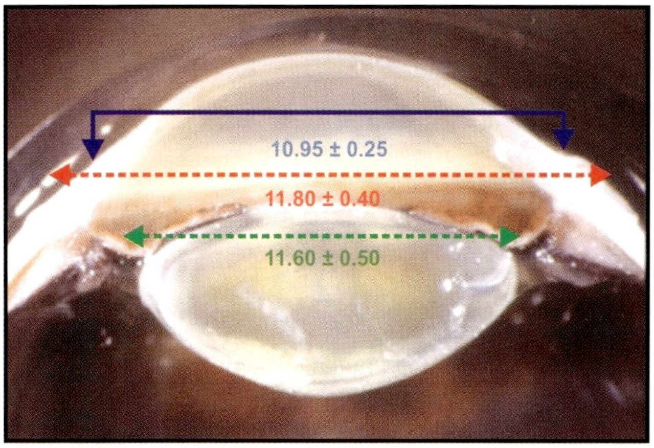

Figure 26.1: Biomechanical relationship of ocular structures *in vivo* White-to-white Anterior chamber diameter Ciliary sulcus diameter

BIOMECHANICAL IMPACT OF AGE-RELATED CHANGES IN OCULAR TISSUE

Biomechanical Dysfunction Hypothesis

The *biomechanical dysfunction hypothesis* postulates that there is a highly-structured inter-relationship in terms of the homeostatic stimuli which are shared in common by different ocular tissues as suggested by the close anatomic and functional relationship which they have evolved from.[1] Biomechanical efficiency relys on: **or ME = W × 100/E – e** *where E is the gross energy output, e is the resting metabolic rate, and W is the external work performed.* Optimal positive work or mechanical efficiency of ocular organ function occurs when this equation is balanced.[10] Every joint has a particular biomechanical arrangement with its associated musculature which is crucial to structure composition and form against gravity (posture) and the coordination of the neuromuscular units of the joint to produce the resultant force necessary to perform movement (function).[11] Restoring normal biomechanical relationships to the aging oculus facilitates the ocular structures to work with gravity in the most efficient way: The *oculociliary joint* is "postured" into optimum position to allow for the maximum potential kinetic energy to perform positive work or anterior acceleration and posterior deceleration of the lens for maximum range of dynamic visual tasks.[12] Biomechanical balance and specificity allows for efficient ocular movement, whereas, biomechanical dysfunction demands compensatory movements (due to over- or inappropriate loading) which will be 'patterned' and eventually interfere with performance. The accommodative mechanism is system of levers, and static contractions are responsible for the discrete adjustments to hold these levers in optimal alignment. The 'posture' of the lens during disaccommodation is an important baseline for determining the functional capacity of the accommodative mechanism.[13] By gaining increasing control over these processes, biomechanical proficiency increases. The LaserACE™ procedure or (Laser Anterior Ciliary Excision) was developed based on the fundamentals of biomechanics, neurophysiology, and kinesiology of the aging eye organ.[14] This procedure effectively and naturally restores the biomechanical inter-relationships of the intraocular structures providing biomechanical efficiency and alleviating biomechanical dysfunction by decreasing anterior global scleral compression load and subsequent subliminal tissue stress, strain and deformation.[15,16]

Scleral Compression Hypothesis

The sclera undergoes a gradual "sclerosclerosis" with age which represents the normal and gradual irreversible changes which occur in all connective tissues as we aged.[17] In addition, increased ocular rigidity has been linearly correlated with age.[18] This sclerotic process imposes staggeringly significant load, stress and strain upon underlying and related ocular and intraocular structures[19,20] (Figure 26.2). Every tissue inter-related with the sclera therefore will respond according to the SAID principle or otherwise respond by Specific Adaptation to Imposed Demands. CT of the ocular organ adapts to stress by compensation, substitution, or overload.[21]

Subsequently, all structures within the ocular organ sustain a 'gradual accumulation of microtrauma' over time. *Aging is a cyclical low-grade inflammatory process ultimately resulting in irreversible changes in tissue. Unless*

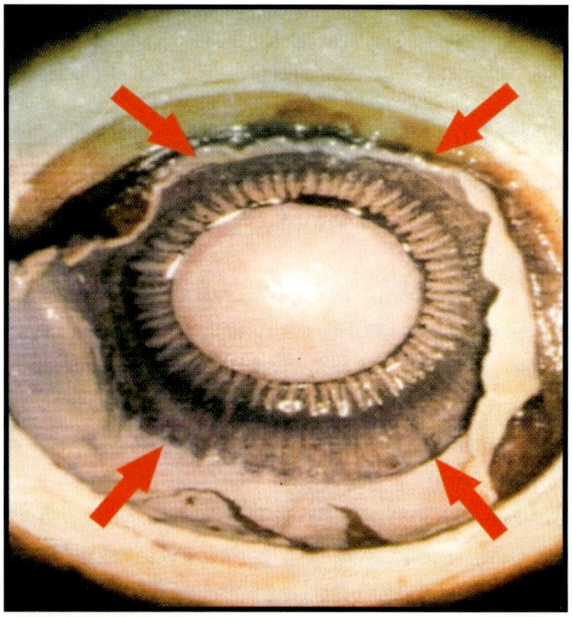

Figure 26.2: Scleral load vectors on underlying structures

the cycle is broken, cell death, organ death, system death and eventually organismal death occurs. Age-related changes in connective tissue of sclera include changes in colla-gen composition of GAGs (glycosaminoglycans), thickness, rigidity, tissue architecture (angle recession and changed biomechanical relationships), and changes homeostatic response.[22-24] Until now, the complex interaction of the sclera and recognition of its huge impact on the internal processing and diffusive mechanism in the eye organ has been considerably overlooked.[25] Age-related changes in the sclera are directly relative, indirectly relative or concomitantly relative to the impairment of the functional performance of the entire eye organ.[26] The majority of the inner anatomical and physiological areas of eye organ function lie beneath 5/6 of the outer tunic or the sclera which makes this structure a critical tissue consideration in terms of age-related changes in CT and its impact on biomechanical function of the eye organ.[27,28] One of the most critical zones is in the area of the limbus at the corneoscleral envelope (Figure 26.3).[29] A primary limiting factor in the ability to respond to near stimulus through the accommodative mechanism is the loss of mobility of the sclera. The magnitude of the response to near stimulus is also limited by the degree of "sclerosclerosis" or age-related fibrosis of the sclera. Muscular imbalance, which develops from biomechanical dysfunction can ultimately involve the whole ocular organ and even body function. All of these underlying structures are impacted by the progressive scleral load either directly or indirectly creating such dysfunction as ONH atrophy, Choroid dysfunction /vascular insufficiency, decreased uveal-aqueous outflow, increased IOP, biomechanical dysfunction of EOM, and ultimately gross disturbances in ICM and ECM metabolic transport. [30-32]

In vivo, CT *mobility* is important for the normal maintenance and turnover of PG (proteoglycan) in healthy tissue. Conversely, tissue *immobilization* or disuse results in atrophy because of a loss of PG from the matrix.[33] However, it is also noted in research that this PG loss following immobilization is *reversible* if normal tissue conditions and more importantly when *mobility* is restored.[34] Age-related effects of connective tissue can have enormous impact specific to overlying sclera shell thickness. "Structure = Function" is at the crux of the VisioDynamic model and is instrumental in the hypothesis and application of the LaserACE™ procedure which is based on restoring the biomechanical relationships of the ocular tunic in critical zones of physiological importance.[35] A state of equilibrium is reached and the internal stress balances the applied load (Figure 26.4). The principal goal of LaserACE™

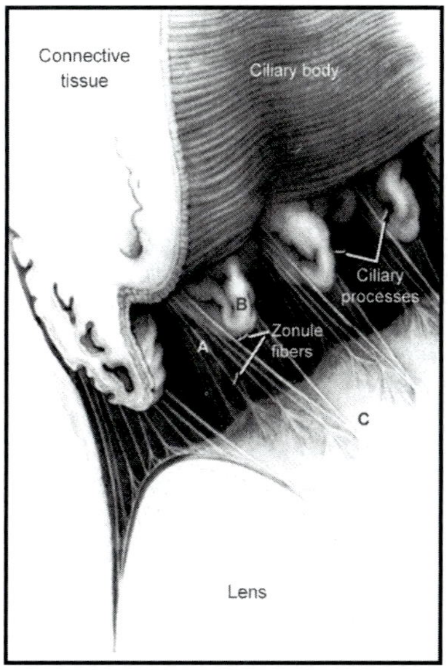

Figure 26.3: Physiology of the limbal structures underlying sclera at corneoscleral envelope

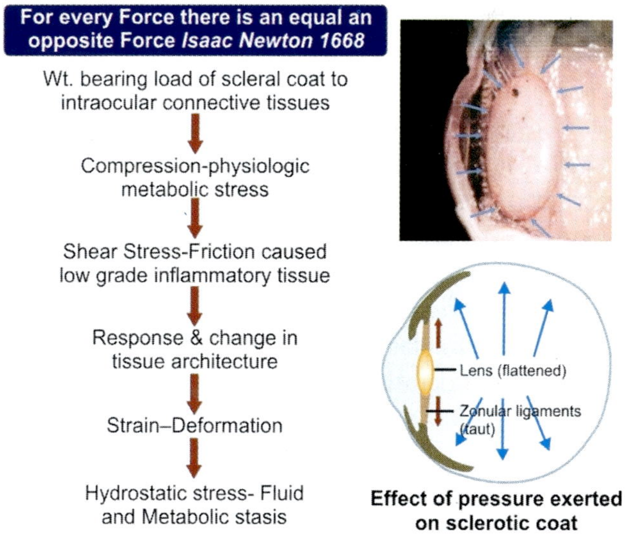

Figure 26.4: Scleral coat load creates an internal stress response of elevated IOP to achieve equilibrium

procedure is to decrease the overall applied load stress by decompression of sclerotic CT load, to restore mobility, to rejuvenate physiological functions in the anterior globe and further retard tissue strain and deformation rates in the aging eye. The fundamental objective is to restore essential biomechanical components which are affected by age-related pathology and promote longevity of the ocular organ.

Principle: Specific Adaptation to Imposed Demands (SAID)

Force and *friction* play a large role in ocular functional capacity. Leonardo da Vinci has the credit to be the first who made quantitative studies on the problem of friction Leonardo defined a friction coefficient as the ratio of the friction divided by the mass of the slider. Experimentally, he found a universal friction coefficient of 0.25 independent of the material. Ocular tissues like other biological tissues like to live in a homeostatic stress/strain range. Therefore, FORCE (mass X acceleration) and friction play a critical role in the ability for aging ocular tissue to function efficiently. Values of stress/strain outside of this range will lead to adaptation and changes in the tissue structure.[36] The *SAID principle* for ocular aging states that: *Age-related changes which occur in connective tissue increase both the static and dynamic coefficient of friction. Constant and gradual increased force and mass of the scleral load on underlying ocular tissues elicits equal and opposite force requirements resulting in intraocular physiological overload. Increased friction and load stress across tissue layers further elicits a cycle of repetitive low-grade inflammatory tissue responses, changes in tissue architecture, connective tissue deformation, and biomechanical dysfunction Specific to Imposed Demands which overall decrease biomechanical efficiency of ocular organ function.* Therefore, there is a constant linear deceleration of intraocular physiological processes concomitant with increased moment of inertia produced by progressive age-related scleral force (load) and friction (stress-strain).

BIOMECHANICAL SOLUTIONS FOR THE AGING OCULAR ORGAN

History of Biomechanical Surgical Solutions

During the mid 1970s in Russia, Fyodorov began treating myopia (near sightedness) in patients using radial or

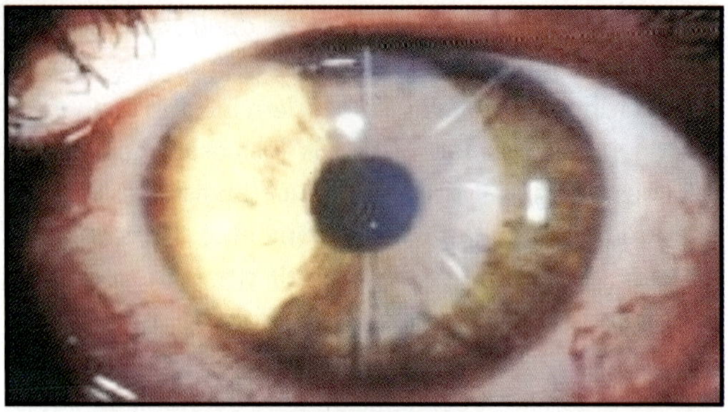

Figure 26.5: Early biomechanical applications in the cornea (RK)

spoke cuts through the cornea to biomechanically flatten its shape.[37] The biomechanics of the RK surgery evolved further to the limbal region and to the sclera after surgeons noticed unanticipated impact on other visual functions (Figure 26.5).

Scleral ablation was first hypothesized as a treatment for presbyopia shortly after RK was brought to the United States (Figure 26.6). Surgeons (particularly a group led by Spencer Thornton, MD) began to notice that some of their patients were not developing presbyopia as expected. It appeared that this was by product of RK surgery when the radial incision went through the limbus.

Dr Thornton organized a group of leading RK surgeons worldwide to perform scleral incisions and test this theory. While the procedure held promise, the results were less dramatic mainly due to regression as the incisional sites healed. Only a small increase in the amplitude of accommodation was observed and .5 D of myopic shift was also recorded.[38] This procedure later

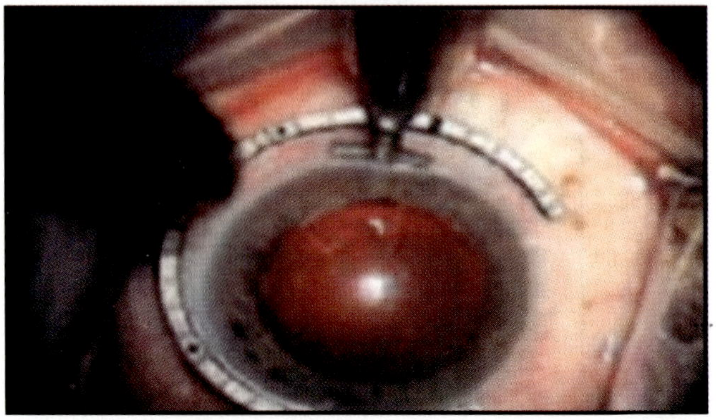

Figure 26.6: Thorntón developed one of the first presbyopic specific procedure using scleral incisions: Anterior ciliary sclerotomy (ACS)

evolved to be combined with silicone plugs having a more impressive and lasting effect. "ACS" is currently in clinical trials.

Schachar hypothesized a new model of accommodation controversial to the Helmholtz theory and performed scleral implants over the ciliary body in order to achieve an increase in accommodative power. (Scleral Expansion Bands "SEB"). He hypothesized that the primary element in achieving the accommodative effect was the increase in the working distance for the ciliary muscle complex.[39]

JT Lin hypothesized that the effect of scleral incisions was not permanent due to the rapid healing response of the body and utilized an Er:YAG laser to make the incisions. Under this technique, LPC or LAPR, near full thickness ablations of the sclera are made in pa allel radial orientation in the four quadrants resulting in an axial length change and anterior globe expansion.[40]

Hipsley introduced VisioDynamic Theory in 2003 based on the effects caused by the age-related changes of CT on the inner structures of critical physiological functional importance and countered that increasing scleral diameter across the globe was not ideal and in fact could superimpose even more biomechanical imbalance and possible instability to an already homeostatically challenged structure.[41] LaserACE™ procedure was developed based upon these fundamental principles of age-related changes on connective tissues and their progress load, stress/strain on subliminal tissues of the eye and imposing biomechanical dysfunction and its effects on ocular function.

LaserACE™ Biomechanical Surgical Solution

Unlike the expansion procedures, LaserACE™ is distinctly different in that it is a *decompression* procedure which emphasizes volumetric excisions in a CT matrix over critical segmental zones of fibrotic sclera in addition to creating a mechanical diaphragm pump in aponeurotic layers of the eye to rejuvenate aqueous outflow and alleviate stress from sensory receptors (Figure 26.7). Restoration of the Biomechanics of Accommodation with LaserACE™ or Laser Anterior Ciliary Excision is performed utilizing the patented VisioLite ophthalmic laser system with optical probe (Figure 26.12A).

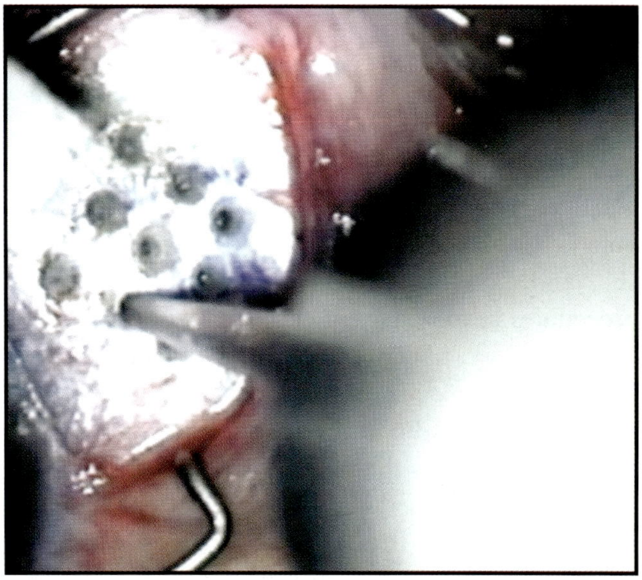

Figure 26.7: LaserACE™ "NeoPore" matrix decompressing fibrotic scleral mass and restoring physiological function

- Since nothing can be done about lenticular hardening on must aim to increase the biomechanical efficiency of oculociliary joint complex.
- Restoration of biomechanical balance requires alleviating restrictions and maximizing intraocular structural functional performance without imposing new biomechanical challenges to the oculus.
- Resultant effects of LaserACE™ allow for a new static oculociliary joint complex resting posture which maximizes the kinetic potential of the neuromuscular system.
- Resultant effects of decompression rejuvenate ocular biotransport mechanisms both indirectly and dynamically.

To distinguish LaserACE™ from scleral expansion procedures: Scleral expansion procedures have been proposed by Thornton ACS (Anterior Ciliary Sclerotomy), Fukusaku, Schachar (Scleral Expansion Bands) and LAPR procedure. Scleral expansion procedures are primarily based on the "Lens Crowding Theory" and strive to achieve improvement of the working distance of the ciliary complex or the circumlental space by inducing a 'pseudomyopic' eye shape with the polar axis longer than the equatorial diameter. Scleral implants are inserted into the superficial tunnels, causing a slight lift or 'myopic roof' in the sclera designed to reduce the crowding of the underlying muscles surrounding the crystalline lens. Alternatively, a radial ablation technique is used to create full thickness expansion of the anterior globe of the sclera producing enough substantial relaxing of the scleral tissue in the anterior globe to effectively change the stability of the anterior globe significantly enough to produce a myopic shift and axial length change. All of the expansion procedures have significant effects on eye shape of the anterior globe as a primary mechanism of action. LaserACE™ is *theoretically* different from the expansion procedures regarding the etiology of loss of ocular function as well as the mechanism and principles of restoration of ocular function. LaserACE™ procedure is based on the VisioDynamic Theory and scleral compression, biomechanical dysfunction, homeostatic, and neuromuscular hypotheses.[1] In this model, the etiology of the loss of accommodation in presbyopia is principally related to the effects of age-related changes of the eye which impact its normal biomechanical functions.[42] Scleral compression ultimately precipitates ocular biomechanical dysfunction leading to increased mechanical load, shear stress and consequential tissue strain.[43] Tissue strain and deformation has effects on micro tissue layer interactions, collagenous integral structure/remodeling and ultimately neuromuscular, physiological and extracellular matrix chemical and nutrient balance and efficiency. LaserACE™ surgical application is fundamentally different from these procedures in that there is no objective for scleral expansion or induced myopia, rather there is a zonal decompression of the connective tissue restriction which eliminates the compression or impingement of subliminal connective tissue, fascal tissue, and biophysiological structures of the eye organ (Figure 26.8).

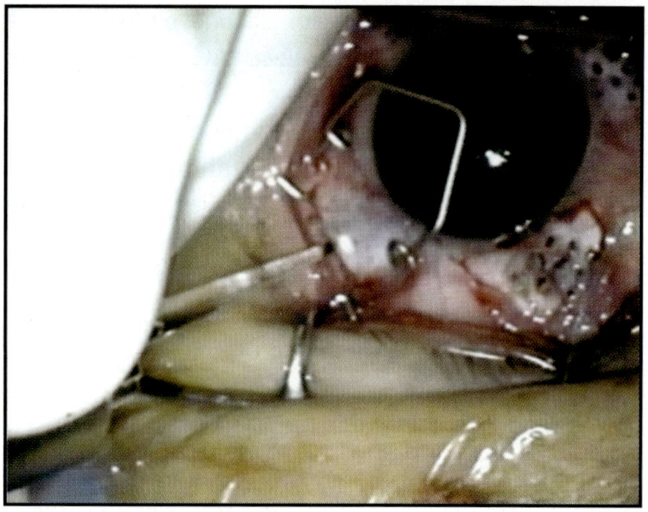

Figure 26.8: LaserACE™ zonal decompression decreases vertical load and creates no expansion

LaserACE™ Strategic Critical Zones of Restoration

LaserACE™ nomogram is based on mathematical calculations in anterior globe sphere specific to three critical zones (Figures 26.9 and 26.10). The key element in the effectiveness of the procedure lies in the ability to decompress the anterior globe with specificity to the key physiological and biomechanical areas of function. It is also critical to create the micro "NeoPores" with respect to the geometry of the sphere and the relative change in scleral thickness, CT characteristics, and rigidity across the globe (Figure 26.9). The cylindrical excisions are made in segmental zones with relativity to the natural physiological shape of the sclera and in tangential quadrants which allows decompression of the functional structures in the physiological planes of the spheroid of the eye globe in three critical zones of anatomical and physiological significance (Figure 26.10).

Critical Zones

- Zone 1: Just distal to the corneal-scleral envelope in the region of the Limbus extending to the pars plana over the girth of the ciliary body/process/complex and particularly the scleral spur 0.5 mm limbal area/tm/ scleral spur/structures of the angle.
- Zone 2: The region of the scleral which is begins just outside of pars plana and represents the largest circumferential diameter of the anterior globe sphere between the equator and the edge of the pars plana.
- Zone 3: The region of the ora serrata and the origin of the anterior radial ciliary muscles.

LASERACE™ NATURAL VISION RESTORATION SURGICAL SOLUTIONS

VisioLite™ Ophthalmic Laser System

The LaserACE™ procedure (Laser Anterior Ciliary Excision) is a revolutionary new technique which is

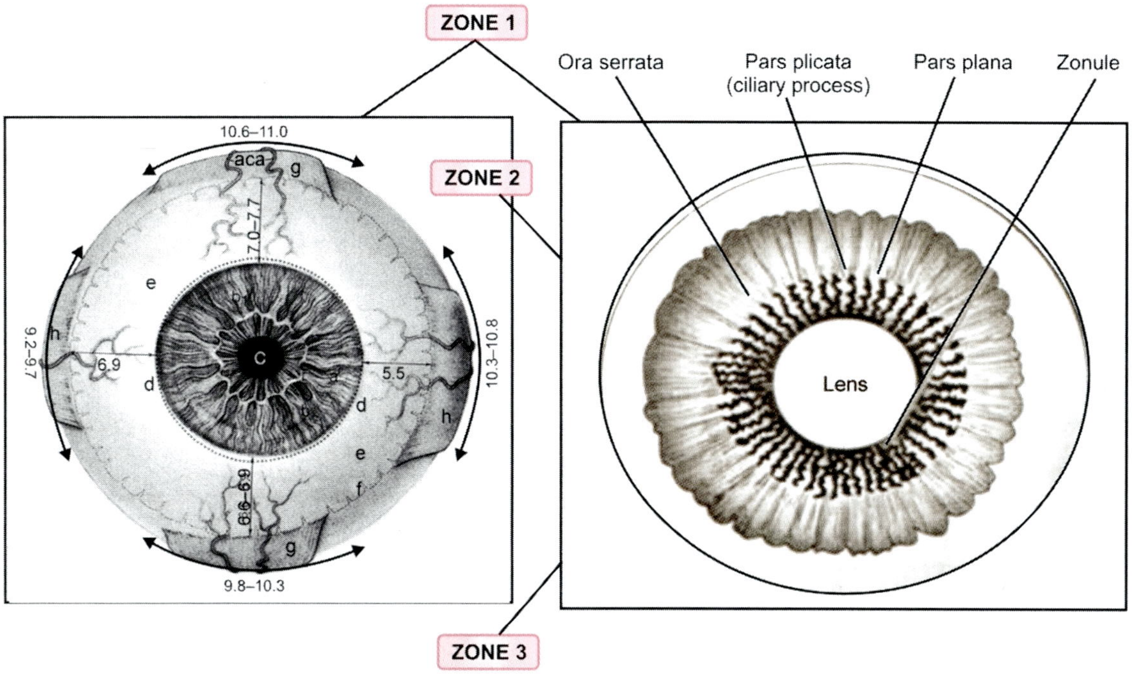

Figure 26.9: LaserACE™ critical zones—anatomy and geometry

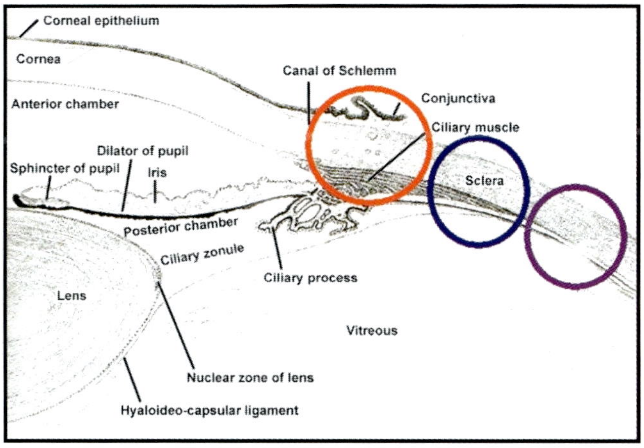

Figure 26.10: LaserACE™ critical zones—physiology

performed with the VisioLite™ Er:YAG laser (Figures 26.11 and 26.12A). The VisioLite™ laser's superior design and ability to control the variations of energy delivered will be the safest laser on the market for low energy soft tissue ablations for microsurgery in the eye. The laser beam of the VisioLite™ is pulsed and at a specific wavelength (2.94 um) that is very highly absorbed by water, as well as anything containing water such as CT. The laser beam causes rapid vaporization, or ablation, in both hard and soft tissues. The efficiency

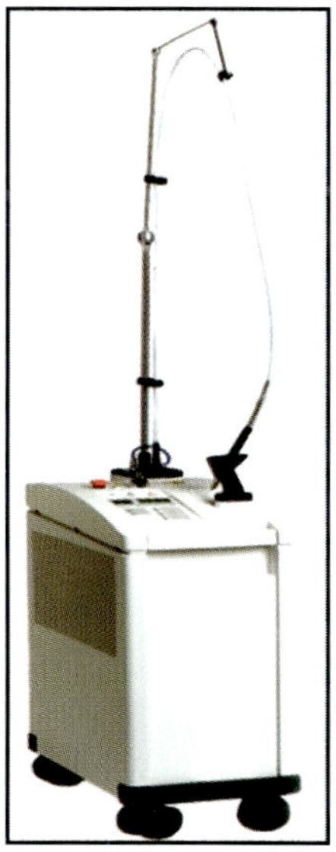

Figure 26.11: VisioLite™ ophthalmic laser system

of tissue removal varies with the available laser beam wavelength, the energy per pulse, the diameter of the pulse at the target, the pulse duration, and the repetition rate of the pulses. The optimum wavelength for energy absorption in water is 2.94 microns which is what the VisioLite™ ophthalmic laser system emits. The laser energy causes a vaporization of the water in the target tissue, causing an expansion of the water volume. The expansion causes the surrounding mineral material to be ejected. This water mediated explosive tissue removal is efficient and *transfers minimal heat to the surrounding tissue.* The unique properties of the Er:YAG laser allow inhibition of tissue healing response therefore preserving the "NeoPores" integrity without tissue regeneration or scarring. In addition to the Er:YAG being the ideal wavelength to create efficient photoablation without significant photocoagulation[44] (Figures 26.12B and C). There are small 'desirable' thermal and mechanical effects that produce stimulation of proprioceptive and vascular tissues in the ciliary complex which facilitate accommodation. It is further proposed that the unique characteristics of the 2.94 Er: YAG laser especially contribute to the 'lasting effects' of the procedure by limiting inflammatory stress and inhibiting tissue remodeling.

How LaserACE Works

- *Excisions in the sclera and globe in critical zones thereby restoring the efficiency to the biomechanics of the accommodative system.*
- *Secondary impact of changing the biomechanics of the relationship of the lens/ciliary oculociliary joint complex mechanism improves mobility to achieve improved accommodative power.*
- *Improves the efficiency of the hydrodynamic system by influencing intraocular pressure and aqueous drainage. Rejuvenation of the trabecular meshwork.*

LaserACE™: Surgical Technique

The aim of the LaserACE™ surgical procedure is the strategic volumetric decompression of scleral tissue outside the limbus over critical zones of the anterior segment of the globe of the eye. The mathematical model for scleral decompression is based on age- related geometric and tissue characteristics. The scleral decompression is accomplished by removing strategic areas of sclera in opposing quadrants of the anterior globe segment whereby a series of zonal connective tissue partitions are created using a non- contact Er: YAG 2.94 um wavelength.

The patient is prepared with 2 percent xylocaine topical drops or subconjunctival anesthesia and draped

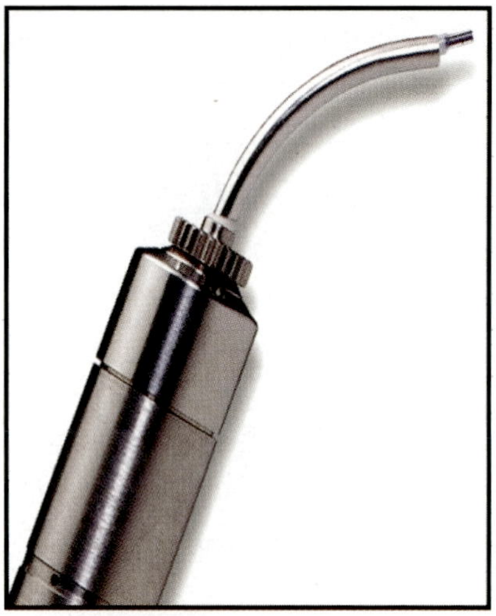

Figure 26.12A: VisioLite patented optical probe and tip

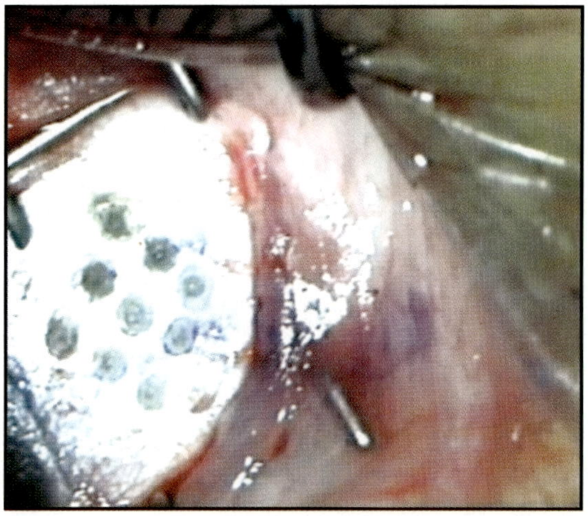

Figure 26.12B: LaserACE™ NeoPores *in vivo*

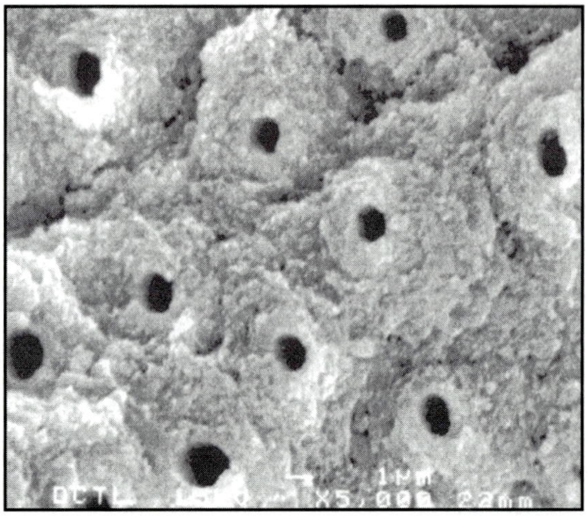

Figure 26.12C: LaserACE™ NeoPores (SEM 5,000 X)

Ideal Eligibility for LaserACE™
Ideal age: 48-65 years
Health patient with no CT diseases or ocular pathology • ±.50 spherical equivalent BCVA 20/25 or better • No more than .50 cylinder • Preferably plano or −.25 to −.50 spherical equivalent prior to LaserACE™ • PRK,RK, LASIK refractive correction can be done either before or after LaserACE™ • Ideally no more than .50 diopters of difference between manifest and cycloplegic refraction
Ideal IOP is 12-20 mm Hg
Normal stereopsis
• No convergence insufficiency or eye teaming deficit, History of fusional problems (phorias and tropias - poor stereopsis) • No excessively large pupils

in usual way as LASIK. One percent povidone-iodine is used to prep lashes and cul-de-sac. Mark 6 O'clock and 12 O'clock meridians with a 26 G needle dipped in gentian violet an opaque "Hover" contact lens is used with Goniosol or other viscoelastic for corneal protection (Figure 26.13A). The Critical Zones are mapped out utilizing custom designed quadrant and matrix markers in the 4 oblique quadrants (Figures 26.13B and C).The surgeon determines method of conjunctival dissection either via flap and conjunctival spreader instrument or transconjunctival excision (Figure 26.13D).

Calipers are used to measure the total length X width parameters of the exicision zone and a gentian violet marker is used to make outer limit guidemarks for the matrix (Figures 26.14A and B).The VisioLite™ laser and patented optical proble/tip is used to create the "NeoPore" excision matrix. Depending on the protocol

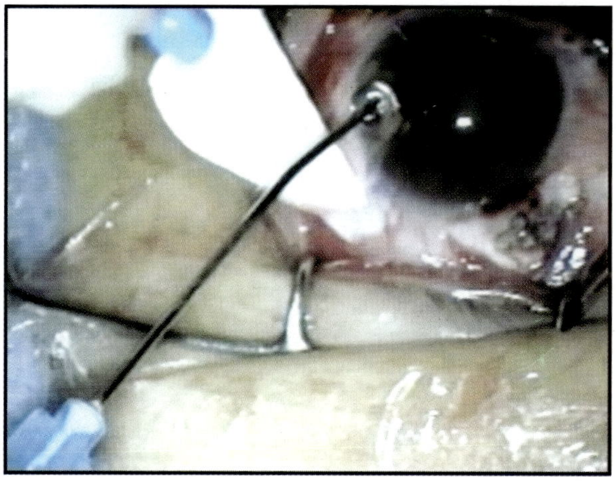

Figure 26.13A: Preparation for quadrant excisions: Visco-elastic and opaque corneal protector Hover lens with topical anesthetic solution

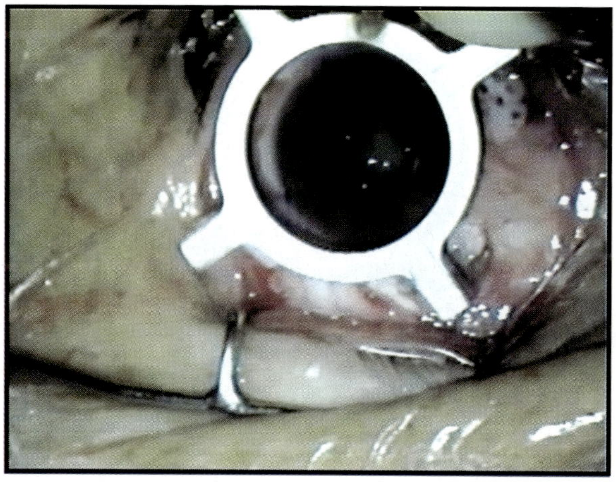

Figure 26.13B: Four point quadrant marker demarcates central segmental guidelines for "NeoPore" matrix

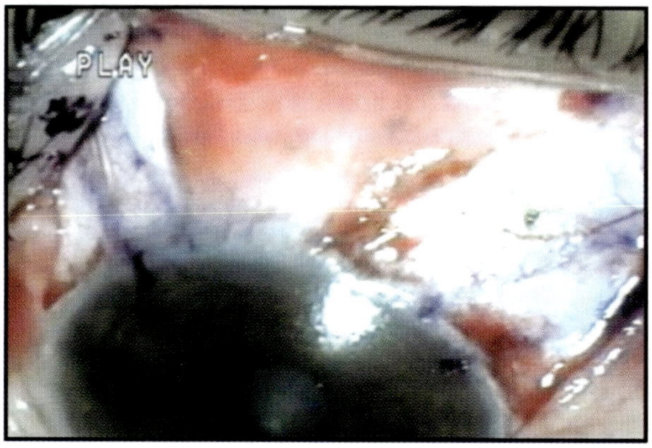

Figure 26.13C: Conjunctiva is opened to expose parameters of the quadrant zones. Zonal guide marks are used for excision matrix pattern

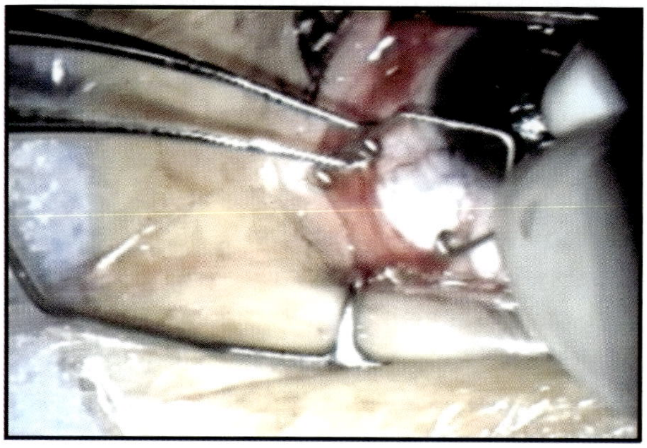

Figure 26.13D: Conjunctival spreader is used for optimal surgical field

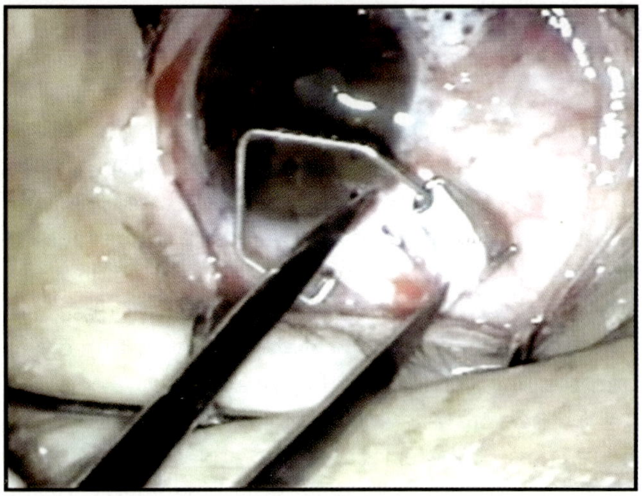

Figure 26.14A: Calipers are used to measure the total length of the excision zone extending from zone 1-3

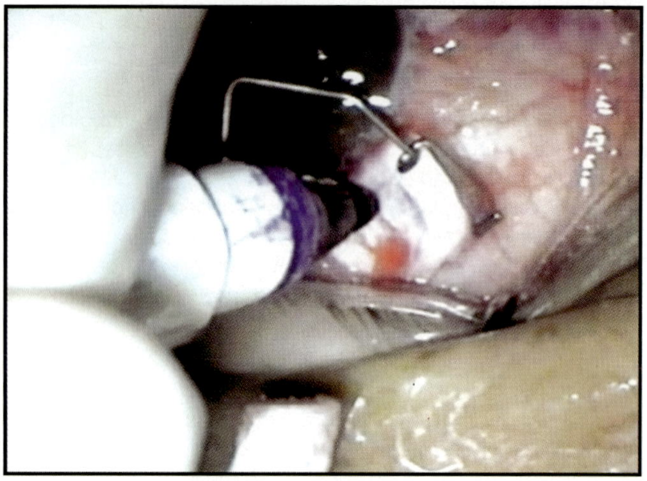

Figure 26.14B: Excision length and total excision surface area are marked

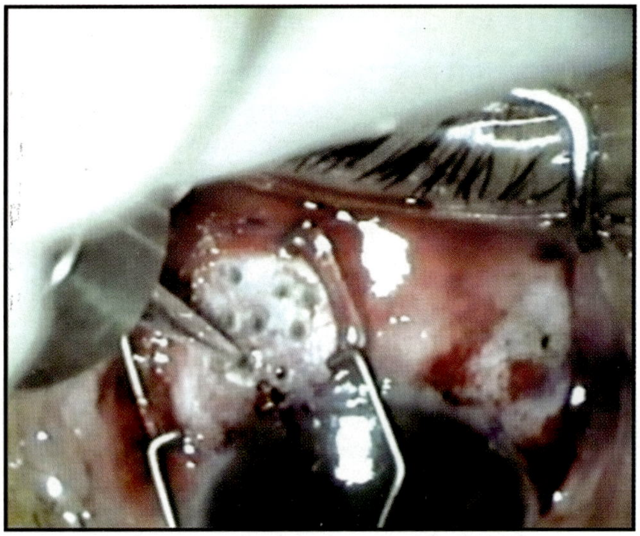

Figure 26.14C: LaserACE™ "NeoPore" excision matrix is made with the VisioLite patented optical probe tip

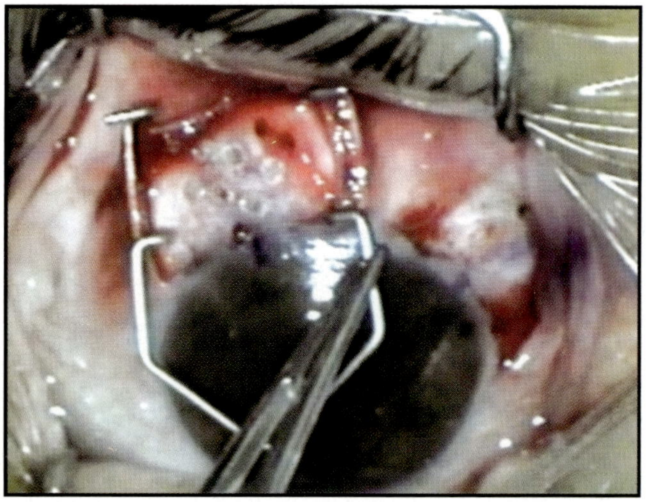

Figure 26.14D: Completed segmental decompression of sclera is stabilized with opaque bioscaffold fill

used, between 9-12 NeoPores are created per quadrant or between 10-12 mm cubic volume of sclerotic sclera is removed. The NeoPore depth is approximately 90-95 percent (Figure 26.14C). The resulting "NeoPores" or 'new pores' can be created in a number of design patterns, however, they must have a critical width which is necessary to inhibit scleral residual tissue approximation thereby inhibiting normal fibroblast activity retarding the connective tissue healing cycle. Collagen reorganization and tissue healing response is further prevented by implantation of a weightless bioscaffold material having very low specific gravity and therefore adding no external loading of the structures beneath and maintaining 'NeoPore' effectiveness (Figure 26.14D). It is believed that this strategic removal of scleral tissue creates a newly formed micro perforated tissue layer at the aponeurosis of the oculus or the subchoroidal lamina within the segmental zone treatment areas. These segmental regions act as biological "flexible diaphragm pumps" or extensible dividing membrane partitions which allow decompression of scleral load and shear stress, rejuvenation of intracellular/extracellular fluid exchange and restoration of biomechanical efficiency in the tissues that are internal to the scleral shell.

The conjunctival spreader is removed after each zone is completed and the conjunctiva is closed with conjunctival glue or alternatively bipolar cautery can be used. Topical anesthetic and steroid drops are placed in the eye following the procedure and are used for one week postoperatively along with biotears. Patient is instructed in VisioFlex™ accommodative exercises immediately.

LaserACE™: Kinesiology Application

The resultant effect of the LaserACE™ procedure is the immediate change in ocular mobility and indirect impact on viscoelastic modulus and rigidity. Enhanced mechanical efficiency of the accommodative mechanism as well as improved aqueous outflow as a result of zonal scleral excisions is demonstrated by an immediate drop in IOP (approximately 3 mm Hg) and ability to respond to near visual stimulus with significant amplitude within a few hours postoperatively. Further implications regarding enhanced metabolic solute transfer in the hydrodynamic system are being studied. It is believed that the culmination of the LaserACE™ decompression results may represent an additional potential prophylactic benefit by producing an improvement of overall eye health and adding the potential effects of increasing the longevity of eye function for satisfactory performance of functional vision ADL with delay of onset of diseased states.

The neuromuscular consequences include a resetting of the oculociliary joint complex in the anterior and posterior chamber, facilitation of the inner scleral wall mobility and choroidal elastic translation of the ciliary ring forces to the lens.[45] The restored biomechanical efficiency may in fact create a positive shift in the AC/C ratio (accommodation convergence/convergence) decreasing the level of effort needed to accommodate.[46] Lens factors still contribute to the overall accommodative deficits but despite this even small changes in vector force translations to the lens produce large functional improvements biomechanical improvements and therefore large functional improvements.[47] This is due to the mass and specific gravity of the lens, compared to mass and specific gravity of the sclera in an aged eye and the postoperative resetting of the ciliary ring lens complex. Even as little as 0.25 mm of anterior translation can contribute a significant change in dioptric power for near response. In addition the increase in specific gravity and central cortex nuclear mass of the lens which accompanies age actually becomes an advantageous mechanical property to allow for an even greater fulcrum with very low requirement in overall force from the ciliary ring in order to move the lens forward to facilitate near vision acuity. Intermediate vision likewise is dramatically improved.

LaserACE™ patient's also experience "overload" to the accommodative mechanism even at rest due to the restoration of functional capacity of the neuromuscular unit until the initial healing phase begins to stabilize and balance the globe. The "NeoPores" remain completely open for approximately 4-6 hours. A thin layer of epithelial cells begin to form in the early healing phase to close the inner fascial layer of the sphere. During this temporary initial phase, over convergence or "super-vision" will occur in for a time period prior to acute stability of the healing anterior globe segment (approx. 10-14 days). This is followed by smaller variations in fluctuation, manifest stability (approx. 6-8 wks), and finally a CNS established end point resting tonus in the accommodative system (approx. 3-6 months). It is critically important during all phases, especially the initial phase for the patient to be compliant in accommodative training exercises in order to maximize potential outcomes. Patients can experience 'overload' and ciliary spasm during prolonged exercise or reading activities especially in the first one or two postoperative months. As the system becomes well trained, accommodative spasm dissipates. It is also imperative for the patient to train the newly activated neuromuscular system in both dynamic burst response and prolonged endurance modes. Accommodative insufficiency is seen more in the myopic eye and underdeveloped neuromuscular systems, whereas, Accommodative spasm is seen more frequently in hyperopic eye type and well- developed accommodative systems. Semi-permanent/permanent stabilization seems to occur at about 6 months post-operative. Safety and preliminary efficacy have been determined by animal studies and *in vivo* treatment of more than 60 human eyes.

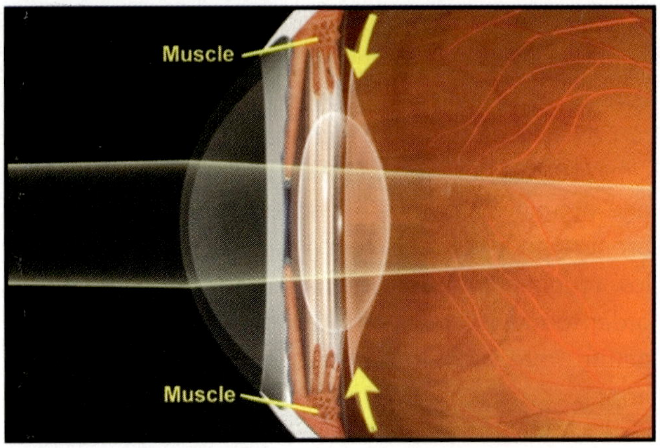

Figure 26.15: Improved VisioDynamic efficiency with natural restoration of accommodative function

LaserACE™ Prospective Clinical Trial: Preliminary Results

In June 2003, clinical surgical validation of the LaserACE™ procedure along with diagnostic proofs for the VisioDynamic theory were initiated in Moscow Russia, with Dr Dimitrii Dementiev (Figure 26.15). A series of aberrometry and evaluative studies were performed as well as evolution of the LaserACE™ nomogram parameters and are ongoing. These early endeavors were pivotal to the efficacy of the volumetric calculations that produce the stable LaserACE™ biomechanical result without compromise of ocular stability or asymmetry. In December 2003, clinical surgical studies began in Juarez Mexico with investigator Dr Bobby Maddox. Clinical surgeries were performed during 2004 on 8 eyes or 16 patients. Results were encouraging with a mean of 3.1 diopters of improvement for accommodative amplitude for near and intermediate vision with no statistically significant change in manifest refraction. In May of 2005 clinical surgical studies began in Valencia, Venezuela with Dr Jose Manuel Vargas. LaserACE™ was performed on 3 eyes recently with similar preliminary results.

Health Canada approved the LaserACE™ procedure for investigative study in October of 2004. Presently ongoing prospective Clinical Trials were initiated with Dr John F Blaylock in British Columbia, Canada. Clinical surgeries were performed during 2004 and 2005 on 20 eyes. The preliminary results represented herein. Patient data demonstrated a good effect in improving near vision and an excellent effect at improving intermediate or "functional" vision. Mean increase for these patients of more than 3.0 diopters. These results include 6 months data for most of the 10 patients, but a minimum of 3 month follow-up on all 10 patients. T test and linear regression analysis were performed and *accommodative amplitude* measured with a 'push-up' and 'pull-up' method utilizing the K-range measurement modified prince rule showed significant increase in accommodative amplitude. Monocular increased by 1.89 ± 1.16 D; (mean ± SD, P= 0.000); Range: –0.1 to +3.8 D and Binocular increased by 3.27 ± 2.38 D; (mean ± SD, P = 0.002); Range: 0.2 to +7.6 D.

LaserACE™
Preoperative and Postoperative Exam

- Medical history
- Visual Function Questionnaire
- Complete eye examination
- Dilated fundus exam
- Video keratography
- Contrast sensitivity
- Manifest and cycloplegic refraction
- Pupillary size
- IOP
- Gonioscopy
- Amplitude of accommodation
- (push-up method)
- Near vision at 35 cm (14")
- Intermediate vision at 60 cm (24")
- Axial length and AC depth (Humphrey Zeiss IOLMaster) Pachymetry

LaserACE™ resulted in significant improvement of both monocular and binocular near uncorrected visual acuity measured at 40 cm (Figure 26.16). Even greater improvements were seen for intermediate visual acuity measured at 60 cm (Figure 26.17). A majority of the patients reported on the patient questionnaire more dissatisfaction and loss of functional ADL (Activities of Daily Living) with loss of intermediate vision or 'functional-arm's length vision'. Therefore, patient satisfaction for functional ADL was over 95 percent.

LaserACE™ results showed a statistically significant reduction for add diopters for 20/20 of near VA (40 cm) after surgery. Monocular add was reduced by 0.68 ± 0.45 D (mean ± SD) (P=0.000); Range: 0.00 to 1.25

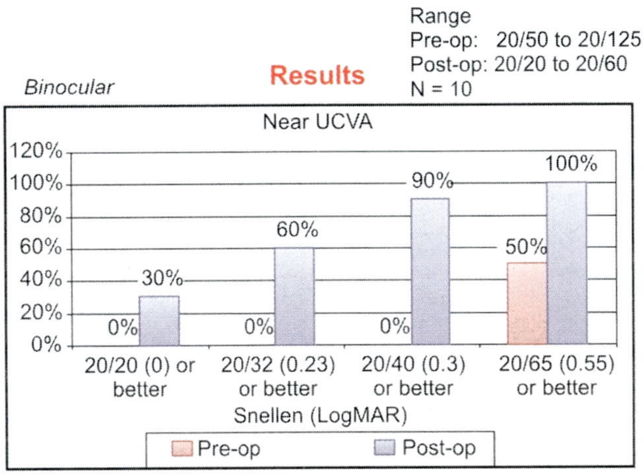

Figure 26.16: Binocular near uncorrected VA (40 cm) showed significant improvement by 0.47 ± 0.27 (log MAR, mean ± SD) (P = 0.000); Range: 0.17 to 0.90

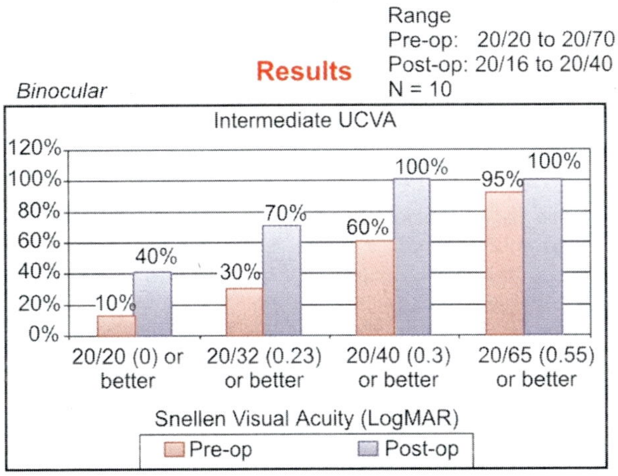

Figure 26.17: Binocular intermediated uncorrected VA (60 cm) showed improvement by 0.21 ± 0.18 (log MAR, mean ± SD) (P = 0.006); Range: 0.00 to 0.53

D. Binocular add was reduced by 0.73 ± 0.53 D (mean ± SD) (P=0.002); Range: 0.25 to 1.75 D (Figure 26.18).

There were minor changes of manifest refraction after surgery, but no statistically significant (P > 0.05); Preoperative spherical refraction equivalent; 0.33 ± 0.31 D (mean ± SD); (Range: –0.25 to +0.75 D). Postoperative spherical refraction equivalent 0.31 ± 0.48 D (mean± SD); (Range: –0.50 to + 1.50 D). No statistically significant change of binocular distance uncorrected visual acuity (UCVA); Preoperative UCVA range: 20/15 to 20/25; Postoperative UCVA range: 20/15 to 20/20; N= 10 patients. There were minor changes of manifest refraction after surgery, but no statistically significant (P > 0.05). Preoperative spherical refraction equivalent 0.33 ± 0.31 D (mean ± SD); (Range: –0.25 to +0.75 D); Postoperative spherical refraction equivalent ± 0.48 D (mean± SD); (Range: –0.50 to + 1.50 D). A-scan showed no statistically significant change of axial length (AL) after surgery (P>0.05). Preoperative AL: 23.57 ± 0.97 mm (mean ± SD).Postoperative AL: 23.56 ± 0.98 mm (mean ± SD). Topography (Humphrey) showed no statistically significant change of corneal curvature after surgery (P > 0.05). Preoperative average K value: 42.92 ±1.57 D; (mean ± SD); Postoperative average K value: 43.12 ± 1.72 D (mean ± SD).

Early outcomes have also shown a small statistically significant improvement in contrast sensitivity (Figure 26.19). Review of preoperative patient questionnaire shows that patient compliance with accommodative

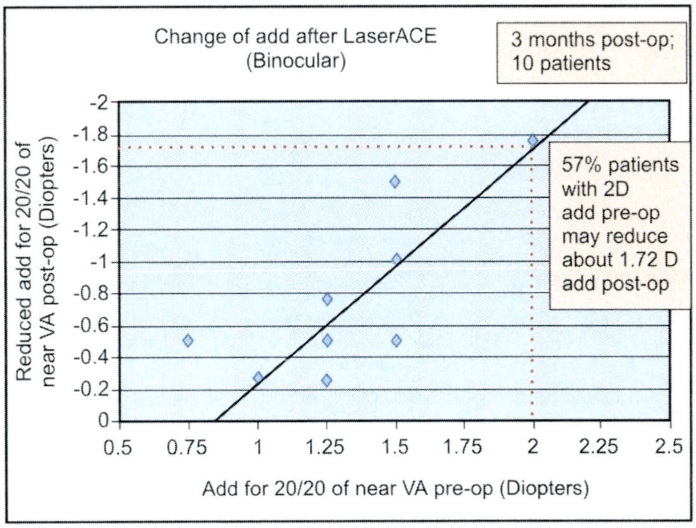

Significantly positive correlation between the add (D) for 20/20 of near VA pre-op (X) and the reduced add (D) for 20/20 of near VA post-op (Y) (P = 0.01)

$Y = -1.29X + 0.86$
$R^2 = 0.57$

Figure 26.18: LaserACE™ statistical correlation between add of near VA

Contrast sensitivity

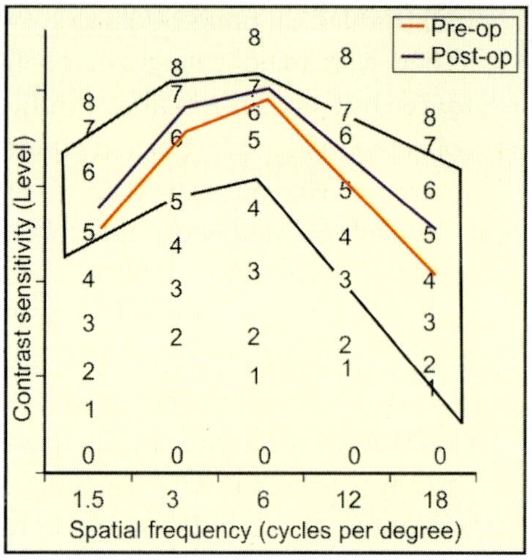

Mean contrast sensitivity level at 5 spatial frequencies before and 3 months after LaserACE

Spatial frequency (cycles per degree)	Mean contrast Sensitivity Level ± SD		P Value
	Pre-op	Post-op	
1.5	5.0 ± 0.6	5.4 ± 0.7	0.06
3	6.1 ± 0.8	6.6 ± 0.9	0.04
6	6.2 ± 1.1	6.8 ± 1.0	0.05
12	4.9 ± 1.0	5.5 ± 1.3	0.06
18	4.0 ± 1.2	5.1 ± 1.6	0.01

Paired samples T test

Figure 26.19: LaserACE™ statistical correlation between mean contrast sensitivity

exercises gives better outcomes as well as patients who read frequently. In patients with previous LASIK or PRK, LaserACE™ appears to be preferred choice for presbyopic solution. Presbyopia with high reading add obtain greater improvement after surgery. Overall preliminary results are promising.

LaserACE™ Complications

Very minor or low complication rate has been reported with the LaserACE™ procedure. No anterior segment ischemia has been reported and no major complications. Patients experience temporary ciliary fimosis initially which can be alleviated by over the counter pain medications. Temporary redness and dryness is alleviated with biotears. Patients have improvement of near and intermediate vision within hours of the procedure.

LaserACE™
Complications

- Two conjunctival cysts
- No ASI
- Subconjunctival hemorrhage
- No dry eye problem
- Temporary redness, and mild to moderate discomfort
- One patient saw shadowing at intermediate VA test in left eye 1 day postoperative and it disappeared within 1 week
- One patient had focusing problem at 20-40 feet 2 weeks postoperative and this disappeared one month postoperative

REFERENCES

1. Hipsley AM. VisioDynamics manuscript. VisioDynamic theory: A biomechanical model for the aging ocular organ 2003.
2. Amile D, Woo SL-Y, Harwood FL, Akeson WH. The effect of immobilization on collagen turnover in connective tissue. A biochemical-biomechanical correlation. Acta Orthop Scand 1982;53:325.
3. Viidik A, Danielsen CC, Oxluind H. Fourth International Congress of Biorheology Symposium on Mechanical Properties of Living Tissues: On fundamental and phenomenological models, structure and mechanical properties of collagen, elastic and glycosaminoglycan complexes. Biorheology 1982;19:437.
4. Sylvie Wendling A1, Patrick CaÑadas , Christian Oddou A1, Alain Meunier A3. Inter-relations Between Elastic Energy and Strain in a Tensegrity Model: Contribution to the Analysis of the Mechanical Response in Living Cells. Computer Methods in Biomechanics and Biomedical Engineering 2002;5(1):1-6.
5. Diamant J, et al. Collagen: Ultrastructure and its relations to mechanical properties as a function of ageing. Proc R Soc Lond (Bio J) 1972;180:293.
6. Dale WC. A composite materials analysis of the structure, mechanical properties, and aging of collagenous tissues. PhD thesis, Case Wetern Reserve University, Cleveland, Ohio 1974.
7. Curtin BJ. "Physiopathological Aspects of Scleral Stress-Strain". Tr Am Opht Soc 1969;67:417-61.
8. Fung YCB. Stress-strain history relations of soft tissues in simpole elongation. In Fung YV, Perrone N, Anliker M (Eds). Biomechanics: Its Foundations and Objectives. Englewood Cliffs, Prentice-Hall 1972;1818-208.
9. Werner L, et al. Correlation between different measurements within the eye relative to phakic intraocular lens implantation. J Cataract Refract Surg 2004;30:1982-88.

10. Fung YCB. Biomechanics: Mechanical Properties of Living tissues, New York: Springer Verlag 1981;222.
11. Hutton RS. Neuromuscular physiology. In Welsh RP, Shephard RJ (Eds): Current Therapy in Sports Medicine. BC Decker. Philadelphia 1985;1985-86.
12. Aura O, Komi PV. Effects of prestretch intensity on mechanical efficiency of positive work and on elastic behaviour of skeletal muscle in stretch-short cycle. Int J Sports Med 1986b;7:137.
13. Craik R. Biomechanics: A neural control perspective. Physical Therapy 1984;64:1810-11.
14. Hipsley AM. VisioDynamics Manucript: Biomechanical Solutions for the Aging Ocular Organ: LaserACE™ Natural Vision Restoration.
15. Arciniegas A, Amaya LE. Mechanical behavior of the sclera. Ophthalmologica 1986;193(1-2):45-55.
16. Paul JP. Approaches to design: Force actions transmitted by joints in the human body. Proc R Soc Lond B 1976; 192,163.
17. Sigal IA, Flanagan JG, Tertinegg I, Ethier RC. Finite Element Modeling of Optic Nerve Head Biomechanics Investigative Ophthalmology and Visual Science. 2004;45: 4378-87.
18. Ioannis G Pallikaris, 1,2 George D Kymionis,1,2 Harilaos S. Ginis,2 George A. Kounis, 2 Miltiadis K. Tsilimbaris1,2. Ocular rigidity in living human eyes. Investigative ophthalmology and visual science 2005;46:409-14.
20. Burgoyne CF, Downs JC, Bellezza AJ, Suh JK, Hart RT. The optic nerve head as a biomechanical structure: A new paradigm for understanding the role of IOP-related stress and strain in the pathophysiology of glaucomatous optic nerve head damage. Prog Retin Eye Res 2005;24(1):39-73.
21. Battaglioli JL, Kamm RD. Measurements of the compressive properties of scleral tissue IOVS: 1984.
22. Rada JA, Achen VR, Penugonda S, Schmidt RW, Mount BA. Proteoglycan composition in the human sclera during growth and aging. Invest Ophthalmol Vis Sci 2000;41(7):1639-48.
23. Rada JA, Achen VR, Rada KG. Proteoglycan turnover in the sclera of normal and experimentally myopic chick eyes. Invest Ophthalmol Vis Sci 1998;39(11):1990-2002.
24. Yamaoka A, Matsuo T, Shiraga F, Ohtsuki H. TIMP-1 production by human scleral fibroblast decreases in response to cyclic mechanical stretching. Opthalmic Res 2001;3(2):98-101.
25. Watson PG, Young, RD. Scleral structure, organisation and disease. A review. Exp Eye Res 2004;78(3):609-23.
26. Julie Albona, Peter P Purslowb, Wojciech SS Karwatowskic, David L Eastyd. Age-related compliance of the lamina cribrosa in human eyes. Br J Ophthalmol 2000;84:318-23.
27. Gong H, Freddo TF, Johnson M. Age-related changes of sulfated proteoglycans in the normal human trabecular meshwork. Exp Eye Res 1992;55(5):691-709.
28. Koretz JF, Rogot A, Kaufman PL. Physiological strategies for emmetropia. Trans Am Ophthalmol Soc 1995;93:105-18; discussion 118-22.
29. Hanna KD, et al. "Computer Simulation of Arcuate and Radial Incisions Involving the Corneoscleral Limbus", Eye 1989;3:227-39.
30. Ross C Ethier, Mark Johnson, Jeff Rubert. Ocular biomechanics and biotransport. Annual Review of Biomedical Engineering 2004;6:249-73.
31. Neacsu A, Tuchila G, Trifu M, Curea M, Boeru G. Biomechanical stress in glaucoma—cause and effect. Oftalmologia 2004;48(4):93-98.
32. Mori F, Konno S, Hikichi T, Yamaguchi Y, Ishiko S, Yoshida A. Factors affecting Pulsatile Ocular Blood Flow. Br J Ophthalmol 2001;85:529-30.
33. Shepherd RJ. Physiology and Biochemistry of Exercise. Praeger, New York 1982.
34. Buckwalter JA. Maintaining and restoring mobility in middle and old age: The importance of the soft tissues. Instr Course Lect 1997;46:459-69.
35. Norton TT, Siegwart JT Jr. Animal models of emmetropization: Matching axial length to the focal plane. J Am Optom Assoc 1995;66(7):405-14.
36. Woo SL-Y, et al. "Nonlinear Material Properties of Intact Cornea and Sclera", Exp Eye Res 1972;14:29-39.
37. Robin JB. Radial keratotomy: Procedures. Indian J Ophthalmol 1990;8(3):103-06.
38. Thornton S. Anterior Ciliary Sclerotomy (ACS), A Procedure to Reverse Presbyopia. In Neal Sher (Ed). Surgery for Hyperopia and Presbyopia 1997;33-37.
39. Schachar RA. Cause and treatment of presbyopia with a method for increasing the amplitude of accommodation. Ann Ophthalmol 1992;24:445-52.
40. Lin JT, Perasso A, Martinez D. A novel device for presbyopia reversal 1999;92.
41. Hipsley AM. Influence of biomechanics on age-related changes of the eye: Clinical implications for refractive surgery. ASCRS 2005.
42. Strenk SA, Semmlow JL, Strenk LM, Munoz P, Gronlund-Jacob J, DeMarco JK. Age-related changes in human ciliary muscle and lens: A magnetic resonance imaging study. Invest. Ophthalmol Vis Sci 1999;40:1162-69.
43. Battaglioli JL, Kamm RD. Measurements of the compressive properties of scleral tissue. IOVS: 1984.
44. Becker PC, Olsson NA, Simpson JR. Erbium-doped fiber amplifiers: Fundamentals and technology. San Diego [etc]: Academic Press Aron Rosa 1999.
45. Friberg TR, Lace JW. A comparison of the elastic properties of human choroid and sclera. Exp Eye Res 1988; 47(3):429-36.
46. Mutti DO, Jones LA, Moeschberger ML, Zadnik K. AC/A ratio, age, and refractive error in children. Invest Ophthalmol Vis Sci 2000;41(9):2469-78.
47. van Alphen GW. Choroidal stress and emmetropization. Vision Res 1986;26(5):723-34.

Section 3

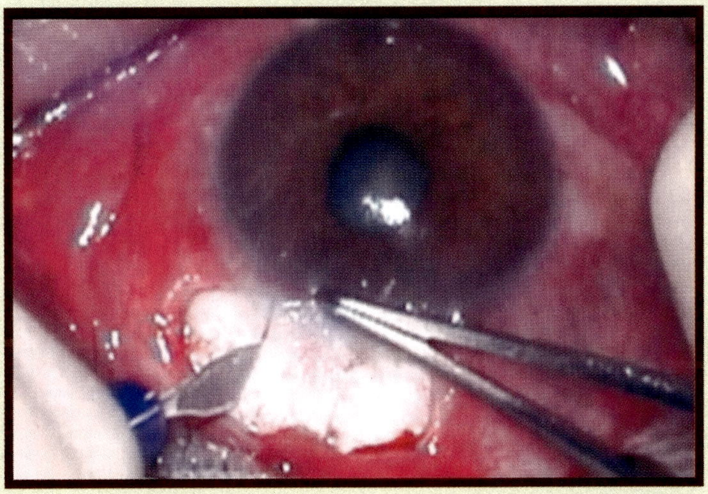

Glaucoma Technologies (Laser & Minimally-Invasive Glaucoma Surgical Techniques)

27

Viscocanalostomy

- MECHANISM OF ACTION
- SURGICAL TECHNIQUE
- INDICATIONS
- RESULTS

Roberto G Carassa (Italy)

INTRODUCTION

In the last years non-penetrating glaucoma surgery achieved great interest as a possible alternative to trabeculectomy. This class of procedures are mainly represented by *"deep sclerectomy"* and by *"viscocanalostomy"* (which was introduced by R. Stegmann in the early nineties), and are based on the original studies by Krasnov[1] and by Zimmerman[2] on "non-penetrating trabeculectomy." Similarly, both procedures are aimed at allowing drainage of the aqueous humor from the anterior chamber not through a patent scleral opening, but by slow percolation through the inner trabecular meshwork and/or Descemet's membrane ("sclerodescemetic membrane"). This avoids sudden IOP drops, hypotonies and flat chambers. The absence of anterior chamber opening and iridectomy limits the risk of cataract and infection. Compared to deep sclerectomy, viscocanalostomy is a step forward. In fact this procedure is aimed not only at taking the advantages of being non-penetrating, as deep sclerectomy, but, most important, in restoring the physiological outflow pathway, thus avoiding any external filtration. This would make the success of the procedure independent of conjunctival or episcleral scarring, leading cause of failure in trabeculectomy, with less indications for wound healing modulation. Moreover, the absence of the filtering bleb avoids related ocular discomfort, and the procedure can be carried out in any quadrant.

MECHANISM OF ACTION

Viscocanalostomy increases the aqueous outflow through different mechanism of action. It creates a by-pass by which aqueous humor can reach Schlemm's canal skipping the trabecular meshwork, which is the site of the increased outflow resistance in open-angle glaucoma. This is obtained by producing a "chamber" inside the sclera which directly communicates both with Schlemm's canal and with the anterior chamber through the "sclerodescemetic membrane." The aqueous enters the "chamber" by percolating through the membrane, and leaves it via Schlemm's canal. A recent experimental study on monkeys also showed the evidence of micro-openings throughout the wall of Schlemm's canal over 360 degrees which may be invoved in the increased aqueous facility.[3] Finally, as in deep-sclerectomy, aqueous humor can also leave the intrascleral chamber through the subconjunctival space and through the supracoroidal space by uveoscleral absorption.

SURGICAL TECHNIQUE

In order to simplify the technique, a specific surgical set, composed by a 0.5 mm diamond knife, a 1 mm round steel bevel-up blade, and a 165 μm blunt needle to cannulate Schlemm's canal (Grieshaber, Switzerland) should be used.

Viscocanalostomy is performed under retrobulbar or peribulbar anesthesia and usually requires 25 to 40 minutes depending on bleeding control. In fact, in order to avoid damage to outflow channels (Schlemm's canal, aqueous veins, collector channels, etc), wetfield cautery is used as little as possible, and bleeding is reduced by frequent irrigation of the surgical area with vasoconstrictive solutions as ornipressin. To provide optimal visualization of the surgical site, a bridle suture should be passed either on the superior rectus or in clear cornea.

The surgical technique can be divided in nine steps:

Conjunctival Flap Dissection

Viscocanalostomy does not require any specific accuracy in the dissection of the conjunctival flap, and can be performed in any quadrant, although the upper and temporal ones are most commonly chosen. The surgical field is prepared by creating a fornix-based conjunctival flap, using as little wetfield cautery as possible.

Outer Scleral Flap Dissection

A 5 × 5 mm parabolic cut approximately 200 μm deep, is made using the diamond knife (the incision can be outlined using a calibrated diamond knife to assure a constant depth of cut). After reaching the correct plane of cut the flap is dissected anteriorly in clear cornea by advancing the incision with the bevel-up spatula which allows easier following of the plane.

Inner Scleral Flap Dissection

A 4 × 4 mm parabolic cut parallel to the outer incision is made beneath the outer flap. The choroidal plane must be almost reached, and this is revealed by the

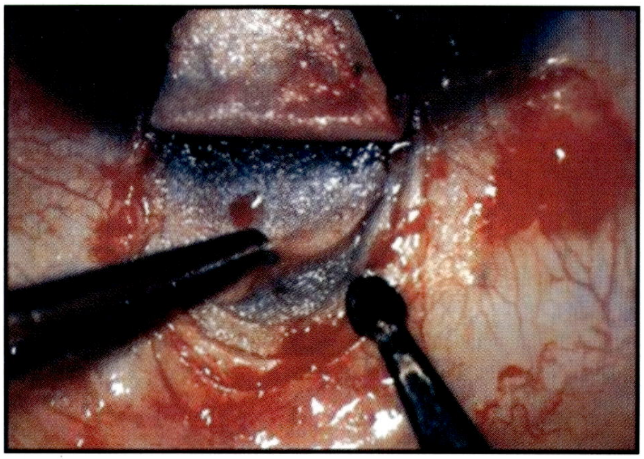

Figure 27.1: Dissection of the internal flap

observation of a dark reflex at the bottom of the cut. Using the specific beaveled spatula a precise dissection is advanced until Schlemm's canal is reached and deroofed leaving two patent openings on the lateral edges of the cut. In order to mantain the same plane of dissection and provide sharp lateral edges, progressive deepening of the lateral cuts is often needed (Figure 27.1).

Paracentesis

A paracentesis should be always made in order to decrease intraocular pressure, to make incannulation of Schlemm's canal easier and to reduce bulging of Descemet's membrane during its cleavage from the corneal stroma, which is at high-risk of tear formation. To avoid external pressure on the eye, the traction on the bridle suture should also be removed.

Cannulation of Schlemm's Canal (Figures 27.2 and 27.3)

Using the specific 165 mm cannula, high molecular weight sodium hyaluronate is slowly injected into Schlemm's canal by cannulating the two ostia at the lateral edges of the inner flap. To avoid damage to the canal endothelium, the insertion of the cannula should not exceed 1 to 1.5 mm from the ostia. The injection of viscoelastic substance allows progressive atraumatic dilatation of Schlemm's canal up to 1 to 2 clock hours from the ostia. Moreover, its hemostatic properties avoid bleeding and fibrin clot formation, thus limiting healing processes and scarring of Schlemm's canal openings.

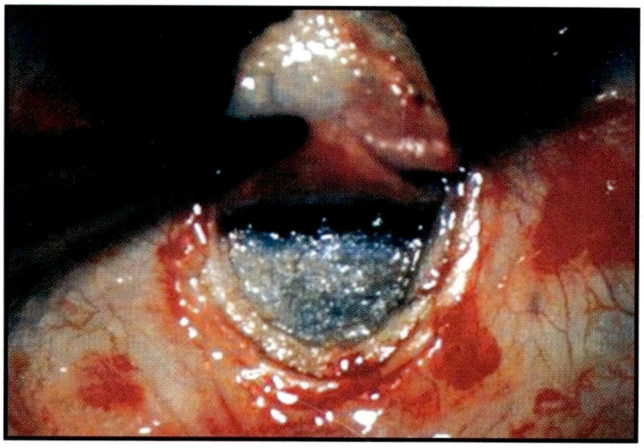

Figure 27.2: Opening of Schlemm's canal

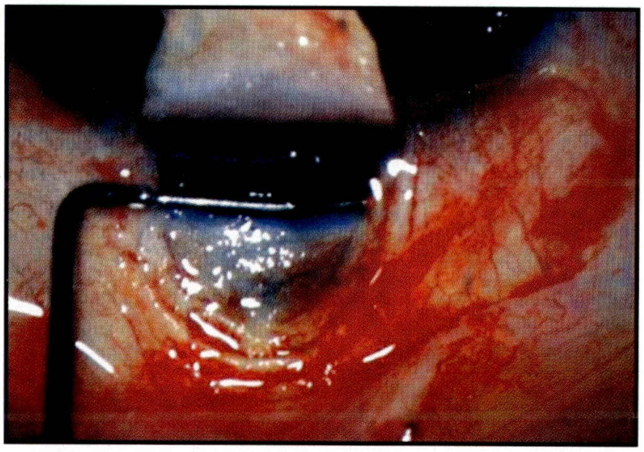

Figure 27.3: Injection of high molecular weight sodium hyaluronate into Schlemm's canal

The slow injection should be repeated 6 to 7 times on each side (Figure 27.4).

Creation of Descemet's Window

The alternative route by which aqueous humor bypasses the trabecular meshwork and reaches Schlemm's canal is a "window" created right anterior to the canal, and represented by the anterior portion of the trabecular meshwork and by the intact Descemet's membrane. The window is realized by gently pulling the inner scleral flap upwards and delicately depressing the floor of the canal and Descemet's membrane with the tip of a cotton swab. By delicately repeating the procedure, the membrane is progressively cleaved from the scleral flap. The flap itself is then advanced in clear cornea for approximately 1 mm by a careful deepening of the lateral cuts with the round bevel-up spatula.

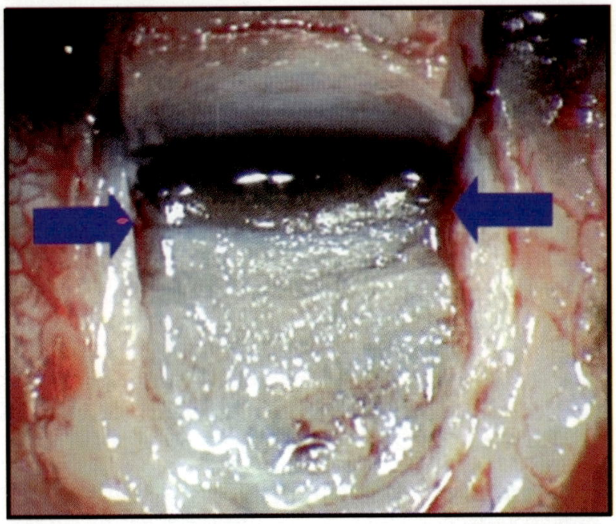

Figure 27.4: Showing sclerodescemetic membrane and the 2 openings of Schlemm's canal

Inner Scleral Flap Excision

The inner scleral flap is then excided using very sharp Vannas' scissors in order to avoid damage to Descemet's membrane.

Outer Scleral Flap Suture

In order to seal the intrascleral "chamber", the outer scleral flap should be tightly sutured by placing 6 or 7 10-0 nylon stitches. The step created by the different size of the two flaps allows a better and tight apposition of the external flap. Finally, in order to minimize bleeding and prevents collapsing and scarring of the intrascleral chamber, high molecular weight sodium hyaluronate is injected underneath the flap.

Closure of the Conjunctiva

The procedure ends by repositioning the conjunctiva with two lateral stitches, and by giving a subconjunctival injection of steroids-antibiotics.

INDICATIONS

Viscocanalostomy has specific indications and contraindications. It cannot be effective when the angle is closed or neovascularized, or when Schlemm's canal is likely to be damaged. This is the case of previously operated eyes where an extensive cautery of the perilimbar area was made. Due to its final results the procedure is indicated in primary open-angle glaucoma when target IOP is not very low (as indicated by the Guidelines for Glaucoma of the European Glaucoma Society). The advantage of the absence (or very reduced) external filtration make the technique safe and particularly indicated in eyes with chronic blepharitis, in lens contact wearer, or when the surgery has to be perform in the lateral or inferior quadrants. Viscocanalostomy was shown effective also in uveitic glaucomas with well-controlled inflammation.[4,5]

RESULTS

Viscocanalostomy seems effective in lowering IOP with a good safety profile. It has low complications, an easy postoperative management and is inducing significant less eye discomfort than trabeculectomy, as could be expected considering the absence of the filtering bleb in the majority of the cases.

When compared with trabeculectomy many of the studies lack to find significant differences between the procedures; nevertheless final IOPs seem higher after viscocanalostomy when compared with trabeculectomy.

A direct comparison between different studies is difficult because criteria for success, length of follow-up and techniques are different.

These can be grouped in retrospective, prospective and randomized-controlled trials.

Retrospective Studies

Stegmann and co-workers[6] reported results of viscocanalostomy in 214 eyes of 157 African patients with open-angle glaucoma and a mean preoperative IOP of 47.4 ± 13.0 mm Hg. After an average follow-up of 35 months, mean IOP was 16.9 ± 8.0 mm Hg; 83 percent of eyes achieved an IOP less than 22 mm Hg off all glaucoma medications.

Two recent studies showed viscocanalostomy a successful procedure in glaucoma secondary to uveitis. Miserocchi et al[4] found a complete and qualified success rate of 54.5 percent and 90.9 percent respectively, after 46 months of follow-up. Final IOP was 18.1+/–11.6 mm Hg.[41] Auer et al [5] after performed NPGDS (including viscocanalostomy) on 14 eyes: complete and qualified success rate were 45.4 percent and 90.4 percent at 12 months. Final IOP was 12.1+/–4.0.(42)

Prospective Studies

Carassa et al[7] reported a series of 23 VCs performed in 23 patients. In four eyes, the procedure was converted to trabeculectomy. Of the 16 eyes with IOP less than 21 mm Hg, mean IOP was 11.6 ± 4.4 mm Hg.

Sunaric-Mégevand et al[8] evaluated the procedure in 67 eyes of 67 consecutive patients with chronic open-angle glaucoma. Complete success was an IOP =<20 mm Hg with 30 percent or greater IOP reduction without ongoing medical or additional surgical treatment. Qualified success was an IOP =< 20 mm Hg with further treatment or an IOP reduction less than 30 percent from preoperative level. The overall success rate was 88 percent at 1 year, 90 percent at 2 years and 88 percent at 3 years. The complete success rate was 68 percent at 1 year, 60 percent at 2 years and 59 percent at 3 years. No serious complications were reported in this series.

Luke et al [9] when comparing viscocanalostomy with and without a SKGel implant showed a success rate (IOP<22 mm Hg without medications) of 40 percent in both groups at 12 months, with a very low complication rate.

Shaarawy et al[10] in a 5-year follow-up study, showed a final IOP of 13.9 mm Hg and a complete success rate with IOP <21 mm Hg in 60 percent of the eyes. Goniopuncture was performed in 37 percent of the cases.

Randomized-Controlled Studies

Jonescu-Cuipers et al[11] in 2001, showed at 6 months, a complete success rate (IOP <20 mmHg) of 0 percent after viscocanalostomy and 50 percent after trabeculectomy on 20 eyes. The same group in 2002,[12] showed an IOP <22 mm Hg without medications in 30 percent with VC and 56.7 after trabeculectomy group at 1 year on 60 patients. Viscocanalostomy showed significant less complications compared with trabeculectomy.

O'Brart et al[13] showed a 1 year success rate (IOP <21 mm Hg on no medications) of 60 percent after viscocanalostomy and of 91 percent after trabeculectomy.

In a 24 month controlled-randomized trial comparing viscocanalostomy with trabeculectomy, Carassa et al,[14] reported similar final IOP levels of 14.1 ± 4.7 mm Hg after viscocanalostomy and 16.3 ± 5.1 mm Hg after trabeculectomy. No significant difference was found between the 2 procedure as for IOP < 21 mm Hg (76% versus 80%) or < 16 (56% versus 72%) on no medications.

A recent study by Yalvac et al[15] on 50 eyes followed for 36 months found similar results. At 3 years, the mean IOP was 17.8 +/– 4.6 mm Hg in the viscocanalostomy group and 16.0 mm Hg +/– 7.07 in the trabeculectomy group (P=0.694). Complete success (IOP 6 to 21 mm Hg without medication) was achieved in 35.3 percent after viscocanalostomy and 55.1 percent after trabeculectomy (P>0.05). Postoperative hypotony and cataract formation occurred more frequently in the trabeculectomy than in the viscocanalostomy group (P=0.002).

O'Brart et al[16] in a 20 month RCT comparing viscocanalostomy with trabeculectomy with adjunctive use of antimetabolites on 50 eyes, found a significantly lower complete success rate (IOP<21 mm Hg) after viscocanalostomy (34%) than after trabeculectomy (68%). Early transient complications such as anterior chamber shallowing and encysted blebs were more common in the trabeculectomy group (p<0.05). Late postoperative cataract formation was similar between the two groups.

CONCLUSIONS

Viscocanalostomy seems a promising surgery for lowering IOP in glaucomatous eyes. It has several potential advantages over trabeculectomy, the major being the absence of external filtration and thus the independence of conjunctival and episcleral scarring. When considering final IOPs between 16 and 21 mm Hg, the rate of failure over time is similar between the 2 procedures. The procedure is affected by few and minor complications, it requires an easy postoperative management and induces significant less eye discomfort than trabeculectomy. Viscocanalostomy is nevertheless technically demanding and requires a long-learning curve.

Results from basic researches aimed at defining the exact mechanism of action will certainly provide improvements in the surgical technique and more appropriate indications.

REFERENCES

1. Krasnov MM. Sinusotomy: foundations, results, prospects. Trans Am Ophthalmol Otolarygol 1972;76:369-74.
2. Zimmerman TJ, Kooner KS, Ford VJ, Olander KW, Mandlekorn RM, Rawlings EF, et al. Trabeculectomy vs non-penetrating trabeculectomy: a retrospective study of two procedures in phakic patients with glaucoma. Ophthalmic Surg 1984;15:734-40.
3. Tamm ER, Carassa RG, Albert DM, Gabelt BT, Patel S, Rasmussen CA, et al. Viscocanalostomy in rhesus monkeys. Arch Ophthalmol 2004;122:1826-38.
4. Miserocchi E, Carassa RG, Bettin P, Brancato R. Visco-canalostomy in patients with uveitis: a preliminary report. J Cataract and Refr Surg 2004;30:566-70.
5. Auer C, Mermoud A, Herbort CP. Deep sclerectomy for the management of uncontrolled uveitic glaucoma: preliminary data. Klin Monatsbl Augenheilkd 2004;221:339-42.
6. Stegmann R, Pienaar A, Miller D. Viscocanalostomy for open-angle glaucoma in black african patients. J Cataract Refract Surg 1999;25:316-22.
7. Carassa R, Bettin P, Fiori M, Brancato R. Viscocanalostomy: a pilot study. Eur J Ophthalmol 1998;8:57-61.
8. Sunaric-Mégevand G, Leuenberger P. Results of viscocanalostomy for primary open angle glaucoma. Am J Ophthalmol 2001;132:221-8.
9. Luke C, Dietlein TS, Jacobi PC, Konen W, Krieglstein GK A prospective randomised trial of viscocanalostomy with and without implantation of a reticulated hyaluronic acid implant (SKGEL) in open-angle glaucoma. Br J Ophthalmol 2003; 87:599-603.
10. Shaarawy T, Nguyen C, Schnyder C, Mermoud A. Five year results of viscocanalostomy. Br J Ophthalmol 2003;87:441-5.
11. Jonescu-Cuypers C, Jacobi P, Konen W, Krieglstein G. Primary viscocanalostomy versus trabeculectomy in white patients with open-angle glaucoma: A randomized clinical trial. Ophthalmology 2001;108:254-8.
12. Luke C, Dietlein TS, Jacobi PC, Konen W, Krieglstein GK. A prospective randomized trial of viscocanalostomy versus trabeculectomy in open-angle glaucoma: A 1-year follow-up study. J Glaucoma 2002;11:294-9.
13. O'Brart DSP, Rowlands E, Islam N, Noury AMS. A randomised, prospective study comparing trabeculectomy augmented with antimetabolites with a viscocanalostomy technique for the management of open-angle glaucoma uncontrolled by medical therapy. Br J Ophthalmol 2002; 86:748-54.
14. Carassa RG, Bettin P, Fiori M, Brancato R Viscocanalostomy versus Trabeculectomy in white adults affected by open-angle glaucoma: a 2-year randomized, controlled trial. Ophthalmology 2003;110:882-7.
15. Yalvac IS, Sahin M, Eksioglu U, Midillioglu IK, Aslan BS, Duman S. Primary viscocanalostomy versus trabeculectomy for primary open-angle glaucoma: three-year prospective randomized clinical trial. J Cataract Refract Surg. 2004;30: 2050-57.
16. O'Brart DP, Shiew M, Edmunds B. A randomised, prospective study comparing trabeculectomy with viscocanalostomy with adjunctive antimetabolite usage for the management of open-angle glaucoma uncontrolled by medical therapy. Br J Ophthalmol. 2004;88:1012-7.

28

Laser Treatment in Glaucomas

- LASER PRINCIPLE AND INTRODUCTION
- LASER IRIDOTOMY
- LASER TRABECULOPLASTY
- LASER PERIPHERAL IRIDOPLASTY
- CYCLOCOAGULATION WITH YAG AND DIODE LASER
- LASER TREATMENTS AFTER FILTERING SURGERY
- SCLEROSTOMIES

Andre Mermoud, Sylvian Roy (Switzerland)

LASER PRINCIPLE AND INTRODUCTION

The word laser was first used in the 60s when light was generated by stimulated emission of radiation. The word LASER is an abbreviation for Light Amplification by Stimulated Emission of Radiation.[9] The physical and wavelength characteristics of the laser light were so specific that they gained rapid interest in the field of medical treatment. Laser light is monochromatic and spatially and temporally coherent. This results in a laser beam that is highly directional with little divergence, thus enabling focusing of the beam into a very small spot of high power per unit area. Monochromaticity means that the laser beam is composed of almost a single wavelength, which has great consequences in the surgical eye treatment. This allows light to be effectively absorbed by the pigments contained in the ocular tissues, e.g. the melanin, hemoglobin or the xanthophyll pigments.[4]

The molecules in biologic tissues are not transparent to wavelength shorter than 300 nm or greater than 100 nm. Between this range, the molecules absorb selectively the light depending on the spectral absorption characteristic of the pigments in the tissues. Laser effects in tissues can be summarized into three groups: photochemical, thermal and ionization effects. The photochemical effect results in photon absorbtion by molecules inducing chemical reactions. A thermal effect is present when photon absorbtion by electrons increases the molecular vibrations to a temperature peak that results in denaturation of proteins in biologic tissues. When the temperature reaches 60°C, the weak van der Waals forces that maintain the molecular bonds are broken and denaturation of the several intracellular proteins occurs.[1] If laser energy is strong enough to tear electrons from the outer orbit, the atoms or molecules become ionized and relax this metastable state by producing mechanical (pressure) waves (photodisruption effect).[7]

The efficiency of laser beam onto biological tissues depend on the absorption spectra of cellular pigments.[5] Melanin best absorbs wavelengths between 400 and 100 nm. Hemoglobin, naturally presents a red appearance that strongly reduces its absorption characteristics in the long wavelengths above 650 nm. Xanthophyll absorbs very well in the short-wavelengths below 500 nm.

The laser delivery systems used in laser glaucoma treatments are divided into two groups: non-contact and contact laser source.[8] The non-contact delivery system produces a beam that is focused onto the area to be treated via a slit-lamp biomicroscope. It may be useful to place a contact lens to stabilize the eye and the lids, to reduce the optical aberrations of the anterior surface of the cornea and to gain access to structures that are otherwise invisible without a contact lens.

The contact delivery system consists of laser source and optical guidance device such as fiberoptic and delivery tip that directly apply onto the tissue to be treated.[10,11] The energy distribution of the laser beam can be set on two different modes.[7] The fundamental mode gives a sharp focus spot with maximum energy at the focus point and minimum energy anterior or posterior to that point. The mode locking produces a series of brief spikes of photon, with a peak of energy that is much higher than the average energy of equivalent photon bursts that are delivered in a continuous flow. It is also possible to modulate the production of the laser light before delivery by placing an electronic shutter that keeps the excited molecules to a high energy level before relaxation. When the shutter opens, an extremely brief pulse (20 ns) of high energy is produced (Q-switch mode).[7]

Several wavelengths are used in ophthalmic laser photocoagulators. Krypton lasers produce red light (647 and 676 nm). Argon lasers produce green light (514.5 nm) and green and blue light (514.5 and 488 nm). Both are used in photocoagulation,[14] whereas Nd:YAG lasers deliver infrared light (1064 nm) which is used with Q-switch mode in photodisruption. Diode lasers deliver red (640 nm) and infrared light (800-820 nm) that can be guided through a fiberoptic device for contact photocoagulation. A new type of laser has recently been developed to enhance the photodissociative effect of the YAG laser in intraocular surgery. It is made by combination of a classic YAG laser on which an erbium component has been added to produce fragmentation effects. The wavelength of 2940 nm is longer than Nd:YAG, thus water absorbs most of the energy with an important water absorption photothermal effect.[6] The transfer of heat to the adjacent tissue is therefore reduced. The beam is directed through a fiberglass tip with a ceramic end. The first attempts have been made in cataract surgery to replace the ultrasonic emulsification currently used.[13] But technical problems regarding the safety of this method in respect to the posterior capsule have not yet been completely solved. New attempts have been made in glaucoma therapy to increase the aqueous outflow by disrupting the trabecular meshwork and inner wall of Schlemm's canal by an ab-interno approach. A quartz fiber contact endoprobe (320 micron core-diameter, 385 micron coating-diameter) applying single neighboring laser pulses (5-7 mJ) to the trabecular meshwork. The procedure was gonioscopically visualized. Although IOP lowering effect of erbium:YAG laser trabecular ablation did not prove as effective as in filtering procedures. LTA might be a valuable alternative in glaucoma surgery especially in order to avoid conjunctival scarring and postoperative hypotony.[3-5] It is not known whether this new technique can be widely used in the field of glaucoma laser surgery to add new prospectives or replace existing and efficient laser technique and procedure that will be explained in more details in the subsequent chapters.

The physical properties of the laser beam are such that safety aspects should always be considered when using or being in close proximity to laser devices. Every laser delivery system protects the operator from direct damages when using the laser by shutting off the beam with a filter. But this is not the case for personnel being nearby and staring at the laser system, for the filter will not prevent hazardous direct or reflected beam from reaching the retina of the observers.[12]

LASER IRIDOTOMY

Laser iridotomy is a laser surgical procedure by which a small aperture through the iris is created to treat several forms of angle-closure glaucomas and more recently pigmentary glaucoma.[25,31] It was introduced in the 80's with the development of laser surgeries.[21] The indication for laser iridotomy is given in the case of acute angle-closure glaucoma when the acute attack has been medically controlled, and the cornea is clear enough to allow sufficient penetration of the laser beam into the anterior chamber without excessive scattering.[5,26] In the case of chronic angle-closure glaucoma, or eyes with peripheral anterior synechia, laser iridotomy may reduce the intraocular pressure (IOP) and allow the angle structures to resume a wider space, by deepening the anterior chamber.[24] Pupillary block may be relief thus allowing a better control of the IOP. In aphakic or pseudophakic eyes, pupillary block from pockets of aqueous behind the iris plane could be relieved by adequate laser iridotomy.[1,6,30] In eyes with intumescent cataracts, or in the fellow eye of an acute angle-closure glaucoma eye, prophylactic laser iridotomy can be performed in order to avoid an attack of angle-closure glaucoma.[30] In eyes with narrow angle, good visualization of the angle structures may be rendered difficult by the geometric disposition of the iris over the angle. This situation could prevent the performance of laser trabeculoplasty in such eyes. To avoid this complication, laser iridotomy can be performed to open a too narrow angle. In the plateau iris syndrome, anteriorly located ciliary processes support the peripheral iris. Variation in the angle values between dark and light are solely related to changes in iris thickness. Pilocarpine produces iris thinning and is an effective method of opening the angle.[18] General disturbance of the geometry of the eye, like in the case of nanophthalmos, have greater risks for developing angle-closure glaucoma. A prophylactic laser iridotomy could reduce the incidence of such complications.

In pigment dispersion syndrome, the iris often presents a marked concavity, forming an inverted pupillary block. Accommodation increases iris concavity in some patients with pigment dispersion syndrome. The most likely explanation is an accommodation-induced relative increase in anterior chamber pressure, secondary to anterior movement of the lens surface. Iridotomy prevents change in the iris profile with accommodation.[19] In this case too, performance of laser iridotomy would reduce the pressure differential between the anterior and posterior plane of the iris, by creating a channel through the iris.[2,4,7,12,22] In the field of refractive surgery, the placement of an intraocular contact lenses (ICL) in the posterior chamber in front of the anterior capsule of the lens reduces the angle and increases the risk for angle-closure glaucoma. Laser iridotomy performed before refractive surgery prevents the likelihood of such complications.[22,35,36] Conversely, in the presence of strong hypermetropic eyes, the current IOL may not have sufficient refractive power for the intended emmetropization. Two intraocular lenses (piggyback) have been placed simultaneously in the capsular bag, thus also reducing the depth of the chamber. In that case too, a laser iridotomy will prevent an attack of angle-closure glaucoma.[14] Laser iridotomy is contraindicated in any situation where the angle-closure is not mechanicaly reversible by deepening the anterior chamber, for instance, a flat anterior chamber, synechial closure of the angle by uveitis, neovascular glaucoma or by iridocorneal endothelial syndrome (ICE). In this situation they are absolute contraindications for laser iridotomy. Any corneal edema or opacities will strongly reduce the quality of the transmission of the laser, and are relative contraindications for the performance of the treatment.

A gonioscopic contact lens, like the Goldmann is placed on the cornea of the patient after topical anesthesia. It sometimes happens that the iris is not contracted enough to present a smooth surface and thin stroma. Only a few shallow crypts are visible. The use of pilocarpine will contract the sphincter iridae and enlarge the angle of view before treatment. In some cases, the IOP rises a few hours after laser iridotomy.[3,27] To prevent the peak of pressure, an alpha agonist such as apraclonidine can be given pre-and perioperatively.[28] The location of the iridotomy should be either the 11 or 1 o'clock positions, so that the upper lid will cover the aperture made by the laser and prevent monocular diplopia (Figure 28.1).[11,16] A crypt should be selected if possible to facilitate the creation of the crater. As laser light is absorbed by ocular pigments, very light iridies are more difficult to perforate than darker. Conversely, very dark pigmented iris have generally thicker stroma and are also difficult to penetrate.[13] Laser energy used will then depend on color and density of irides pigments. Current power level for argon type laser ranges from 500 upto 1500 mW for a duration of 0.1 sec. Spot size is set at 50 μm. Nd:YAG laser energy level is set between 2.0 and 8.0 mJ with single burst mode. Small bubbles form around the spot site and, in case of dark brown pigmented iris, some pigments will be released into the anterior chamber. This can severely reduce visibility of the treated area and preclude the completion of the treatment. In such case, a break between laser applications should be made. When passing through the posterior plane of the iris, clouds of pigments burst in the iridotomy crater may appear. As soon as the iris stroma has been totally penetrated, a flow of aqueous humor "leaks" through the aperture and the iris stroma moves slightly backwards. Retroillumination through the pupil will reveal a red reflex via the iridotomy. Care should be exercised not to be overconfident in the patency of the iridotomy, as red reflex is not enough to ensure complete burn of iris stroma. Some very thin transparent membranes could still be present, preventing aqueous from freely flowing through the iridotomy. Gonioscopy should always be performed in doubtful cases. Ultrasound biomicroscopy will show an increase in the iridocorneal angle after completion of a successful iridotomy (Figure 28.2).

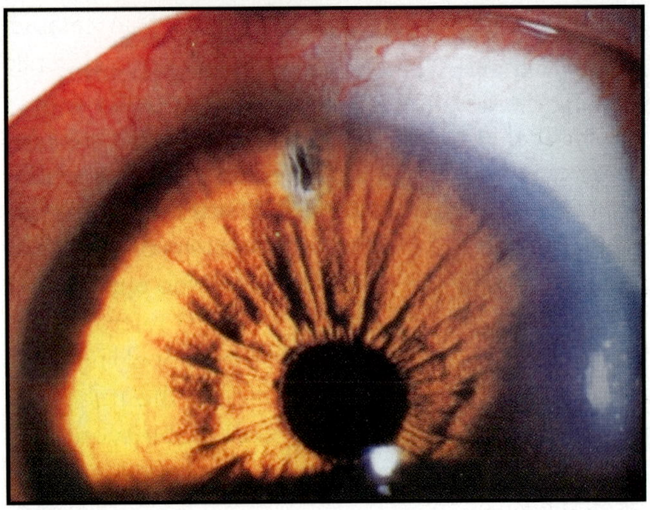

Figure 28.1: Iris aspect after Nd:YAG laser iridotomy located at 12 o'clock position. Note the depigmentation of the anterior surface of the stroma around the aperture

Corneal edema and epithelial erosion can occur when performing laser iridotomies. Such complications generally resolve in a few days. Endothelial cell can be affected by Nd:YAG laser, caused by the shock waves produced during the treatment. Endothelial cells count have shown that proper application of laser burn with Nd:YAG laser does not significantly increase the endothelial cells lost.[15,17,23] Nevertheless, caution should be exercised not to focus the laser beam onto the Descemet's membrane. The iris stroma is strongly vascularized by arteries from the major iris circle, and injury to arterioles cause instant

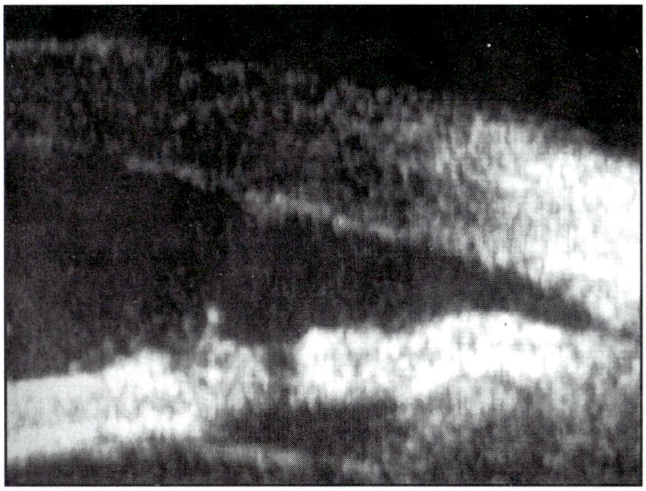

Figure 28.2: Ultrasound biomicroscopy of the anterior chamber angle after patent iridotomy through the iris stroma, the angle is wider

bleeding in the anterior chamber. When this complication occurs, a gentle pressure with the contact glass will temporarily increase the IOP and promote hemostasis. Dramatic hyphema have been reported after such laser procedures.[29] Argon laser, or Nd:YAG laser set on multimode iridotomy, generally prevent such complications, as the thermal effect of the laser burns coagulates the vessels and avoids bleeding when hitting a vascular branch.[13] The stroma and iris pigment epithelium dispersion phenomena observed during completion of laser iridotomies increase the amount of particles in the anterior chamber. Inflammation and anterior uveitis are generally present after the procedure. To prevent extension and persistence of this inflammation, topical steroids are given and tapered in a few days. Posterior synechiae may develop as a result of prolonged inflammation.[10] As mentioned before, the IOP rises in the next few hours after laser therapy. Close monitoring of the IOP is mandatory and adequate medication given in case of persistent elevated values. Some case of damages to the lens have been reported as the result of excessive laser application to the capsule behind the iris plane.[32,33] Care should therefore be exercised when applying laser energy on an patent iridotomy.

LASER TRABECULOPLASTY

When laser burns are applied on the trabecular meshwork, persistent IOP reduction is followed.[30,31] The pathophysiology of the laser burns on the trabecular meshwork was hypothesized as follows: thermal effect of the burns induces collagen shrinkage and scarring of the meshwork. This leads to mechanical traction on the adjacent intertrabecular space that becomes open, thus increasing the outflow facility.[5,27] Argon blue-green laser (488 nm) was the laser of choice for this procedure. This has been named argon laser trabeculoplasty (ALT). It can be used in several forms of open-angle glaucoma. A Nd:YAG laser trabeculoplasty (YLT) has also been used as an alternative to the ALT. In case of hypopigmented trabeculum meshwork, YLT is a safe and effective alternative technique to perform laser trabeculoplasty, which is especially useful in poorly-pigmented angles where ALT is known to be less effective.[14]

Slit-lamp, is used for the ALT procedure. To gain access to the entire angle structure, a contact lens with a gonioscopic mirror (CGI from LASAG, Bern, Switzerland) is placed on the cornea of the patient after topical anesthesia. In some cases, when the angle is too narrow to allow a good visibility of the trabecular meshwork, use of pilocarpine may enlarge the angle to enable the treatment. Laser spot parameters are set commonly with 50 mm spot size, 0.1 sec. of duration and 800 mW of power. The correct effect of the laser burns should be a blanching of the trabecular meshwork. When too much power is applied, a bubble will form and intense blanching and scarring will result. The power should then be reduced just enough to get blanching with minimal bubble creation. The amount of power required to get this result may vary with the degree of pigmentation of the trabecular meshwork.[20] It is important to readjust the power setting throughout the laser session to get homogenous treatment all over the treated quadrants. The laser beam spot must be kept on focus over the entire portion of the treated zone. The spots should be placed evenly over the anterior half portion of the trabecular meshwork (Figure 28.3). Attention should be paid not to burn adjacent structures of the meshwork such as the ciliary body, the iris processes or the cornea. Correct placement of the spot minimize the possibility of early postoperative IOP rise[25] and peripheral anterior synechiae formations.[23] Should hemorrhage occur during the laser treatment, it could

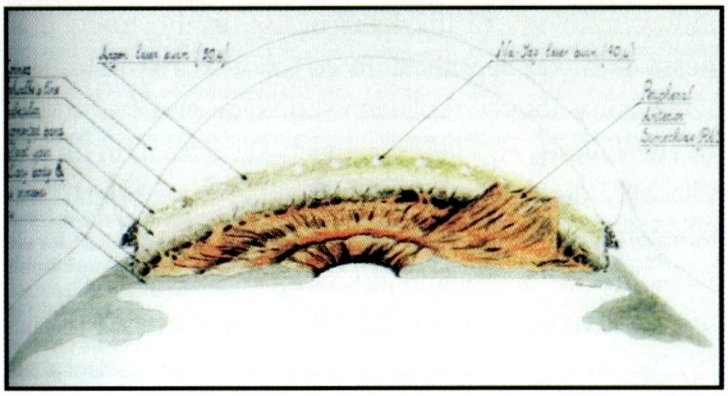

Figure 28.3: Artist's view of gonioscopic aspect of laser burns after argon and Nd:YAG laser trabeculoplasty, and complication of peripheral anterior synechiae (Courtesy: Dr A Mermoud)

be kept under control by gently applying a slight pressure to the globe through the contact lens. This relatively rare event might be the result of an inadvertent burn of a peripheral iris vessel from the ciliary circle. Caution should also be exercised not to damage the structure of the cornea. The corneal epithelium may be inadvertently removed when placing or moving the contact lens. The resulting corneal abrasion will heal within hours often without treatment. Corneal endothelium lesions are of greater importance and may lead to permanent corneal lesions. Corneal edema results from insult to the corneal endothelium and may persist for several months, severely impairing the visual outcome of the patient. Pre-existent endothelial pathology such as Fuch's endothelial dystrophy or cornea guttata have greater risks to induce complications of the corneal endothelium.[28]

Care should be given not to treat too many areas of the trabecular meshwork. An experimental glaucoma model in rhesus monkey has been created by giving a large number of long duration laser burns.[8] Postoperative IOP rise peak may also depend on the number of burns.[25] Generally, 50 to 70 burns over 180 degree are enough to create a sustained consistent IOP drop overtime.[13,26] It should be kept in mind that the long-term overall outcome of ALT is about 50 percent after 5 years.[18,19] Most of the patients will probably require other types of treatment, for instance a filtration surgery. In order not to compromise the result of further filtrating surgery, it is advisable not to treat the upper quadrant, and to leave the trabecular meshwork untouched.

It is not uncommon to encounter some pressure spike after argon ALT. To prevent or avoid the extension of such pressure rise, α-2 agonist may be given before and/or just immediately after the laser treatment.[17] Apraclonidine or brimonidine are the therapy of choice.[1,2,4] Even with an adequate postoperative therapy, the IOP sometimes remains elevated several weeks after the ALT. It should be emphasized that the ALT produces or enhance inflammation in the anterior chamber and over the trabecular meshwork.[15] Inflammatory cells and inflammation products collect into the trabecular meshwork and dramatically reduce the outflow facility, resulting in persistent IOP elevation. This inflammatory reaction is thought to be the result of transient breakdown of the blood-aqueous barrier and is correlated with the type of glaucoma. Pigmentary and pseudoexfoliative glaucoma show the greatest inflammatory reaction after ALT compared with chronic open-angle glaucoma.

Beside the inflammatory reaction, the ALT can also induce other reactions or changes in the anterior chamber. Laser burns placed too posteriorly result in creation of peripheral anterior synechiae.[19] This complication does not happen when burns are placed in the anterior trabecular meshwork. It is still unclear whether peripheral anterior synechiae play a role in the long-term outcome of ALT or not.[12]

The long-term results of the ALT is relatively modest. A mean success rate of 45 percent 5 years after ALT has been reported in several studies.[3,6,18,19] Despite this rate, the ALT might be indicated in patients where classical filtrating surgeries cannot be performed for general health state reasons, for ophthalmological reasons, or because of nonmotivated patients.[7,9,11,29] Primary ALT gives a long-lasting and favorable effect in chronic open-angle glaucoma where 2/3 of the eyes were still managed without additional medication for 8 years. The success in pseudoexfoliation glaucoma was even higher the first 3 years, and stayed above 50 percent for 10 years.[3,16,22] In young patients below 50 years, the overall results without additional medication is even higher.[10] Some variations in the efficiency of the ALT may be seen between individuals having different intensity in the pigmentation of the trabecular meshwork. The caucasian patients have generally less-pigmented meshwork in comparison to the black African patients, and the former may respond poorly to the ALT.[21,24]

LASER PERIPHERAL IRIDOPLASTY

Not every angle-closure glaucoma may be relieved by laser iridotomy. Structural modifications of the anterior chamber angle, like appositional angle-closure in the plateau-iris syndrome, peripheral anterior synechiae or attacks of severe acute angle-closure glaucoma with corneal edema, anterior chamber flattening and inflammation, will prevent laser iridotomy to be effective.[4,5] In case of narrow anterior chamber angle induced by lens intumescence or anterior chamber crowding as the result of short anteroposterior axis eyes (hypermetropia or nanophthalmos), the trabecular meshwork might be also difficult to see through the gonioscopic mirror. In such situations, alternative laser procedures on the iris could be performed to open the angle.[5,7,10]

Localized heat application onto biological tissues induces protein coagulation and shrinkage around the burn spot. This produces contractions of the tissue fibers and can be used as mechanical retractors. The argon laser peripheral iridoplasty consists of using the thermal effect of argon laser burns of large spot size, long duration and low power applied at the iris periphery to promote contractions of the iris stroma that will retract the iris root and open the angle.[8,6,10,11]

The treatment is performed with a contact lens under topical anesthesia. In order to have maximum efficiency, the iris surface should be as smooth as possible. To stretch the iris stroma, pilocarpine 4 percent is given one hour before initiating the procedure. Alpha-agonist is also recommended to avoid postoperative rise of the IOP. The laser is set at 500 mm, 0.5 sec and 400 mW of power, depending on the irides coloration. Excess power results in bubble formation and pigment dispersion. In that case, power should be reduced. Enough power should be applied to produce a noticeable stromal contraction. Lighter irides require more power than darker, as pigments are less dense in the former and absorb less power at a time. Location of the burns must be at the most peripheral part of the iris to produce better results. Should the burns be placed less peripherally, the contraction would not be acting directly against the iris root and the resulting effect would be much less effective. For instance, placement of burns in the mid-periphery would lead to failure of this procedure. The effect of laser burns on tissues is almost immediate and iris stroma shrinkage is followed by local opening of the anterior angle and local deepening of the anterior chamber. The spots are placed around the circumference of the iris over 360 degrees with two to three spot diameters inbetween.

Postoperative treatment consists of an alpha-agonist like apraclonidine given once just after the laser session and topical steroids 3 times a day for a week. Caution should be given to the IOP rise in the early hours and adequate medication be administered accordingly. Complications are relatively seldom and consist in mild iritis lasting no longer than a few days. Corneal burns and endothelial decompensation might occur as the laser beam strikes the iris plane with a narrow angle in the case of plateau iris and shallow anterior chamber. Contrary to laser iridotomy, the iris is not cut through the entire stromal portion and the lens or retina will not suffer from damages linked to laser application.[2,3,9] A case of malignant glaucoma has been reported.[1]

CYCLOCOAGULATION WITH YAG AND DIODE LASER

The intraocular pressure can be lowered not only by enhancing the outflow through the trabeculum meshwork, but also by reducing the production of aqueous humor from the ciliary body.[1,18,21] During the era when laser techniques were not currently used, cyclodestruction was made by applying either an intense and focal heat onto the ciliary body, a procedure called cyclodiathermy, or by freezing the ciliary processes with the help of a cryoprobe applied close to the limbus.[3,19]

The laser technique used to destroy the ciliary body belongs to the group of cyclophotocoagulation, a way of reducing the activity of the ciliary body by the means of light as a vector of energy. Nd:YAG laser and diode laser are both used to achieve this goal. The laser delivery system can be of contact or non-contact type, if the laser beam has to be directed through a fiberoptic end probe or applied through the air to the globe via the optic devices of a slit lamp. The latter has the advantage that the end part of the delivery system does not carry the risk of transmitting infectious diseases and does not need to be sterilized, while the former can be more compact and easier to use on a patient in a bed. The energy delivery mode can be set on a pulse mode, whereas during short time intervals a predetermined burst of energy is emitted, or the beam is continuously emitted from the laser source during a preset time.

The Nd:YAG laser produces a laser beam of 1064 nm, that is well below the lowest visible wavelengths. The pulse-wave mode creates a mechanical photodisruption that is concentrated in the pigment epithelium of the ciliary body. The continuous wave mode gives a very high level of energy that is mostly absorbed thermally over the ciliary body and partially absorbed in the sclera.[16] The effects of Nd:YAG laser application onto the ciliary body result in destruction of tissue, inflammation fibrosis and coagulation necrosis. At the end stage, the production of aqueous humor is markedly reduced, thus lowering the IOP.[12,20]

The patient is given a retrobulbar injection of anesthetic to reduce the pain induced by the laser treatment and to avoid unexpected eye movements during the procedure. With a non-contact delivery system, the patient is seated in front of a slit-lamp. The laser beam is set with the maximum offset value to separate the aiming beam from the Nd:YAG beam. The energy is set between 5 and 10 J/pulse, the duration of the continuous mode is 20 ms. The beam is pointed between 1 and 2 mm from the limbus and burns are made around evenly spaced. The number of burns varies between 20 and 40. When using a contact delivery system, the probe is placed at less than 1 mm from the limbus and the energy level limited to 5 J.

The diode laser produces a laser beam of 810 nm which is slightly lower than the lowest visible wavelength.[15,22] There is only one mode, the continuous-wave mode. Two delivery systems can equally be used, the contact and non-contact, in the same way the Nd:YAG laser is being used (Figure 28.4). The effects on the ciliary body are mostly due to the thermal action of the laser beam absorbed by the melanin pigments of the ciliary epithelium. Coagulation necrosis and tissue shrinkage are the main changes observed after diode laser cyclophotocoagulation.[8] The patient is prepared according to the same protocol used for the Nd:YAG treatment. The power level for non-contact diode treatment is set between 1000 and 2000 mW, the duration is 2 sec, and the spot size varies between 150 and 500 μm.[9] In the contact mode, the duration is slightly longer, giving a power level of 2000 mW.[17] The laser beam or the diode probe are placed 1 mm behind the limbus and 20 to 40 burns are made over the entire 360 degrees of the limbus (Figure 28.5).[7,10,13]

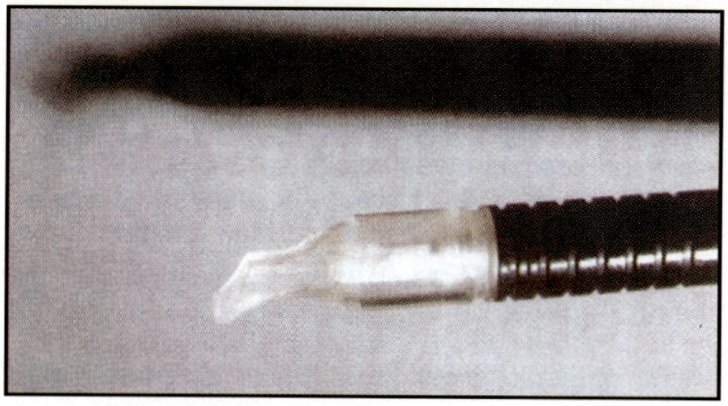

Figure 28.4: Diode cyclophotocoagulation probe for contact cyclocoagulation

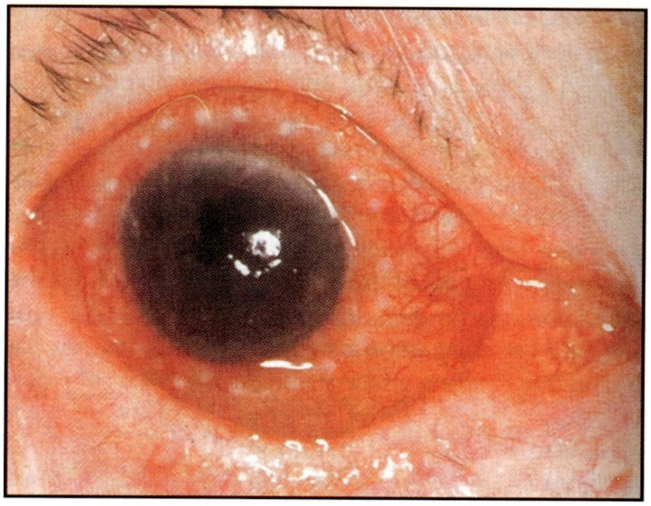

Figure 28.5: Inflammation is noticeable after Nd:YAG cyclophotocoagulation, with mixed perilimbal conjunctival injection. The laser burns are clearly visible around the limbus as white scars evenly spaced

A new technique for controlling refractory glaucoma has been developed that acts directly from inside the eye instead of acting through the sclera. One reason for failure of trans-scleral cyclophotocoagulation, particularly in congenital glaucoma, may be the displacement of the ciliary processes. This displacement does not permit the indirect treatment to reach the appropriate area. Because endoscopic laser cyclophotocoagulation allows direct visualization of the processes, treatment can be accurately applied to the very individual ciliary processes.[6,14] Endoscopic cyclophotocoagulation treatment encompassed 180 to 360 degrees of the ciliary body circumference and is performed through a limbal incision. An 810 nm pulsed continuous-wave diode laser capable of 1.2 W output is being used. Generally, 800 mW are being used for less than 1 second, for a total of 0.8 J per treatment. Early results suggest that endoscopic cyclophotocoagulation is a safe and effective therapeutic modality for refractory glaucomas.[11]

The postoperative care of patients undergoing cyclophotocoagulation consists of patching the eye for one day with topical steroids to control the postoperative inflammatory stage (Figure 28.5). The steroids are gently tapered and antiglaucoma medication adjusted according to the postoperative examinations. The conjunctiva is frequently burned and uveitis is present after every laser treatment but subsides with steroids application. The pain might be moderate to severe, generally lasting no longer than a few days. The most severe complication implies prolonged hypotony and phthisis bulbi, a feared event that had already occurred in several cases after cyclocryocoagulation.[5] These complications tend to be less frequent when using the diode laser cyclophotocoagulation.[2]

The pressure lowering effect of laser cyclophotocoagulation is variable but values of 15 to 30 mm Hg might be achieved, and results overtime remain quite stable. Nd:YAG and diode laser cycloablations are relatively safe and effective at controlling IOP in eyes with advanced refractory glaucoma in the short and medium term.[4] Glaucoma medications are generally also reduced after one or more laser sessions. Repeated treatments are nevertheless required in some patients when the intended lowering effect is not reached at the first session.

LASER TREATMENTS AFTER FILTERING SURGERY

After classical filtering surgery that has been performed without complications, it may happen that filtration progressively decreases. The IOP rises again to values measured before surgery. **The main cause for such failure is an overscarring of the filtration bleb.**

The trabeculectomy technique requires a good closure of the scleral flap to prevent excessive aqueous outflow resulting in hypotony and shallow anterior chamber. But a too tight closure of the scleral flap may result in excessive elevation in IOP in the postoperative period. To prevent prolonged elevation in the IOP, it is possible to selectively cut some sutures to release the tension of the scleral flap.[7,9] Scleral flap sutures are made of nylon or polypropylene sutures that are either black or deep blue. The thermal effect of argon laser is efficient in lysis of such material through the conjunctiva. Technically, the procedure is performed with a contact glass applied to the conjunctiva, using the Hoskins or the Ritch lens.[4,11] This allows a better visualization of the suture by flattening the Tenon and conjunctiva layers. It is better not to perform ocular massage immediately before the laser lysis, as the massage brings some subconjunctival fluid that will scatter laser light and reduce visibility and accessibility to the suture. The laser setting is 50 μm for the spot size, with a duration of 0.1 sec and power of 300 to 500 mW. The laser beam is focused on the suture and shots are applied until the suture is being cut. Intraocular pressure is then measured to ascertain the degree of efficiency reached. Gentle massage of the globe might also be performed to promote the outflow. Caution should be exercised not to excessively treat by cutting too many sutures resulting in hypotony, shallow anterior chamber, choroidal effusion, optic disk and macular edema.[1] The ideal time to perform suture lysis is 1 to 2 weeks after surgery in case of elevated IOP. After this period, the result is less prone to be efficient, probably because of scarring of the scleral flap.[3] Other causes of elevated pressure like iris incarceration into the internal sclerostomy or malignant glaucoma, should be investigated and eliminated accordingly.

Overfiltration on the other hand is a troublesome complication that requires efficient treatment. Overfiltrating bleb can be brought to a less effective size by enhancing the fibrosis. Invasive techniques like autologous blood injection in the bleb have been reported to be efficient. Noninvasive methods using laser techniques can also be developed to prevent persistent hypotony and create some local subconjunctival bleeding. By applying gentle laser spots onto the conjunctiva with a Nd:YAG laser, the conjunctival vessels are disrupted and bleeding occurs.[2] The idea is to create adhesion scars between the conjunctival bleb and the Tenon shield that reduce the size and efficiency of the bleb. It is also possible to physically promote scarring of the subconjunctival space and Tenons and mechanically tighten the two layers. To achieve this goal, several burns are made at the edge of the bleb by using the Hoskins or the Ritch lens to depress the conjunctiva. The spot size is set between 50 and 100 μm, with a duration of 0.1 sec, a power of 200 to 400 mW. The beam is focused on the Tenon or slightly deeper to avoid perforation of the conjunctiva, and the spots are evenly spaced all around the bleb. Power should not be excessive as this will result in conjunctival buttonhole or formation of subconjunctival bubbles that will increase the bleb size instead of helping scar formation.[6]

Laser treatment in the postoperative period can also be used in conjunction with other surgical techniques used to treat refractory glaucoma. In this case, drainage devices are being used to create an effective outflow from the anterior chamber to the subconjunctival and sub-Tenon's space. But this technique requires an adequate control of the outflow that can be achieved by placing a stent suture around the tube. In the postoperative period, the IOP is monitored and the suture may be released should the pressure be elevated.[8] It may also happen that the tube opening in the anterior chamber becomes blocked by fibrin clots and this results in failure of the shunt technique. Nd:YAG laser membranectomy will clean the tube and thus restore a patent drainage to the external plate.[12]

In the new non-perforating techniques, like deep sclerectomy with collagen implants or viscocanalostomy, the trabecular meshwork remains untouched and only the inner wall of Schlemm's canal and the juxtacanalicular meshwork are removed.[5,13] A very thin membrane prevents the anterior chamber to collapse during the filtering surgery. But after a few weeks or months, the trabeculodescemetic membrane may become fibrotic because of elevated IOP and should be open to allow better outflow. This procedure is called goniopuncture, and can easily be done with a Nd:YAG laser. The goal of this technique is to perforate the remaining trabecular meshwork at the surgery site by performing an internal trabeculotomy or descemetomy. A gonioscopic contact glass is set on the eye of the patient after topical anesthesia to gain access to the anterior chamber angle. The trabecular meshwork at the surgery site appears as a thin less-pigmented membrane, some light from the sclerectomy being transmitted through the wall (Figure 28.6). The laser beam is pointed to this membrane and several impacts are shot. The power level is set at 5 mJ. Some air-bubbles may be generated during the treatment. It is sometimes difficult to ascertain the patency of the trabeculotomy, as the perforation diameter is very small, being less than 70 μm and the edge barely distinguishable from the surrounding poorly-pigmented trabecular tissue. In such case, it is best advisable to measure the pressure a few days later and perform a second session if necessary. The postoperative treatment consists of topical corticosteroids three times a day, tapered in a few days. The hypotensive medication if required before goniopuncture, should be continued or stopped after laser treatment according to the IOP lowering effect achieved.[10]

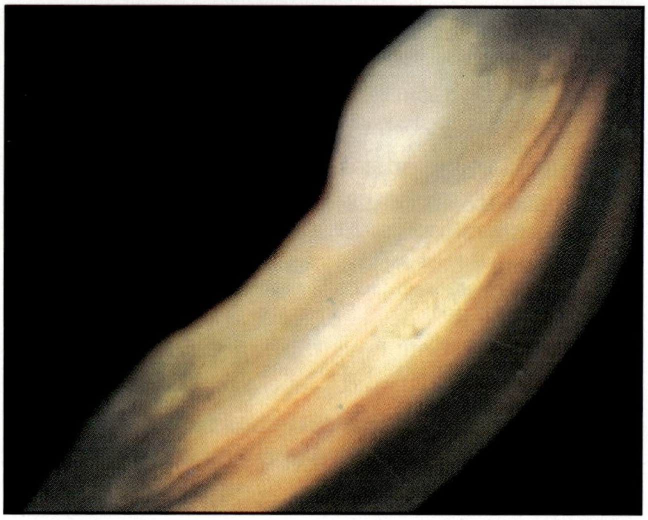

Figure 28.6: Gonioscopic view of the anterior chamber, and inner aspect of the trabeculodescemetic membrane after Nd:YAG goniopuncture. Note the black suture used to secure the collagen implant

SCLEROSTOMIES

The technical approach of glaucoma surgery is based on the creation of a fistula that drains into a filtering bleb. Mechanical techniques that involve the use of cutting blades, blunt dissection, tissue removal and titrated sutures promote inflammatory responses that will modulate the healing and scarring processes. Overacting fistulas or inefficient filtering blebs result from variation of standard procedure and lead to the need of complementary surgery or adjunctive treatment. Laser, by its physical property, is a very useful tool that can provide calibrated beams at various energy levels. By developing adequate delivery systems to the trabecular meshwork, it is possible to perform a direct fistula through the tissue, a so-called sclerostomy.[7] The advantages of such techniques are that the fistula diameter can be better predicted, tissue trauma could be less-extended, especially regarding the development of the filtering bleb.[3]

Three methods have been developed to achieve this goal. All are based on the kind of delivery system being used to apply laser energy to create a channel through the sclera and trabecular meshwork. Basically, there are two approaches possible, from outside the eye, the ab-externo procedure, or from inside, the ab-interno procedure. The latter can further be divided into two categories, invasive or non-invasive procedure.

To perform a non-invasive ab-interno sclerostomy, a modification of the current laser technique has to be made before completion of the treatment. A pulse-dye laser is used to get a beam for the non-contact delivery system connected to the slit-lamp. A gonioscopy lens is applied on the eye to allow good visualization of the angle structures. The laser produces a beam at 660 nm, set at 200 μm spot size, 10 μsec duration and 200 to 400 mJ energy level. In order to get the most effects from the beam at that wavelength, the site of sclerostomy must be dyed with methylene blue dye with an iontophoresis marker.[14] The beam is then directed to the blue patch that is visible in the gonioscopic lens. Shots are given repetitively until the whole sclera has been drilled and the anterior chamber shallows and the conjunctival bleb develops.[8] The invasive ab-interno sclerostomy consists of introducing an endolaser probe in the anterior chamber to deliver laser beam directly to the trabecular meshwork.[11] The main advantage consists of leaving the conjunctiva untouched avoiding scar formation. Disadvantages of this technique are those related to any intraocular approach; the infectious risks, trauma to the endothelium, the iris structures and the lens. Thermal damages due to accumulation of heat at the impact site are also related to this technique. To introduce the endolaser probe, a paracentesis is performed on the cornea and the anterior chamber is filled with a viscoelastic agent. The fiberoptic probe is introduced and the tip is brought into perpendicular contact with the corneoscleral tissue, taking care to avoid the posterior trabecular meshwork. Laser beam is actuated and tissue ablation begins. The probe is moved forward as ablation removes tissue leaving space for further ablation. The end of the procedure is determined when the tip is seen through the conjunctiva, and the aqueous humor and viscoelastic agent flow into the bleb.[1]

The ab-externo sclerostomy consists in creating a channel through the sclera to the anterior chamber.[12,13] A contact probe is placed at the limbus to guide the laser beam. The conjunctiva is cut 15 mm away from the intended treatment site to allow the probe to be placed correctly, thus allowing an adequate contact with the sclera. A holmium:YAG laser is used to produce the energy required to ablate the tissue. The energy level is set at 100 mJ/pulse. The beam is applied to the sclera and can be seen through the cornea into the anterior chamber. Progression of creation of the channel can therefore be monitored until completion. At that stage, aqueous humor flows through the fistula into the subconjunctival space.[10] After removal of the probe, the conjunctival incision is closed with a single suture and topical antiinflammatory medication given.[2,5,6,9]

REFERENCES

Laser Principle and Introduction

1. Birngruber R. Thermal modeling in biological tissues. In: Hillenkamp F, Praetesi R, Sacchi CA (Eds): Laser in Biology and Medicine Plenum: New York, 1980.
2. Dietlein TS, Jacobi PC, Krieglstein GK. Ab-interno infrared laser trabecular ablation: preliminary short-term results in

patients with open-angle glaucoma. Graef's Arch Clin Exp Ophthalmol 1997;235(6):349-53.
3. Dietlein TS, Jacobi PC, Krieglstein GK. Erbium: YAG laser trabecular ablation (LTA) in the surgical treatment of glaucoma. Lasers Surg Med 1998;23(2):104-10.
4. Hillenkamp F. Interaction between laser radiation and biological systems. In: Hillenkamp F, Praetesi R, Sacchi CA (Eds): Laser in Biology and Medicine. Plenum: New York, 1980.
5. L'Esperance FA Jr. Ophthalmic Laser: Photocoagulation, Photoradiation and Surgery (3rd edn): Mosby: St. Louis 1989.
6. Loertscher H, Shi WQ, Grundfest WS. Tissue ablation through water with erbium: YAG lasers. IEEE Trans Biomed Eng 1992;39:86-8.
7. Mainster MA, Sliney DH, Blecher CD, et al. Laser photodisruptors: damage mechanisms, instrument design and safety. Ophthalmology 1983;90:973-91.
8. Mainster MA, Ho PC, Mainster KJ. Argon and krypton laser photocoagulators. Ophthalmology 1983;90:48-54.
9. Ready JF. Industrial Applications of Lasers. Academic Press: New York, 1978.
10. Schuman JS, et al. Experimental use of semiconductor diode laser in contact transscleral photocoagulator in rabbits. Arch Ophthalmol 1990;108:1152-7.
11. Schuman JS, et al. Energy levels and probe placement in contact transscleral semiconductor diode laser cyclophotocoagulation in human cadaver eyes. Arch Ophthalmol 1991; 109:1534-8.
12. Sliney DH, Mainster MA. Potential laser hazards to the clinician during photocoagulation. Am J Ophthalmol 1987;103:758-60.
13. Wetzel W, Brinkmann R, Koop N, et al. Photofragmentation of lens nuclei using the Er: YAG laser: preliminary report of an in vitro study. Ger J Ophthalmol 1996;5(5):281-4.
14. Wieder M, Pomerantzeff O, Schnieder J. Retinal vessel photocoagulation: a quantitative comparison of argon and krypton laser effects. Invest Ophthalmol Vis Sci 1981; 20:418-24.

Laser Iridotomy

1. Anderson DR, Forster RK, Lewis ML. Laser iridotomy for aphakic pupillary block. Arch Ophthalmol 1975;93:343-6.
2. Breingan PJ. Esaki K, Ishikawa H, et al. Iridolenticular contact decreases following laser iridotomy for pigment dispersion syndrome. Arch Ophthalmol 1999;117(3):325-8.
3. Brooks AMV, Harper CA, Gillies W. Occurrence of malignant glaucoma after iridotomy. Br J Ophthalmol 1989;73:617-20.
4. Carassa RG, Bettin P, Fiori M et al. Nd:YAG laser iridotomy in pigment dispersion syndrome: an ultrasound biomicroscopic study. Br J Ophthalmol 1998;82(2):150-3.
5. Fleck BW, Wright E, Fairley EA. A randomised prospective comparison of operative peripheral iridectomy and Nd:YAG laser iridotomy treatment of acute angle closure glaucoma: 3- year visual acuity and intraocular pressure control outcome. Br J Ophthalmol 1997;81(10):884-8.
6. Forman JS et al. Pupillary block following posterior chamber lens implantation. Ophthalmic Laser Ther 1987;2:85-8.
7. Gandolfi SA, Vecchi M. Effect of a YAG laser iridotomy on intraocular pressure in pigment dispersion syndrome. Ophthalmology 1996;103(10):1693-5.
8. Janiec S, Rzendkowski M, Bolek S, et al. The effect of Nd:YAG laser iridotomy on irido-corneal angle width assessed with ultrasound biomicroscopy in patients with primary open angle glaucoma. Klin Oczna 1998;100(1):15-8.
9. Kim YY, Jung HR. Dilated, miotic-resistant pupil and laser iridotomy in primary angle-closure glaucoma. Ophthalmologica 1997;211(4):205-8.
10. Kraemer C, Gramer E. Posterior synechiae after Nd:YAG laser iridotomy. A clinical study. Ophthalmologe 1998; 95(9):625-32.
11. Kublin J, Simmons RJ. Use of tinted soft contact lenses to eliminate monocular diplopia secondary to laser iridectomies. Ophthalmic Laser Ther 1987;2:111-3.
12. Lagreze WD, Mathieu M, Funk J. The role of YAG-laser iridotomy in pigment dispersion syndrome. Ger J Ophthalmol 1996;5(6):435-8.
13. Lim L, Seah SK, Lim AS. Comparison of argon laser iridotomy and sequential argon laser and Nd:YAG laser iridotomy in dark irides. Ophthalmic Surg Lasers 1996; 27(4):285-8.
14. Masket S. Piggyback intraocular lens implantation. J Cataract Refract Surg 1998;24(4):569-70.
15. Meyer KT, Pettit TH, Straatsma BR. Corneal endothelium damage with neodymium: YAG laser. Ophthalmology 1984; 91:1022-8.
16. Murphy PH, Trope GE. Monocular blurring: a complication of YAG laser iridotomy. Ophthalmology 1991;98:1539-42.
17. Panek WC, Lee DA, Christensen RE. The effects of Nd:YAG laser iridotomy on the corneal endothelium. Am J Ophthalmol 1991;111:505-7.
18. Pavlin CJ, Foster FS. Plateau iris syndrome: changes in angle opening associated with dark, light, and pilocarpine administration. Am J Ophthalmol 1999;128(3):288-91.
19. Pavlin CJ, Macken P, Trope GE et al. Accommodation and iridotomy in the pigment dispersion syndrome. Ophthalmic Surg Lasers 1996;27(2):113-20.
20. Pesando PM, Ghiringhello MP, Tagliavacche P. Posterior chamber collamer phakic intraocular lens for myopia and hyperopia. J Refract Surg 1999;15(4):415-23.
21. Pollack IP. Use of argon laser energy to produce iridotomies. Ophthalmic Surg 1980;11:506-15.
22. Potash SD et al. Ultrasound biomicroscopy in pigment dispersion syndrome. Ophthalmology 1994;101:332-9.
23. Power WJ, Collum LMT. Electron microscopic appearances of human corneal endothelium following Nd:YAG laser iridotomy. Ophthalmic Surg 1992;23:347-50.

24. Quigley HA. Long-term follow-up of laser iridotomy. Ophthalmology 1981;88:218-24.
25. Ritch R, Podos SM. Argon laser treatment of angle-closure glaucoma. Perspect Ophthalmol 1980;4:129-34.
26. Ritch R, Solomon IS. Glaucoma surgery. In L'Esperance FA (Ed): Ophthalmic Lasers (3rd edn): Mosby: St Louis, 1989.
27. Robin AL. Intraocular pressure rise after iridotomy (letter). Arch Ophthalmol 1986;104:1117.
28. Robin AL, Pollack IP, DeFaller JM. Effects of topical ALO 2145 (p-aminoclonidine hydrochloride) on intraocular pressure rise following argon laser iridotomy. Arch Ophthalmol 1987;105:1208-11.
29. Rubin L, Arnett J, Ritch R. Delayed hyphema after argon laser iridectomy. Ophthalmic Surg 1984;15:852-3.
30. Samples J et al. Pupillary block with posterior chamber intraocular lenses. Am J Ophthalmol 1987;105:335-7.
31. Schwartz LW et al. Argon laser iridotomy in the treatment of patients with primary angle-closure or pupillary block glaucoma: a clinicopathologic study. Ophthalmology 1978; 85:294-309.
32. Wollensak G, Eberwein P, Funk J. Perforation rosette of the lens after Nd:YAG laser iridotomy. Am J Ophthalmol 1997;123(4):555-7.
33. Zadok D, Chayet A. Lens opacity after neodymium: YAG laser iridectomy for phakic intraocular lens implantation. J Cataract Refract Surg 1999;25(4):592-3.
34. Zaldivar R, Davidorf JM, Oscherow S. Posterior chamber phakic intraocular lens for myopia of ~8 to ~19 diopters. J Refract Surg 1998;14(3):294-305.

Laser Trabeculoplasty

1. Barnebey HS, et al. The efficacy of brimonidine in decreasing elevation in intraocular pressure after laser trabeculoplasty. Ophthalmol 1993;100:1083-8.
2. Barnes SD, Campagna JA, Dirks MS, et al. Control of intraocular pressure elevations after argon laser trabeculoplasty: comparison of brimonidine 0.2% to apraclonidine 1.0%. Ophthalmology 1999;106(10):2033-7.
3. Bergea B, Bodin L, Svedbergh B. Primary argon laser trabeculoplasty vs pilocarpine. IV Long-term effects on optic nerve head. Acta Ophthalmol Scand 1995;73(3):216-21.
4. Brown RH, et al. ALO 2145 reduces the IOP elevation after anterior segment surgery. Ophthalmol 1988;95:378-84.
5. Brubaker RF. Liesegang TJ. Effect on trabecular photocoagulation on the aqueous humor dynamics of the human eye. Am J Ophthalmol 1983;96:139-47.
6. Chen TC, Wilensky JT, Viana MA. Long-term follow-up of initially successful trabeculectomy. Ophthalmology 1997; 104(7):1120-5.
7. Damji KF et al. Selective laser trabeculoplasty v argon laser trabeculoplasty: a prospective randomised clinical trial. Br J Ophthalmol 1999;83(6):718-22.
8. Gaasterland D, Kupfer C. Experimental glaucoma in rhesus monkey. IOVS 1974;13:455-7.
9. Guzey M, et al. Effects of frequency-doubled Nd:YAG laser trabeculoplasty on diurnal intraocular pressure variations in primary open-angle glaucoma. Ophthalmologica 1999;213(4):214-8.
10. Jacobi PC, Dietlein TS, Krieglstein GK. Primary trabeculectomy in young adults: long-term clinical results and factors influencing the outcome. Ophthalmic Surg Lasers 1999; 30(8):637-46.
11. Jampel HD. Initial treatment for open-angle glaucoma-medical, laser, or surgical? Laser trabeculoplasty is the treatment of choice for chronic open-angle glaucoma. Arch Ophthalmol 1998;116(2):240-1.
12. Koller T, Sturmer J, Reme C, et al. Membrane formation in the chamber angle after failure of argon laser trabeculoplasty: analysis of risk factors. Br J Ophthalmol 2000; 84(1):48-53.
13. Lustgarten J, et al. Laser trabeculoplasty: a prospective study of treatment parameters. Arch Ophthalmol 1984;102:517-9.
14. Mermoud A, Herbort CP, Schnyder CC, et al. Comparison of the effects of trabeculoplasty using the Nd-YAG laser and the argon laser. Klin Monatsbl Augenheilkd 1992;200(5): 404-6.
15. Mermoud A, Pittet N, Herbort CP. Inflammation patterns after laser trabeculoplasty measured with the laser flare meter. Arch Ophthalmol 1992;110:368-70.
16. Odberg T, Sandvik L. The medium and long-term efficacy of primary argon laser trabeculoplasty in avoiding topical medication in open angle glaucoma. Acta Ophthalmol Scand 1999;77(2):176-81.
17. Robin AL. Argon laser trabeculoplasty medical therapy to prevent the intraocular pressure rise associated with argon laser trabeculoplasty. Ophthalmic Surg 1991;22:31-7.
18. Shingelton BJ et al. Long-term efficacy of argon laser trabeculoplasty. Ophthalmol 1987;94:1513-9.
19. Schwartz AL, Love DC, Schwartz MA. Long-term follow-up of argon laser trabeculoplasty for uncontrolled open angle glaucoma. Arch Ophthalmol 1985;103:1482-4.
20. Schwartz LW et al. Variation of techniques on the results of argon laser trabeculoplasty. Ophthalmol 1983;90:781-4.
21. The Advanced Glaucoma Intervention Study (AGIS): 4. Comparison of treatment outcomes within race. Seven-year results. Ophthalmology 1998;105(7):1146-64.
22. Ticho U, Nesher R. Laser trabeculoplasty in glaucoma. Ten-year evaluation. Arch Ophthalmol 1989;107(6):844-6.
23. Traverso CE, Greenidge KC, Spaeth GL. Formation of peripheral anterior synechiae following argon laser trabeculoplasty: a prospective study to determine relationship to position of laser burns. Arch Ophthalmol 1984;102:861-3.
24. Varma R. Trabeculoplasty, trabeculectomy, and race: is there a difference in response to treatment between blacks and whites? Ophthalmology 1998;105(7):1135-6.
25. Weinreb RN, et al. Immediate intraocular pressure response to argon laser trabeculoplasty. Am J Ophthalmol 1983; 95:279-86.
26. Weinreb RN, et al. Influence of the number of laser burns administered on the early results of argon laser trabeculoplasty. Am J Ophthalmol 1983;95:287-92.

27. Wickham MG, Worthen DM, Binder PS. Physiologic effects of laser trabeculectomy in rhesus monkey eyes. IOVS 1977;16:624-8.
28. Wilensky JT, Jampol L. Laser therapy for open-angle glaucoma. Ophthalmol 1981;88:213-7.
29. Wise JB: Ten year results of laser trabeculoplasty. Does the laser avoid glaucoma surgery or merely defer it? Eye 1987;1(Pt 1):45-50.
30. Wise JB, Witter SL. Argon laser therapy for open angle glaucoma: a pilot study. Arch Ophthalmol 1979;97:319-22.
31. Wise JB: Status of laser treatment of open angle glaucoma. Ann Ophthalmol 1981;13:149-50.

Laser Peripheral Iridoplasty

1. Fourman S. "Malignant" glaucoma post laser iridotomy. Ophthalmology 1992;99(12):1751-2.
2. Karjalainen K, Laatikainen L, Raitta C. Bilateral non-rhegmatogenous retinal detachment following neodymium-YAG laser iridotomies. Arch Ophthalmol 1986;104:1134.
3. Karmon G, Savir H. Retinal damage after argon laser iridotomy. Am J Ophthalmol 1986;101:554-60.
4. Lai JS, Tham CC, Lam DS. Limited argon laser peripheral iridoplasty as immediate treatment for an acute attack of primary angle closure glaucoma: a preliminary study. Eye 1999;13(Pt 1):26-30.
5. Lam DS, Lai JS, Tham CC. Immediate argon laser peripheral iridoplasty as treatment for acute attack of primary angle-closure glaucoma: a preliminary study. Ophthalmology 1998;105(12):2231-6.
6. Ritch R, Liebmann JM. Argon laser peripheral iridoplasty. Ophthalmic Surg Lasers 1996;27(4):289-300.
7. Ritch R. Plateau iris is caused by abnormal positioned ciliary processes. J Glaucoma 1992;1:23-7.
8. Sassani JW et al. Histopathology of argon laser peripheral iridoplasty. Ophthalmic Surg 1993;24:740-5.
9. Shapiro A, Tso MO, Goldberg MF. Argon laser-induced cataract. Arch Ophthalmol 1984;102:579-83.
10. Verma N, Fromberg G. Combined argon laser iridoplasty and trabeculoplasty in the management of open angle glaucomas. Indian J Ophthalmol 1986;34:221-3.
11. York K, Ritch R, Szmyd LJ. Argon laser peripheral iridoplasty: indications, techniques and results. IOVS 1984; 25(Suppl):94.

Cyclocoagulation with YAG and Diode Laser

1. Albaugh CH, Dunphy EB. Cyclodiathermy. Arch Ophthalmol 1942;27:543.
2. Azuara-Blanco A, Dua HS. Malignant glaucoma after diode laser cyclophotocoagulation. Am J Ophthalmol 1999; 127(4):467-9.
3. Bietti G. Surgical intervention on the ciliary body: new trends for the relief of glaucoma. JAMA 1950;142:889.
4. Bloom PA, Tsai JC, Sharma K, et al. "Cyclodiode". Trans-scelral diode laser cyclophotocoagulation in the treatment of advanced refractory glaucoma. Ophthalmology 1997; 104(9):1508-19.
5. Brindley G, Shields MB. Value and limitation of cyclocryotherapy. Graefe's Arch Clin Exp Ophthalmol 1986;224:545-8.
6. Chen J, Cohn RA, Lin SC, et al. Endoscopic photocoagulation of the ciliary body for treatment of refractory glaucomas. Am J Ophthalmol 1997;124(6):787-96.
7. Detry-Morel M, Gilon B. Treatment of refractory glaucoma with trans-scleral cyclophotocoagulation using a diode laser. Bull Soc Belge Ophthalmol 1999;272:45-52.
8. Hennis HL, Stewart WC. Transcleral cyclophotocoagulation using a semiconductor diode laser in cadaver eyes. Ophthalmic Surg 1991;22:274-8.
9. Kida K, et al. Non-contact transscleral semi-conductor diode laser cyclophotocoagulation for refractory glaucoma. IOVS 1992;33(Suppl):1267.
10. Linsen MC, Mannes C, Zeyen T. Diode laser cyclophotocoagulation in refractory glaucoma. Bull Soc Belge Ophthalmol 1998;270:69-73.
11. Mora JS, et al. Endoscopic diode laser cyclophotocoagulation with a limbal approach. Ophthalmic Surg Lasers 1997;28(2):118-23.
12. Nassise MP, et al. Inflammatory effects of continuous-wave Nd:YAG laser cyclocoagulation. IOVS 1992;33:2216.
13. Oguri A, Takahashi E, Tomita G, et al. Transscleral cyclophotocoagulation with the diode laser for neovascular glaucoma. Ophthalmic Surg Lasers 1998;29(9):722-7.
14. Plager DA, et al. Intermediate-term results of endoscopic diode laser cyclophotocoagulation for pediatric glaucoma. J AAPOS 1999;3(3):131-7.
15. Schlote T, Kreutzer B, Kriegerowski M, et al. Diode laser cyclophotocoagulation in treatment of therapy refractory glaucoma. Klin Monatsbl Augenheilkd 1997;211(4):250-6.
16. Schubert HD, Agarwal A. Quantitative CW Nd:YAG pars plana transscleral photocoagulation in postmortem eyes. Ophthalmic Surg 1990;21:835-9.
17. Schuman JS, et al. Energy levels and probe placement in contact transscleral semiconductor diode laser cyclophotocoagulation in human cadaver eyes. Arch Ophthalmol 1991; 109:1534-8.
18. Stocker FW. Response of chronic simple glaucoma to treatment with cyclodiathermy puncture. Arch Ophthalmol 1945;34:181.
19. Vogt A Versuche zur intraokularen Druckherabsetzung mittels Diathermieschadigung des corpus ciliare (Zyklodiatermiestichelung) Klin Monatsbl Augenheilkd 1936;97:672.
20. Weekers R, et al. Effects of photocoagulation of ciliary body upon ocular tension. Am J Ophthalmol 1961;52:156.
21. Weve H. Die Zyklodiatermie das corpus ciliare bei Glaukom Zentralbl Ophthalmol 1933;29:256.
22. Wong EY, Chew PT, Chee CK, et al. Diode laser contact transscleral cyclophotocoagulation for refractory glaucoma in Asian patients. Am J Ophthalmol 1997;124(6):797-804.

Laser Treatments After Filtering Surgery

1. Bardak Y, Cuypers MH, Tilanus MA, et al. Ocular hypotony after laser suture lysis following trabeculectomy with mitomycin C. Int Ophthalmol 1997-98;21(6):325-30.
2. Bettin P, Carassa RG, Fiori M, et al. Treatment of hyper-filtering blebs with Nd:YAG laser-induced subconjunctival bleeding. J Glaucoma 1999;8(6):380-3.
3. Chopra H, et al. Early postoperative titration of bleb function: argon laser lysis and removable sutures in trabeculectomy. J Glaucoma 1992;1:54.
4. Hoskins HD Jr, Migliazzo C. Management of failing filtering blebs with the argon laser. Ophthalmic Surg 1984;15:731.
5. Karlen ME, Sanchez E, Schnyder CC, et al. Deep sclerectomy with collagen implant: medium term results. Br J Ophthalmol 1999;83(1):6-11.
6. Lanzl IM, Katz LJ, Shindler RL, et al. Surgical management of the symptomatic overhanging filtering bleb. J Glaucoma 1999;8(4):247-9.
7. Lieberman MF. Suture lysis by laser and goniolens. Am J Ophthalmol 1983;95:257.
8. Liebmann J, Ritch R. Intraocular suture ligature to reduce hypotony following Molteno seton implantation. Ophthalmic Surg 1992;23:51.
9. Macken P, Buys Y, Trope GE. Glaucoma laser suture lysis. Br J Ophthalmol 1996;80(5):398-401.
10. Mermoud A, Karlen ME, Schnyder CC, et al. Nd:YAG goniopuncture after deep sclerectomy with collagen implant. Ophthalmic Surg Lasers 1999;30(2):120-5.
11. Ritch R, Potash SD, Liebmann JM. A new lens for argon laser suture lysis. Ophthalmic Surg 1994;25:126.
12. Singh K, Eid TE, Katz LJ, et al. Evaluation of Nd:YAG laser membranectomy in blocked tubes after glaucoma tube-shunt surgery. Am J Ophthalmol 1997;124(6):781-6.
13. Stegmann R, Pienaar A, Miller D. Viscocanalostomy for open-angle glaucoma in black African patients. J Cataract Refract Surg 1999;25(3):316-22.

Sclerostomies

1. Berlin MS, Rajacich G, Duffy M, et al. Excimer laser photoablation in glaucoma filtering surgery. Am J Ophthalmol 1984;103:713-4.
2. Friedman DS, Katz LJ, Augsburger JJ, et al. Holmium laser sclerostomy in glaucomatous eyes with prior surgery: 24-month results. Ophthalmic Surg Lasers 1998;29(1):17-22.
3. Haring G, Behrendt S, Wetzel W. Evaluation of laser sclerostomy fistulas using ultrasound biomicroscopy. Int Ophthalmol 1997-98;21(5):261-4.
4. Iwach AG, Hoskins HD Jr. Laser sclerostomy for the management of glaucoma. Curr Opin Ophthalmol 1993; 4(2):85-92.
5. Iwach AG, Hoskins HD Jr, Drake MV, et al. Subconjunctival THC:YAG ("Holmium") laser thermal sclerostomy ab externo. a one-year report. Ophthalmol 1993;100:356-65.
6. Jacobi PC, Dietlein TS, Krieglstein GK. Prospective study of ab externo erbium: YAG laser sclerostomy in humans. Am J Ophthalmol 1997;123(4):478-86.
7. Kendrick R, Kollarits CR, Khan N. The results of ab interno laser thermal sclerostomy combined with cataract surgery versus trabeculectomy combined with cataract surgery 6 to 12 months postoperatively. Ophthalmic Surg Lasers 1996;27(7):583-6.
8. Latina MA, Melamed S, March WF, et al. Gonioscopic ab interno laser sclerostomy: a pilot study in glaucoma patients. Ophthalmol 1992;99:1736-44.
9. Luntz MH, Fliegler RD, Mastrobattista J. Subconjunctival THC:YAG laser sclerostomy under a partial thickness flap. Eur J Ophthalmol 1996;6(3):268-72.
10. Mannino G, et al. Ultrasound biomicroscopy in the clinical evaluation of ab externo holmium: YAG laser sclerostomies. Ophthalmic Surg Lasers 1998;29(2):157-61.
11. Melamed S, Neumann D. Internal sclerostomy with laser: a new approach to glaucoma surgery. Lasers Surg Med 1991; 11(5):440-4.
12. Onda E, Ando H, Jikihara S, et al. Holmium YAG laser sclerostomy ab externo for refractory glaucoma. Int Ophthalmol 1996-97;20(6):309-14.
13. Spiegel D, Wetzel W, Birngruber R. Ab externo erbium YAG laser sclerostomy versus conventional trabeculectomy. Treatment of glaucoma patients. Ophthalmologe 1998; 95(8):537-41.
14. Wang Y, Cohen RE, Schuman JS. Iontophoresis of indocyanine green and monastral blue B for gonioscopic diode laser sclerectomy. Ophthalmic Surg Lasers 1996;27(6):484-7.

29

Trabecular Meshwork Ablation as an Alternative to Invasive Glaucoma Surgery

Mona Pache, Jens Funk (Germany)

INTRODUCTION

Open-angle glaucoma is the second leading cause of blindness in the world.[1,2] Glaucomatous optic neuropathy (GON) is characterized by a loss of retinal ganglion cells and their axons, associated by a tissue remodeling both of the optic nerve head (ONH) and the retina leading to the characteristic ONH cupping. Many glaucoma patients present with elevated intraocular pressure (IOP), most often caused by reduced outflow capacity of aqueous humor. The outflow resistance is localized at the level of the trabecular meshwork, or, more precisely, at the juxtacanalicular meshwork and the inner wall of Schlemm's canal.

Data from several major studies available on this topic, such as the OHTS,[3] EGPS,[4] CIGTS,[5] EMGT[6] and the AGIS[7] suggest that both development and progression of glaucomatous damage can be mitigated by lowering IOP. Moreover, the NTGS has clearly demonstrated that lowering of the IOP can slow down the progression of the disease even in patients with normal-tension glaucoma (NTG).[8]

Topical IOP-lowering medication is often the first-line therapy for glaucoma, even though it harbors potential disadvantages such as local and systemic side effects, tachyphylaxis, and, probably most important, compliance problems. Friedman and coworkers recently examined a cohort of 1712 glaucoma suspects and 3623 diagnosed glaucoma patients and found that a large proportion of individuals requiring treatment are falling out of care and are being monitored at rates lower than expected from recommendations of published guidelines because they do not come for follow-up visits and do not ask for a refill of their prescribed glaucoma medication.[9] Apart from this disappointing information, it has to be added that local medication is also not always sufficient if a very low individual target IOP is required. The CNTGS has shown that a 30 percent reduction in IOP is often only reached by surgical intervention. Another point is that the costs of medical control over a lifetime might also be prohibitive for some glaucoma patients.

Glaucoma surgery includes nowadays a number of potential therapies all aiming either to increase the outflow of aqueous humor or to decrease its production. Argon laser trabeculoplasty (ALT), for example, increases the conventional outflow through the trabecular meshwork and is easy to perform. The procedure has however a limited efficacy and duration of effect, as ALT produces thermal effects with coagulation of the trabecular meshwork. A successfully performed trabeculectomy shows a much better efficacy, however, a number of potential complications such as hypotony, suprachoroidal hemorrhage, and bleb failure exist. Patients often find the conjunctival bleb uncomfortable, moreover it can become thin and avascular, thus increasing the risk of bleb leaks, blebitis and endophthalmitis. In case of surgery failure, repeated operations can become necessary, however the chances for success decrease as both sclera and conjunctiva are subjected to repeated surgical insults. Glaucoma drainage devices (tube shunts) have a relatively high success rate in experienced hands, however, the patients are at greater risk for complications.

In 1996, Vogel and coworkers reported a new IOP-lowering operation technique: Using an excimer laser, they managed to ablate trabecular meshwork tissue with minimal thermal effects and necrosis, thus resulting in only minimal scar formation. The authors assumed that it should be possible to create an open connection between the anterior chamber and Schlemm's canal. The group treated 6 patients with open-angle glaucoma. In 4 cases intraocular pressure was reduced by 11 mm Hg over a follow-up time of 5 months. In 2 cases IOP rose by 2 mm Hg in spite of medication.[10]

ERBIUM-YAG GONIOTOMY

Also in 1996, an endoscopic erbium-YAG laser system allowing effects on trabecular tissue comparable to those produced by a 308 nm excimer laser became available. In the following years we could demonstrate a reduction in IOP with this laser system that was comparable to the excimer laser.[11] We performed combined cataract surgery and erbium-YAG goniotomy in 24 eyes and compared the IOP results to a control group that underwent cataract surgery. In the combined surgery group, mean IOP dropped from 21.8 to 15.5 mm Hg. IOP regulation was successful in 88 percent of these cases. In eyes that underwent only cataract surgery, the IOP reduction was less pronounced (mean IOP preoperative 20.0, postoperative 17.4, success rate 35%). The follow-up in this preliminary study was 4 months (mean 6.5 months, max. 12 months).[12]

In another non-randominized clinical trial with a 3-year follow-up, we treated 20 eyes of 20 patients suffering from both glaucoma and cataract with combined phacoemulsification and erbium-YAG goniotomy and compared them to a control group that underwent cataract surgery. Main outcome variables were IOP, visual acuity, and number of antiglaucomatous drugs 1 year after surgery. The mean IOP dropped by 30 percent (23.5 to 16.3 mm Hg) after 12 months in the laser-treated group and by 9 percent (19.8 to 18.1 mm Hg) in the control group. After 3 years, the mean IOP in the laser group was 15.0 mm Hg. The mean number of antiglaucomatous drugs needed decreased significantly from 1.6 to 0.5 in the laser group and from 1.0 to 0.8 in the control group. Anterior chamber hemorrhage occurred in 12 eyes after laser treatment and resolved within 72 hours in all but 1 patient who was on warfarin sodium therapy. There were no cases of hypotony in either group.[13]

We also aimed to compare the efficacy of erbium-YAG goniotomy to trabeculectomy, with both methods as adjuncts to cataract surgery. Fifty-nine eyes of 59 glaucoma patients with coexistent cataract underwent combined phacoemulsification and erbium-YAG goniotomy. We compared this prospective treatment arm to a retrospective inclusion-matched control group treated by trabeculectomy and cataract surgery in a single procedure. Primary endpoints were IOP, number of antiglaucomatous drugs, postoperative complications, hospitalization time and visual acuity 1 year after surgery. In the laser-treated group, the mean IOP dropped by 30 percent from 23.4 mm Hg to 16.3 mm Hg after 12 months. Without reoperation, treatment was successful in 71 percent of these eyes. In the control group, the IOP decreased by 33.5 percent from 22.7 mmHg to 15.1 mm Hg. The success rate without reoperation was 46 percent. The number of antiglaucomatous drugs needed decreased from 1.48 to 0.48 in the laser-treated group and from 2.0 to 0.39 in the controls. Postoperative complications were more frequent in the control group, and postoperative visual acuity was as well. Hospitalization time was shorter in the laser group. It can be concluded from these data that the IOP-lowering effect of combined erbium-YAG goniotomy and cataract surgery is comparable to that of combined trabeculectomy and cataract surgery. Moreover, due to fewer postoperative complications, erbium-YAG goniotomy seems to be superior to standard fistulation surgery as the primary approach.[14] To date, 3 years follow-up data of a small pilot group that underwent combined erbium-YAG goniotomy and cataract surgery are available; and the IOP-lowering effect has not diminished over this follow-up period.[15]

EXCIMER-LASER-TRABECULOTOMY (ELT)

Background

In the meantime, the CE-certified AIDA excimer laser (TuiLaser AG, Germering, Germany) has become commercially available (Figure 29.1). We therefore switched from the erbium-YAG system prototype to the certified laser, assuming that it should have a comparable effect. Like the erbium-YAG laser, the AIDA excimer laser reestablishes the outflow of aqueous humor through conventional drainage pathways. By excising a defined area of trabecular meshwork, juxtacanalicular tissue, and the inner wall of Schlemm's canal via a fiberoptic probe delivering 308 nm XeCL excimer laser energy, aqueous outflow is reestablished.[16] The creation of the openings through the trabecular meshwork and the inner wall of Schlemm's canal is accomplished by using the fiberoptic delivery system LAGO 200 or LAGO 200 ENDO. In detail, the fiberoptic system is positioned across the anterior chamber to contact the trabecular meshwork. Laser pulses remove tissue to create a fistula into Schlemm's canal. Direct viewing for positioning of the fiber is performed with either a goniolens or an endoscope. The small size of the delivery system (external diameter 0.5 mm for the LAGO 200, 1.3 × 0.95 mm for the LAGO 200 ENDO, coaxial endoscope) ensures access through a self sealing clear cornea incision (Figures 29.2 and 29.3). Twenty laser pulses are

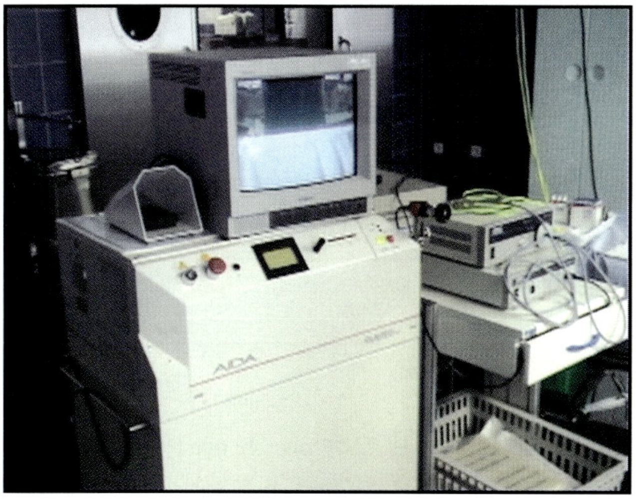

Figure 29.1: AIDA laser

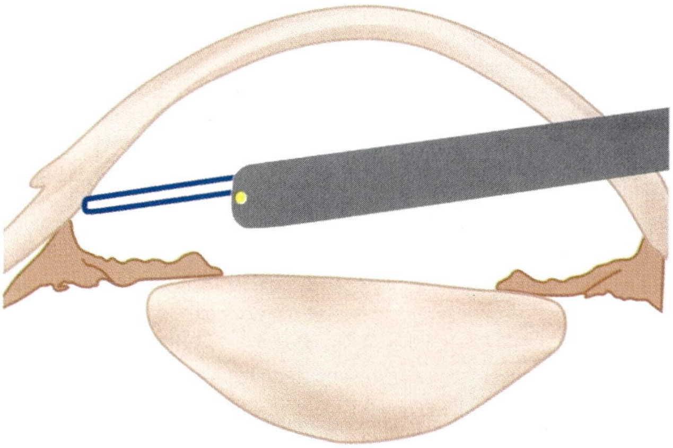

Figure 29.2: Photomontage

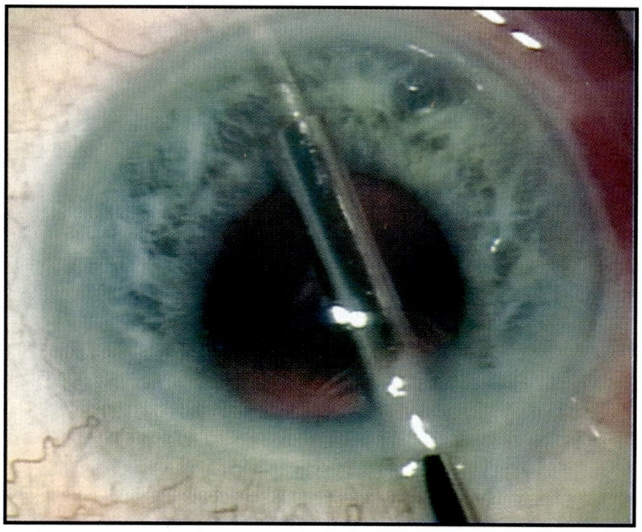

Figure 29.3: Operative setting

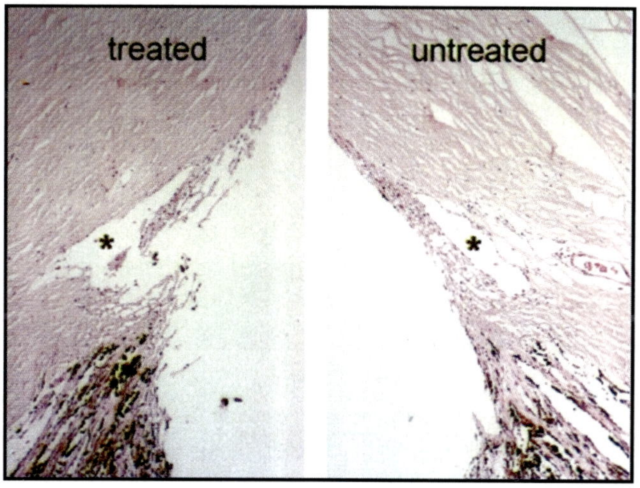

Figure 29.4: Histology

adequate to create a permanent opening into Schlemm's canal. Once the corneal incision is prepared, the actual procedure requires about three minutes. The procedure can easily be combined with cataract surgery. The wavelength of the AIDA laser 308 nm has been found to ablate the trabecular meshwork without inducing thermal damage, thereby minimizing fibrous tissue healing reactions[17-19] (Figure 29.4).

Surgical Procedure

ELT can easily be performed through a clear cornea tunnel incision as used for cataract surgery. We constrict the pupil with topical pilocarpine 2 percent or intracameral injection of acetyline chloride (i. e. Miochol®), then inject a viscoelastic gel (i.e. Healon) into the anterior chamber and insert the laser probe. We then advance the probe to the opposing chamber angle under gonioscopic or endoscopic visualization. The application of the laser pulses can be controlled when the probe tip is in contact with the trabecular meshwork (Figures 29.5 and 29.6). The probe tip is then repositioned such that ten trabecular meshwork perforations are created to the inferior 180°. Following removal of the probe (and endoscope), the viscoelastic is exchanged by BSS. Postoperatively, all eyes are treated with topical steroids 4x/d tapered over 3 weeks. In case of a persistent fibrin reaction, atropine 1 percent eye drops 2x/d can be added. In case of combined cataract + ELT procedure,

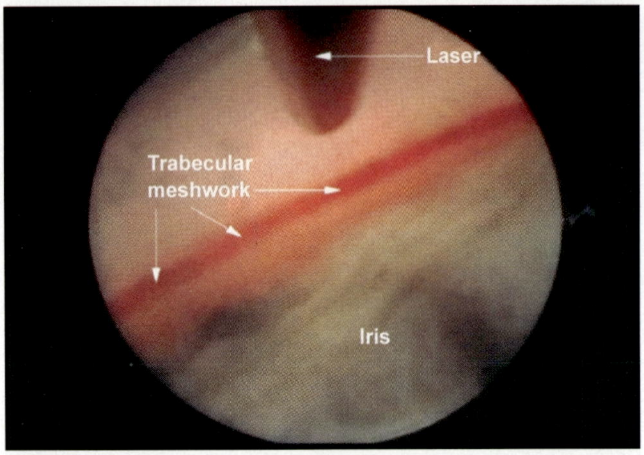

Figure 29.5: ELT view 1

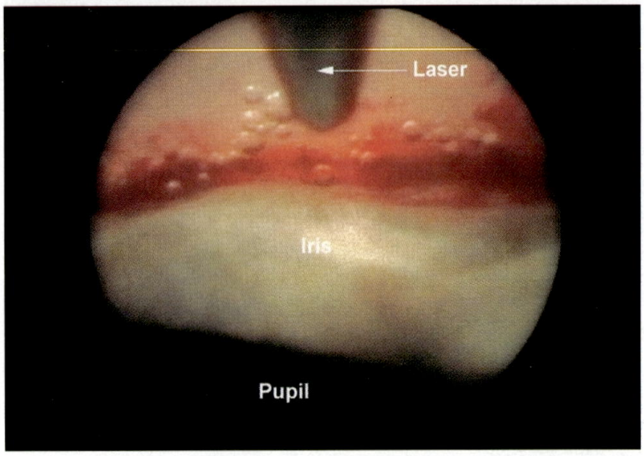

Figure 29.6: ELT view 2

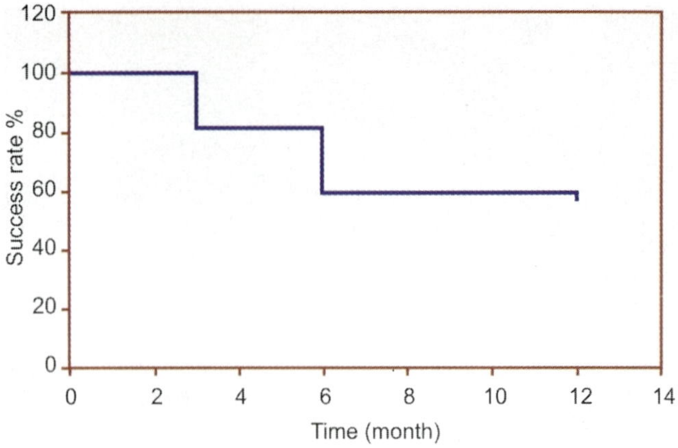

Figure 29.7: ELT IOP over 22 mm Hg Kople

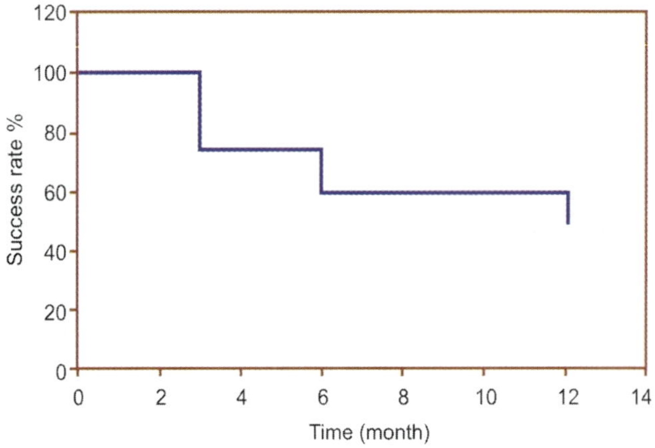

Figure 29.8: ELT IOP below 22 mm Hg Kople

we first perform cataract surgery followed by the ELT procedure, which takes about three minutes longer than cataract surgery alone.

Study Results

Pooled data from a number of study groups have demonstrated that ELT is a safe and sufficient IOP-lowering procedure that can easily be combined with cataract surgery.[20]

In our own clinic, we have retrospectively studied a group of 135 patients with open-angle glaucoma (n = 128) and ocular hypertension (n = 7) that were divided into two groups: a) ELT as a stand-alone procedure (n=75), b) combined cataract and ELT procedure (n= 60). Both groups were further divided into 2 subgroups: 1. Preoperative IOP > 22mm Hg, 2. Preoperative IOP = 22 mm Hg. Kaplan-Meier survival curves were calculated. Success criterion was 20 percent decrease of IOP in combinaton with IOP = 21 mm Hg and postoperative IOP-lowering medication = preoperative IOP-lowering medication. Follow-up time was 1 year. For group a) ELT, 1. Preoperative IOP > 22 mm Hg, 2. Preoperative IOP = 22 mm Hg: Kaplan-Meier survival curves showed a success rate of 57 percent in subgroup 1 and of 41 percent in subgroup 2 (Figures 29.7 and 29.8) For group b) Combined cataract and ELT procedure, 1. Preoperative IOP > 22 mm Hg, 2. Preoperative IOP = 22 mm Hg: Success rate was 91 percent in subgroup 1 and 52 percent in subgroup 2 (Figures 29.9 and 29.10).

Side effects of the ELT were rare: In two cases, an iris adhesion at the tunnel occurred, in 3 cases there was

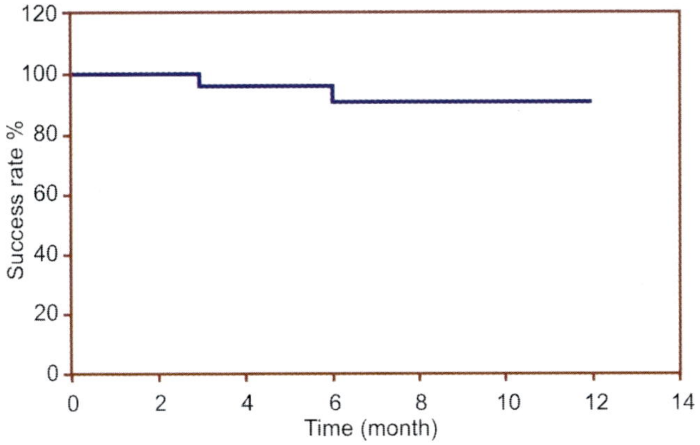

Figure 29.9: ELT phako IOP over 22 mm Hg Kopie

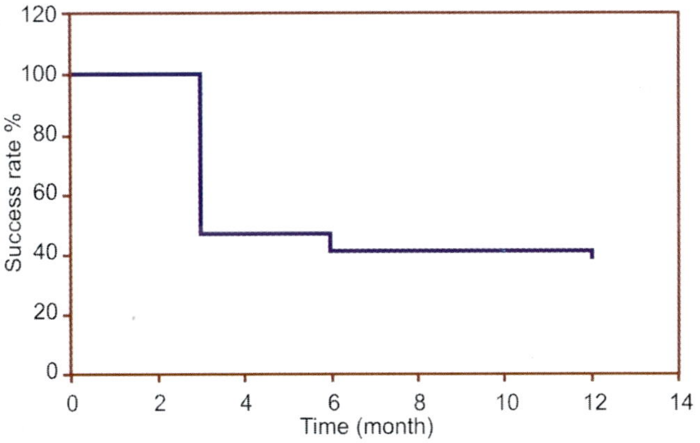

Figure 29.10: ELT phako IOP below 22 mm Hg

a fibroid reaction that responded very well to topical steroids. One patient developed an occlusion of the central retinal vein 5 month after surgery. IOP however was well-controlled at that time, indicating that there was no connection between the CRVO and the ELT procedure.

Our data indicate that ELT is not only a safe and efficient IOP-lowering procedure, but also that it is most effective in patients with a high preoperative IOP. The 2-year follow-up data are now available for many patients, and it seems obvious that the IOP-lowering effect of ELT is conserved also after this longer period of time. We have a prospective multi-center study ongoing in this field and are looking forward to its result.

Due to its sufficient IOP-lowering effect and the minimal invasiveness of the procedure, ELT has become the therapy of choice for patients who suffer from cataract and glaucoma. We recommend the combined procedure in all cataract patients with an IOP of more than 22 mm Hg without therapy. ELT as a stand-alone procedure is performed in patients whose IOP is above 22 mm Hg despite maximally tolerated therapy. In patients with low preoperative IOP, such as patients with normal-tension glaucoma, ELT has proven to be less powerful. We assume that in such cases, the episcleral venous pressure limits the chances of success and prefer a trabeculectomy instead.

CONCLUSION

Excimer-Laser-Trabeculotomy is a promising IOP-lowering technique both as a stand-alone procedure and in combination with cataract surgery. It is especially suitable for patients with high preoperative IOP levels and can easily be combined with cataract surgery.

REFERENCES

1. Quigley HA. Proportion of those with open-angle glaucoma who become blind. Number of people with glaucoma worldwide. Ophthalmology 1999;106(11):2039-41.
2. Quigley HA. Number of people with glaucoma worldwide. Br J Ophthalmol 1996;80(5):389-93.
3. Kass MA, Heuer DK, Higginbotham EJ, Johnson CA, Keltner JL, Miller JP, et al. The ocular hypertension treatment study: a randomized trial determines that topical ocular hypotensive medication delays or prevents the onset of primary open-angle glaucoma. Arch Ophthalmol 2002;120(6):701-13; discussion 829-30.
4. Miglior S, Zeyen T, Pfeiffer N, Cunha-Vaz J, Torri V, Adamsons I. Results of the European glaucoma prevention study. Ophthalmology 2005;112(3):366-75.
5. Feiner L, Piltz-Seymour JR. Collaborative initial glaucoma treatment study: a summary of results to date. Curr Opin Ophthalmol 2003;14(2):106-11.
6. Heijl A, Leske MC, Bengtsson B, Hyman L, Hussein M. Reduction of intraocular pressure and glaucoma progression: results from the early manifest glaucoma trial. Arch Ophthalmol 2002;120(10):1268-79.
7. The advanced glaucoma intervention study (AGIS): 7. The relationship between control of intraocular pressure and visual field deterioration.The AGIS Investigators. Am J Ophthalmol 2000;130(4):429-40.
8. Comparison of glaucomatous progression between untreated patients with normal-tension glaucoma and patients with therapeutically reduced intraocular pressures. Collaborative Normal-Tension Glaucoma Study Group. Am J Ophthalmol 1998;126(4):487-97.

9. Friedman DS, Nordstrom B, Mozaffari E, Quigley HA. Glaucoma Management among Individuals Enrolled in a Single Comprehensive Insurance Plan. Ophthalmology 2005.
10. Vogel M, Lauritzen K, Quentin CD. Punktuelle Ablation des Trabekelwerks mit dem Excimer-Laser beim primären Offenwinkelglaukom. Ophthalmologe 1996;93(5):565-8.
11. Funk J, Schlunck G. Endoskopisch kontrollierte Erbium-YAG-Laser-Goniotomie. Erste präklinische Versuche. Ophthalmologe 1998;95(1):33-6.
12. Funk J, Feltgen N, Asbeck D. Augendrucksenkung durch endoskopisch kontrollierte Erbium: YAG-Goniotomie. Ophthalmologe 2000;97(7):473-7.
13. Feltgen N, Mueller H, Ott B, Frenz M, Funk J. Combined endoscopic erbium:YAG laser goniopuncture and cataract surgery. J Cataract Refract Surg 2003;29(11):2155-62.
14. Feltgen N, Mueller H, Ott B, Frenz M, Funk J. Endoscopically controlled erbium:YAG goniopuncture versus trabeculectomy: effect on intraocular pressure in combination with cataract surgery. Graefes Arch Clin Exp Ophthalmol 2003;241(2):94-100.
15. Philippin H, Wilmsmeyer S, Feltgen N, Ness T, Funk J. Combined cataract and glaucoma surgery: endoscope-controlled erbium:YAG-laser goniotomy versus trabeculectomy. Graefes Arch Clin Exp Ophthalmol 2005.
16. Walker R, Specht H. Theoretical and physical aspects of excimer laser trabeculotomy (ELT) ab interno with the AIDA laser operating at 308 nm. Biomedizinische Technik 2002;47(5):106-10.
17. Berlin MS. Perspectives on new laser techniques in managing glaucoma. Ophthalmology Clinics of North America 1995;8(2):341-63.
18. Berlin MS. We need a trabecular meshwork procedure that works. American Glaucoma Society Annual Meeting, San Jose 2002.
19. Berlin MS. ELT Eximer Laser Trabeculostomy: Update 2003. ASCRS 2003.
20. Berlin MS, Funk J, Pache M, Wilmsmeyer S, Giers U, Kleineberg L, et al. Excimer laser trabeculostomy. A new, minimally-invasive surgical procedure for the treatment of open-angle glaucoma. Glaucoma Today 2004;2-6.

30

Selective Laser Trabeculoplasty

Mordechai Goldenfeld, Shlomo Melamed (Israel)

INTRODUCTION

Since the introduction of the concept that laser treatment can be used in order to lower intraocular pressure (IOP) in open-angle glaucoma[1] by Krasnov in 1973, and the evolution into the currently used Argon Laser Trabeculoplasty (ALT), as described initially by Wise and Witter in 1979,[2] Argon Laser Trabeculoplasty (ALT) has become a standard method of treatment for medically-uncontrolled open-angle glaucoma. However, the precise mechanism of this pressure reduction remains unclear. The efficacy of ALT in open-angle glaucoma was demonstrated by the Glaucoma Laser Trial.[3] The Glaucoma Laser Trial authors concluded that initial ALT is at least as effective as initial treatment with topical medication. Anderson and Parrish[4] discovered that selectively absorbed laser by the Pigmented Trabecular Cells, can alter the structure of the Trabecular Meshwork (TM), and gave the basis for the mechanical theory of action of ALT. Their findings revealed that precise focusing of the laser beam unnecessary because it is possible to use the tissue properties (absorbing only a specific wavelength), in order to provide target selectivity. Melamed et al, suggested an important role for modified biological activity triggered by ALT,[5] their studies of ALT in monkeys have shown increased phagocytic activity of trabecular cells in the acute phase, followed by structural trabecular alterations and accumulation of inflammatory cells in the long-term. Regions adjacent to 'lasered' regions have shown more vacuolizations into the Schlemm's canal and more permeability to flow, as detected by cationized ferritin perfusion. According to the mechanical theory, ALT causes coagulative damage to the TM, which results in collagen shrinkage and subsequent scarring of the TM. Tightening the meshwork in the area of each beam, thus and reopening the adjacent, untreated intertrabecular spaces[2,6,7] (Figure 30.1). The cellular theory proposes that in response to coagulative necrosis induced by the laser, there is migration of macrophages, which phagocytose debris and thus clear the TM.[8] Recently, an addition to the cellular theory has been suggested. This theory employs facts described by Wang et al,[9] who demonstrated that the TM endothelium shares similar response to oxidative

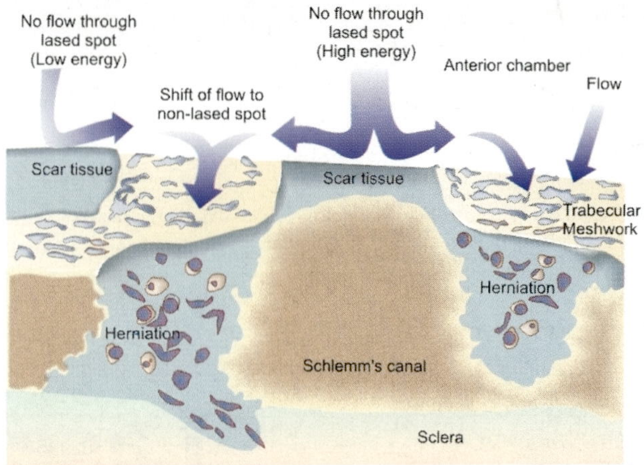

Figure 30.1: Schematic view of ALT coagulation damage. Note the arrows indicating areas of no flow, stretching and reopening the adjacent, untreated intertrabecular spaces

insults as the systemic endothelial cells, and that inflammatory cytokines can play a role in glaucoma. Wang et al demonstrated that in response to a sublethal stress in glaucoma, specifically performed to the trabecular meshwork, cytokines, such as endothelial leukocyte adhesion molecule-1 (ELAM-1), can be released into the aqueous and influence glaucomatous aqueous outflow pathways. Signals, such as laser radiation, can promote oxidative stress. The gene for ELAM-1 has receptors in its promoter region that could respond to this kind of stress, and release and activate inflammatory cytokines, such as interleukin-1 (IL-1), which could in turn increase the formation of ELAM-1. Bradley et al[10,11] have demonstrated that IL-1 increases outflow facility and showed that IL-1β and Tumor Necrotizing factor-α, (TNFα), mediate ALT-induced MMP expression. For the first time it was shown that humoral pathway can be as important as the mechanical one. Although the Glaucoma Laser Trial demonstrated the efficacy of ALT,[3] in follow-up studies,[12,13] it was shown that after a mean follow-up of 7 to 10 years , only 20 to 32 percent of the patients remained controlled. The need for repeat laser therapy was evident, but he fact that ALT creates a scar in the treated TM (Figure 30.2), limited the possibility of repeated treatment. Selective Laser Trabeculoplasty (SLT) was developed in order to employ the fact that cellular and humoral mechanisms, can effect the out-flow facility without

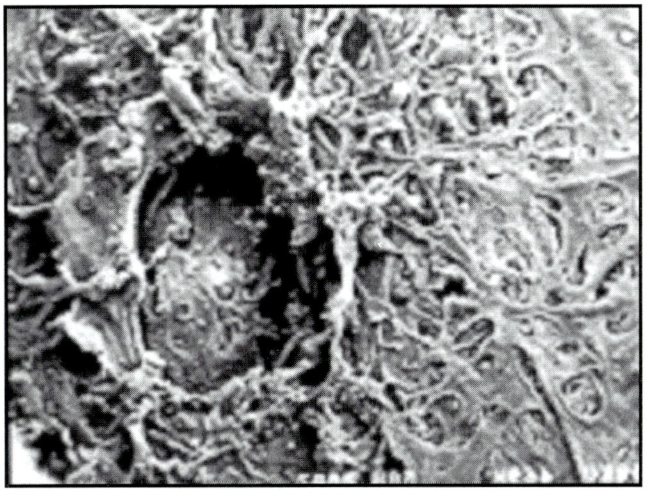

Figure 30.2: ALT laser burn SEM

creating a permanent scar in the TM.[8-11] The energy delivered by the SLT is mostly absorbed by pigmented cells and is, therefore, spatially confined to the pigmented TM cells. SLT uses a Q-switched, frequency-doubled 532 nm Nd:YAG laser with a short-pulse duration of 3 nanoseconds. This modality limits the conversion of energy to heat, further minimizing the collateral tissue damage[14] (Figure 30.3). Histological studies,[14] (Figure 30.4) in human cadaver eyes after SLT reveal no evidence of coagulative damage or disruption of the corneoscleral or uveal trabecular beam structure. Because of the minimal cytologic damage, SLT offers two theoretical advantages; one is that it may be repeatable and two, it may have a higher safety profile.[15] Latina et al,[16] were the first to establish the efficacy and safety of SLT by demonstrating a 70 percent response rate and a 5.8 mm Hg (23.5%) IOP lowering effect of SLT, in addition, they demonstrated that SLT can be repeated after failed ALT without the risk of post-laser IOP spike. Other studies confirmed his findings.[18-20] Melamed et al treated newly diagnosed glaucoma patients with SLT and demonstrated a mean IOP reduction of 7.7 mm Hg (30%). He also reported that the incidence of postoperative pressure spikes was very low.[21] Chen E et al,[22] reported that the IOP lowering effect of SLT was independent of previous ALT and that there is no difference between the effects of 25 spots on 90 degrees of TM vs. 50 spots on 180 degrees of TM. SLT was also reported to cause significantly less pain

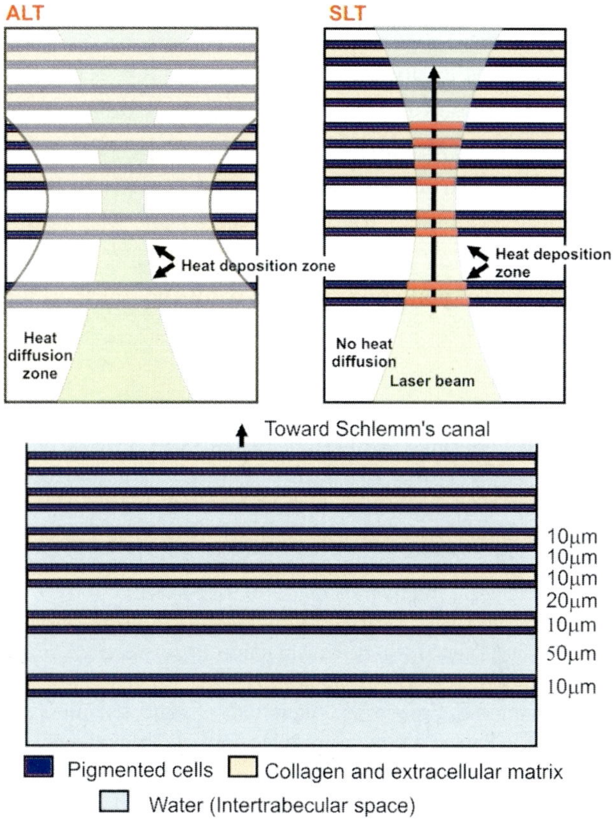

Figure 30.3: Multilayer optical model of trabecular meshwork effect of ALT vs SLT (Modified from Manns et al). Note the difference in the heat-diffusion zone, minimizing the collateral tissue damage

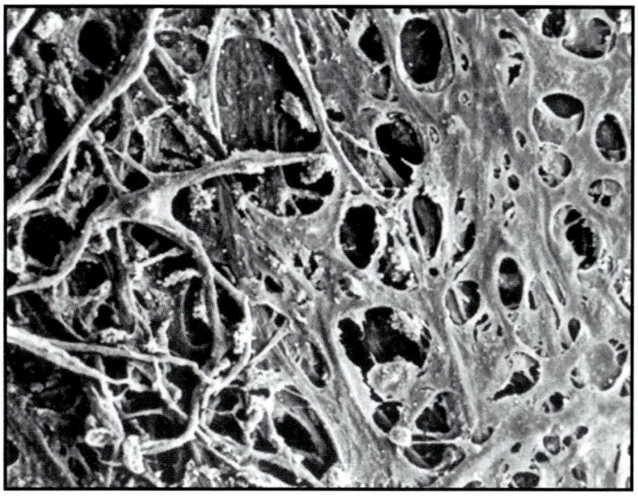

Figure 30.4: SLT - No visible scar SEM

and flare than ALT.[23] To date, no remarkable postoperative complications have been reported with SLT.

CONCLUSION

SLT is at least as good as ALT regarding IOP reduction. SLT may be safer than ALT because it delivers less energy to the TM, causing less post-therapy IOP spikes. The lack of structural damage to the TM offers re-treatment possibility following failed ALT. SLT should be considered as either a first or second line treatment in open-angle glaucoma patients with uncontrolled IOP.

REFERENCES

1. Krasnov MM. Laser puncture of anterior chamber angle in glaucoma. Am J Ophthalmol 1973;75:674-8.
2. Wise JB, Witter SL. Laser. Therapy for open-angle glaucoma: a pilot study. Arch Ophthalmol 1979:97:319-22.
3. The Glaucoma Laser Trial Research Group. The glaucoma laser trial (GLT), results of laser trabeculoplasty vs. topical medicines. Ophthalmology 1990;97:1403-13.
4. Anderson RR, Parish HA. Selective photothermolysis: Precise microsurgery by selective absorption of pulsed radiation. Science 1983;220:524-47.
5. Melamed S, Epstein DL. Alterations of aqueous humor outflow following argon laser trabeculoplasty in monkeys. Br J Ophthalmol 1987;71:776-81.
6. Reiss GR, Wilensky IT, Higginbotham El. Laser trabeculoplasty. Surv Ophthalmol I991;35:407-28.
7. Weinreb RN, Tsai CS. Laser trabeculoplasty. In Ritch R, Shields MB, Krupin T (Eds). The glauomas: glauoma theropy (2nd edn). Missouri: Mosby-Year Book, 1996;111: 1575-90.
8. Damji KF, Shah KC Rock WJ, et al. Selective laser trabeculoplasty v argon laser trabeculoplasty: a prospective randomized clinical trial. Bj J Ophthalmol 1999;83:718-22.
9. Wang N, Chintala SK, Fini ME, Schuman JS. Activation of a tissue-specific stress response in the aqueous outflow pathway of the eye defines the glaucoma disease phenotype. Nat Med 2001;7(3):304-9.
10. Bradley JM, Vranka J, Colvis CM, Conger DM, Alexander JP, Fisk AS, et al. Effect of matrix metalloproteinases activity on outflow in perfused human organ culture. Inves Ophthalmol Vi Sci 1998;39:2649-58.
11. John MB Bradley, Ann Marie Anderssohn, Christine M Colvis, Dorothy E Parshley, XiangHong Zhu, Michael S. Ruddat, et al. Mediation of laser trabeculoplasty–induced matrix metalloproteinase expression by IL-1β and TNF. Inves Ophthalmol Vis Sci 2000;41:422-30.
12. The Glaucoma Laser Trial (GLTFS) AJO 1995;120:718.
13. Bradford JS, Richter CU, Dharma SK, et al. Long-term efficacy of argon laser trabeculoplasty. Ophthalmol 1993;100(9):1324-9.
14. Latina MA, Park C. Selective targeting of trabecular meshwork cells: In vitro studies of pulsed and CW laser interactions. Exp Eye Res 1995;60:359-72.
15. Huck A Holz, Michele C Lirn. Glaucoma lasers: a review of the newer techniques Curr Opin Ophthalmol 2005;16:89-93.
16. Latina MA, Sibayan SA, Shin DH, et al. Q switched 532 nm Nd:YAG, laser trabeculoplasty (selective laser trabeculoplasty). A multicenter pilot cinical study. Ophthalmol 1998;105(11):2082-8.
17. Damji KF, Shah KC, Rock WJ, et al. Selective laser trabeculoplasty v argon laser trabeculoplasty: a prospective randomized clinical trial. Br J Ophthalmol 1999;83:718-22.
18. Mermound A, Herbort CP, Schnyder CC, et al. Comparison of the effects of trabeculoplasty using the Nd:YAG laser and argon laser. Klin Monatsbl Augenheilkd 1992;200:4046.
19. Tabak S, de Waard PWT, Lemij HG, et al. Selective laser ttabeculoplasty in glaucoma. Invst Ophthalmol Vis Sci 1998;39:S472.
20. Pirnazar JR, Kolker A, Wax M, et al. The efficacy of 532 nm laser trabeculoplasty. Invest Ophthalmol Vis Sci 1998;39:S5.
21. Melamed S, Ben Simon GJ, Levkovitch-Verbin H. Selective laser trabeculoplasty as primary treatment for open-angle glaucoma. Arch Ophthalmol 2003;121:957-80.
22. Chen E, Golchin S, Blomindahl S. Comparison between 90 degrees and 180 degrees selective laser trabeculoplasty. J Glaucoma 2004;13:62-5.
23. Martinez-de-Ia-Gasa JM, Garcia-Feijoo J, Castillo A, et al. Selective vs argon laser trabeculoplasty: hypotensive efficacy, anterior chamber inflammation, and postoperative pain. Eye 2004;18:498-502.

31

Milling Trabeculoplasty: A New Technique for Non-penetrating Glaucoma Surgery

José L Rodriguez-Prats, Jorge L Alió, Ahmed Galal (Spain)

INTRODUCTION

Trabeculectomy has been the operation of choice for glaucoma since its introduction in 1961 and as a full-thickness operation it had its complications. Guarded filtration procedures were developed to reduce these risks such as hypotony, and infections.[1-3] In the standard trabeculectomy, as reported by Cairns, the trabecular block is excised anterior to the scleral spur or alternatively from the posterior side as proposed by Watson.[2] The success rate of trabeculectomy is influenced by several factors including patient's characteristics, type of glaucoma and wound healing processes.[1-4] Other important factors that might reduce the success of this surgery include tissue scarring, anterior segment neovascularization, active uveitis, aphakia, previous ocular surgery and chronic conjunctival inflammation.[1-5]

Over the past 10 years new modalities in glaucoma surgery have been introduced as possible alternatives to trabeculectomy. Krasnov and Zimmerman have identified those procedures into deep scleretomy and viscocanalostomy.[3] The non-penetrating glaucoma surgeries aim to allow drainage of the aqueous humor by slow percolation through the inner trabecular meshwork and/or Descemet membrane (trabeculo-descemetic membrane) rather than through a patent scleral opening, as in standard trabeculectomy. This avoids sudden reductions in IOP, hypotony and flat chambers. Performing such a non-penetrating glaucoma surgeries has great advantages are the absence of anterior chamber opening and iridectomy, the facts that limit the risk of cataract and infection.[6-9] In the past 10 years new non-penetrating modalities in glaucoma surgery were introduced as possible alternatives to Trabeculectomy. Krasnov and Zimmerman have proposed these procedures as deep sclerotomy and viscocanalostomy.[3] The non-penetrating glaucoma surgeries aim to allow drainage of the aqueous humor by slow percolation through the inner trabecular meshwork and/or trabeculo-descemetic membrane rather than a patent trabeculo-scleral opening, as in standard trabeculectomy. This avoids sudden reductions in IOP, hypotony and flat chambers. Non-penetrating glaucoma procedures have important potential advantages mainly the absence of anterior chamber opening and iridectomy, the fact that limits the risk of cataract and infection.[6-9]

One of the important targets while performing trabeculectomy or non-penetrating glaucoma surgeries is to minimize the stimulation of fibroblast proliferation that might reduce the success rate of the procedure. The cutting, spreading, and tearing of tissue should be kept to a minimum. In addition, the surgeon should strive to keep the incisions linear, rather than multilaminate, to maintain as small and localized incisional scars as possible.[9-11]

Milling trabeculoplasty is considered a variation of deep sclerectomy with more refining. The technique of milling trabeculopasty provides the opportunity to perform a non-penetrating glaucoma surgery with greater attention for the dissection of the deep scleral flap or the deroofing of the Schlemm's canal with the addition advantage that is being much faster.[12]

INDICATIONS

Eyes with primary open-angle glaucoma are the best candidates for the milling surgery. However, all indications of deep sclerectomy are cases of milling procedure.

PATIENT PREPARATION

Preoperative Examination

Before surgery, each patient had manifest refraction, slit lamp biomicroscopy with measurement of IOP by using Goldman tonometry, gonioscopy and computerized perimetry.

Preoperative Medications

Medications included Ciprofloxacin 0.3 percent eye drops 3 times/ day for a week. The topical antiglaucoma therapy was stopped 3 days before the surgery.

Anesthesia

Peribulbar anesthesia in the form of combination of 8 ml of 0.75 percent Bupivacaine and 2 percent Lidocaine was injected. Intravenous sedation was used when necessary. A light compression with the Honnan balloon was applied 15 minutes prior to surgery for 5 minutes to insure diffusion of the anesthetic agent.

MILLING SURGICAL PROCEDURE

Instruments

Milling drill (Katena Inc, Denville, NJ USA) is the main instrument necessary to perform this procedure. The mode of action of the drill is similar to that used to burr the nasal bone in dacryocystorhinostomy (DCR) surgery or that used to polish the bed after removing corneal foreign bodies. The drill used in our milling procedure is handheld 150-mg weight equipment and made of autoclaveble material (Figure 31.1). Following the concept of refined tissue removal would decrease the rate of postoperative fibrosis, a high frequency and velocity motorized drill tip could be able to polish (no cutting method) the remaining scleral thickness with minimal tearing and smaller more localized scars at the end of the procedure.

The high speed Milling drill (6000 RPM) allows easy (Figure 31.2), quick and more controlled refining of the remaining scleral thickness by using sharp- metallic tip first to refine the sclera and later on as the tissue became thinner another notched hemispherical metallic tip was used to polish and not cut the remaining scleral thickness (Figure 31.3). A new tip covered with diamond powder is also needed for more delicate maneuvers as removing debris making the technique ideal to have an extremely smooth bed (Figure 31.4). In both Groups the procedure started as the initial steps of deep sclerotomy[13] then the

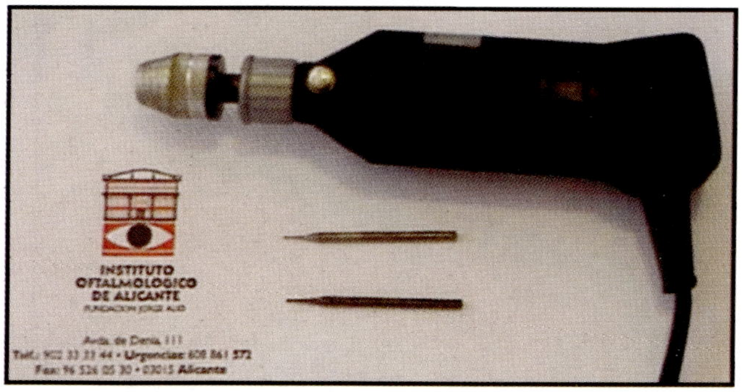

Figure 31.1: Milling drill with the tips used in the surgery of milling

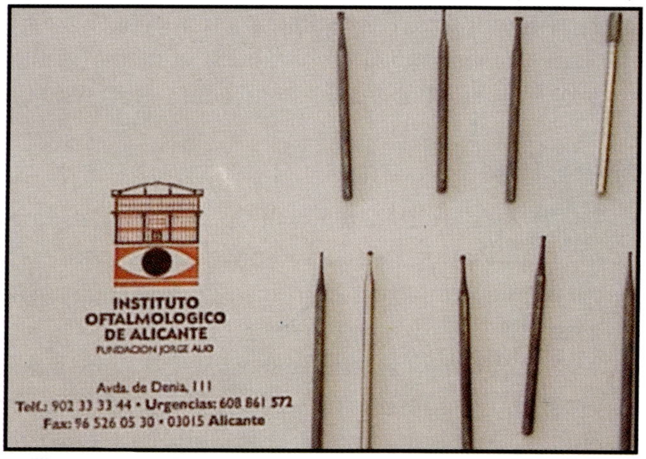

Figure 31.2: The drill held with the tip unassembled just before the surgery

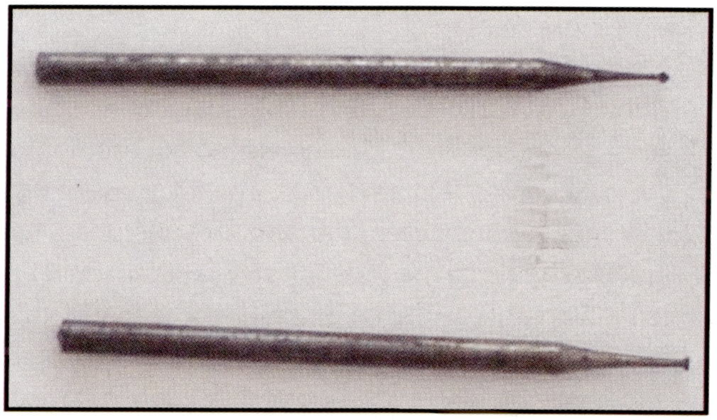

Figure 31.3: Milling set of metallic tips. The set includes tips for cutting, other for refining

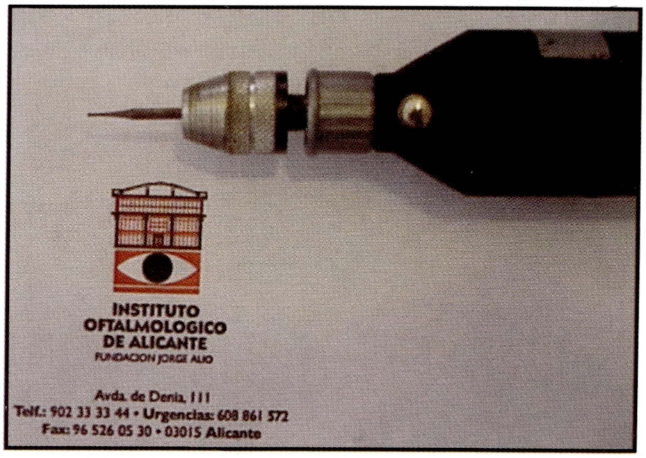

Figure 31.4: The notched hemispherical metallic tips to polish but not cut the remaining scleral thickness

specific steps of milling surgery were continued. In Group II, the milling procedure is carried out until Schlemm's canal is identified. Thereafter, phaco is performed (through a separate clear corneal incision) and after the IOL was implanted, the milling procedure was finished.

Surgical Steps

1. The eyelids are sterilized with ophthalmic Betadine solution (Purdue Frederick, Norwalk, CT), and after the sterile drape was placed, a lid speculum was inserted.
2. An 8 mm fornix-based conjunctival flap is prepared superiorly and Tenon's capsule was retracted. Bipolar cautery is then applied sparingly to cauterize individual limbal vessels one by one to achieve homeostasis preserving as much as possible the episcleral vessel.
3. A superficial scleral flap of 4 × 4 mm hinged at the limbus was designed using ultra sharp mini blade such as the No. 7511 Beaver, extending 1 mm into the clear cornea (Figure 31.5A). The thickness of the flap should be between 200 and 250 microns. The incision should be made definitively, without multiple tentative strokes (Figure 31.5B). The edge of the scleral flap was then grasped with Hoskins forceps and gently retracted. The scleral dissection is carried out using a crescent-style blade extending the lamellar dissection anterior tell the blue limbal zone then more anteriorly until 1 or 2 mm of a clear cornea is reached and the iris details can be seen through the deep layers of corneal tissue (Figures 31.5C to E).

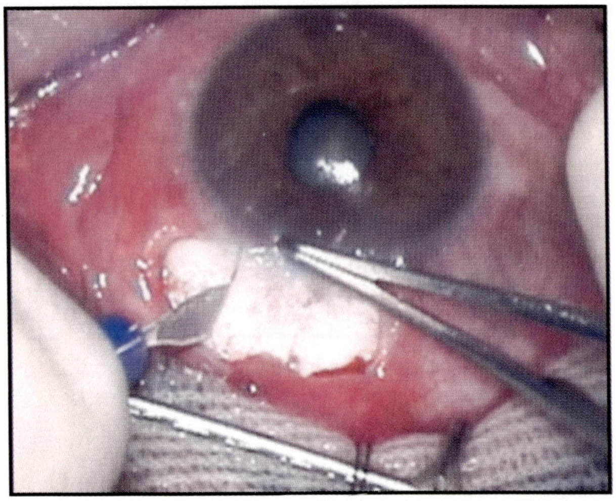

Figure 31.5A: Fashioning of the scleral flap size and site

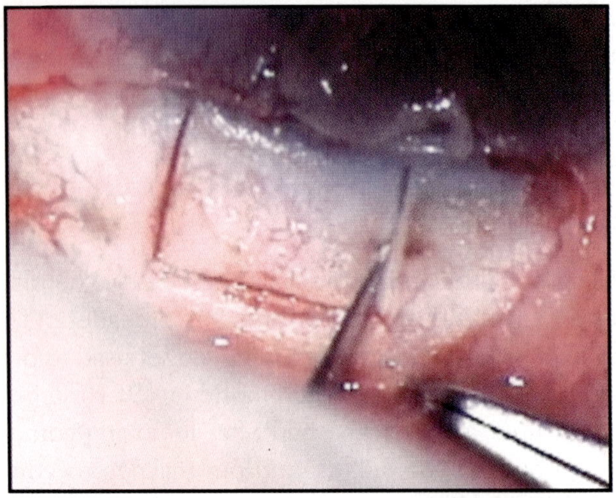

Figure 31.5B: The scleral incision as being completed

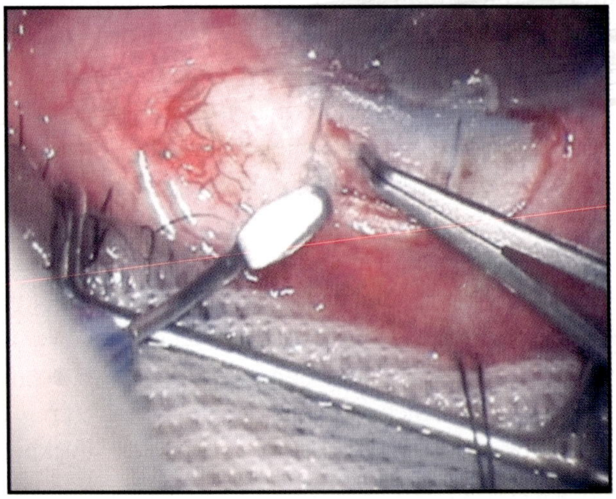

Figure 31.5C: Beginning of the lamellar dissection

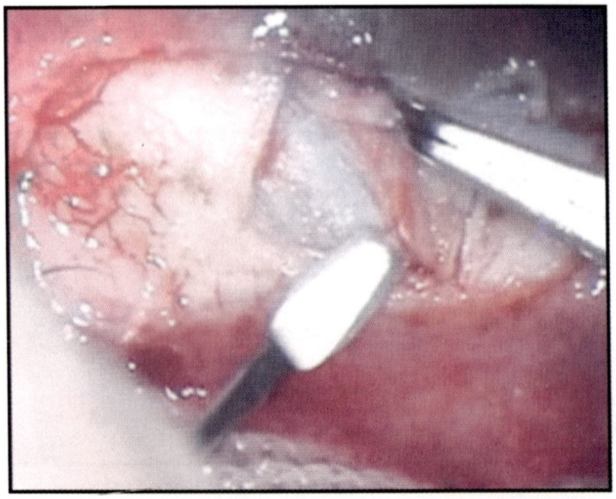

Figure 31.5D: Lamellar dissection of the scleral flap

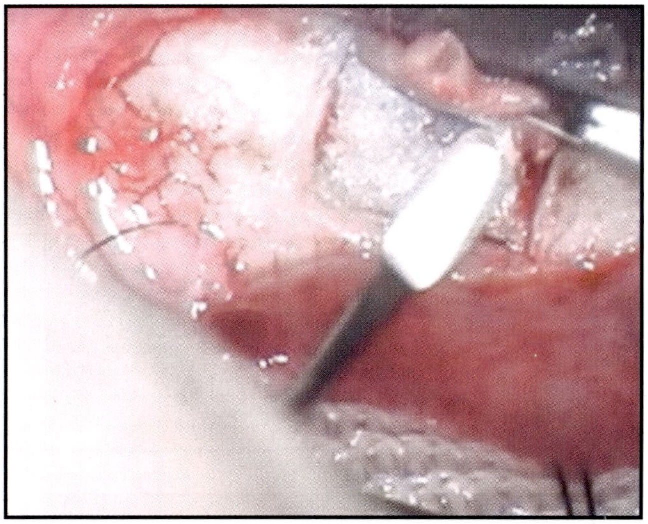

Figure 31.5E: Completion of the lamellar dissection

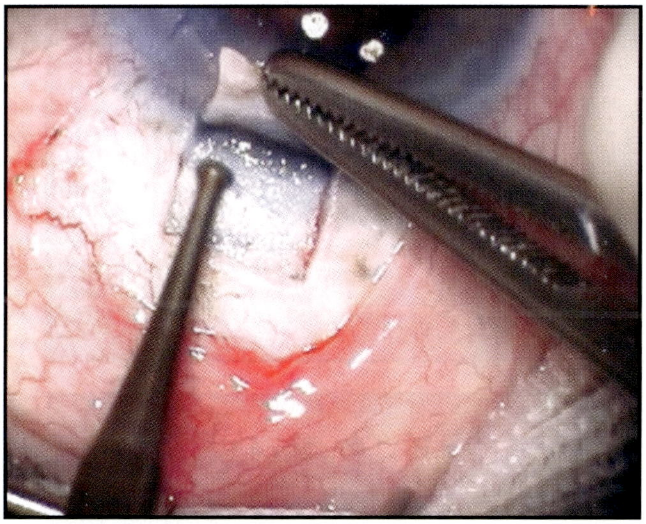

Figure 31.6: The scleral bed refined and grazed using the milling motorized drill in dry field through the remaining scleral thickness in a linear pattern to leave a thin layer of sclera below and a width of 3.5 mm

4. Under high magnification, a rectangular dry area of the scleral bed about 3 × 3 mm inside the superficially created flap is selected to start milling and the milling motorized drill was applied without pressure allowing to drill and refine the remaining scleral thickness in a linear pattern to leave a thin layer of sclera underneath (Figure 31.6). The site of milling should be applied at the surgical limbus in order to expose the canal of Schlemm. The refining is carried anteriorly and downwards until the blue-gray color

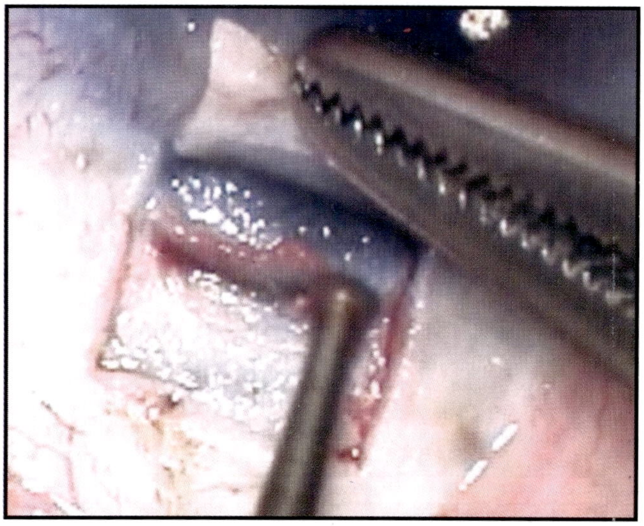

Figure 31.7: The refining is carried anteriorly and down until the roof of Schlemm's canal can barely be visible

of the choroid should appear through the residual scleral fibers (Figure 31.7). When reaching the appropriate depth, the canal openings are identified by passing a hook though them (Figures 31.8A and B).

5. The process of "Unroofing" of the canal is automatically done using the motorized milling drill but care should be taken not to apply any pressure (maintaining the high velocity) and leave the drill to refine the tissues. After being unroofed, the inner wall of Schlemm's canal appears as a dark line, just anterior to the scleral spur. The milling is continued anteriorly towards the cornea to remove the sclerocorneal trabecular meshwork (T.M), which typically exhibits a granular texture. If phacoemulsification is combined with the procedure,- the superficial corneal flap is reposted and a clear corneal incision is prepared then the phaco is performed. After the phaco has been completed the milling is carried out anteriorly and 1 to 2 mm of Descement´s membrane is exposed by milling anterior to the canal till clear corneal tissue is reached and iris details could be identified though the remaining thin sheet of T.M. Another alternative to create the descemtic window is using a mini-blade starting with down-up incision at one of the two opening of the canal then with a shaving movement a block of tissue is excised moving

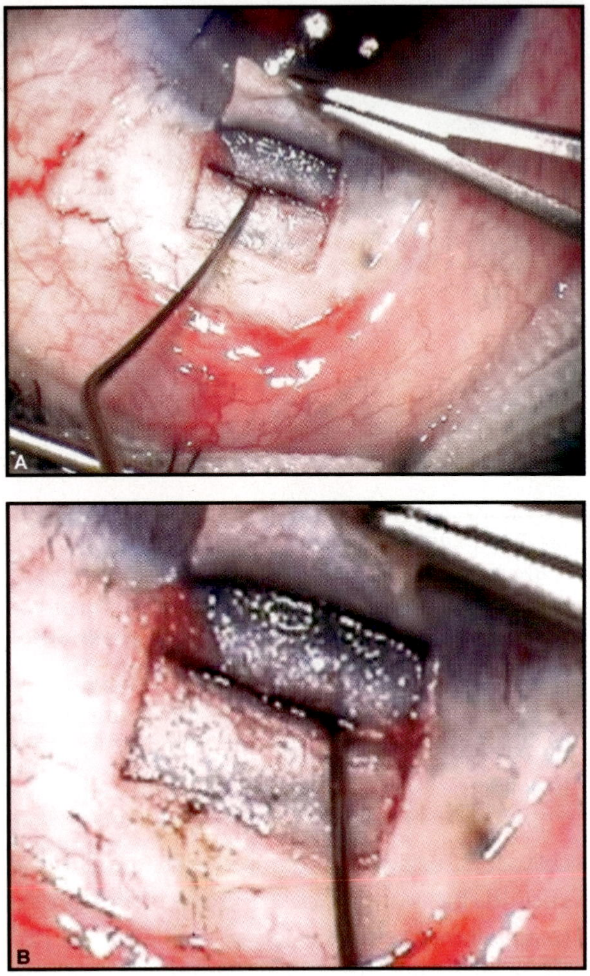

Figures 31.8A and B: A hook is passed though the opening of the canal to insure adequate level of dissection and milling

towards the other opening of the canal (Figures 31.9A to C).

6. At this stage of the procedure, aqueous humor should be seen percolating through the trabeculo-descemetic membrane. If still there is reduced outflow, stripping the inner wall of Schlemm's canal was done (Figure 31.10) to increase aqueous outflow and then further milling is carried out to smoothen the surface (Figure 31.11). Ultimately, only the trabeculodescemetic membrane remains intact. Visible filtration of aqueous through the thin trabeculodescemetic membrane should be obtained. Dilatation of Schlemm's canal could be also done by inserting a cannula into the canal for 0.5 or 1 mm.

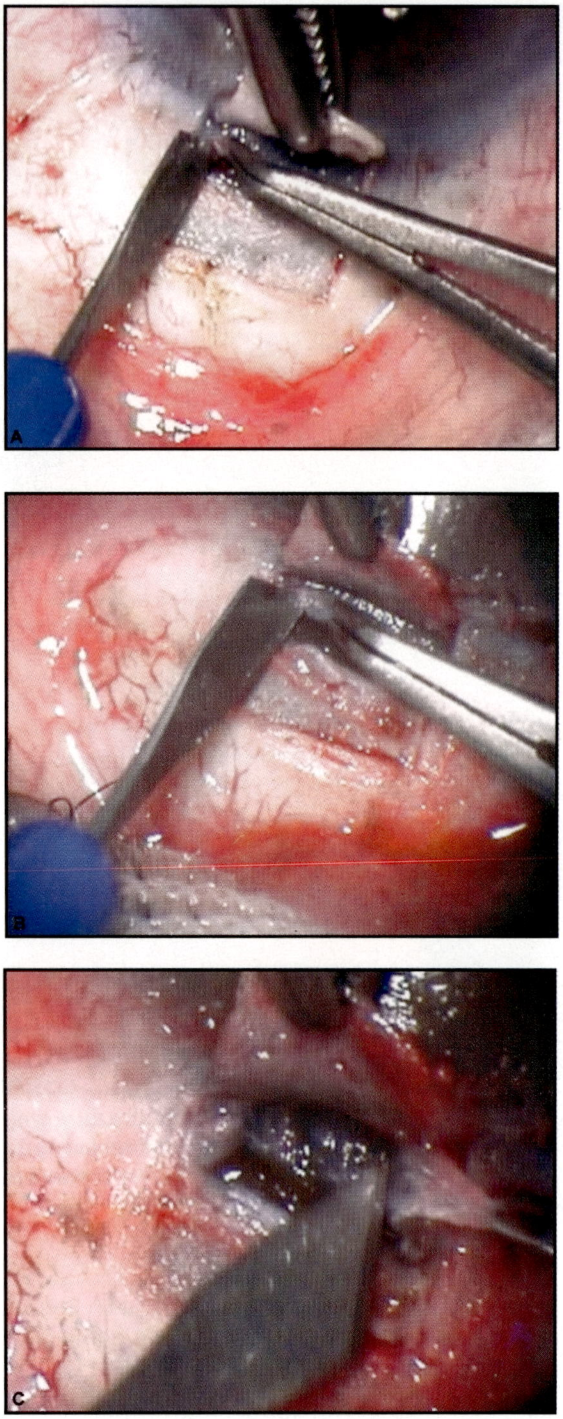

Figures 31.9A to C: Deroofing of Schlemm's canal is done: **A.** Two incisions are created at both sides starting from the opened Schlemm's canal and anteriorly tell reaching the clear corneal under the flap. **B.** The site of incision is checked again and repeated on the other side. **C.** The roof of the canal is removed using the surgical knife

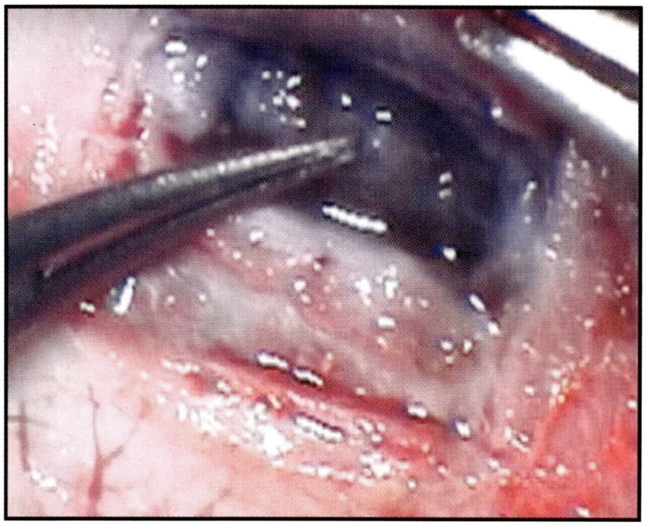

Figure 31.10: Stripping of the floor of the canal is done if insufficient filtration is found

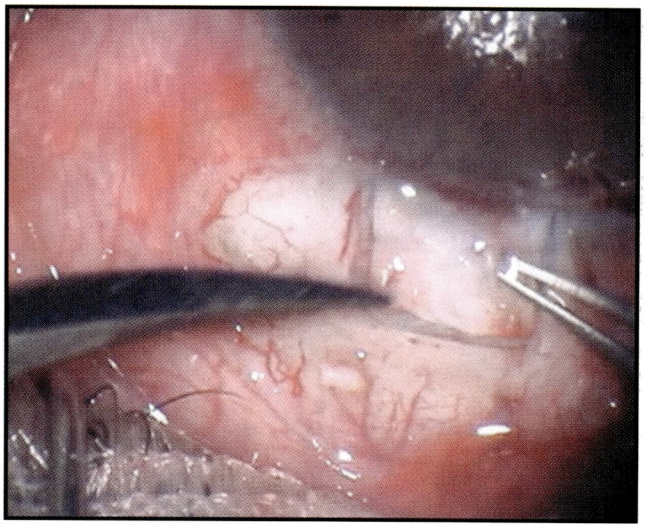

Figure 31.12: The scleral flap is reposted at the end of the surgery

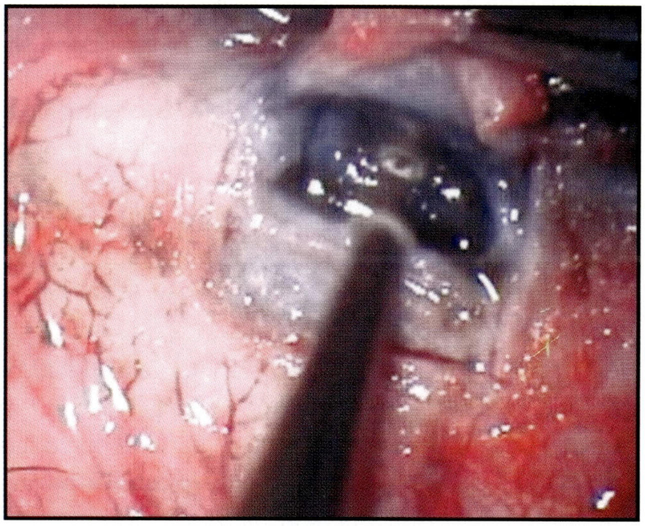

Figure 31.11: Refining the descement window is done using the drill and the milling is done applying no pressure

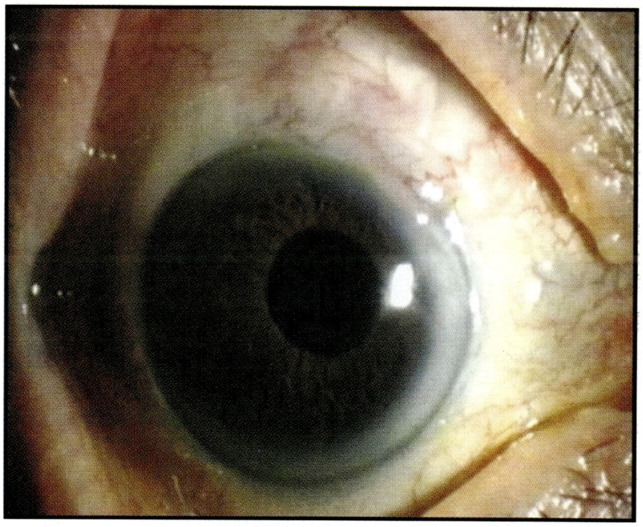

Figure 31.13: Slit-lamp photo of the postoperative bleb obtained at 6 months in group I

7. In case of glaucoma implant the implant should inserted at this level of the surgery and sutures to sclera as in conventional deep sclerectomy.[14]
8. The flap is gently laid in its normal anatomic position (Figure 31.12). Two 10-0 nylon stitches were placed at both edges of the superficial flap and tied fairly (not very tight and not very loose). The suture ends were cut and the knots were parried to prevent the suture tips from eroding the conjunctiva. After closing the scleral flap repositioning of the conjunctiva was then done with 2 lateral 10/0 nylon stitches (Figures 31.13 to 31.15).

POSTOPERATIVE FOLLOW-UP

Treatment

Antibiotic-steroidal combination; Tobradex® (Lab Alcon Cusi, Inc. Barcelona. Spain) eye drops were instilled postoperatively 4 times daily for 1 week and slowly withdrawn over one month period. No viscoelastics was

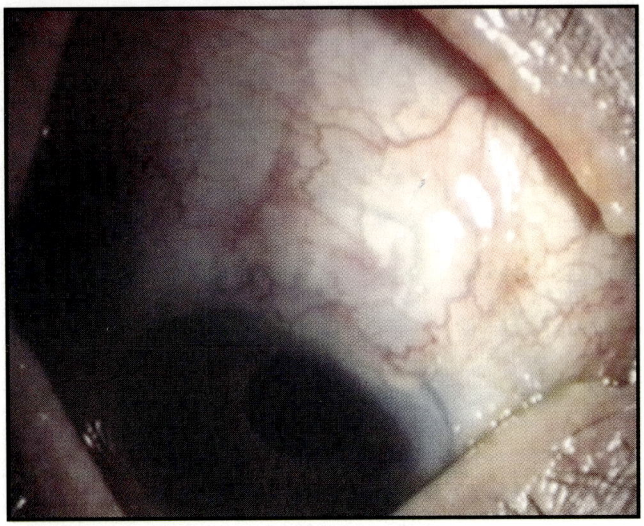

Figure 31.14: Slit-lamp photo of the postoperative bleb obtained at 6 months in group II (Phaco-milling)

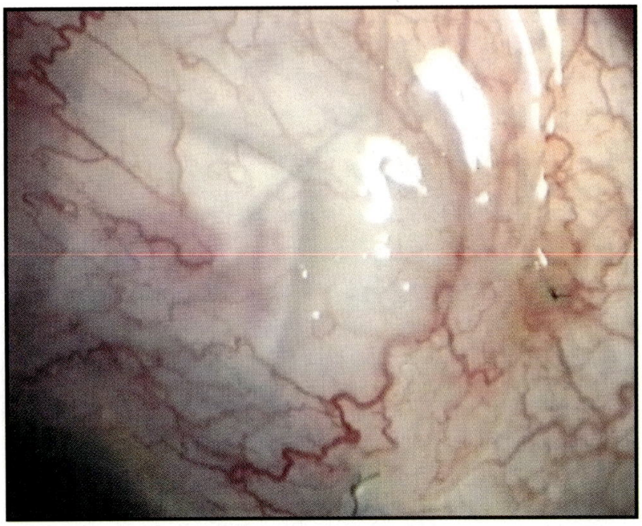

Figure 31.15: The diffuse filtering bleb as appeared at the end of the 6th month in group II

injected into the Schlemm canal, and the procedure was completed without the use of collagen device or mitomycin C at any stage of the surgery in our series.

Follow-up

Patients were scheduled for follow-up visits at 1 day, 1 week then 1, 3 and 6 months after surgery. The post-operative evaluation included the IOP, presence of functioning bleb, gonioscopy, visual acuity status and possible surgical and postoperative complications.

RESULTS

The study performed by the authors included 41 eyes (41 patients). The mean age of the patients was 67.9 ± 10.9 (range 50 to 80) years. The preoperative diagnoses had confirmed that all eyes have medically uncontrolled primary open-angle glaucoma. The mean pre-operative cup/disc ratio was 0.7 ± 0.25. The mean angle grading as reported by gonioscopic findings was 3.6 ± 0.61 according to shaffer grading system.

The eyes were divided into 2 groups: group I (20 eyes) underwent milling procedure and group II (21 eyes) underwent combined procedure, milling and phacoemulsification procedures. In both groups the milling procedure was done without the use of collagen device or MMC. The other eye of each patient was operated by conventional deep sclerectomy and combined phaco and deep sclerectomy and their results are behind the scope of this chapter.

The past medical history of the patients included hypertension in 36 percent patients, and one patient had history of diabetes mellitus. Among the eyes included in the study, 23.7 percent had history of cataract extraction and IOL implantation, 7.2 percent had history of previous glaucoma surgery (deep sclerectomy). Preoperative history of anti-glaucoma therapy is shown in Figures 31.16A and B.

The study included 16 eyes (10 right and 6 left) of 13 patients. The mean age of the patients was 67.9 ± 10.9 (range 50 to 80) years. The patients included female, and 8 male. All eyes were diagnosed as having primary open angle glaucoma medically uncontrolled. Only one eye 1/16 (6.25%) had a previous unsuccessful glaucoma surgery (deep sclerectomy). The data of the 6th month postoperative visits are available for 100 percent of the eyes, and those for the 1st year follow up visits are available only for 37.5 percent of the eyes.

Group I (Milling Procedure)

Visual results and refractive results of this group: refer to Table 31.1. Intraocular pressure (IOP) and its results during the study are shown in Table 31.2. Figure 31.17 shows the IOP results of both groups during the follow-up period of the study.

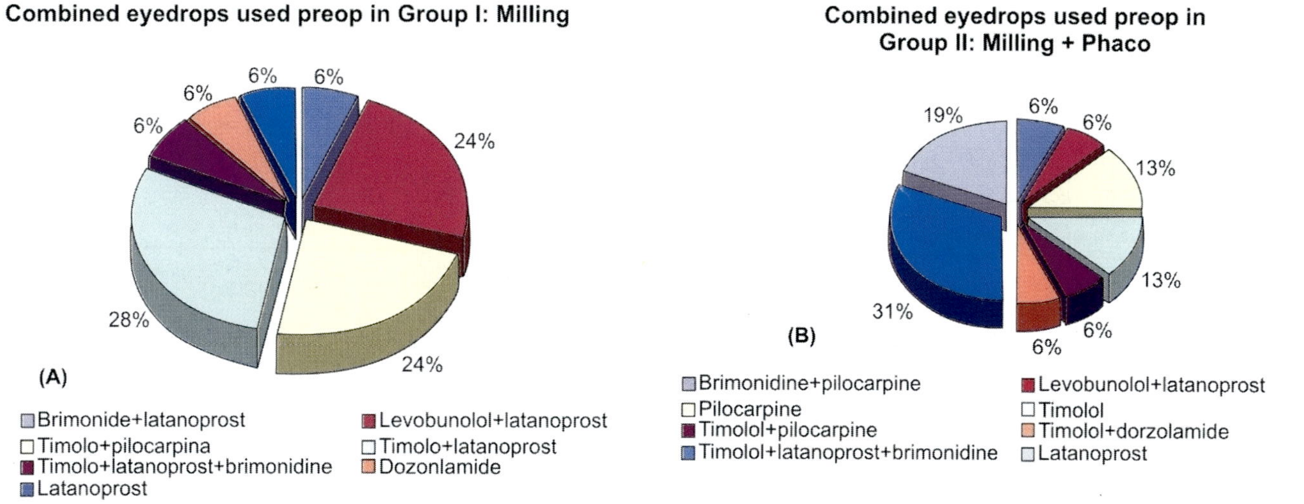

Figures 31.16A and B: Graph showing the percent of pre-op combination of anti-glaucoma treatment in (A) GI and (B) GII

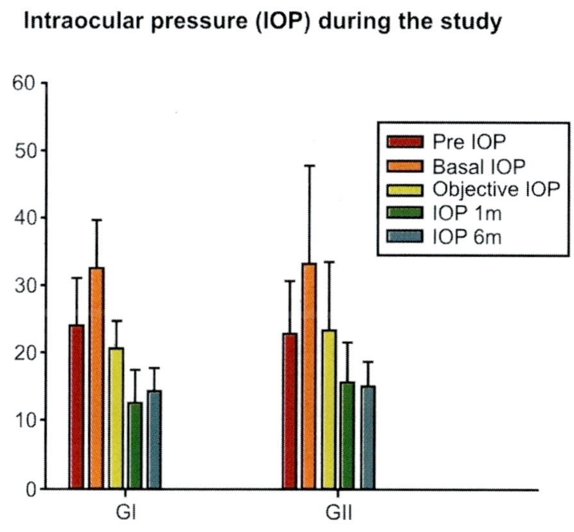

Figure 31.17: Graph showing the IOP changes during the follow-up period in both groups

Group II (Milling Procedure Combined with Phaco)

Visual results and refractive results of this group: refer to Table 31.3. Intraocular pressure (IOP) and its results during the study are shown in Table 31.4. Figure 31.17 shows the IOP results of both groups during the follow up period of the study.

DISCUSSION

Non-penetrating glaucoma surgeries including visco-canalostomy and deep sclerectomy are difficult to perform, need a high learning curve and time consuming. In both non-penetrating glaucoma surgeries and milling surgery, both the postoperative recovery and follow up are faster and the level of IOP reduction achieved is satisfactory when compared with the results of trabeculectomy.

Milling trabeculoplasty in this prospective, pilot study on 41 eyes has showing good results as it led to a 30 to 40 percent reduction of IOP in both groups operated with the technique. The percent of success of surgery at the 6th month without the use of collagen device or MMC was 60 percent for group I and 80 percent for group II (Figure 31.18). The rate of postop

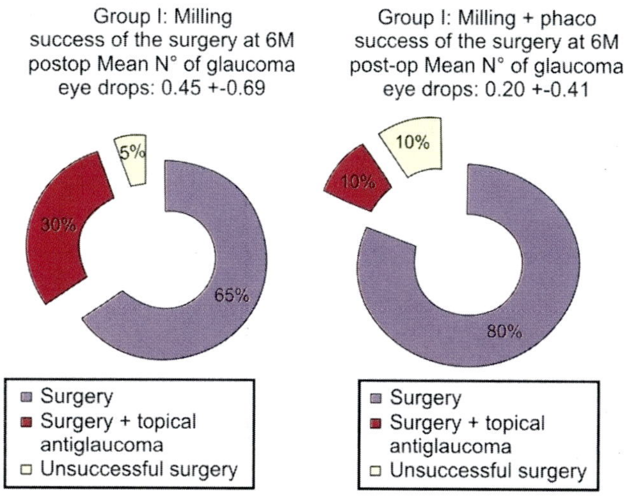

Figure 31.18: Graph showing the percent of success of milling surgery and milling-phaco after 65 months, the percent of eyes that had to use topical treatment and eyes that had to go back to treatment as the target pressure was not reached

Table 31.1: Shows the results of group I, milling trabeculoplasty

Group 1: Milling trabeculoplasty		*N*	*Mean ± SD*	*Standard error*	*Range*	
					Maximum	*Minimum*
Pre-op refraction	BCVA		0.828 ± 0.279	0.0624	1	0.05
	Sphere		0.025 ± 0.648	0.145	1.5	−1.5
	Cylinder	20	−0.675 ± 1.067	0.239	0	−4
	SE		−0.313 ± 0.512	0.115	0.5	−1.5
	Defocus equivalent		0.725 ± 0.786	0.176	2.500	0.000
Post-op refraction at 1M	BCVA		0.792 ± 0.258	0.0578	1	0.05
	Sphere		−0.025 ± 0.858	0.192	1.25	−2
	Cylinder	20	−0.0875 ± 2.507	0.561	10	−3
	SE		−0.069 ± 1.302	0.291	4.5	−2.25
	Defocus equivalent		0.713 ± 0.762	0.170	2.500	0.000
Post-op refraction at 6M	BCVA		0.835 ± 0.262	0.0587	1	0.05
	Sphere		0.1 ± 0.357	0.0799	1	−0.5
	Cylinder	20	−0.713 ± 0.964	0.216	0	−4
	SE		−0.257 ± 0.336	0.0752	0.13	−1
	Defocus equivalent		0.625 ± 0.750	0.168	3.000	0.000

Table 31.2: Shows the results of IOP in group I, milling trabeculoplasty

Variable	*N*	*Mean ± SD*	*Standard error*	*Range*	
				Maximum	*Minimum*
Initial IOP	20	23.9 ± 7.166	1.602	50	16
Basal IOP	20	32.640 ± 7.151	1.599	50.0	22.0
Objective IOP	20	20.650 ± 3.99	0.894	26.60	14.4
IOP at 1m	20	12.65 ± 4.945	1.106	22	2
Reduction IOP at 1 m	20	−7.994± 5.853	1.309	6.50	−15.95
% Reduction IOP at 1 m	20	47.205 ± 15.039	3.282	88.89	19.23
IOP at 1m	20	14.45 ± 3.379	0.756	24	10
Reduction IOP at 6 m	20	−6.200± 4.148	0.928	1.5	−14.6
% Reduction IOP at 6 m	20	36.821 ± 17.252	3.765	64	−5.26

bleb fibrosis and the use of postop anti-glaucoma therapy was found to be similar to that found with deep sclerectomy.

The followings are the potential advantages of the Milling trabecuoloplasty over the non-penetrating glaucoma surgeries:

1. Facilitate the surgical procedure of non- penetrating technique as the refining is carried anteriorly and down until the roof of Schlemm's canal can barely be visible. Unlike deep non-penetrating sclerectomy, this technique does not require any specific accuracy in the dissection of the deep sclera.
2. To reduce the wound healing as a determinate factor for the IOP outcome as the diamond powder tip is available for more delicate maneuvers like removing debris, making the technique ideal and leaving an extremely smooth bed.
3. Offers less complications than deep sclerectomy and it prevents the "double-cut" sclera and hazards.
4. The economic coast of the drill.

Table 31.3: Shows the results of group II, milling trabeculoplasty plus phacoemulsification at the same session

Group I1: Milling + Phaco		*N*	*Mean ± SD*	*Standard error*	*Range*	
					Maximum	*Minimum*
Pre-op refraction	BCVA		0.298 ± 0.217	0.0473	0.8	0.01
	Sphere		–2.821 ± 5.946	1.298	2.5	–16
	Cylinder	21	–1.012 ± 1.1	0.24	0.5	–3.25
	SE		–3.328 ± 6.17	1.346	1.25	–17.5
	Defocus equivalent		4.024 ± 6.339	1.383	19.000	0.000
Post-op refraction at 1M	BCVA		0.571 ± 0.313	0.0682	1	0.01
	Sphere		–0.464 ± 1.004	0.219	1.5	–2.5
	Cylinder	21	–1.179 ± 1.151	0.251	0	–4.5
	SE		–1.055 ± 1.247	0.272	0.5	–4.75
	Defocus equivalent		1.714 ± 1.603	0.350	7.000	0.000
Post-op refraction at 6M	BCVA		0.636 ± 0.304	0.0663	1	0.05
	Sphere		–0.238 ± 0.835	0.182	1.5	–1.5
	Cylinder	21	–1.19 ± 0.898	0.196	0	–3
	SE		–0.835 ± 0.867	0.189	0.5	–3
	Defocus equivalent		1.524 ± 1.006	0.220	4.500	0.000

Table 31.4: Shows the results of IOP in group II, milling trabeculoplasty plus phacoemulsification at the same session

Variable	*N*	*Mean ± SD*	*Standard error*	*Range*	
				Maximum	*Minimum*
Initial IOP	21	22.952 ± 7.619	1.663	42	10
Basal IOP	21	33.310 ± 14.487	3.161	65.1	13.0
Objective IOP	21	23.319 ± 10.154	2.216	25.2	6
IOP at 1m	21	15.762 ± 5.761	1.257	38	10
Reduction IOP at 1m	21	–7.546 ± 9.047	1.974	6.9	–27.9
% Reduction IOP at 1m	21	25.906 ± 28.22	6.017	56.67	-60
IOP at 1m	21	15.19 ± 3.473	0.758	23	10
Reduction IOP at 6m	21	–8.11± 8.607	1.878	6.9	–24.8
% Reduction IOP at 6m	21	27.91 ± 26.897	5.734	56	-60

5. Saves time as this technique has an easier approach to the trabeculodescemetic membrane.
6. No need for the use of high expensive surgical set.

CONCLUSION

Milling trabecuoloplasty is an evolving technique for easy scalpel-free non-penetrating glaucoma surgery. The milling surgery seems to be a promising technique for surgical management of POAG glaucoma. Milling trabeculoplasty is a fast, safe, effective technique to perform non-penetrating glaucoma surgery with low coast and simple instruments. Milling trabeculoplasty is a potential alternative to deep sclerectomy providing comparable results to conventional deep sclerectomy mainly the low level of IOP together with minimal intra and postoperative complications.

REFERENCES

1. Carassa RG. Non-penetrating surgery. In: Weinreb RN, Kitazawa Y, Krieglstein GK, (Eds). Glaucoma In the 21st century. Philadelphia: Harcourt Health Communications, 2000;249-56.
2. Watson PG, Grierson I. Early trabeculectomy in the treatment of chronic open-angle glaucoma in relation to histological changes. In: Zimmerman TJ, Monica ML, (Eds): Controversies in glaucoma. Int Ophthalmol Clin 1984;24: 13-32.
3. Zimmerman TJ, Kooner KS, Ford VJ, et al. Trabeculectomy vs. non- penetrating trabeculectomy: a retrospective study of two procedures in phakic patients with glaucoma. Ophthalmic Surg 1984;15:734-40.
4. Mermoud A. La sclerectomie profonde. Technique chirurgicale [Deep sclerectomy: surgical technique]. J Fr Ophtalmol 1999;22:781-6.
5. Bas JM, Goethals MJ. Non-penetrating deep sclerectomy preliminary results. Bull Soc Belge Ophtalmol 1999;272:55-9.
6. Carassa RG, Bettin P, Fiori M, Brancato R. Viscocanalostomy: a pilot study. Eur J Ophthalmol 1998;8:57-61.
7. Hara T. Deep sclerectomy with trabeculotomy ab externo: one-stage procedure. Ophthalmic Surg 1989;20:406-9.
8. Demailly P, Lavat P, Kretz G, Jeanteur-Lunel-MN. Non-penetrating deep sclerectomy (NPDS) with or without collagen device (CD) in primary open-angle glaucoma: middle-term retrospective study. Int Ophthalmol 1996-97; 20:131-40.
9. Demailly P, Jeanteur-Lunel MN, Berkani M, Ecoffet M, Kopel J, Kretz G, et al. La sclerectomie profonde non-perforante associee a la pose d'un implant de collagene dans le glaucome primitif a angle ouvert. Resultats retrospectifs a moyen terme (Non-penetrating deep sclerectomy combined with a collagen implant in primary open-angle glaucoma. Medium-term retrospective results). J Fr Ophtalmol 1996;19:659-66.
10. Chiou AG, Mermoud A, Hediguer SE, Schnyder CC, Faggioni R. Ultrasound biomicroscopy of eyes undergoing deep sclerectomy with collagen implant. Br J Ophthalmol 1996;80:541-4.
11. Tixier J, Dureau P, Becquet F, Dufier JL. Sclerectomie profonde dans le glaucome congenital. Resultats preliminaries (Deep sclerectomy in congenital glaucoma. Preliminary results). J Fr Ophtalmol 1999;22:545-8.
12. Rodriguez Prats JL, Alio JL, Galal A. Milling trabeculoplasty for non-penetrating glaucoma surgery. J cataract Refract Surg 2004;30:1507-16.
13. Goldsmith JA, Ahmed IK, Crandall AS. Non-penetrating glaucoma surgery. Ophthalmol Clin North Am 2005; 18:443-60.
14. Dahan E. Long-term results of deep sclerectomy with collagen implant. J Cataract Refract Surg 2005;31:868-9.

32

Sclerothalamotomy ab interno: A Minimally-invasive Surgical Option for Glaucoma

Bojan Pajic (Switzerland)

INTRODUCTION

The ongoing devote on recent developments in glaucoma surgery reflects that an ideal solution is not available which would promise long-term IOP reduction and eliminate the necessity of supplementary pressure-reducing medication at low complication rates. Trabeculectomy, first described in the sixties,[3,9,30] is probably the most widespread approach in glaucoma surgery presently. The intention of trabeculectomy is to bypass the resistance of trabecular meshwork by channelling aqueous humor directly to the Schlemm's canal. In literature the success rate of trabeculectomy ranges between 32 to 96 percent.[1,4,9,12,14,16-18,21-23,30,32-35] On the other hand, postoperative complications like hypotony and choroidal detachment are reported up to 24 percent.[6] Variation of success rates may be explained by different criteria of surgical indications, selection of cases, various diagnoses, the various degrees of surgical experience and variations in postoperative medical treatment. Failure of pressure regulations is associated with the assence of a filtering bleb and depends on the duration of follow-up involved. It has become evident that successful reduction in IOP following trabeculectomy is clearly related to the presence of a filtering bleb.[26]

The more recent method of non-penetrating deep sclerectomy, was first described by Fjodorov in the eighties.[8] This techniques tries to achieves an improved uveoscleral outflow, and therefore, is not depending on the presence of a filtering bleb. Koslov[13] expanded this method by introducing a collagen implant. Literature on non-penetrating deep sclerectomy indicates a success rate of 58 to 74 percent without collagen implant and 74 to 90 percent with collagen implantation.[5, 24]

In 1976, Benedikt[2] described that the exposure of the ciliary body (i.e. a form of penetrating sclerectomy) was leading to successful long-term IOP regulation in 27 of 38 cases involving hemorrhagic, aphakic and irreversible angle-closure glaucoma after initially failed filtering surgery. This technique was the basis for later development of perforating deep sclerectomy, a method which has been used since 1985 was described previously[20] as "*sclerothalamectomy.*" Bypassing of the trabecular meshwork is an alternative for aqueous humor outflow from the anterior chamber to the Schlemm's canal. It is the principal mechanism for non-penetrating glaucoma surgery, in particular, for deep sclerectomy and visco-canalostomy. These surgical procedures provide effective IOP reduction as well as the elimination of typical filtration bleb complications.[7,15,31] So far clinical application of these procedures has been limited by technical difficulties to perform this kind of surgery and a poor predictability of pressure reduction.

The concept of trabecular meshwork bypass as a surgical principle for glaucoma treatment evolved from the discovery that pathologic outflow resistance is caused primarily by the juxtacanicular conjunctive tissue of the trabecular meshwork and, in particular, by the inner wall of the Schlemm's canal.[10, 11] A further publication in this area indicates that 35 percent of the outflow resistance arises distally to the inner wall of the Schlemm canal.[25]

Spiegel et al[29] have described a new surgical technique involving the use of an implanted tube, the so-called trabecular meshwork bypass tube shunt, which should provide a direct connection between Schlemm canal and the anterior chamber. This surgical technique avoids technical difficulties of non-penetrating deep sclerectomy, especially the delicate microperforation of the trabecular meshwork in order to ensure the permeability of the Descemet's membrane. Furthermore, these techniques avoid the disadvantages of filtration blebs.

All surgical procedures for glaucoma involving the creation of external access may be complicated by the risk of fibroblast proliferation and failure of filtration. The novel procedure published offers a chance to avoid some of the above-mentioned disadvantages. We refer to this technique as *sclerothalamotomy ab interno.*[19]

PATIENTS AND METHODS

Before beginning the clinical study phase, the tips used for the STT ab interno procedure were developed using a large number of pigs' eyes. The high-frequency diathermic technique was already very well known in the application for capsulorhexis in cataract surgery. It was important to create a design for optimal application of the STT probe in the iridocorneal angle and to evaluate the charcteristic of the achieved deep sclerotomy. By virtue of this results the STT ab interno probe development as describe below.

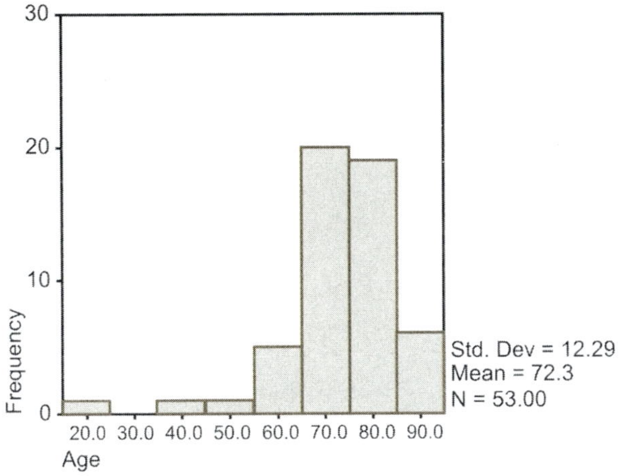

Figure 32.1: Mean age

Fifty-three sclerothalamotomies ab interno in 53 patients were carried out in primary open-angle glaucoma between 1 April 2002 and 31 July 2002. Main inclusion criterion into this study was an insufficient response to medical treatment of IOP. Data was documented according to a prospective study protocol. Mean age of patients was 72.3 ± 12.3 years (range: 15-92 years) (Figure 32.1). Seventeen patients (32%) were female, 36 patients (68%) male. In 25 cases (47.4%) the right eye in 28 cases (52.6%) the left eye was treated. There was no patient who received bilateral surgery. Snellen visual acuity was 0.7±0.3 (range 0.1 to 1.0) preoperatively. In 5 cases a moderate cataract was observed which didn't have influence on the visual acuity.

A complete ophthalmologic status check was carried out in each patient prior to surgery including: uncorrected and best-corrected visual acuity, IOP applanation tonometry, biomicroscopy of anterior segment, funduscopy (in particular, stereoscopie evaluation of the optic nerve head) and computerized visual field testing (Octopus 101, program G2).

Complete ophthalmologic follow-up examinations were carried out postoperatively at day 1, 2, 3 and 4, after 1, 2 and 4 weeks, and 2, 3, 6, 12, 15, 18, 21, 24, 27, 30, 33 and 36 months.

In a pilot study with at least of 24 months follow-up, 5 patients with therapy-resistant juvenile glaucoma were treated.

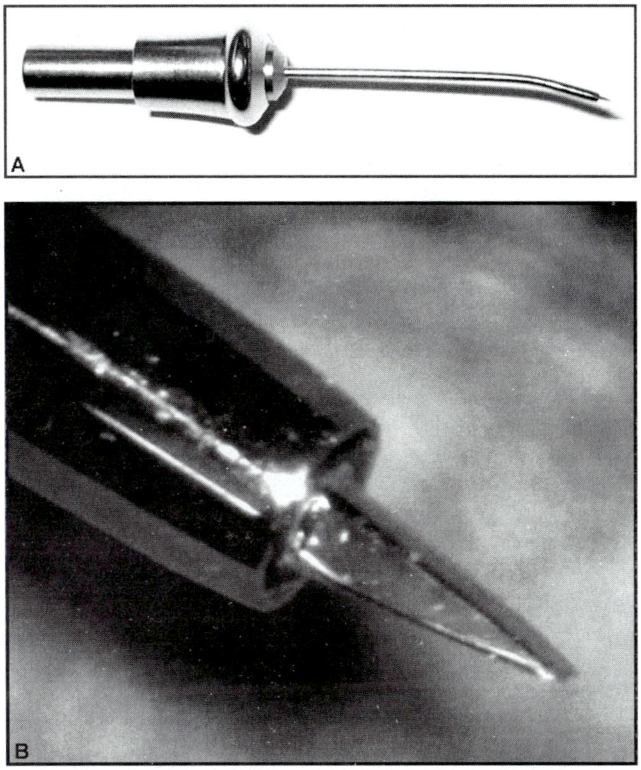

Figures 32.2A and B: STT glaucoma tip (Oertli Reference VE 201750)

HIGH-FREQUENCY DIATHERMIC PROBE

The high-frequency diathermic probe consists of an inner platinum electrode which is isolated from the outer coaxial electrode. The platinum probe tip is 1 mm in length, 0.3 mm high and 0.6 mm width and is bent posteriorly at an angle of 15° (Figures 32.2A and B). The external diameter of the probe measures 0.9 mm. Modulated 500 kHz current generates a temperature of approximate 130°C at the tip of the probe. The setup provides high frequency power dissipation in close vicinity of the tip. As a result, heating of tissue is locally very limited and is applied as a rotationed ellipsoid.

SURGICAL PROCEDURE

A clear cornea incision (1.2 mm wide) was placed in the temporal upper quadrant using a diamond knife. A second corneal incision was performed 120° apart from the first followed by injection of Healon GV. The high-frequency diathermic probe (Oertli) was inserted through

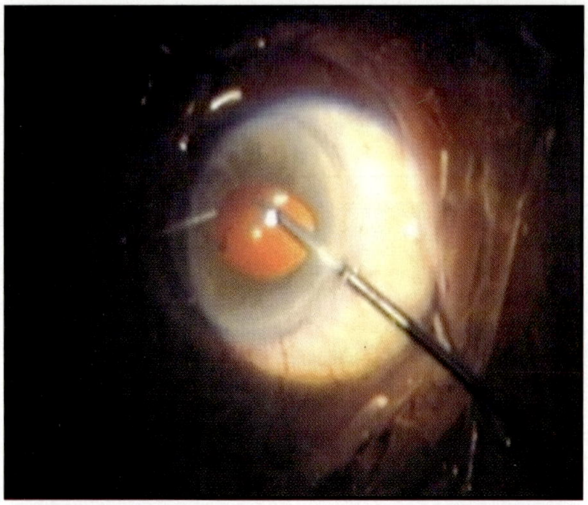

Figure 32.3: Insertion of the high-frequency diathermic probe (Oertli) through the temporal corneal insertion

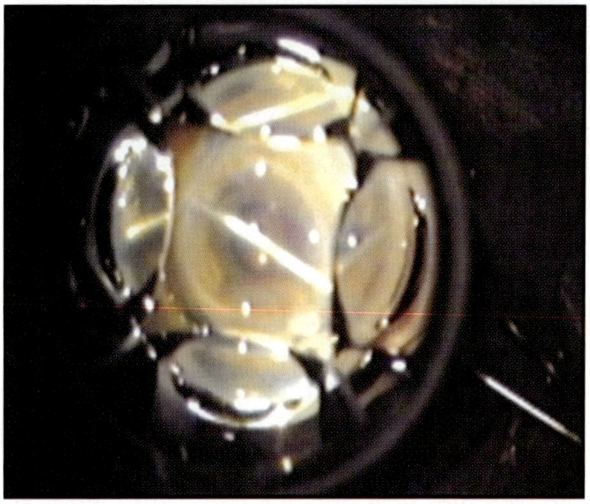

Figure 32.4: Visual inspection of the target zone (opposite iridocorneal angle) by a 4-mirror gonioscopic lens

the temporal corneal insertion (Figure 32.3). Visual inspection of the target zone (opposite iridocorneal angle) was observed by a 4-mirror gonioscopic lens (Figure 32.4). The high-frequency tip penetrates up to 1mm nasal into the sclera through the trabecular meshwork and Schlemm canal, forming a deep sclerotomy (i.e. "thalami") of 0.3 mm high and 0.6 mm width (Figures 32.5 and 32.6). This procedure was repeated 4 times within one quadrant. Healon GV was evacuated from the anterior chamber with bimanual irrigation/aspiration (Figure 32.7). Tobramycin/Dexamethason eye drops were then applied 3X daily for 1 month and Pilocarpin 2 percent eye drops 3X daily for 10 days.

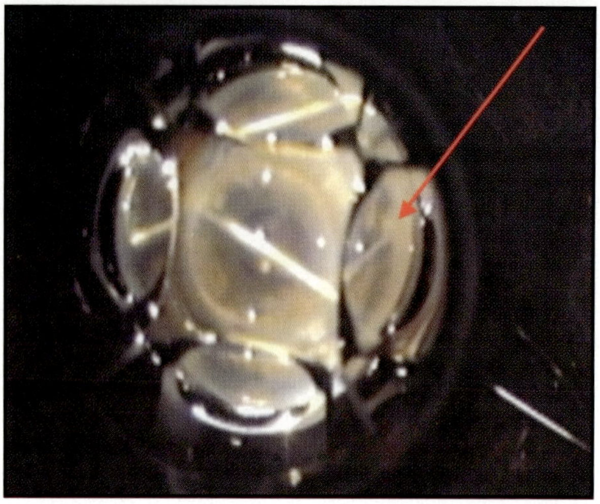

Figure 32.5: Penetration of the high-frequency tip

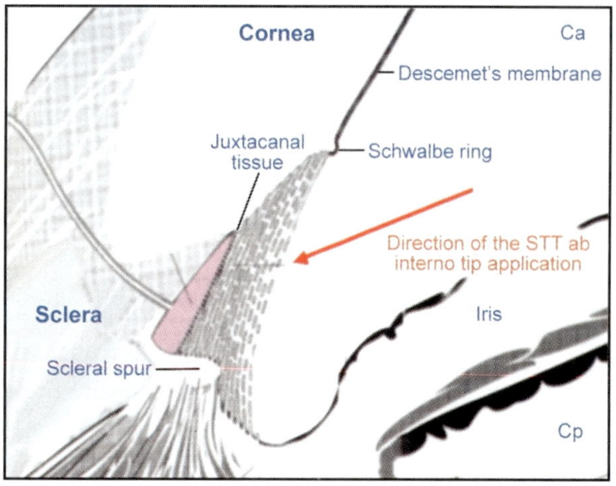

Figure 32.6: Penetration up to 1 mm nasal into the sclera through the trabecular meshwork and Schlemm's canal

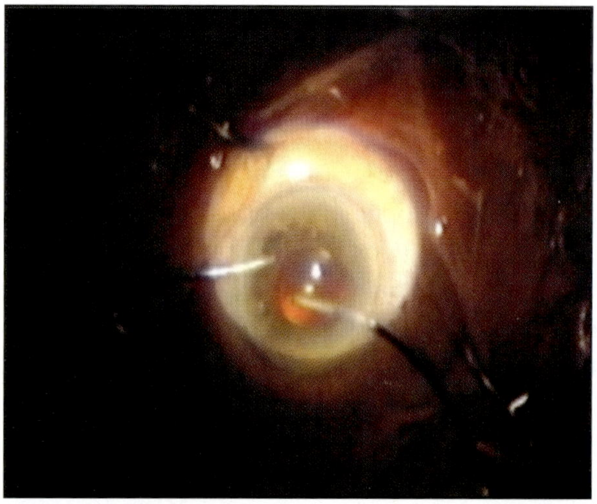

Figure 32.7: Healon GV was evacuated from the anterior chamber with bimanual irrigation/aspiration

EVALUATION OF THE RESULTS

Statistical evaluation of results was calculated with SPSS Program Version 10. Two-tailed Student t-test was used for statistical evaluation of parametric data. The unit of significance was set at a critical p value of <0.05, including Bonferroni correlation for repetitive use of data sets.

RESULTS

Mean preoperative IOP in the study population of 53 patients with primary open-angle glaucoma was 25.6 ± 2.3 mm Hg (range18 to 48 mm Hg). Average IOP was 17.6 ± 2.7 mm Hg (range 2 to 36 mm Hg) after a follow-up period of 1 day, 14.9 ± 2.4 mm Hg (range 2 to 30 mm Hg) after 2 days, 15.7 ± 2.4 mm Hg (range 4 to 28 mm Hg) after 3 days, 16.0 ± 2.6 mm Hg (range 4 to 36 mm Hg) after 4 days, 19.0 ± 2.6 mm Hg (range 12 to 39 mm Hg) after 7 days, 16.9 ± 2.5 mm Hg (range 9 to 44 mm Hg) after 1 month, 15.1 ± 1.8 mm Hg (range 11 to 20 mm Hg) after 3 months, 14.7 ± 1.7 mm Hg (range 11 to 20 mm Hg) after 6 months, 14.8 ± 1.7 mm Hg (range 10 to 20 mm Hg) after 9 months, 14.7 ± 1.7 mm Hg (range 10 to 20 mm Hg) after 12 months, 15.5 ± 1.7 mm Hg (range 11 to 20 mm Hg) after 15 months, 14.1 ± 1.6 mm Hg (range 11 to 20 mm Hg) after 18 months, 16.5 ± 1.7 mm Hg (range 12 to 22 mm Hg) after 21 months, 15.0 ± 1.6 mm Hg (range 11 to 20 mm Hg) after 24 months, 14.7 ± 1.7 mm Hg (range 11 to 20 mm Hg) after 27 months, 14.7 ± 1.7 mm Hg (range 10 to 20 mm Hg) after 30 months, 15.5 ± 1.7 mm Hg (range 11 to 20 mm Hg) after 33 months and 14.6 ± 1.7 mm Hg (range 10 to 20 mm Hg) after 36 months a result which, at p<0.005, is statistically highly significant (Figure 32.8). Pressure reduction at any time of standardised follow up was statistically significant compared to preoperative data at a level of a<0.03 (Bonferroni corrected). For all patients the follow-up was 36 months.

At month 36, 54.7 percent of patients had an IOP<15 mm Hg, 77,4 percent had an IOP<18 mm Hg and 83 percent had an IOP<21 mm Hg (Figure 32.9). After 36 months, 86.8 percent achieved >20 percent reduction in IOPs and 77 percent of treated patients achieved >30 percent reductions of the IOP. The complete success rate, defined as an IOP lower than 21 mm Hg without medication, was 83 percent at 36 month. Qualified success rate, defined as an IOP lower than 21 mm Hg with medication, was 100 percent at 36 month (Figure 32.10).

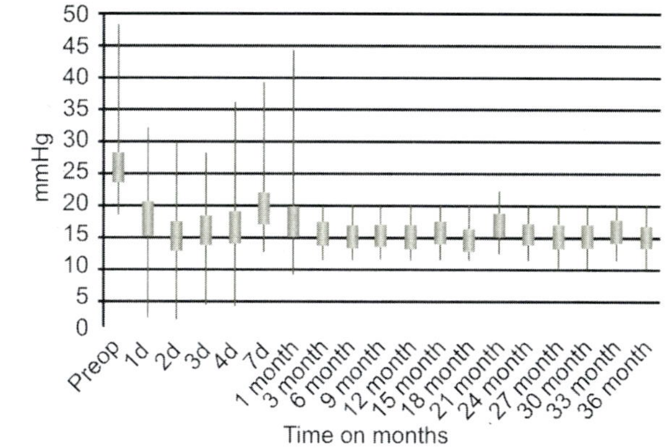

Figure 32.8: Average level of intraocular pressure (IOP) after Sclerothalamotomy (STT) ab interno surgery for all 53 cases at the time of scheduled examination

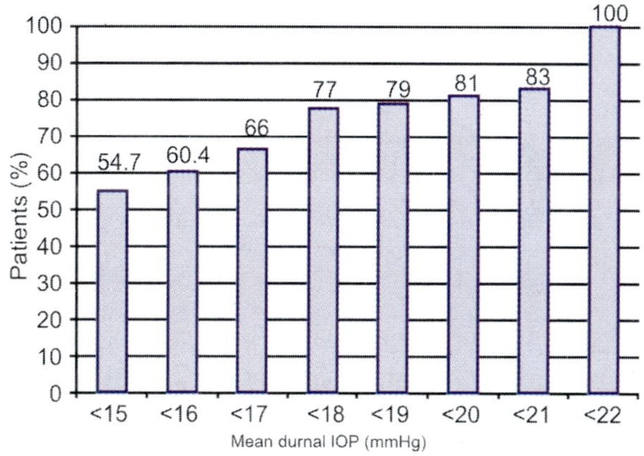

Figure 32.9: Percentages of patients reaching specified intraocular pressure (IOP) levels

The average preoperative administration of pressure-reducing eye agents was 2.6 ± 1.0. Following surgery, this value was decreased to 0.45 ± 0.72 after 1 month, 0.38 ± 0.60 after 3 months 0.38 ± 0.69 after 6 months, 0.19 ± 0.52 after 12 months, 0.21 ± 0.53 after 24 months and 0.50 ± 0.90 after 36 months (Figure 32.11). After 36 months, it was necessary to administer IOP reducing medication in only 9 eyes, a figure which corresponds to 17 percent of all cases.

Average visual acuity after treatment was 0.69 ± 0.31 (range 0.05 to 1.0). In 6 eyes (11.3%) moderate cataract

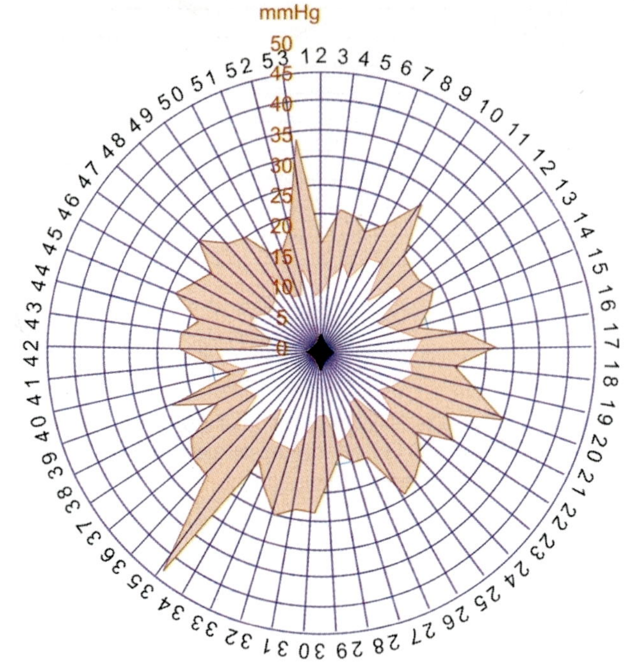

Figure 32.10: Preoperative and postoperative level of IOP 36 months of follow-up

development after surgery which was without influence of visual acuity. Another 3 eyes (5.7%) developed cataract with decreased visual acuity of one Snellen line. There is no significant difference regarding the cup/disc ratio at baseline with 0.65±0.18 and at 36 months with 0.66±0.19 (p=0.11) (Figures 32.12A and B).

There is no significant changes comparing the visual field at baseline with mean defect MD 9.45±2.32, loss variance LV 30.0±5.11 and at 36 months with MD 9.29±2.59, LV 31.4±5.66 (p=0.78 for MD, p=0.96 for LV) (Figure 32.13).

Temporary IOP elevation higher than 21 mm Hg was observed in 12 of 53 eyes (22.6%). These patients responded well to pressure-reducing treatment with one agent and medication could gradually be withdrawn in all of these patients. A single case of hypotension (1.9%) that lasted for 3 days after surgery was observed. Hyphema was present in 6 cases (11.4%) which disappeared within the first 2 weeks after surgery. One eye (1.9%) exhibited transient fibrin formation at pupillary level. Fibrin was cleared within one day after frequent application of topical Dexamethason (Figure 32.14).

In a pilot study 5 patients with therapy-resistant juvenile glaucoma were treated. We observed an IOP reduction from 41 ± 6.4 mm Hg prior to surgery to 12 ± 2.6 mm Hg after surgery, a result that has remained stable without any additional pressure-reducing therapy for 24 months.

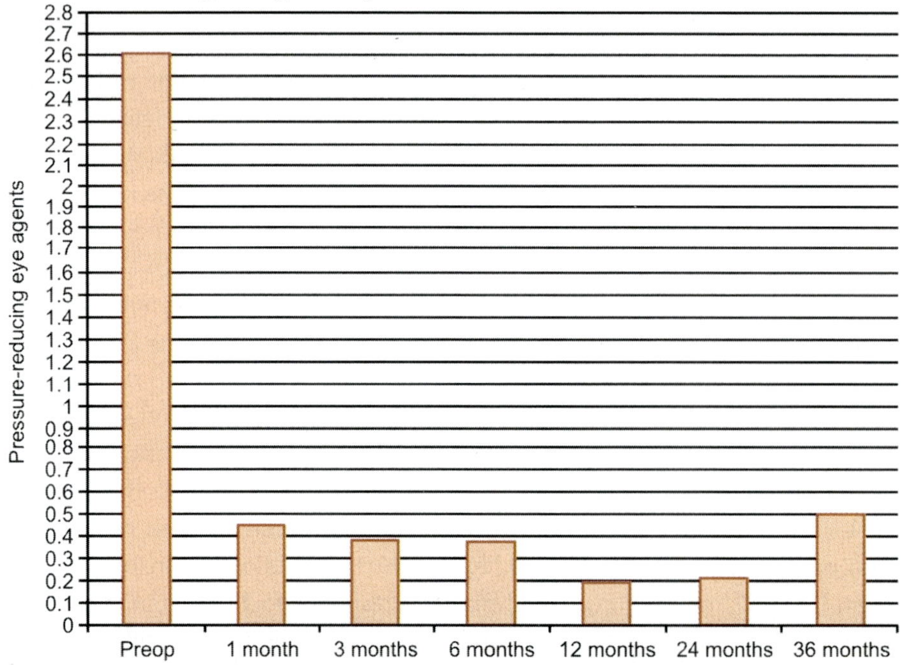

Figure 32.11: Administration of pressure-reducing eye agents during 36 months

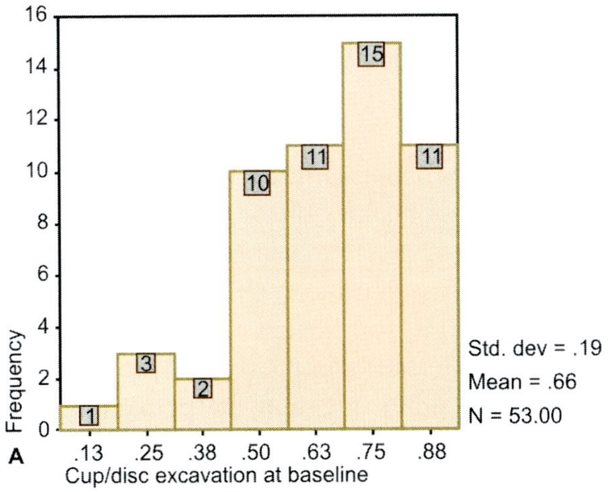

Figure 32.12A: Cup/disc ratio at baseline

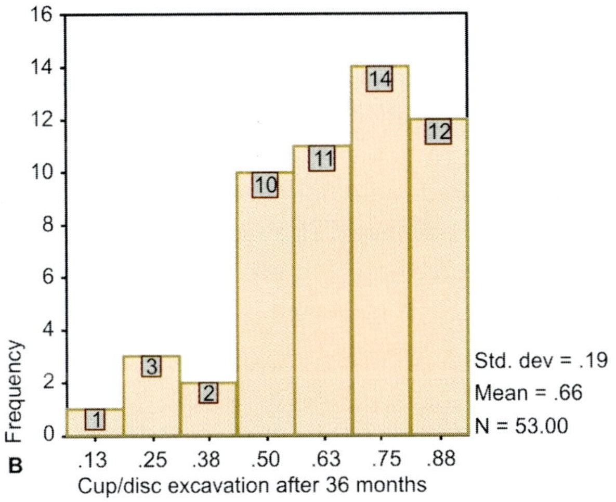

Figure 32.12B: Cup/disc ratio at 36 months

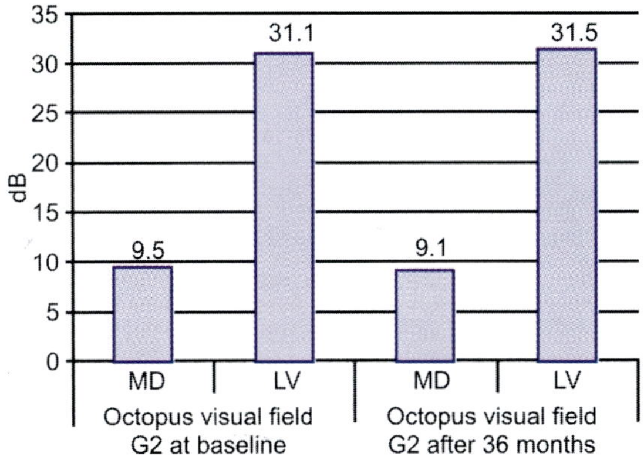

Figure 32.13: Visual field analysis

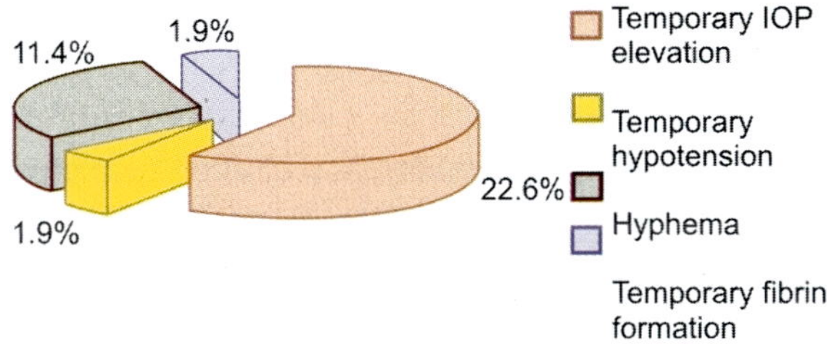

Figure 32.14: Complications after sclerothalamotomy (STT) ab interno surgery

DISCUSSION

This study reports long-term results of a new surgical technique for treating open-angle glaucoma. The STT ab interno method intends the creation of a direct channel between the anterior chamber and the Schlemm's canal. Persistence of the sclerotomy can be investigated with a 3-mirror Lens (Goldmann 903). The STT ab interno tip creates a deep sclerotomy with subsequent access of aqueous to the scleral layer. Both aspects may facilitate a bypass effect of aqueous outflow. In light of the fact that about 85 percent of the aqueous humor drains (in physiological terms) transtrabecularly, we suspect an additional route for aqueous humor absorption in the case of elevated IOP. There is evidence in literature that such bypass effects may be present after surgical intervention which do not lead to the formation of filtering blebs. In a previous study,[20] it was ascertained that eyes without filter bleb exhibited very stable long-term IOP regulation postoperatively. In addition to the bypassing of trabecular outflow resistance caused by STT ab interno treatment, outflow resistance may be further reduced by scleral thinning at the base of the thalamus. In addition to that aqueous humor could perhaps be absorbed by the ciliary body.[20,27] After early postoperative reduction, the average IOP continued to decline gradually over a period of 6 months before reaching a relatively a constant level. It can be speculated that newly formed blood vessel and lymph vessel close to the surgical site, may contribute to the decrease of IOP level during follow up.[2]

In literature the success rate range for trabeculectomy ranges between 57 percent and 96 percent,[1,4,9,12,14-18,21-23,30,32-35] for deep sclerectomy without collagen device between 57 percent and 74 percent, and for deep sclerectomy with collagen device between 58 percent and 90 percent.[1,5,15,24] The STT ab interno technique with a complete success rate of 90.6 percent is comparable with other so far published surgery methods.

Advantages of the STT ab interno method, compared with trabeculectomy and perforating and non-perforating deep sclerectomy seem to be a rate of postoperative complications and a constant level of reduced IOP. Hypotension, a frequent finding in trabeculectomy, perforating deep sclerectomy and non-perforating deep sclerectomy, is a relatively rare postoperative complication. The most frequent early complications in trabeculectomy are hyphaema (24.6%), shallow anterior chamber (23.9%), hypotony (24.3%), wound leak (17.8%) and choroidale detachment (14.1%). The most frequent late complications are cataract (20.2%), visual loss (18.8%), iris incarceration (5.1%) and encapsulated bleb (3.4%). After STT ab interno cataract development was seen in 17 percent with only 5.7 percent loss of one line of visual acuity after 36 months. Compared with other techniques STT ab interno seems to be a relatively save surgical technique.[1,5,6,7,15,16]

Transient IOP elevation after STT ab interno may occur in the first 6 weeks and can be effectively brought under control with the use of a topical medication. In most cases, IOP-reducing therapy could be gradually withdrawn after 3 weeks post surgery. It was necessary to continue pressure-reducing therapy in 5 of 53 eyes, in all this cases medication was effective in controlling IOP.

Problems of scarring to the Tenon's capsule, fibroblast proliferation and secondary occlusion associated with trabeculectomy which are induced by the surgical procedure itself may the reason behind the practice of antimetabolites applications (Mitomycin C at concentration of 0.2-0.4 mg/ml for 1-5 minutes). Although this practice was conceived to modulate wound healing and thus to counteract scar formation, it often resulted in serious complications, such as scleral necrosis and an increased incidence of avascular filter bleb and their late complications.[28] The surgical procedure applied in this study avoids stimulation of episcleral and conjunctival proliferations and may therefore be related with less secondary cell invasion at the filtrating bypass.

Preliminary histological investigations of post mortem human eyes following STT ab interno did not indicate signs of indirect necrosis in cell layers adjacent to the thalamus formed by high-frequency diathermy. It is yet unknown, if the inner surface of the thalamus will be covered by endothelial cells of corneal or trabecular origin, and whether the thalamus and its function will remain intact on a much longer time scale.

Avantages to STT ab interno include the comparative simplicity and quickness of the surgical procedure itself.

This study point out, that the performance of 4 thalami has so far proved sufficient, what corresponds to a resorption surface area of 2.4 mm^2. The number of 4 thalami was defined empirical. Regarding the results of this study the creation of 4 thalami seems to provide a sufficient long-term decrease of IOP as a low rate of postoperative complications. For a further potentiality of IOP decreasing effect we recommend to perform up to 6 thalami.

A randomized multicentre study will be conducted in the future to compare STT ab interno, trabeculectomy, and deep sclerectomy for the surgical treatment of primary open-angle glaucoma.

REFERENCES

1. Akafo SK, Goulstine DB. Long-term post-trabeculectomy intraocular pressure. Acta Ophthalmologica 1990;70:312–6.
2. Benedikt O, Hiti H. Die Ziliarkörperfreilegung. Eine neue Operationsmethode zur Behandlung des irreversiblen Winkelblockglaukoms und des Aphakieglaukoms. Klin Monatsbl Augenheilkd 1976;169:711-6.
3. Burian HM. A case of Marfan's syndrome with bilateral glaucoma. With a description of new type of operation for developmental glaucoma (trabeculotomy ab externo). Am J Ophthalmol 1960;50:1187-92.
4. Cairns JE. Trabeculectomy. Preliminary report of a new method. Am J Ophthalmol 1968;66:673-9.
5. Demailly P, Lavat P, Kretz G, et al. Non-penetrating deep sclerectomy with or without collagen device in primary open-angle glaucoma: middle-term retrospective study. Int Opthalmol 1997;20:131-40.
6. Edmunds B, Thompson JR, Salmon JF, et al. The National Survey of Trabeculectomy. III. Early and late complications. Eye 2002;16:297-303.
7. El Sayyad F, Helal M, El-Kholify H, et al. Nonpenetrating deep sclerectomy versus trabeculectomy in bilateral primary open-angel glaucoma. Ophthalmology 2000;107:1671-4.

8. Fjodorov SN, Loffe DI, Ronkina TI. Deep sclerotomy: technique and mechanism of new glaucomatous procedure. Glaucoma 1984;6:281-3.
9. Fronimopoulos J, Lambrou N, Pelekis N, et al. Elliot's trepanation with scleral cover (procedure for protecting the fistula in Elliot's trepanation with a lamellar scleral cover). Klin Monatsbl Augenheilkd 1970;156:1-8.
10. Grant WM. Experimental aqueous perfusion in enucleated human eyes. Arch Ophthalmol 1963;69:738-801.
11. Johnson DH, Johnson M. How does nonpenetrating glaucoma surgery work? Aqueous outflow resistance and glaucoma surgery. J Glaucoma 2001;10:55-67.
12. Konstans AGP, Jay JL, Marshall GE, et al. Prevalence, diagnostic feature, and response to trabeculectomy in exfoliation glaucoma. Ophthalmology 1993;100:619-27.
13. Kozlov VI, Bagrov SN, Anisimova SY, et al. Non penetrating deep sclerectomy with collagen. Ophthal Surg 1990;3:44-6.
14. Mermoud A, Salmon JF, Barron A, et al. Surgical management of posttraumatic angle recession glaucoma. Ophthalmology 1993;100:634-42.
15. Mermoud A, Schnyder CC, Sickenberg M, et al. Comparison of deep sclerotomy with collagen implanta and trabeculectomy in open-angle glaucoma. J Cataract Refract Surg 1999;25:323-31.
16. Mills KB. Trabeculectomy: a retrospective long-term follow-up of 444 cases. Br J. Ophthalmol 1981;65:790-95.
17. Molteno ACB, Bosma NJ, Honours BSc, et al. Otago glaucoma surgery outcome study. Ophthalmology 1999;106: 1742-50.
18. Morell AJ, Searle AET, O'Neill EC. Trabeculectomy as an introduction to intraocular surgery in an ophthalmic training program. Ophthalmic Surg 1992;23:38-9.
19. Pajic B, Pallas G, Gerding H, Böhnke M. A novel technique of ab interno glaucoma surgery: follow-up results after 24 months. Graefes Arch Clin Exp Ophthalmol 2005;19:1-6.
20. Pallas G, Pajic B 1999. Die Sklerothalamektomie (STE): Stabile postoperative Augendruckregulierung beim Offenwinkel- und Kapselhäutchenglaukom. Klin Monatsbl Augenheilkd 2000;216:256-60.
21. Popovic V, Sjöstrand J. Long-term outcome following trabeculectomy: Visual field survival. Acta Ophthalmologica 1991;69:305-9.
22. Roth SM, Spaeth G, Starita RJ, et al. The effects of postoperative corticosteroids on trabeculotomy and the clinical course of glaucoma: Five-year follow-up study. Ophthalmic surg 1991;22:724-9.
23. Saiz A, Alcuaz A, Maquet JA, et al. Pressure-curve variations after trabeculectomy for chronic primary open-angle glaucoma. Ophthalmic Surg 1990;21:799-801.
24. Sanchez E, Schnyder CC, Sickenberg M, et al. Deep sclerectomy: Results with and without collagen implant. Int Ophthalmol 1997;20:157-62.
25. Schuman JS, Chang W, Wang N, et al. Excimer laser effects on outflow facility and outflow pathway morphology. Invest Ophthalmol Vis Sci 1999;40:1676-80.
26. Schwartz AL, Anderson DR. Trabecular surgery. Arch Ophthalmol 1974;92:134-8.
27. Schwenn O, Dick B, Pfeiffer N. Trabekulotomie, tiefe Sklerektomie und Viskokanalostomie. Ophthalmologe 1998;95:835-43.
28. Singh J, O'Brien C, Chawla HB. Success rate and complications of intraoperative 0.2 mg/ml Mitomycin C in trabeculectomy surgery. Eye 1995;9:460-66.
29. Spiegel D, Kobuch K. Trabecular meshwork bypass tube shunt: initial case series. Br J Ophthalmol 2002;86:1228-31.
30. Starita RJ, Fellmann RL, Spaeth GL, et al. Short- and long-term effects of postoperative corticosteroids on trabeculectomy. Ophthalmology 1985;92:938-46.
31. Sunaric-Megevand G, Leuenberger PM. Results of viscocanalostomy for primary open-angle glaucoma. Am J Ophthalmol 2001;132:221-8.
32. Tanihara H. Surgical effects of trabeculectomy ab externo on adult eyes with primary open angle glaucoma and pseudoexfoliation syndrome. Arch Opthalmol 1993;111: 1653-61.
33. Vernon SA, Spencer AF. Intraocular pressure control following microtrabeculectomy. Eye 1995;9:299-303.
34. Watson PG, Barnett F. Effectiveness of trabeculectomy in glaucoma. Am J Ophthalmol 1975;74:831-45.
35. Watson PG. When to operate an open angle glaucoma. Eye 1987;1:51-4.

33

Open-Angle Filter Surgery for Glaucoma Deep Sclerocanalostomy (DSC): A New Technique

- HISTORY
- ANATOMO-PHYSIOLOGY
- SURGICAL TECHNIQUE IN OUTPATIENT SURGERY
- MANAGEMENT
- COMPLICATIONS

Jerome Bovet (Switzerland)

HISTORY

The goal of all surgery for glaucoma is to lower the ocular pressure in order to reduce postoperative risk as much as possible.

Surgical techniques using perforation have several postoperative disadvantages.

A certain number produce complications such as hyphema, flat anterior chamber, choroid detachment, cataract, and endophtalmitis,

Non-penetrative surgical techniques do not have the post-operative complications of the first, penetrative, surgery, but they are more difficult to carry out. An exact knowledge of the microanatomy of the region is important and a learning curve necessary.

The main drawbacks with these new techniques are that they are less effective with weak hypertensions, and, importantly, they increase the number of times the operation needs to be performed due to poor healing and flap collapse.

1909 Elliott's trepanation

1960 Burian's trabeculectomy,[7] Sugar 1961[26]

1968 Cairn's trabeculectomy for open angle glaucoma[8]

1962 Krasnov's Sinusotomy: this technique aims to remove the external wall of the Schlemm Canal[15]

1984 Zimmermann: Non-penetrating trabeculectomy[28]

1984 Fiodorov and Koslov suggest the term 'non-penetrating deep sclerectomy' (NPDS)[12]

1990 Koslov improves his technique by adding a collagen implant into the base of the flap. At the same time, many others tried different types of implants to increase the duration of the drainage life of the aqueous humour.[14]

1991 Arenas: *Archila Trabeculotomy ab externo*. Areans uses the same technique but employs the help of a trepan to open the Schlemm Canal[1]

1999 Stegman: *Viscocanalostomy* The author proposes a dissection and an injection of viscous fluid into the Schlemm's canal.[20]

ANATOMO-PHYSIOLOGY

Goldman[13] demonstrated by using manometric experiments, the main point of resistance to the drainage of the aqueous humour was situated between the anterior chamber and the Schlemm's canal.[23] Nowadays, it is generally accepted that 75 percent of drainage resistance is situated at the level of the endothelium of the Schlemm's canal and of the trabeculum network.[21]

New techniques: The new techniques of filtering non-perforating are all connected with dissection or injection of the Schlemm's canal.

Krasnov[15] proposes the sinusotomy removing the endothelium of the Schlemm's canal using micro-dissection: The principle of deep sclerectomy is to dissect the internal wall of the Schlemm's canal where the greatest resistance to drainage of the aqueous humor is situated, thus allowing a physiological filtration, since the external wall is kept intact.

The technique of using high viscosity to widen the Sclemm's canal, allows better filtration of aqueous humor.

The biggest drawback of these techniques, above all deep sclerectomy, is the formation of fibrous tissue on the sclerotic flap.

Numerous authors have described a multitude of implants that would keep the space of the second flap free.[10,11,14,16,18,19,24]

We submit a new surgical technique which allows a synthesis of the three main surgical techniques for non-penetrative filter surgery. This reduces the risks of each, whilst increasing the long-term chances of success.[4]

SURGICAL TECHNIQUE IN OUTPATIENT SURGERY[17]

Local Anesthetic[5]

This anesthetic technique has been described in the previous chapter.

Let us remember that this local anesthetic allows—thanks to the patient's ability to participate—exposure of the operative field for dissection and its best, and variable angles of work.

Choices for Dissection

The path of dissection and flap's localisation are chosen to spare the penetrating vessels and to search for the zone that is the most avascular.

The draining vessels are on the surface, as shown by Stegmann.[21]

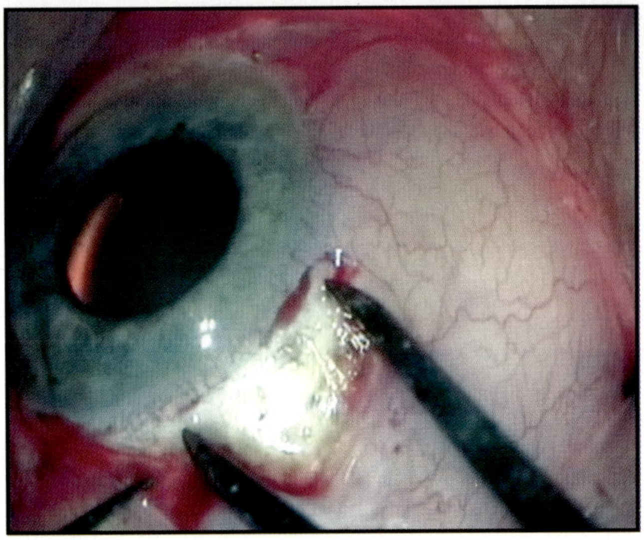

Figure 33.1A: Measure, the width being of less importance than the length

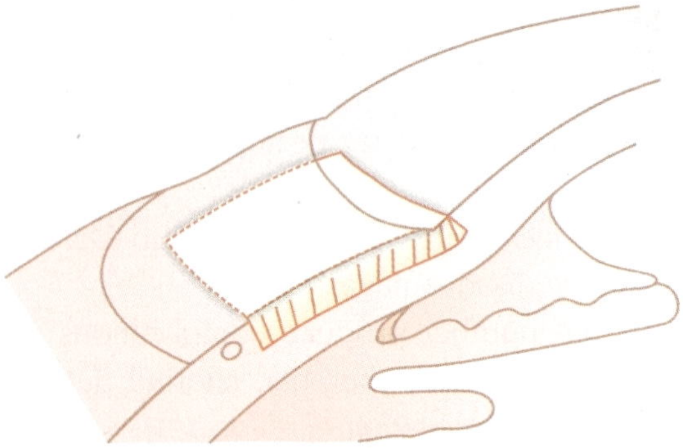

Figure 33.1B: The path of dissection and flap's localization are chosen to spare the penetrating vessels-Conjonctival flap at the limbus L shape

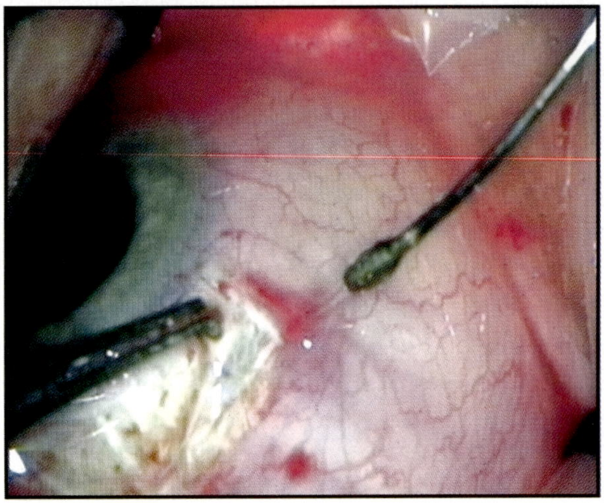

Figure 33.2A: Dissecting the first flap

The choice of the best place for the flap to spare the penetrating vessels to find the most avascular zone, one must not forget that the draining vessels are on the surface, as shown by Stegmann in his film.

Conjunctival Shutter with Limb

Stages are as follows:

- Dissection of the conjunctival shutter with limb, not less than 10 mm, with Vescoat scissors. Dissection in an L shape allowing the conjunctival flap to relax in the opening
- Exposing the sclera by dissecting Tenon's capsule with care (Figures 33.1A and B)
- Use the lightest possible electro coagulation in order to spare the draining vessels as much as possible.

1st Scleral Flap

Incision of the scleral flap (Figures 33.2A and B)

- 6 mm × 4 mm, the width being of less importance than the length
- Depth of 300 microns, cut with a 30° diamond (Meyco Switzerland) or with a diamond for KR (Meyco, Switzerland) up to the lames corneostromales.

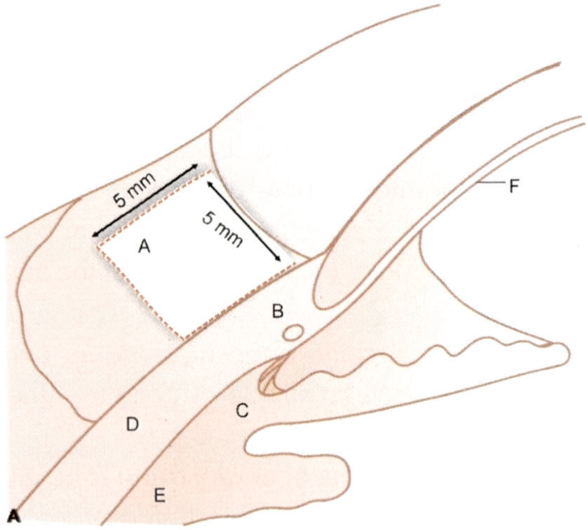

Figure 33.2B: A. First scleral flap 6 x 4 mm x 300 micron; B. Schlemm's canal; C. Scleral spur; D. Sclera; F. Descemet's membrane

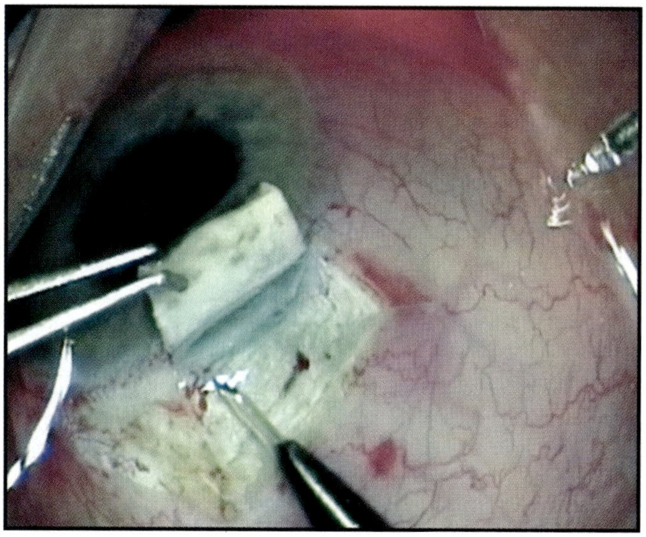

Figure 33.3: First flap's dissection to the stromal lamellae

It is important to make a flap which is thick enough not to tear when one arrives in the corneal stroma[6] (Figure 33.3).

It is important to dissect the lames corneennes, starting from the limb, the cut allowing more room when making the incision of the second flap.

2nd Scleral Flap

Five mm dissection, with a 30° diamond (Meyco, Switzerland), of the length of the second triangular flap of all the depth of the sclera leaving some lamelles sclerales in order to just reveal the choroidien tissue. This allows getting exactly at the scleral spur, at the beginning of Descemet's membrane (Figures 33.4A and B).

Dissection, holding on to the second flap, au tampon triangulaire pour repousser le stroma. Thus, we free Descemet's membrane. Those who practice deep lamellar keratoplasty ("keratoplastie lamellaire") operations will have no difficulty in finding the plane of dissection.

Separation of the Descemet from the stromal tissue is quite easy, so long as one is in the right plane.

The 1.5 mm incision in Descemet's membrane is made in order that the Sclemm's canal is not covered at the time of the cutting of the flap (Figure 33.5).

On this level, each side, in the scleral tissue, a slight bleeding can be seen at the cut in the drainage vein of the Schlemm canal (Figure 33.6).

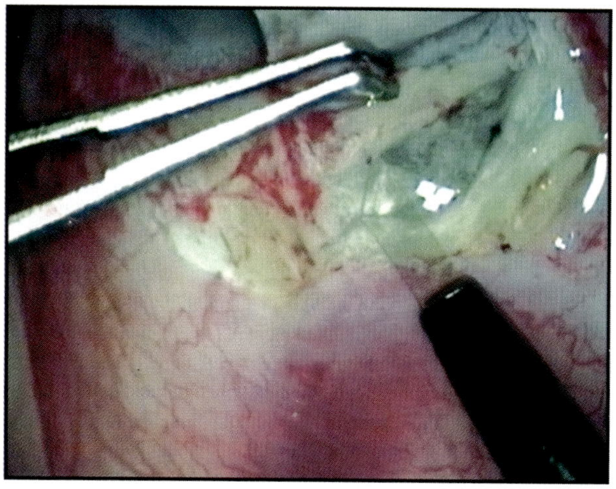

Figure 33.4A: Second flap's dissection

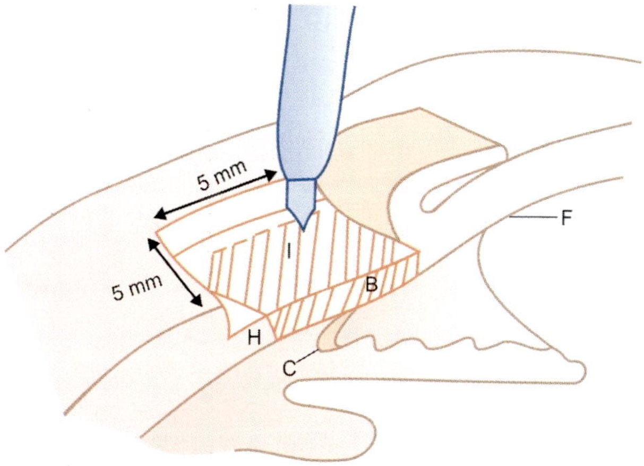

Figure 33.4B: Second triangular flap of all the depth of the sclera

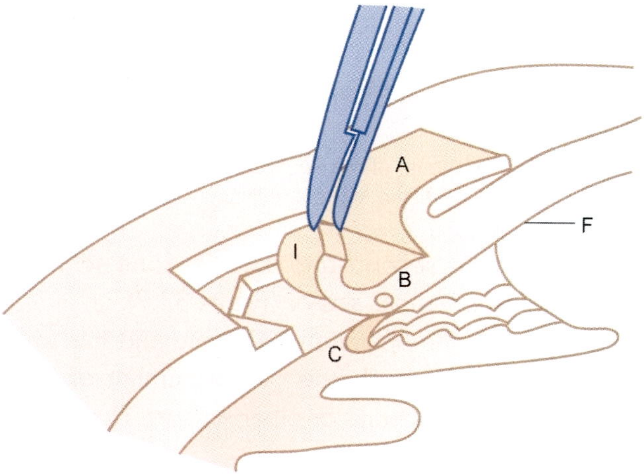

Figure 33.5: Second flap as to be deep enough. This allows getting exactly at the scleral spur, at the beginning of Descemet's membrane

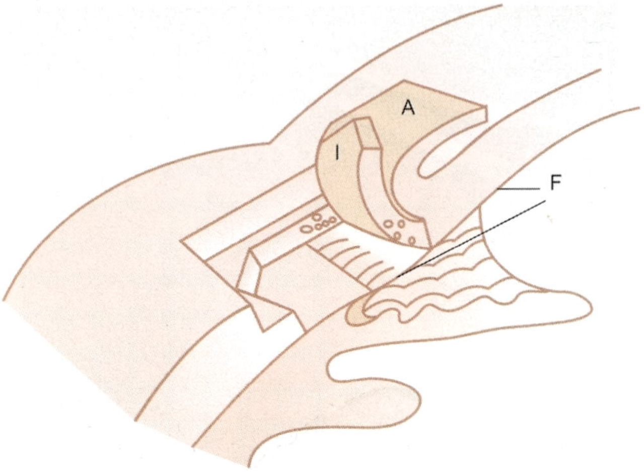

Figure 33.6: A slight bleeding can be seen at the cut in the drainage vein of the Schlemm's canal

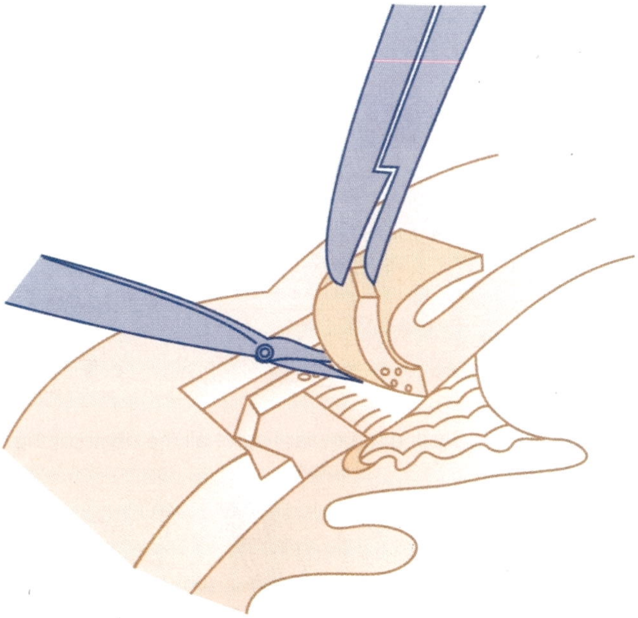

Figure 33.7: Removal of the second flap with the diamond or the Vannas scissor

Removal of the second flap This is done with the diamond or the Vannas scissor (Figure 33.7).

This part of the operation is delicate and has to be done with great care. Because, on a number of occasions, when using Vannas or other scissors, Descemet's membrane has been torn.

Cut up the scleral flap in half One-half is soaked for 5 minutes in 0.04 percent mytomicin, then rinsed.

Schlemm's canal dissection (Figures 33.8A and B).

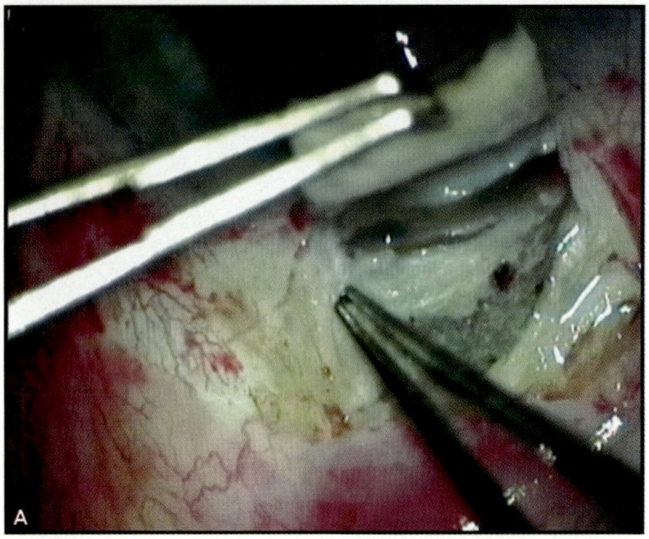

A

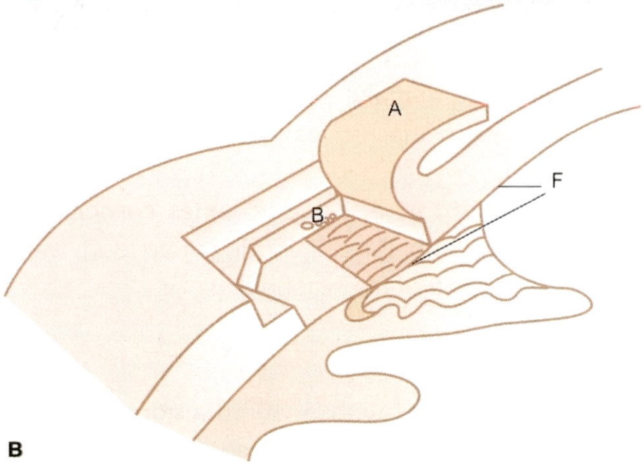

B

Figures 33.8A and B: Schlemm's canal dissection

Using Bonn forceps with microteeth, a 5 mm dissection of the interior wall of the Sclemm's canal is made, allowing us to see some seepage of the aqueous humor.

Canalostomy

The Schlemm's canal vein gives the location of the Sclemm canal. Introduction of an extra-fine Grieshaber cannula on both sides of the sclera of the Sclemm's canal until some resistance is felt. Slow injection of high viscosity viscous fluid (Healon, G V *AMO*) whilst removing the microcatheter (Figures 33.9 and 33.10).

Implant/Mitomycin C

Put in place, in the bed of the second flap, the previously prepared implant, the implant having been, beforehand, soaked in mitomycine and rinsed before being used.

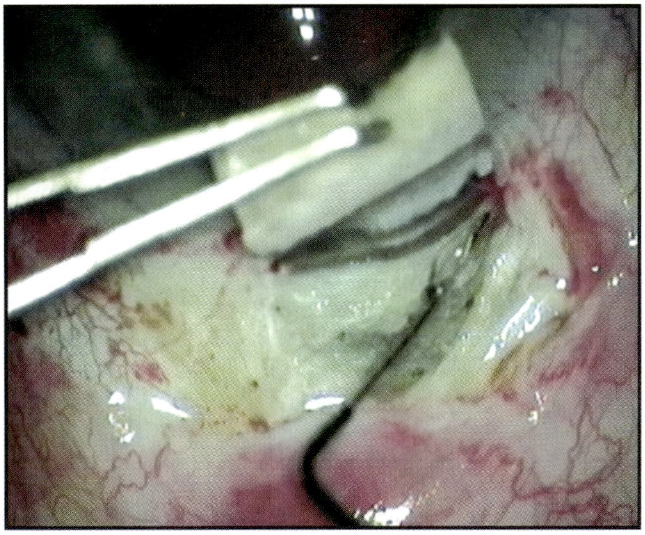

Figure 33.9: Canalostomy

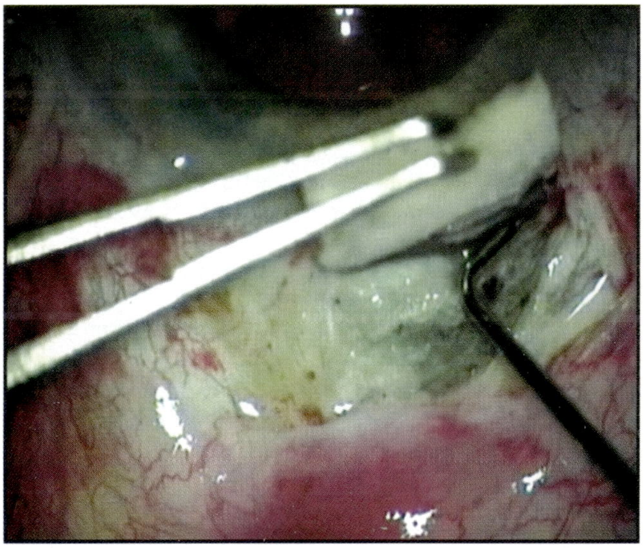

Figure 33.10: Introduction of an extra-fine Grieshaber cannula

Close the first flap with inverted stitches using nylon 10.0, at each corner of the flap pulling the stitches tight)Figure 33.11).

Close the conjunctive with 3 inverted stitches using 9.0 reabsorbable thread.

MANAGEMENT

Postoperative Treatment

As this operation is extraocular, done with ambulatory surgery and local anesthetic, there is no need to cover the eye with a dressing.

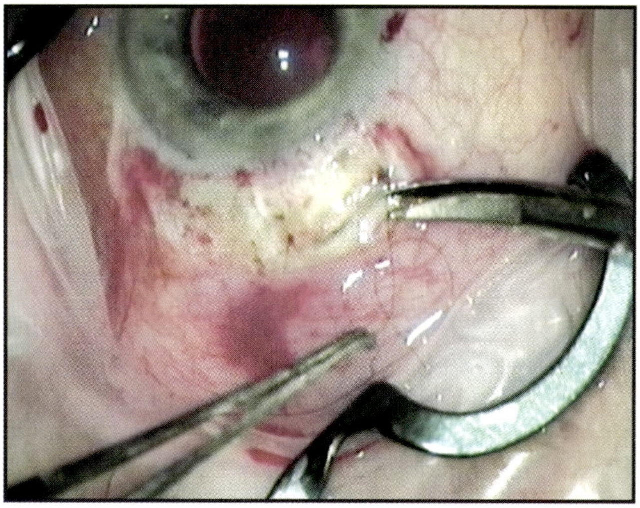

Figure 33.11: Closing the first flap

Patients are treated using eyedrops of cortisone and antibiotics.

The dose is 1 drop 3 x a day for 3 weeks.

Postoperative Checkups

The postoperative follow-up must be rigorous,

The patient is checked, one hour after the operation, before leaving the clinic, after 1 day, 1 week, and 1 month.

Usually, all eye hypotensor treatments are stopped, even if it's necessary for them to be re-introduced at a later date.

The filtration bubble that is found when trabectomy is used, does not exist using this technique. As a result, the patient has to be checked controlling the ocular tension in both the eyes. If possible, the measure has to taken each time at the same hour, in order to avoid obtaining distorted results because of the curve of the nychthemeral ocular pressure.

Patients who are cortisone respondant need particularly special attention.

Continuous checkups to control post-operative pressure are necessary in cases of glaucoma.

It is extremely important to check the pre- and post-operative pressures in the two eyes at the same times.

COMPLICATIONS

Perioperative Complications

The most frequent complication is rupture of the Descemet's membrane when dissecting the second scleral flap: the rupture happens after the scleral spur and, especially, after the removal with diamond or Vannas scissors.

If this happens, it will be necessary to convert the deep sclerectomy into trabeculectomy without viscocanalostomy, whilst not forgetting to make an iridectomy.

When the canalostomy is done, the viscous fluid can leak into the anterior chamber. In the hours following the operation, this will cause a rapid increase in the intraocular pressure. The operation will have to be reviewed, by carrying out a paracentesis, emptying the viscous fluid and rinsing the anterior chamber.

The other possible complication is the perforation of the choiroid, which has no postoperative importance.

Postoperative Complications

The most frequent complication from using this technique is increased postoperative pressure, more or less long-term, due to the collapse or closing up healing of the scleral flap on the bed of the operation. This is the reason why many authors have proposed different types of implants which very in the rapidity of their reabsorbtion.

Our technique uses an autograft from the sclera, soaked in mitomycin C^2 which inhibits all fibrocyte proliferation. This produces the best results in the long term and the lowest costs. When, after this operation, pressure increases occur rarely, they can still happen after 3 to 4 years.

If there is a recurrance, nowadays we favour repeating the procedure in a more favorable quadrant. We have never had to repeat this operation more than twice.

We have stopped doing trabeculopasty au YAG for patients who have increased pressure after three weeks, this technique not having brought the expected results.

We do no longer convert our deep sclerocanalostomy into a trabeculectomy, because the complications were too important.

REFERENCES

1. Arenas E.Trabeculectomy ab externo. Highlights of Ophthamol.World Atlas Series 1993;1:216-8.
2. Arenas E. The routine use of mytomycine in trabeculectomy ab externo using a modified drill technique. Highlights of Ophthamol. World Atlas Series 1993;2:236-7.
3. Baumgartner JM, Bovet J, Baumgartner A. Etude de la stabilisation de la plaie opŽratoire et de la rapidité de la récupération fonctionnelle dans la chirurgie de la cataracte: Comparaison des résultat entre quatre techniques chirurgicales différentes. Ophtalmologie 1995;9:624-5.
4. Bovet J. Deep lamellar sclerectomy, what's new. Eye Advance Mumbay India (abstract). Chairmann Keiki Metha August 2004.
5. Bovet J, Baumgartner JM, Bruckner JC, Ilic V, Achard O. L'anesthésie topique en chirurgie oculaire et sa préparation. In Safran AB, Landis T, Dayer P (Eds): Les Dimensions de la douleur en ophtalmologie. Paris Masson, 1998;166-73.
6. Bovet J, Molnar I, Baumgartner JM, Failla F, Tabatabay C. combined glaucoma and cataract surgery (phacotrabeculectomy). European Ophtalmic Society (abstract), SOE 1997, Budapest.
7. Burian HM, Allen L. Trabeculotomy ab externo. A new glaucoma operation : technique and results of experimental surgery. Amer J Ophthalmol 1962;53:19-26.
8. Cairns JE. Trabeculectomy; prelimminary report of a new method. Amer J Ophthalmol 1968;66:673.
9. Chiou AGY, de Courten C, Bovet J. Pseudophakic ametropia managed with a phakic posterior chamber intraocular lens. J Cataract Refract Surg 2001;27:1516-8.
10. Chiou AGY, Mermoud A, Underahl PJ, Schnyder CC. An ultrasound biomicroscopic study of eyes after deep sclerectomy with collagen implant. Ophtalmology 1998;105(4):104-8.
11. Demailly P, Jeanteur-Lunel MN, Berkani M, et al. Non penetrating deep slerectomy associated with collagen device in primary open angle glaucoma. Middle term retrospective study. J Fr Ophtalmol 1996;19(11):659-66.
12. Fyodorov SN, Ioffe DI, Ronkina TI. Deep sclerectomy: technique and mechanism of a new glaucomatous procedure. Glaucoma 1984;6:281-383.
13. Goldmann H. Drainage of aqueous in man. Ophthalmologica 1946;112:11-146.
14. Koslov VI and all. Non-penetrating.deep sclerectomy with collagen. IIRTC Eye Microsurgery. RSFSR Ministry of Public Health,Moscow 1990;3:44-6.
15. Krasnov MM. Externalization of Schlemm's canal (sinusotomy) in glaucoma. Brit J Ophthalmol 52:157-61.
16. Kershner RM. Nonpenetrating trabeculectomy with placement of collagen drainage device. J Cataract Refract Surg 1995;21(6):608-11.
17. Krasnov MM. Externalisation of Schlemm's canal (sinusotomy) in glaucoma. Br J Ophtalmol 1968;52:157-61.
18. Lebuisson DA, Bovet JJ. Le concept opératoire pour patients ophtalmologiques ambulants in Laroche L, Lebuisson DA, Montard M Chirurgie de la cataracte chap 6 ed Masson 1996;61-74.

19. Massy J, Gruber D, Muraine M, Brasseur G. Nonpenetrating deep sclerectomy: collagen implant and viscocanalostomy procedures. Bylsma S Int Ophtalmol Clin Summer; 1999;39(3):103-19.
20. Kozlov VI, Bagrow SN, Anisimova SY, et al. Deep sclerectomy with collagen. Eye Microsurgery 1990;3:44-46.
21. Stegmann RC. Viscocanalostomy: a new surgical technique for open angle glaucoma. An Inst Barraque, Spain 1995; 25:229-32.
22. Stegmann R, Piennaar A, Milller D. Viscocanalostomy for open-angle glaucoma in black African patients. J Cataract Refract Surg 1999;25(3):316-22.
23. Sampaolesi R. Glaucoma, 2n edition, 1991;525-26. Editorial Médica Panamericana, Buenos Aires, 1991.
24. Perkins ES.Pressure in the canal of Schlemm. Brit J Ophthalmol 1955;39:215-9.
25. Sourdille P, Santiago PY, Villian F, et al. Reticulated hyaluronic acid implant in nonperforating trabecular surgery. J Cataract Refract Sur 1999;25:332-9.
26. Sugar HS. Experimental trabeculotomy in glaucoma. Amer J Ophtalmol 1961;54:623-7.
27. Tanibara H, Negi A, Akimoto M, et al. Surgical effects of trabeculectomy ab externo on adults eyes with primary open angle glaucoma and pseudoexfoliation syndrome. Arch Ophtalmol 1993;111:1653-61.
28. Verges C, Llevat E. Non-penetrating deep sclerectomy (NPDS) with an Er: YAG laser.Clinical results after 16 months follow up ASCRS abstracts 2000;201.
29. Zimmerman ThJ, et al. Trabeculectomy vs. non penetrating trabeculectomy. A retrospective study of two procedures in phakic patients with glaucoma. Ophthalmic Surgery 1984;15:734-40.

34

Customized Laser-assisted Filtration Surgery (CLAFS) Using a Solid-State UV Laser

- NPDS: AN EVOLUTIONARY TECHNIQUE
- LASER-ASSISTED TECHNIQUE FOR THE FUTURE
- CUSTOMIZED LASER-ASSISTED FILTRATION SURGERY (CLAFS) WITH THE PR-270

JT Lin (USA), Vivek Kadambi (India)

INTRODUCTION

The aim of surgical management of open-angle glaucoma is to create an alternate channel for drainage of aqueous humor from the anterior chamber of the eye by surgical techniques collectively called "Filtration Microsurgery," or to open previously blocked trabecular meshwork with the help of lasers.

Many surgical procedures have been devised for chronic open-angle glaucoma. These include:

1. **Trabeculectomy (Figure 34.1):** This is the most commonly performed surgical technique and it involves making a surgical opening into the anterior chamber under a partial thickness scleral flap through which the excess fluid drains into the subconjunctival space.
2. **Argon/Diode (Thermal) Laser Trabeculoplasty:** 50- to 100 micron laser spots are aimed at the trabecular meshwork. The laser application results in a biological and mechanical reaction in the trabecular meshwork to open the previously blocked meshwork and increases the flow of aqueous fluid from the eye.
3. **Selective Laser Trabeculoplasty:** Reduces intraocular pressure by enhancing drainage of excess aqueous fluid. The laser increases drainage by selectively treating certain cell tissue of the trabecular meshwork.
4. **Non-penetrating Deep Sclerostomy (Viscocanulostomy):** This is a modification of trabeculectomy, wherein a full-thickness hole in the eye is avoided. Instead, a very deep dissection is performed in the sclera and trabecular meshwork.
5. **Tube-shunt:** These are synthetic drainage devices particularly useful in neovascular glaucoma, aphakic glaucoma and advanced developmental glaucoma. In most cases the treatment is palliative.

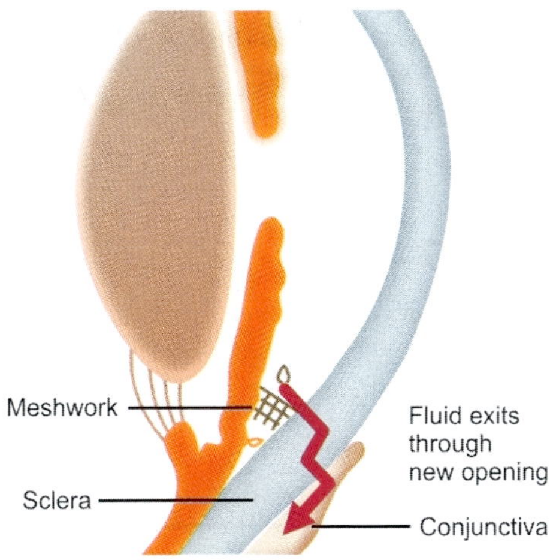

Figure 34.1: Aqueous drainage through sclerostomy and then via subconjunctival route in trabeculectomy

NPDS: AN EVOLUTIONARY TECHNIQUE

The ideal glaucoma surgery is that which can create adequate drainage to enable a controlled reduction of IOP without the risk of over-filtration while ensuring long-term patency of the filtration channel. Hence, we believe that the model around which all glaucoma surgeries should be conceptualized is the Non-penetrating deep sclerectomy (NPDS) or viscocanalostomy.[1-4] In this procedure the intraocular pressure is lowered as fluid oozes through a permeable thin layer of tissue, the trabeculo-Descemet's membrane. A bleb may be formed, but it is usually smaller than one that would be formed following trabeculectomy. The main advantage of this procedure is that it minimizes the chances of over-filtration. This avoids the complications of filtration blebs and the shallow anterior chamber seen after trabeculectomy.[17] In viscocanalostomy, the cut ends of the Schlemm's canal are expanded with sodium hyaluronate. However, the IOP lowering capacity of this procedure is less than that of conventional trabeculectomy and the chances of closure are high. Some surgeons place a lake of viscoelastic such as sodium hyaluronate or a collagen implant[5,6] under the scleral flap to reduce the chance of closure due to the natural process of healing.

The NPDS is fast gaining popularity among surgeons due to decreased incidence of postoperative complications when compared with conventional trabeculectomy. However, most surgeons find dissection of the trabecular meshwork and the scleral bed difficult to perform. The meticulous tissue excision is challenging even to the most skillful and experienced surgeon. Additionally, it is commonly reported by surgeons, that once aqueous percolation starts to occur during the course of tissue dissection, a significant amount of hypotony sets in, making the excision of tissue even more difficult. From the variable reports of clinical success, it is clear that this technique has a long-learning curve. Nevertheless, the potential opportunity to create a filtration procedure which successfully controls intraocular pressure in the absence of a prominent bleb is prompting innovators to improve upon the technique of NPDS.

Accelerated advancement in laser technology in the late 90's has been responsible for the widespread use of this hi-tech modality in ophthalmology and it's no surprise that investigators are aggressively exploring the potential of lasers to help evolve a more reliable version of NPDS. Technically, lasers with predominant *ablative* properties have the advantage of helping the surgeon remove precise amount of tissue with relative ease. This appears to be the critical factor responsible for ensuring consistency in the surgical technique.

LASER-ASSISTED TECHNIQUES FOR THE FUTURE

Many investigators evaluated the use of of the Holmium laser,[7] Nd: YAG,[8,9] Erbium YAG laser[10-12] and the Excimer laser[13-15] in an attempt to create a minimally-invasive controlled glaucoma procedure. The technique of non-penetrating filtering procedure, called sinusotomy was first introduced by Krasnov in 1969.[1,2] Zimmerman et al investigated non-penetrating trabeculectomy in 1984 and demonstrated a success rate of 83.7 percent after 1 year.[3,4] An increased success rate was demonstrated with collagen implants or sodium hyaluronate.[1-4] Injection of sodium hyaluronate into the canal of Schlemm was recommended to make the procedure more effective and the procedure was called viscocanalostomy.[16,17] Non-penetrating techniques reported lower rate of complications[1-4]as compared to conventional trabeculectomy or sclerostomies. However, it has been observed that most surgeons require extensive experience to master the technique of accurate dissection of the trabacular meshwork and the scleral bed. It is also difficult to control the amount of tissue to be excised even with the aid of specially designed surgical instruments. A pulsed laser, capable of ablating ocular tissue with high precision, is the obvious tool that can overcome this challenge. The laser should have cutting properties ideally-suited for corneal and scleral tissues and should be preferably available to the surgeon at the tip of an ergonomically designed hand piece.

Partial excimer laser sclerostomy and trabeculectomy has not gained wide acceptance due to inconsistent scleral ablative properties and lack of control arising from the non-availability of a suitable delivery system through a surgical hand piece. Pulsed Erbium: YAG laser was used to ablate scleral and corneal tissue layer by layer to create filtration channels.[18,19] Our own experience with the Er:YAG laser (unpublished studies) showed that the laser did produce significant co-lateral thermal damage. This would often lead to formation of coagulum at the tip of the fiber in the contact mode thus reducing the efficiency of subsequent ablation.

CUSTOMIZED LASER-ASSISTED FILTRATION SURGERY (CLAFS) WITH THE PR-270

The PR-270 pulsed laser (Figure 34.2) uses as it's source, the Nd:YAG laser crystal and nonlinear crystals to generate the 4th-harmonic at a UV wavelength of 266

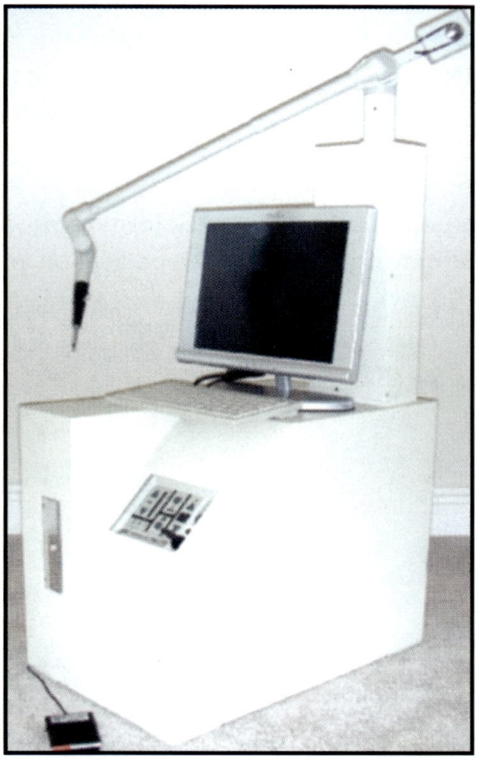

Figure 34.2: Picture of PR-270 UV laser with the "articulated arm" delivery system

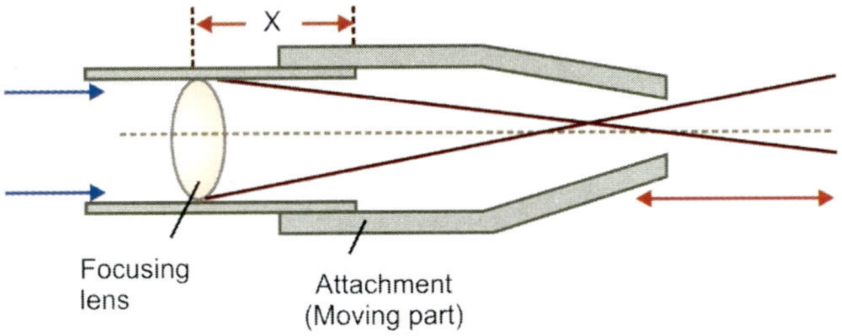

Figure 34.3: Schematics of the handpiece design for adjustable spot size on the treated surface by adjusting the distance of the attaching front end. "X" is the distance between the attached end piece and the position of the focal length

nm. It is very efficient in ablating tissues with high water content such as cornea and sclera. The laser is delivered through a specifically designed articulated arm coupled to a handpiece which delivers the UV laser energy via a focusing lens (Figure 34.3). The 5-nanosecond short-pulsed laser is focused to a spot size of about 0.6 mm on the treated area with energy per pulse of 5 to 7 mJ and operates at 10 to 20 Hz. Both, the pulse energy and frequency, are adjustable. We note that this 5 ns frequency of the laser is much shorter than the typical excimer laser (about 10 to 20 ns), Ho:YAG laser (about 200 microsecond) or Er:YAG (about 500 microsecond). Therefore it offers minimal thermal damage with effective tissue ablation. Furthermore, the focused UV laser spot may be as small as 0.3 mm if needed, an attribute which is not available with IR lasers. Being *non-contact* in its operation the laser overcomes two major disadvantages of the *contact fiber-based* lasers. Firstly, unlike contact ablative systems, one does not encounter progressive decrease in the efficiency of ablation due to accumulation of coagulum at the end of the fiber tip. Secondly, there is no apprehension about damage to the tips which, in the fiber based system, adds significantly to running cost.

Depending on the initial IOP and the target IOP we recommend different ab externo techniques of ablation:

1. **Linear radial sclerostomy (Figure 34.4A):** After creating a conjunctival flap, preferably fornix-based, a pair of linear ablative scleral grooves is created about 85 percent of scleral depth. The starting point of the groove is about 0.5 mm from the limbus and is about 4mm in length. The limbal end of the groove is deepened in a controlled fashion until aqueous percolates. This provides an open non-penetrative aqueous drainage pathway via the subconjunctival space. The expected reduction in intraocular pressure is between 2 to 4 mm Hg.
2. **Extended linear radial sclerostomy:** The opposite end of the groove is deepened until a small brownish dot, about 1 mm in size, appears indicating exposure of underlying choriodal tissue. This will provide additional suprachoroidal drainage for the aqueous. The IOP lowering effect of this modification is expected to be about 4 to 6 mm Hg.

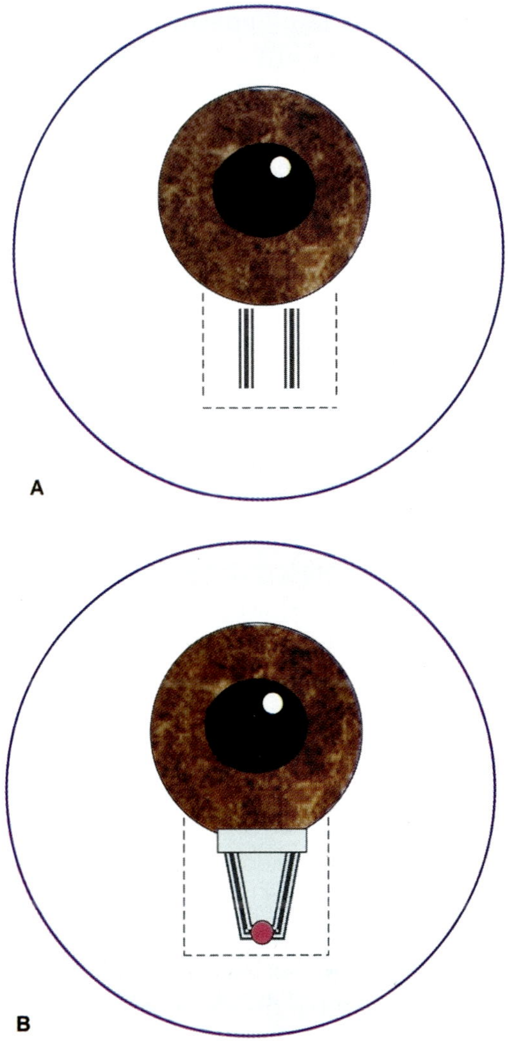

Figures 34.4A and B: CLAFS (A) Linear Laser radial sclerostomy (B) Non-penetrating deep laser sclerostomy providing multiple drainage channels

3. **Laser-assisted non-penetrating deep sclerostomy (Figure 34.4B):** The initial steps are same as that of the surgical NPDS procedure. After an initial 5 mm x 5 mm partial thickness scleral flap, the scleral bed overlying the canal of Schlemm is ablated in order to "De-roof" the canal. This ablative excision is carried on anteriorly as a partial trabeculectomy and further anteriorly to expose the Descemet's membrane. The endpoint is the percolation of aqueous. This procedure may be combined with collagen implants sutured to the bed under the partial thickness scleral flap or a lake of sodium hyaluronate may be placed under the flap. Viscocanalostomy using sodium hyaluronate may also be for carried out for additive effect. Judicious use of sponge soaked in 5-FU or mitomycin placed over the scleral bed is advocated in select cases or at the discretion of the operating surgeon. The expected IOP lowering capacity of this procedure is between 4 to 10 mm Hg and more.
4. **Extended laser-assisted non-penetrating deep sclerostomy:** An additional step of ablative dissection in the posterior part of the scleral bed in order to expose a small dot of brown choroidal tissue would be useful in providing additional suprachoroidal drainage for the percolating aqueous humour. The IOP lowering capacity of this modification in expected to be about the same as 3. However, the chances of short term as well as long term success are expected to be better.
5. **Combination procedure:** The procedure described above may be combined in a single operation or separately for additive effect.
6. **Modified scleral bed ablation:** In order to facilitate the drainage of the percolated aqueous under the flap, the surgeon can conveniently create ablative grooves connecting the trabeculectomized regions to the posterior parts. Creation of such multiple drainage channels will also decrease the chances of closure of the drainage channel and the grooves will facilitate fixation of the collagen implant.
7. **Penetrating filtration Procedure:** Any of the above mentioned procedures can be converted to penetrating trabeculectomy combined with iridotomy if desired.

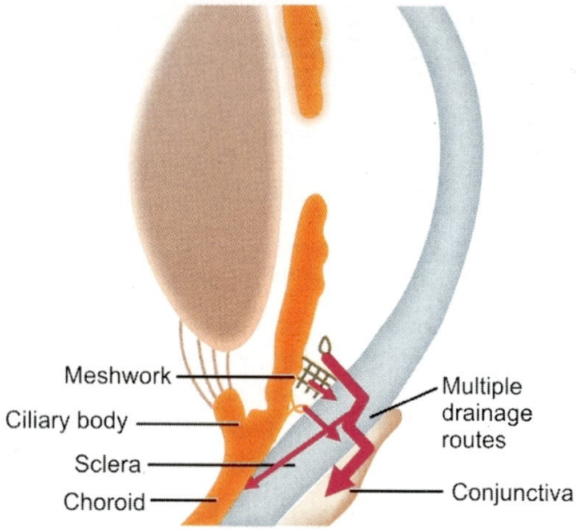

Figure 34.5: CLAFS–Aqueous drainage through trabeculo-Descemet's membrane and then via subconjunctival as well as through suprachoroidal spaces

From the above description it can be appreciated that the surgeon can customize the type of ablative excisions to suit the requirement of individual cases. Hence we propose the name "Customized Laser-Assisted Filtration Surgery" (CLAFS) to encompass all the variation of the procedures described. The multiple filtration channels are well-illustrated in Figure 34.5. The procedure is preferably carried out under peribulbar anesthesia, although, topical anesthesia with subconjunctival infiltration over the surgical site is also possible.

As shown in Table 34.1, the PR-270 using a solid-state UV laser has the advantages of minimal thermal effects, small energy per pulse and intermediate range power required for efficient ablation. The unique feature of beam spot adjustable of 0.2 to 0.8 mm also offers better controllable precise ablation. One of the major innovations employed in the new laser unit is an optical delivery system through an articulated arm in place of a fiber-based system. Any fiber-based delivery system inherently demonstrates a fairly early and consistent deterioration of energy output due to progressive fiber damage during usage. Moreover, the beam spot size in such a system is limited by the size of the fixed fiber core. In contrast, the optic-based system gives a fairly steady output even during prolonged usage.

In argon laser trabeculoplasty (LTP), focal burns with an argon laser beam of 50 micron spot size and 1000 mW power for 0.1 seconds causes contraction of the

Table 34.1: Comparison of laser candidates for glaucoma treatment

	Argon-ion	Excimer	IR (Er:YAG)	UV-266
Laser	CW gas	Gas (XeCl)	Solid-state	Solid state
Wavelength	488/514 nm	308 nm	2940 nm	266 nm
Pulse width	CW	200 ns	500 microsec	5 ns
Operation mode	CW	long-pulse	long-pulse	Q-switched
Energy/pulse	Varies	4-5 mJ	10-15 mJ	5-8 mJ
Average power	Few W	0.3–0.4 W	0.1 - 0.2 W	0.1–0.2 W
Ablation efficiency	Low	Medium	High	High
Thermal effects	All thermal	Partial	Partial	Minimal
Beam delivery	Fiber/contact	Same	Same	Non-contact
Beam spot size	Fixed	Fixed	Fixed	Adjustable
Treating area	Trabeculum	Trabeculum	Sclera	Sclera, cornea, Trabeculum [Customized]

meshwork tissues. This cause separation of the adjacent trabecular sheets to increase the outflow of aqueous. Additionally the laser burns induce alteration in phagocytic activity of the trabecular cells.[20] LTP does succeed in lowering the IOP in 70 to 75 percent of patients with open-angle glaucoma.[21] Over time the effectiveness good intraocular pressure control.[22] Basically, the type of filtration channel created by tissue ablation of UV or IR laser differs little from that created by surgical Trabeculectomy or NPDS. Preliminary studies indicate good initial IOP reduction. The main advantage of CLAFS is that the ablation pattern can be tailor-made to suit the target pressure. There appears to be adequate justification to expect that the long-term results of this minimally-invasive procedure is likely to be the same or better than that of the more invasive, conventional filtration procedures (Figure 34.6).

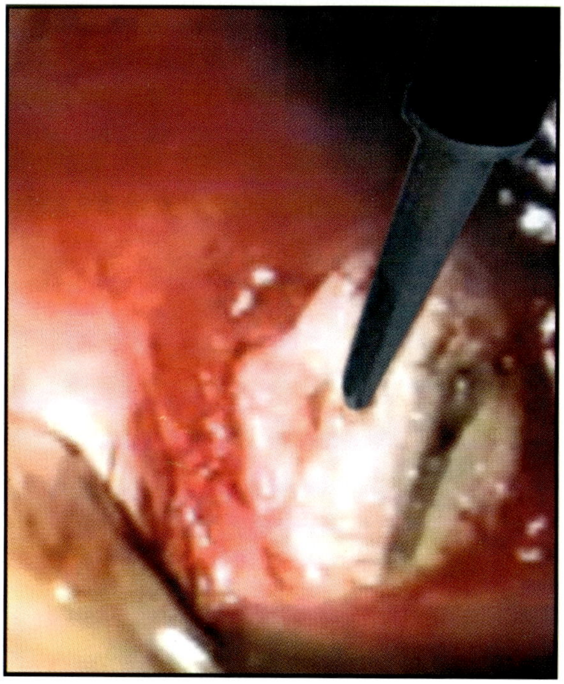

Figure 34.6: Picture of linear radial laser sclerostomy

REFERENCES

1. Krasnov M. Microsurgery of glaucoma: indications and choice of technique. AmJ Ophthalmol 1969;67:857-64.
2. Krasnov MM. Current technic of sinusotomy (externalization of Schlemm's canal) without resection of the sclera. Vestn Oftalmol 1988;104:102-4.
3. Zimmerman TJ, Kooner KS, Ford VJ et al. Trabeculectomy vs nonpenetrating trabeculectomy: a retrospective study of two procedures in phakic patients with glaucoma. Ophthalmic Surg 1984;15:734-40.
4. Zimmerman TJ, Kooner KS, Ford VJ et al. Effectiveness of nonpenetrating trabeculectomy in aphakic patients with glaucoma. Ophthalmic Surg 1984;15: 44-50.
5. Delarive T, Mermoud A, Uffer S, Rossier A. Histological findings of deep sclerectomy with collagen implant in animal model. Proceedings of the First International Congress on Non-penetrating Glaucoma Surgery. Lausanne, February 2001.
6. Sourdille P, Saniago PY, Ducourneau Y. Non-perforating surgery of the trabeculum with reticulated hyaluronicacid implant. J Fr Ophthalmol 1999; 22:794-7.

7. Schuman JS, Stinson WG, Hutchinson BT et al. Holmium laser sclerectomy. Success and complications. Ophthalmology 1993;100:1060-65.
8. March WF, Gherezghiher T, Koss MC, Nordquist RE. Experimental Y AG laser sclerostomy. Arch Ophthalmol 1984;102:1834-6.
9. March WF, Gherezghiher T, Koss MC, et al. Histologic study of a neodymium-YAG laser sclerostomy. Arch Ophthalmol 1985;103:860-63.
10. Wetzel W, Haring G, Brinkmann R, Birngruber R. Laser sclerostomy ab externo using the Erbium:Y AG laser: first results of a clinical study. Ger J Ophthalmol 1994;3:112-25.
11. Wetzel W, Otto R, Falkenstein W et al. Development of a new Er:YAG laser conception for laser sclerostomy ab externo: experimental and first clinical results. Ger J Ophthalmol 1995;4:283-8.
12. Wetzel W, Schmidt ED, Haring G, et al. Laser sclerostomy ab externo using two different infrared lasers: a clinical comparison. Ger J Ophthalmol 1995;4:1-6.
13. Brooks AM, Samuel M, Carroll N et at. Excimer laser filtration surgery. Am J Ophthalmol 1995;119:40-47.
14. Campos M, Lee PP, Trokel SL, et al. Transconjunctival sinusotomy using the 193nm excimer laser. Acta Ophthalmol Copenh 1994;72:707-11.
15. Traverso CE, Murialdo D, Di LG, et al. Photoablative filtration surgery with the excimer laser for primary open-angle glaucoma: a pilot study. Int Ophthalmol 1992;16:363-5.
16. Stegmann RC. Viscocanalostomy: a new surgical technique for open-angle glaucoma. An Inst Barraquer Spain 1995; 25:229-32.
17. Stegmann R, Pienaar A, Miller D. Viscocanalostomy for open-angle glaucoma in black African patients. J Cataract Refract Surg 1999; 25:316-22.
18. Klink T, Lieb W, Grehn F. Erbium :YAG laser-assisted deep sclerectomy. Invest Ophthalmol Vis Sci 1999;40:272.
19. Klink T, Lieb W, Grehn F. Erbium:YAG laser-assisted preparation of deep sclerectomy. Grafes Arch Clin Exp Ophthalmil 2000; 238:792-6.
20. Ticho U, Cadet JC, Mahler J, Sekelese, Bruchin A. Argon laser trabeculotimies in Primates: evaluation by histological and perfusion studies. Invest Ophthalmol Vis Sci 1978;17:667.
21. Grinich NP, van Buskirk EM, Samples JR. Three-year efficacy of argon laser trabeculoplasty. Ophthalmology 1987;94:858.
22. Shingleton BF, Richter CU, Bellows AR, Hutchinson BT, Glynn RJ. Long-term efficacy of argon laser trabeculoplasty. Ophthalmology 1987;94:1513.

Section 4

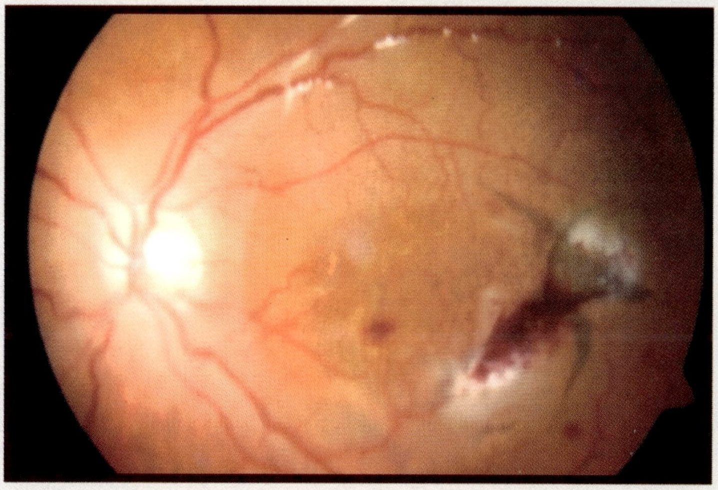

Miscellaneous Technologies (Pharmacotherapeutics, Retina, Lacrimal and New Research Modalities)

35

Optical Coherence Tomography

- PRINCIPLE
- BASIS FOR INTERPRETATION OF OCT IMAGES
- APPLICATIONS
- INTERPRETATION OF ABNORMAL OCT IMAGING
- OCT METHODOLOGY
- OCT IN MACULAR DISEASES
- LIMITATIONS

Kamal Nagpal, Manish Nagpal, Narendra GV, PN Nagpal (India)

INTRODUCTION

Optical coherence tomography (OCT) is an optical technique for high resolution, cross-sectional imaging of tissue. It is analogous to computed tomography, which uses X-rays, magnetic resonance, which uses spin resonance and ultrasound B scan, which uses sound waves. OCT uses a superluminescent diode as its light source. It can perform micron resolution ($\leq$10 microns) cross-sectional or tomographical imaging in biological tissues.

PRINCIPLE

OCT is based on the principles of low coherence interferometry. Low coherent superluminiscent diode light is directed onto a partially-reflective mirror (splitter), whereby two beams are created—measurement and reference beams. The measurement beam is directed into the subject's eye. Here, it gets reflected from the boundaries between the microstructures and scattered differently from tissues with different optical properties. The reference beam is reflected from the reference mirror at a known, variable position. Both beams are combined resulting in a phenomenon called interference. This interference is measured by the means of a photosensitive detector. The echo time delay of the measurement and reference beams is compared. Several data points over 2 mm of depth are integrated by the interferometer to construct a tomogram of retinal structures. Image thus produced has an axial resolution of $\leq$10 microns and a transverse resolution of 20 microns. The operating wavelength of OCT probe beam is typically in the near infrared (800 nm) and thus minimally-visible to the patient.

The tomogram is displayed in either grey scale or false color on a high resolution computer screen. It allows measurement of retinal thickness from the tomograms by means of computer image-processing techniques. Diagnostic applications in ophthalmology are made easy because of simplicity of optical access to the anterior and posterior segments of the eye. These features help yield powerful diagnostic information, complementary to conventional fundus photography and flourescein angiography. The scale of resolution in OCT provides an in vivo alternative to histopathology (Figures 35.1A and B).

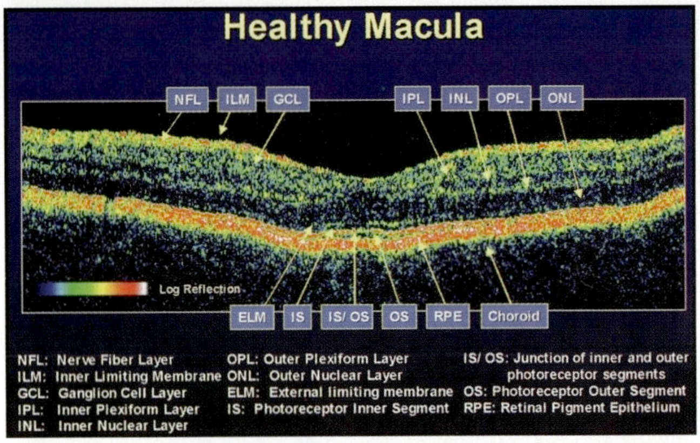

Figure 35.1A: Normal OCT

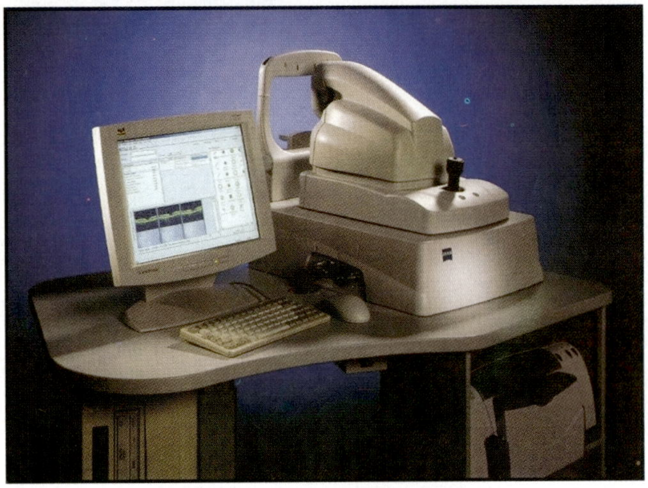

Figure 35.1B: OCT machine

BASIS FOR INTERPRETATION OF OCT IMAGES

The physical basis of imaging depends on the contrast in optical reflectivity between different tissue microstructures. The proportion of incident light which is directly back scattered by a tissue structure defines the reflectivity of that structure. The OCT signal from a tissue layer is a combination of its reflectivity and the absorption and scattering properties of the overlying layers. On this basis, cross-sectional images of reflectivity in tissues are obtained that can differentiate internal tissue structure.

APPLICATIONS

OCT permits simultaneous viewing of the position on the ocular structure being scanned as well as its tranverse cross-section. It can be used either in real time to diagnose characteristic morphologies or to create a diagnostic record similar to fundus photography. The rapid acquisition time of OCT images permits many images to be acquired on different cross-sectional planes. Furthermore, OCT images contain quantitative information on dimensions of intraocular structures with the potential to stage disease progression or response to therapy. Its clinical applications can be summarized as:

a. Follow-up of the clinical course, understanding the pathogenesis of the disease.
b. For assessing the response to medical /surgical/ laser therapy
c. For documentation and explaining the prognosis of a particular disease

These applications are valid for most disease processes affecting the posterior segment of the eye and an endless discussion can ensue. However, we are providing a brief outline of the potential applications. For greater details readers are referred to the list of reading material, suggested at the end of this chapter.

OCT Imaging of Normal Anterior Eye Structures

The strongest reflected signals arise from epithelial surface of the cornea and the highly scattering sclera and the iris. Other clearly identifiable structure is anterior capsule of lens. Structures in the angle region like trabecular meshwork and canal of Schlemm are not clearly visualized in the tomogram since the incident and backscattered light is highly attenuated after traversing the overlying scleral tissue.

OCT Imaging of Normal Retina

The optic nerve head can be identified on the basis of its contour—central depression of the cup and the stalk, behind being the anterior part of the nerve. The vitreous being non-reflective is seen as a dark space. The vitreoretinal interface is demarcated by the contrast between the non-reflective vitreous and the backscattering surface of the retina. The inner margin of retina shows area of bright back scattering, a red layer that corresponding to the retinal nerve fiber layer (RNFL). Its thickness increases from the macula to the optic disc. A highly reflective red layer delineates the posterior boundary of the retina and corresponds to retinal pigment epithelia (RPE) and choriocapillaries. A dark layer indicative of minimal reflectivity appears just anterior to choriocapillaris layer and represents the outer segment of retinal photoreceptors. The intermediate layers exhibit moderate back scattering. Below choriocapillaries, relatively weak scattering returns from the deep choroid and sclera, due to attenuation of the signal after passing through the overlying layers. Fovea is identifiable by the characteristic thinning of the retinal layers.

Tomograms at Disc, Peripapillary Region, Including RNFL

The points at which choriocapillaris terminates at lamina cribrosa determines the disc boundaries. Extrapolation of these points to retinal surface defines a line segment which measures disc diameter. Documentation of nerve fiber layer thickness and degeneration in the peripapillary region is important, apart from optic disc cupping, in diagnosis and treatment of glaucoma and other neurodegenerative diseases. The RNFL in peripapillary region is assessed by imaging the cylindrical tissue sections centered around optic disc. The RNFL, RPE/choriocapillaris in peripapillary region are imaged as highly backscattering anterior and posterior layers respectively. The inferotemporal and supertemporal nerve fiber bundles are evident in both tomograms as localized thickenings in both the RNFL and retina. The observation of depressions from both anterior and posterior margins is a helpful indicator of RNFL thinning.

Retinal Thickness

OCT is uniquely suited for measurement retinal thickness—an important parameter in assessment of macular diseases by virtue of high axial resolution combined with well defined contrasts in reflectivity at the anterior and posterior boundaries of retina. Retinal edema causes increased retinal thickness and a change in the scattering properties of the tissue. Retinal edema may be differentiated from retinal traction by identification of cystic spaces within the retina or by the visualization of posterior hyaloid or epiretinal membrane causing traction. Decreased retinal thickness occurs with atrophy or scarring and may be either focal or diffuse.

INTERPRETATION OF ABNORMAL OCT IMAGING

Reflectivity pattern of the scanned images is used to interpret abnormal findings as follows:

- *Hyper-reflectivity:* Can be caused by inflammatory infiltrate into any layer of retina, fibrosis like disciform or other scar, hard exudates, and hemorrhages. Thin hemorrhages appear as thin, highly reflective bands with little effect on underlying tissue. Thick hemorrhages completely attenuate reflections from underlying structures.
- *Hypo-reflectivity:* Decreased reflectivity may be caused by retinal edema, serous fluid, hypopigmentation of RPE. These morphological causes of reduced back scattering must be distinguished from alterations in the incident light caused by dense cataracts, cloudy media, astigmatism, decentred lens implant or poor alignment of OCT instrument at imaging.
- *Nature of fluid:* Distinction between blood, serous fluid and exudate is made on the basis of reflectivity. Serous fluid is optically transparent, blood has both enhanced reflectivity and increased attenuation of the incident light. Exudate typically has intermediate appearance between blood and serous fluid on OCT images.
- *Detachments of neurosensory retina and RPE:* OCT is extremely useful for evaluating detachments of neurosensory retina and RPE. Neurosensory detachment appears as a shallow elevation of the retina, with an optically clear space between the retina and RPE. The backscattering from the normally minimally reflective photoreceptors is increased, resulting in a well defined fluid-retina boundary. On the other hand, serous detachments of pigment epithelium show the reflective band corresponding to the RPE focally elevated over an optically-clear space. The detached RPE is more reflective than normal, perhaps due to a refractive index difference between serous fluid and the choriocapillaris or due to decompensation and morphological changes in the RPE cells themselves. The angle of detachment is also more acute in a pigment epithelial to a neurosensory detachment, because of the tight adherence of RPE cells to the basement membrane at the edge of the detachment, which supports an increased fluid pressure.

OCT METHODOLOGY

OCT imaging employs software that allows customized cross sectional optical cut sections to suit to a particular subject for the disease under study.

Thus, for macular disorders the following protocols may be applied:

1. Fast macular scan
2. Macular scan
3. Line scan
4. Repeat scan
5. Raster lines scan
6. Macular thickness scan
7. X-line scan

For studying glaucoma, the following protocols may be applied:

1. Optic disc scan
2. Concentric 3 rings scan
3. Nerve head circle scan
4. Fast optic disc scan
5. RNFL map scan
6. RNFL thickness scan
7. Fast RNFL thickness scan
8. Proportional circle scan
9. Radial lines scan
10. Cross hair scan

OCT IN MACULAR DISEASES

Macular Hole and Vitreomacular Traction

OCT can effectively distinguish lesions that ophthalmoscopically resemble various stages of macular hole development like lamellar macular hole, macular cysts, foveal detachments of neurosensory retina or pigment epithelium, and epiretinal membranes with macular pseudoholes. It also effectively stages idiopathic macular holes according to the criteria developed by GASS, which may be important in evaluating surgical intervention. **Stage 1**, impending macular holes may be distinguished by a reduced or absent foveal pit and

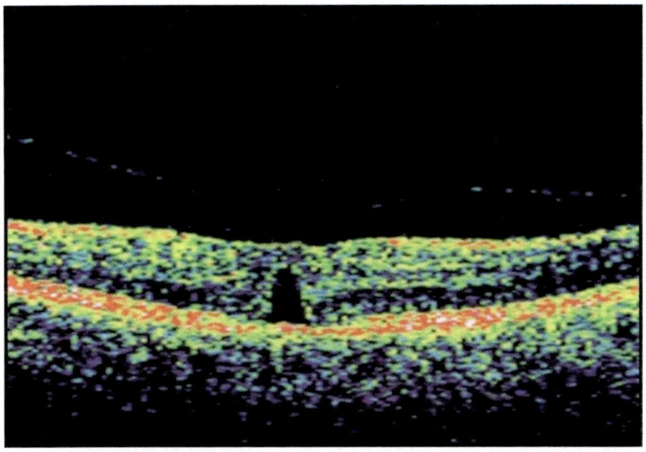

Figure 35.2A: Grade 2 mac hole OCT

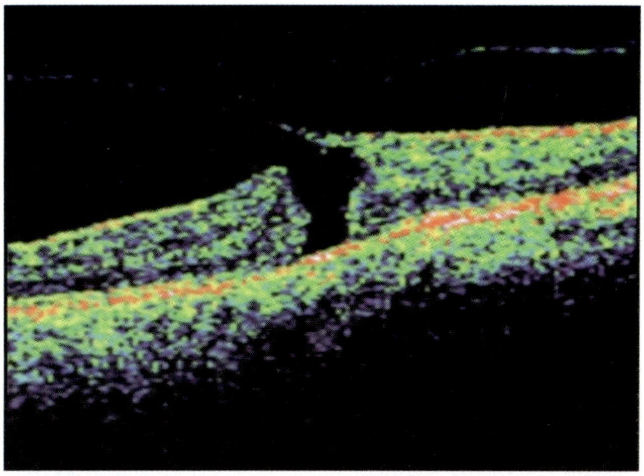

Figure 35.3A: Grade 3 mac hole OCT

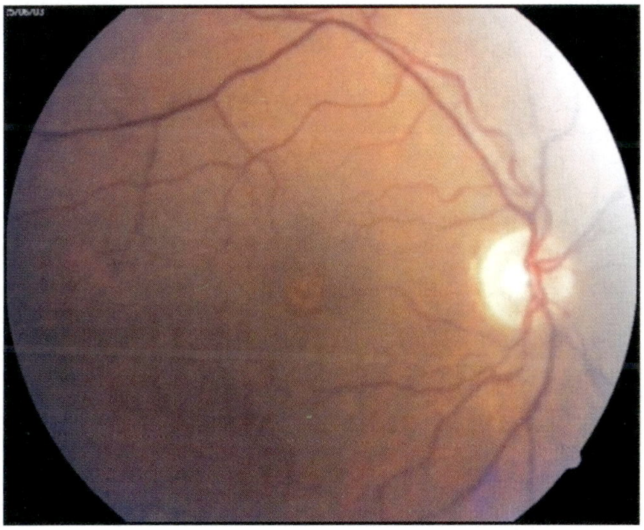

Figure 35.2B: Grade 2 mac hole OCT

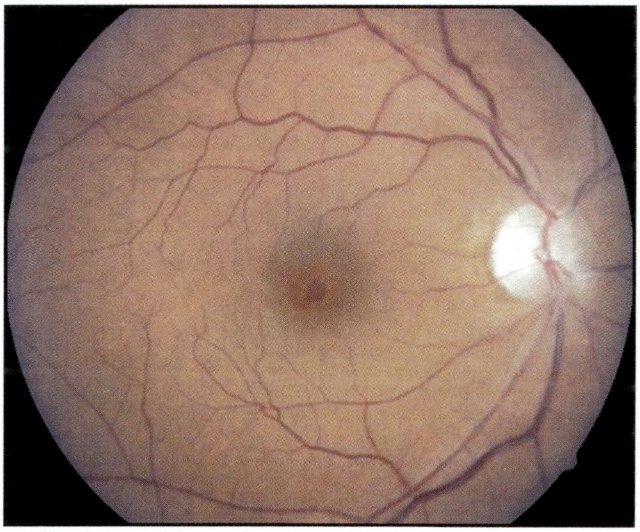

Figure 35.3B: Grade 3 mac hole photo

presence of optically-clear space beneath fovea suggestive of foveolar detachment. **Stage 2** holes have an attached operculum corresponding to a partial break in the outer retinal tissue. A full thickness retinal dehiscence with a complete break in the outer retinal tissue and variable amounts of surrounding macular edema is observed in **Stage 3** hole. An operculum may be present and is completely separated from edges of the hole. **Stage 4** holes are characterized by complete loss of tissue and a detachment of the posterior hyaloid involving the fovea and optic disc (Figures 35.2 to 35.4).

Vitreomacular traction has been implicated in the pathogenesis of hole formation. OCT can assess the status of vitreoretinal interface which is useful in evaluating the risk of hole formation, especially in the fellow eyes of patients with a unilateral macular hole. Vitreous detachment has a protective value in preventing hole formation. OCT tomograms identify a detached vitreous by presence of a faint membrane anterior to the retina corresponding to the posterior hyaloid. Fellow eyes with a high-risk of progression to a full thickness hole display a perifoveal vitreous detachment with foveal adhesion and loss of normal pit contour. This heralds the onset of stage 1 hole and emphasizes the role of vitreous traction. With OCT tomograms, quantitative information may be directly extracted including—

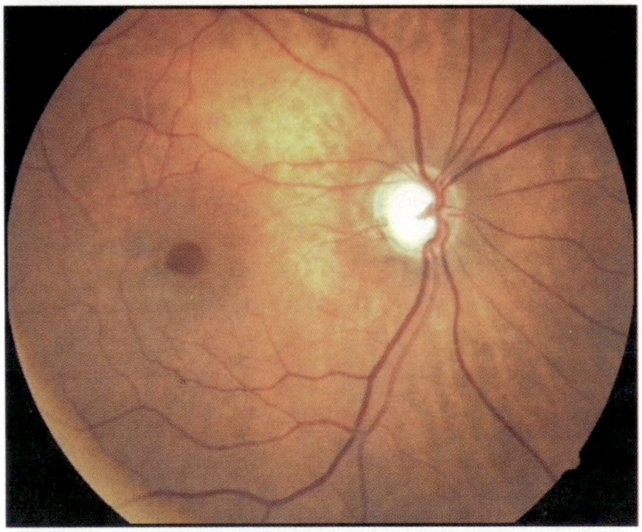

Figure 35.4A: Grade 4 mac hole photo

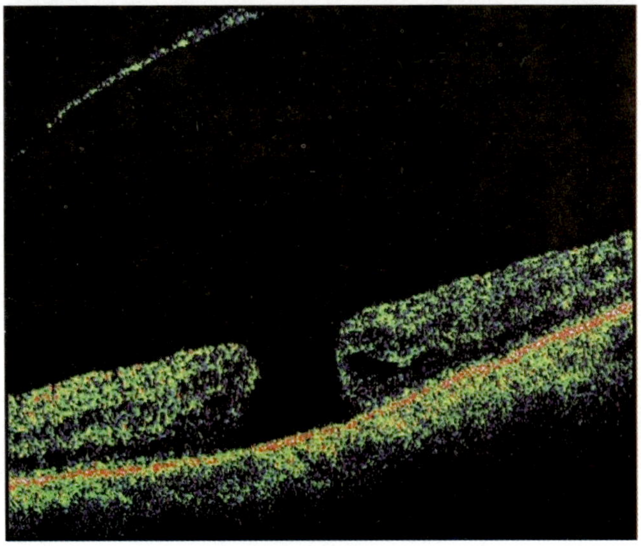

Figure 35.4B: Grade mac hole OCT

diameter of hole, the extent of surrounding subretinal fluid accumulation.

Epiretinal Macular Membranes

OCT images confirms the diagnosis of faint, diaphanous membranes and provides a cross-sectional assessment of factors contributing to vision loss, such as membrane opacity, retinal distortion or tractional detachment and macular oedema. The thickness and reflectivity of membrane on tomogram gives information on membrane opacity. It has a higher reflectivity than underlying retinal tissue and more thickness and differences in contour than detached posterior hyaloid. A macular pseudohole associated with an epimacular membrane displays a steepened foveal pit contour on OCT, simulating a full thickness hole but without a full thickness retinal dehiscence (Figures 35.5 and 35.6).

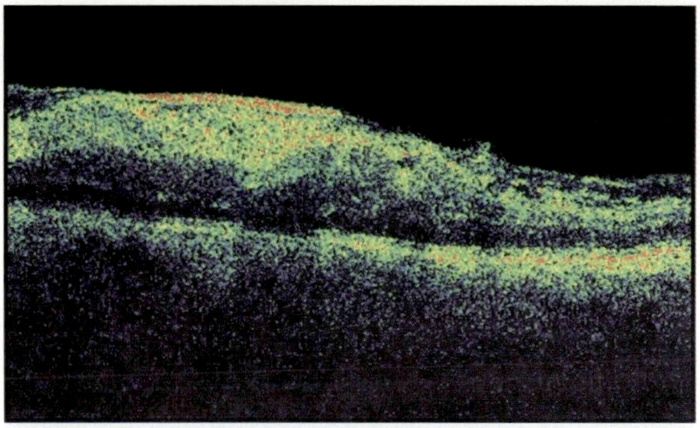

Figure 35.5A: ERM OCT

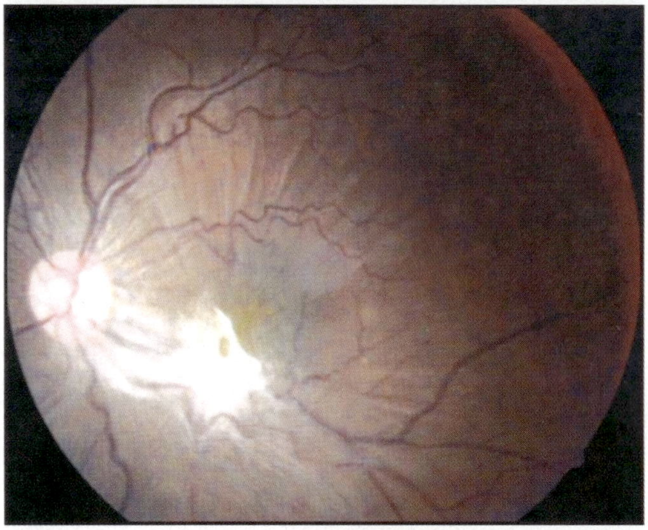

Figure 35.5B: ERM OCT

Retinal Vascular Disorders

Retinal Venous Occlusions (BRVO/CRVO)

The OCT image findings include macular thickening, intraretinal fluid accumulation, serous retinal detachment, cystoid macular edema, lamellar macular hole formation and papilledema. OCT is useful in quantitatively monitoring the development of macular edema and its resolution following treatment (Figures 35.7 and 35.8).

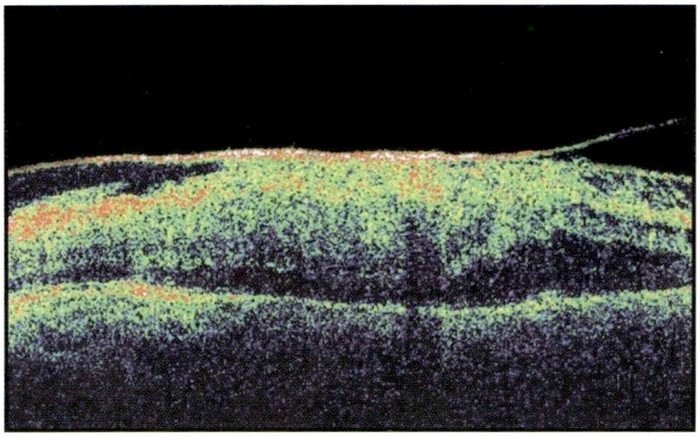

Figure 35.6A: ERM OCT 1

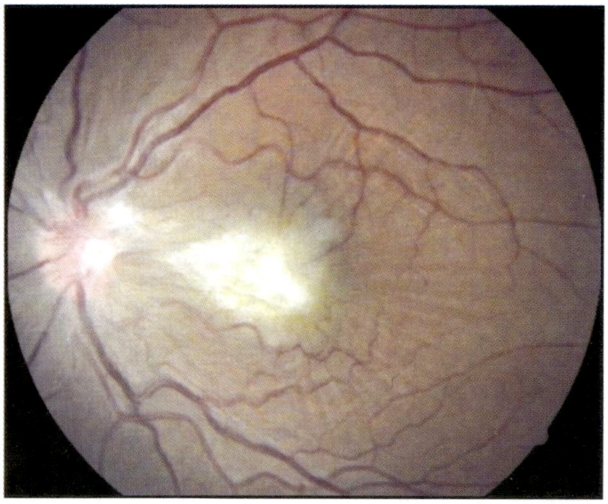

Figure 35.6B: ERM photo 1

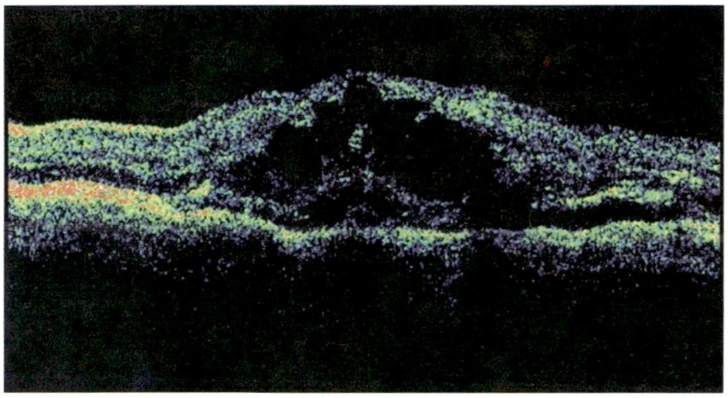

Figure 35.7A: BRVO OCT

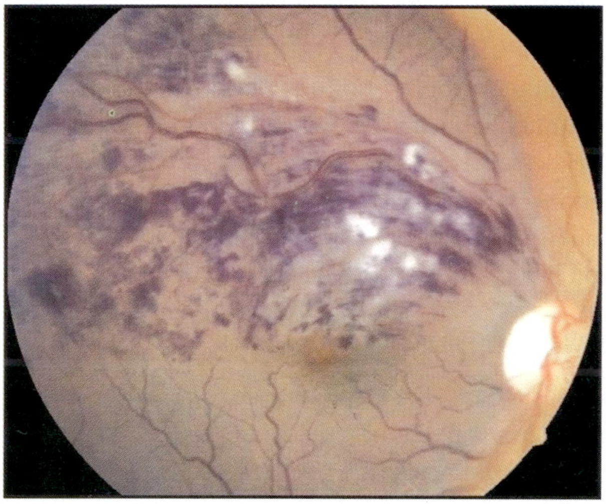

Figure 35.7B: BRVO photo

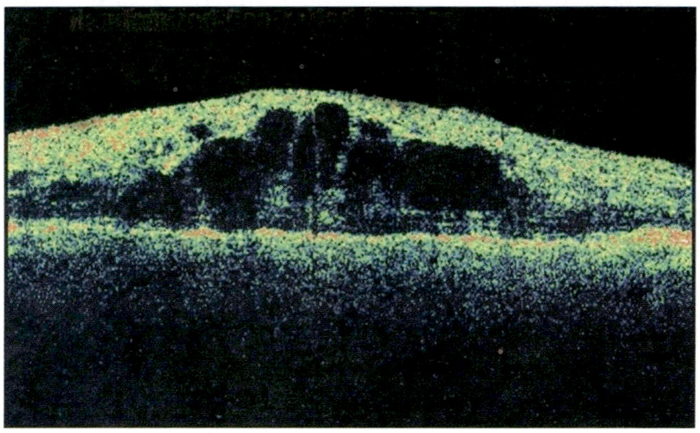

Figure 35.8A: CRVO OCT

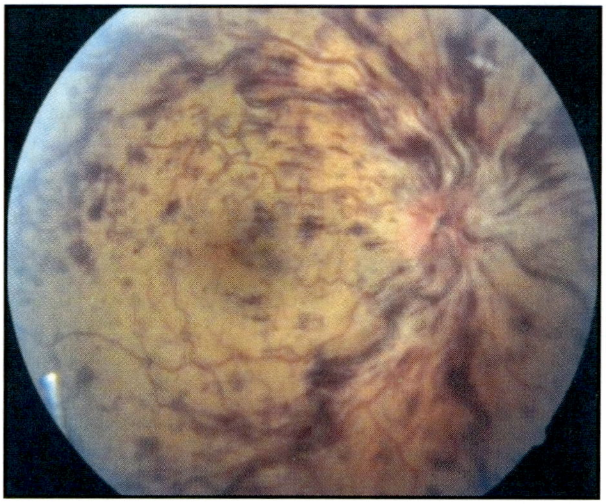

Figure 35.8B: CRVO photo

Macular thickening due to BRVO with chronic macular edema and ischemic CRVO may be measured at one or many points on identically placed tomograms to accurately track the intraretinal or subretinal fluid accumulation with high resolution. OCT is valuable in evaluating the presence of serous retinal detachment secondary to a branch vein occlusion, seen as hypo-reflective intraretinal cavities in cross sectional scans radiating from the center of macula. It can demonstrate optic disc traction syndrome (vitreopapillary traction) associated with central retinal vein occlusion, due to traction from detached posterior hyaloid or from vitreopapillary membrane.

Retinal Arterial Occlusion (CRAO)

Cases of CRAO exhibit acute macular edema followed by retinal atrophy, both of which may be assessed quantitatively on OCT by measurements of retinal thickness. The retinal pallor that accompanies ischemic retinal injury is visible on the OCT tomograms as enhanced reflectivity from the retinal nerve fiber layer and inner neurosensory retina.

Diabetic Retinopathy

Macular edema is a leading cause of treatable vision loss in patients with diabetic retinopathy. OCT is effective in quantifying macular thickness. Measurements of central foveal thickness with OCT correlate with visual acuity and provide indication of relative contribution of macular edema. Sequential tomograms allow accurately tracking changes in retinal thickness. Macular edema is seen as decreased intra-retinal reflectivity corresponding to cystic changes and fluid accumulation; and reduced back scattering obvious in outer retinal layers. Lamellar macular hole may form due to chronic cystoid macular oedema, evident as partial thickness loss of retinal tissue and abnormal retinal contour suggesting cystic rupture. Hard exudates are seen as focal area of high intraretinal backscatter and complete shadowing of reflection from neurosensory retina. Cotton wool spots appear as regions of increased reflectivity of retinal fiber layer and inner neurosensory retina. Preretinal membranes in proliferative diabetic retinopathy are visible as thin, reflective bands anterior to the retina; traction can also be quantified. OCT has excellent reproducibility and is able to detect sight threatening macular edema with great reliability.

Defining the Disease Pattern

By conventional techniques of retinal examination, we see diabetic macular edema as a two dimensional pathology. The OCT almost gives the in vivo histopathology of the retinal layers that helps in the better understanding and pathogenesis of the disease process. OCT is a useful tool in monitoring response to an intervention in clinically significant macular edema (CSME).

Diabetic macular edema has been found to have 5 distinct OCT patterns: (Figures 35.9 to 35.12)

- Sponge-like retinal thickness
- Cystoid macular edema
- Subfoveal serous retinal detachment
- Foveal tractional retinal detachment
- Taut posterior hyaloid membrane.

OCT findings, which mostly complement fluorescein angiography may have a role towards indicating treatment of diabetic macular edema. Pattern 1, i.e. sponge like thickening can be considered an indication for focal/grid laser photocoagulation. Pattern 2, i.e. cystoid macular edema shows good response to intravitreal triamcinolone injection, where OCT also helps in close monitoring following the injection. Pattern 3, i.e. subfoveal serous retinal detachment could be laser induced or caused by associated traction, the latter being an indication for vitrectomy. Patterns 4 and 5, i.e. tractional foveal detachment and taut posterior hyaloid membrane (TPHM) either alone or in conjunction with patterns 2 and 3 constitute an indication for surgical intervention.

Central Serous Retinopathy (CSR)

Longitudinal examinations with OCT are able to track the resolution of small elevations of neurosensory retina because of clear difference in optical reflectivity between retinal tissue and serous fluid. OCT differentiates CSR from occult form of choroidal neovascularisation which

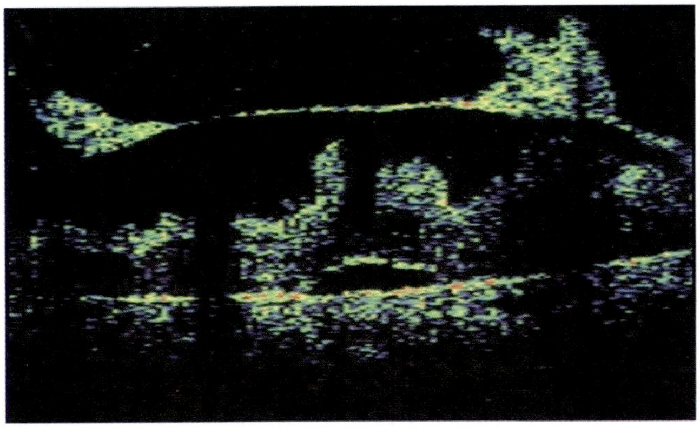

Figure 35.9A: PDR OCT

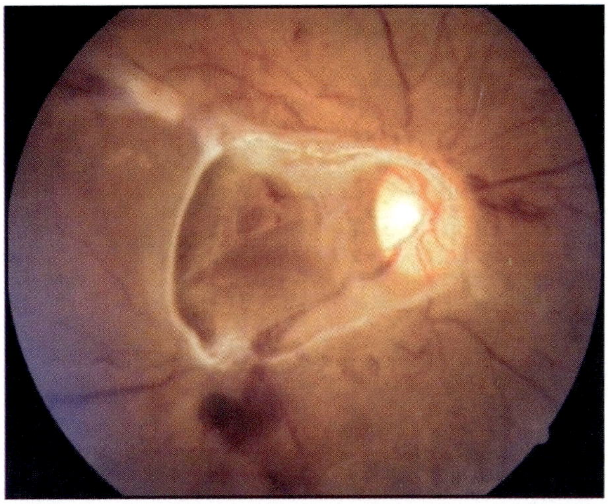

Figure 35.9B: PDR photo

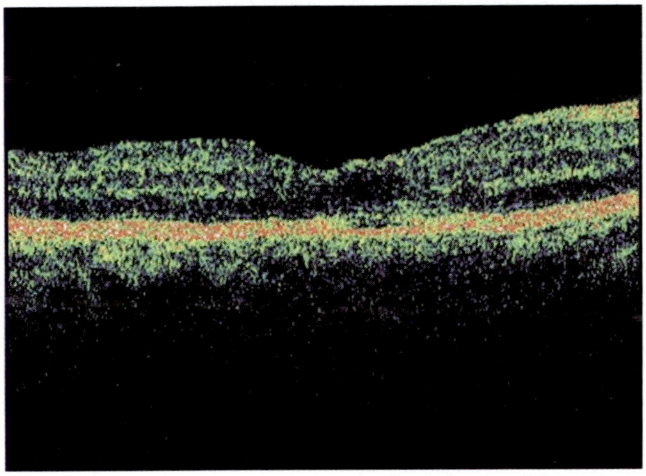

Figure 35.10A: CME OCT

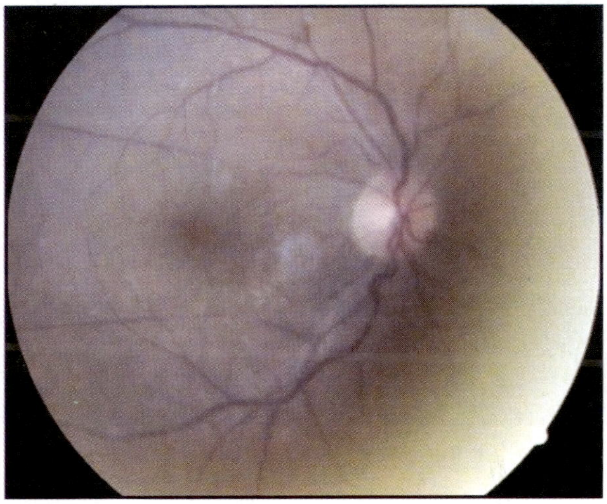

Figure 35.10B: CME photo

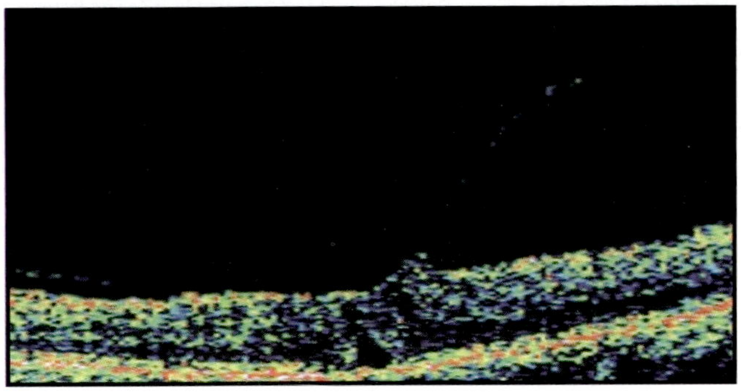

Figure 35.11A: Vitreofoveal traction OCT

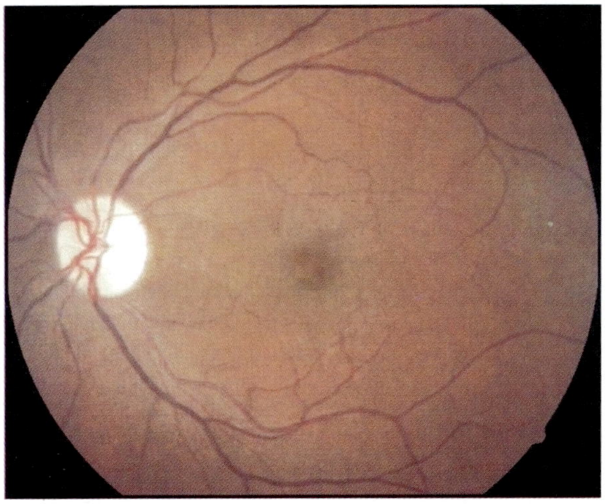

Figure 35.11B: Vitreofoveal traction photo

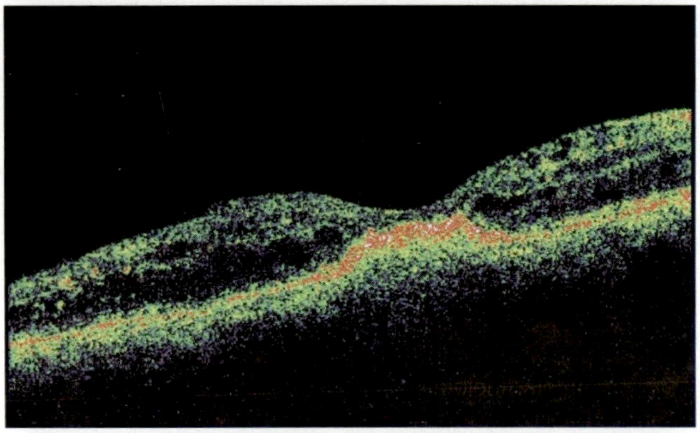

Figure 35.12A: Maculopathy OCT

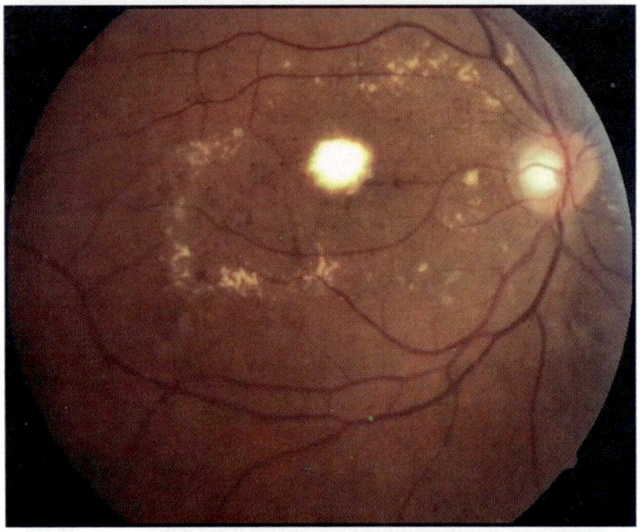

Figure 35.12B: Maculopathy photo

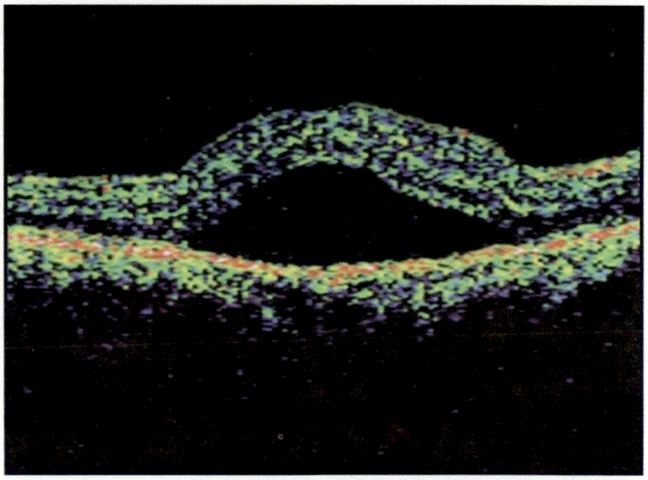

Figure 35.13: CSR OCT

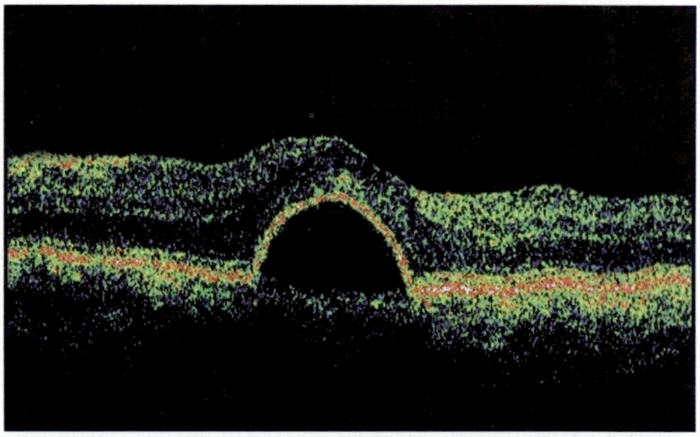

Figure 35.14A: PED OCT

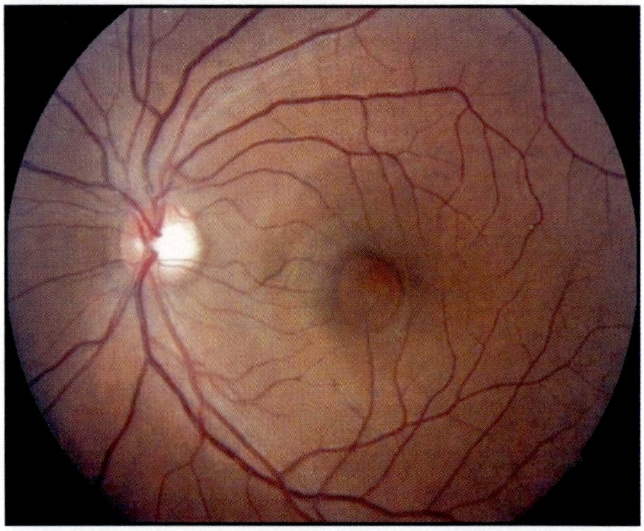

Figure 35.14B: PED photo

may show similar angiographic appearance when a focal leakage point is present. Neurosensory detachments exhibit well defined reflection at fluid-RPE interface, whereas elevation of RPE reflection above an optically clear space occurs when the pigment epithelium is detached (PED) (Figures 35.13 and 35.14).

Age-related Macular Degeneration (ARMD)

OCT can cross-sectionally image the morphological changes in non exudative ARMD and aids in the diagnosis and management of exudative ARMD. Many eyes with choroidal neovascularisation lack the flourescein angiographic features required for treatment eligibility according to macular photocoagulation study guidelines. OCT may represent a new technique for visualizing angiographically occult CNV. OCT is effective in identification and quantification of subretinal, intraretinal and sub-RPE fluid and is particularly useful in evaluating possible foveal involvement of fluid collection. Retinal thickness measurement by OCT provides objective means of following edema and subretinal fluid in a patient through successive examination. OCT detects occult membranes, identifies type I and II membranes, and detects various types of PED – serous, hemorrhagic and fibrovascular. In brief, the appearance of tomogram in the following conditions is given:

1. **Soft drusen**—Mild back scatter extending from RPE to choroids.
2. **Geographic atrophy**—Increased choroidal signals, thin retina.
3. **Subretinal neovascular membrane (SRNVM)**—Fragmentation and thickening of posterior reflection and may be associated with thickening of neurosensory retina (Figures 35.15 and 35.16).
4. **RPE hyperpigmentation**—Increased reflectivity, shadowing of backscattering from choroid.
5. **Pigment epithelial detachment (PED)**—serous detachments have clear cavity with focally elevated reflective band corresponding to RPE over it; while hemorrhagic detachment have brighter back scatter.
6. **Classic SRNVM**—Definite boundaries and localized disruption or fusiform thickening of RPE/chorocaplliaris complex.
7. **Occult SRNVM**—Fibrovascular PED:
8. Well-defined elevation of RPE with mild back scattering due to fibrous proliferation; no shadowing of choroidal reflection similar to soft drusen, unlike serous or hemorrhagic PED.
9. **Disciform scar**—Like laser scars,they appear on OCT as highly reflective and well demarcated lesions art the chorioretinal interface.

Chorioretinal Inflammatory Diseases

OCT can provide dynamic images of the inflammatory process, localizing the infiltrate to specific retinal layers and providing a means to track the extent of inflammation following treatment. Vision loss in uveitis due to macular edema can be followed with tomograms in assessment of retinal thickness. OCT is useful in assessing the density of infiltrate, the morphological changes like edema, and atrophy. OCT image in inflammation shows increase in reflectivity as the inflammatory cells scatter the rays. In a case of sympathetic ophthalmitis (Figures 35.17A to E) and Vogt-Koyanagi-Harada syndromes, OCT scans reveal increased retinal thickness comprising of multiple sub-sensory retinal cystic spaces. A course of pulse intravenous methyl prednisolone therapy in a case of sympathetic ophthalmitis shows remarkable diminution the edema and serous detachments. Premature termination of treatment (oral steroids) may precipitate a recurrence. Thus monitoring on OCT over a period of time may be useful in guiding the treatment endpoint.

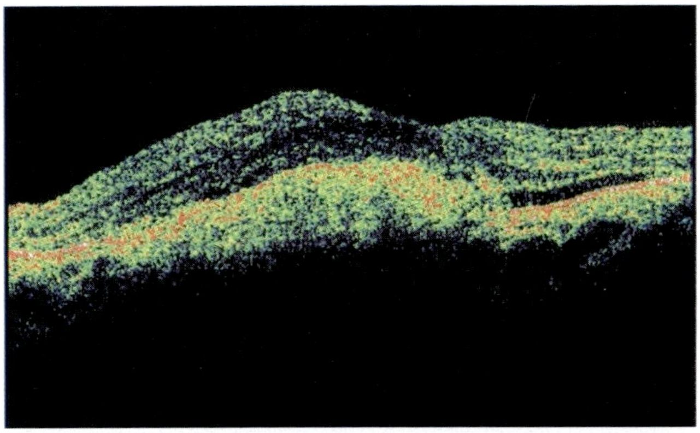

Figure 35.15A: SRNVM OCT

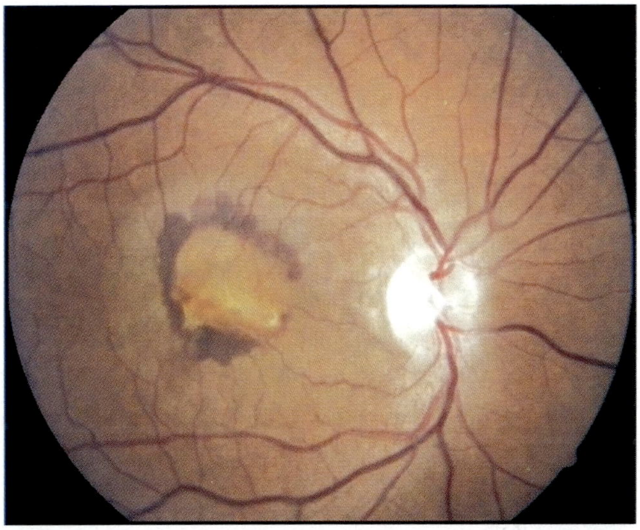

Figure 35.15B: SRNVM photo

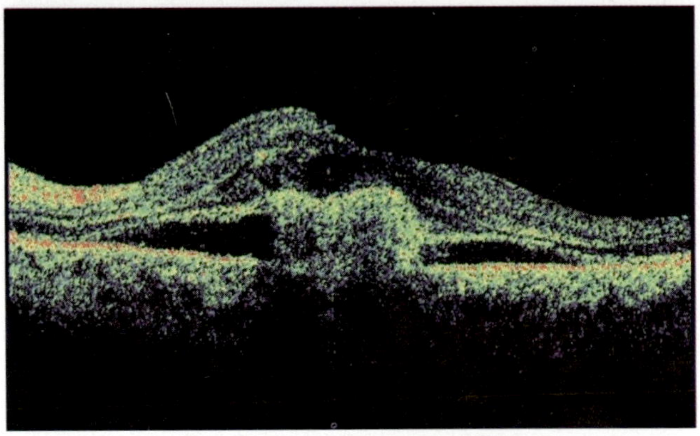

Figure 35.16A: SRNVM 2 OCT

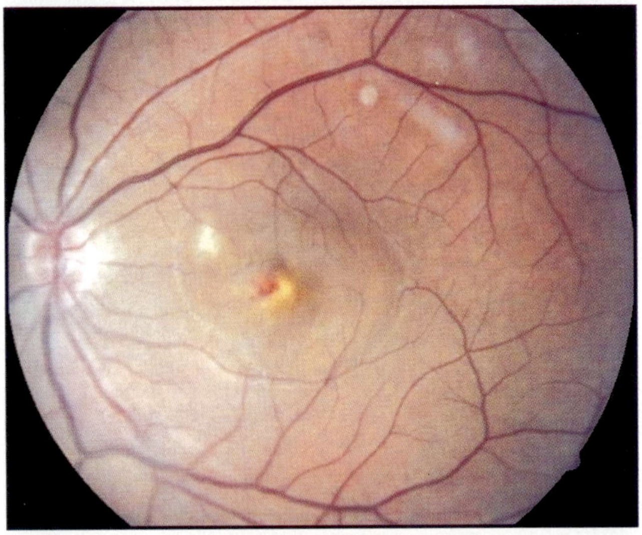

Figure 35.16B: SRNVM 2 photo

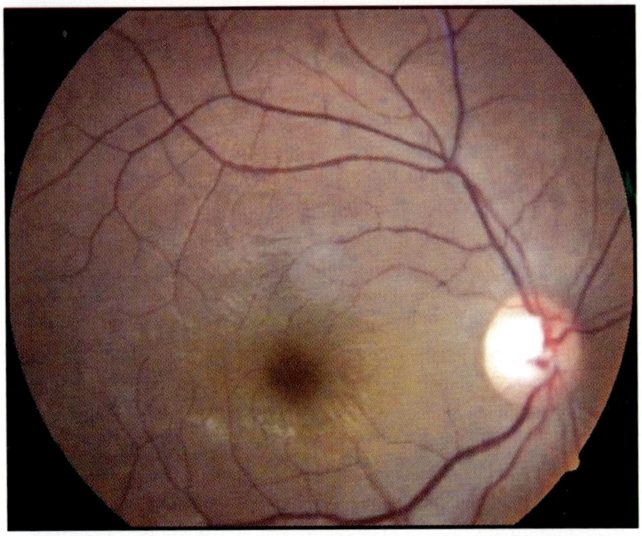

Figure 35.17A: Sympathetic ophthalmia pre-treatment

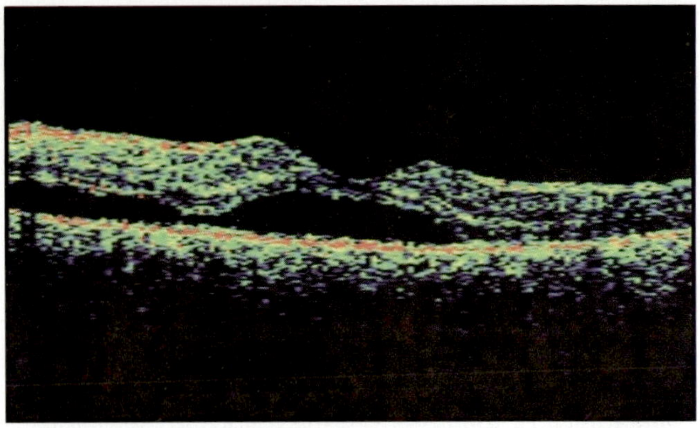

Figure 35.17B: Sympathetic ophthalmia post treatment

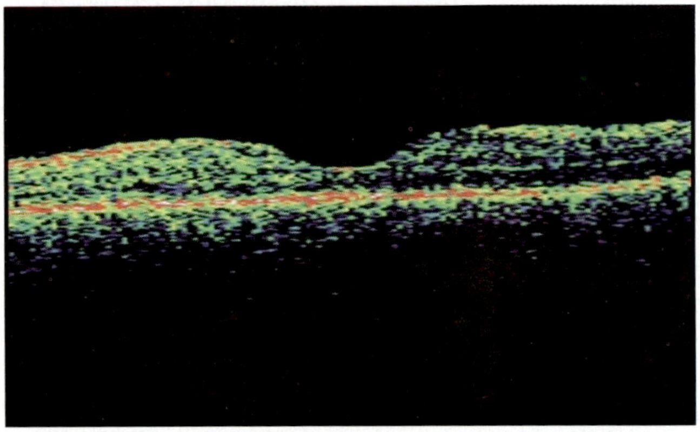

Figure 35.17C: Sympathetic ophthalmia post-treatment

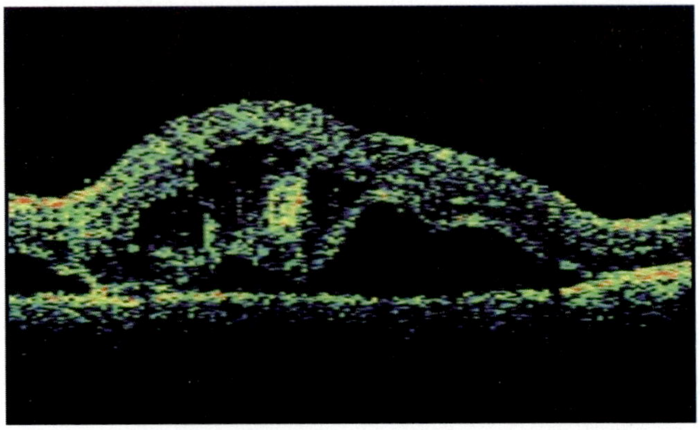

Figure 35.17D: Sympathetic ophthalmia post-treatment

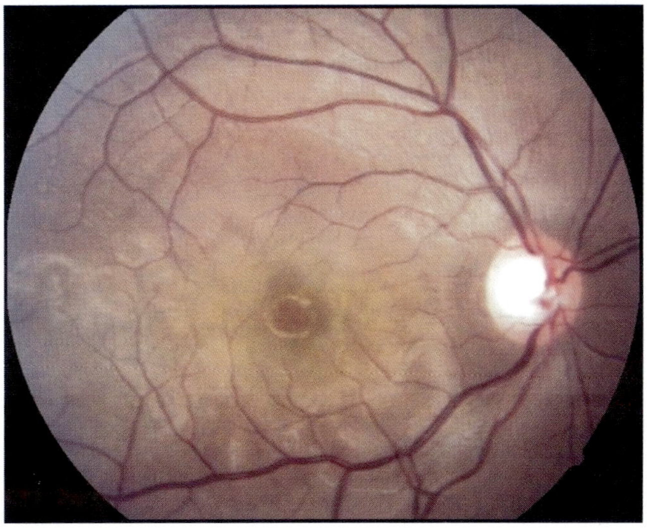

Figure 35.17E: Sympathetic ophthalmia pre treatment

LIMITATIONS

Presence of conditions like asteroid hyalosis, cloudy media, high astigmatism, decentred lens implant and dense cataracts can compromise the quality of the tomograms.

SUGGESTED READING

1. Michael Jumper. Features of macular hole closure in the early postoperative period using optical coherence tomography. Retina 2000;20:232-7.
2. Gupta V, Gupta A, Dogra MR. Inflammatory diseases of retina-choroid. In Atlas Optical Coherence Tomography of Macular Diseases, Jaypee Bros. Med. Publishers (P) Ltd. 2004;241-52.
3. Michael S, Brad J Baker. Anatomical outcomes of surgery for idiopathic macular hole as determined by OCT, Arch Ophthalmol 2002;120:29-35.
4. Michael N. Apostolopoulos, Evaluation of successful macular hole surgery by OCT and Multifocal ERG. Am J Ophthalmol 2002;134:667-74.
5. Tanner V. Optical coherence tomography of the vitreoretinal interface in macular hole formation. Br J Ophthalmol 2001; 85:1092-7.
6. Haruhiko Yamada. Spontaneous closure of traumatic macular hole. Am J Ophthalmol 2002;134:340-47.
7. Reika Sou. Optical coherence tomographic evaluation of a surgically treated traumatic macular hole secondary to Nd: Yag laser injury. Am J Ophthalmol 2003;135:537-39.
8. Richard F Spaide. Optical coherence tomography of branch retinal vein occlusion. Retina 2003;23:343-47.
9. Shimon Rumelt. Optic disc traction syndrome associated with central retinal vein occlusion. Arch Ophthalmol 2003; 121:1093-7.
10. Antonio Polito. Comparision between retinal thickness analyser and OCT for assessment of foveal thickness in eyes with macular disease. Am J Ophthalmol 2002;134:240-51.
11. Isabel Pires. Retinal thickness in eyes with mild NPDR in patients with type 2 diabetes mellitus–comparision of measurements obtained by retinal thickness analysis and OCT. Arch Ophthalmol 2002;120:1301-06.
12. Winfried Goebel. Retinal thickness in diabetic retinopathy-study using OCT. Retina 2002;22:759-67.
13. Teiko Yamamoto. Early Postoperative retinal thickness changes and complications after vitrectomy for diabetic macular oedema. Am J Ophthalmol 2003;135:14-9.
14. Pascale Massin. OCT for evaluating diabetic macular oedema before and after vitrectomy. Am J Ophthalmol 135:169-77.
15. Yumiko Yamaguchi. Resolution of diabetic cystoid macular edema associated with spontaneous vitreofoveal separation. Am J Ophthalmol 2003;135:116-8.
16. Carl H Park. Macular translocation surgery with 360-degree peripheral retinectomy following ocular photodynamic therapy of choroidal neovascularization. Am J Ophthalmol 2003;136:830-5.
17. Daniel Ting T. Decreased visual acuity associated with cystoid macular oedema in neovascular age related macular degeneration. Arch Ophthalmol 2002;120:731-7.
18. Lvisa Pierro. Optical coherence tomography findings in adult onset foveomacular vitelliform dystrophy 2002;134:675-80.
19. Jose Garcia-Arumi. Vitreoretinal surgery for cystoid macular oedema associated with retinitis pigmentosa. Ophthalmology 2003;110:1164-9.
20. Wolfgang Drexler. Enhanced visualization of macular pathology with use of ultra-high resolution OCT. Arch Ophthal 2003;121:695-706.
21. Richard J Antcliff. Comparision between OCT and FFA for detection of CME in uveitis patients. Ophthalmology 2000; 107:593-9.
22. Norikazu Hagimura. OCT of the neurosensory retina in rhegmetagenous retinal detachment. Am J Ophthalmol 2000;129:186-90.
23. Norikaza Hajimura. Persistent foveal RD after successful rhegmetogenous retinal detachment surgery. Am J Ophthalmol 2002;133:516-20.
24. Takayuki Baba. Prevalance and characteristics of foveal retinal detachment without macular hole in high myopia. Am J Ophthalmol 2003;135:338-42.
25. Vincent J Hoye. OCT demonstrates subretinal macular edema from papilledema. Arch Ophthalmol 2001;119: 1287-90.
26. Panagiotis G Theodossiadis. Retinal disorders in preeclampsia studied with OCT. Am J Ophthalmol 2002;133:707-9.
27. Alfonso Giovannini. OCT in the assessment of RPE tear; Retina 2000;20:37-40.
28. Naoichi Horio. Progressive change of optical coherence tomography scans in retinal degeneration slow mice. Arch Ophthalmol 2001;119:1329-32.

36

Quick Look Complete Ocular Therapeutic Information

- ANTIBACTERIALS
- COMBINATION ANTIBIOTICS
- ANTI-INFLAMMATORY DRUGS
- TOPICAL STEROID–ANTIBIOTIC COMBINATIONS
- ANTIVIRAL THERAPY
- ANTIFUNGAL THERAPY
- ANTI-ALLERGY THERAPY
- ANTIGLAUCOMA THERAPY
- LOCAL ANESTHETIC AGENTS
- MYDRIATICS AND CYCLOPLEGICS
- OPHTHALMIC VISCOSURGICAL DEVICES (OVD) AND SURGICAL ADJUNCTS
- OPHTHALMIC DYES
- LUBRICANTS AND ARTIFICIAL TEAR SOLUTIONS
- TOPICAL IMMUNE THERAPY
- TOPICAL HYPEROSMOTIC AGENTS
- CONTACT LENS CARE PRODUCTS
- NON SURGICAL ADJUNCTS
- DISINFECTIVE AND ANTISEPTIC AGENTS IN OPHTHALMOLOGY

Ashok Garg (India)

Drug name (Generic)	Dosage form/strength	Commercial packing
ANTIBACTERIALS		
Aminoglycosides		
Gentamicin sulfate	Solution 0.3% (3 mg/ml)	In 5 and 10 ml dropper vials
	Ointment 3 mg/g	3.5 g and 5 g tubes
Tobramycin	Solution 0.3% (3 mg/ml)	In 3 and 5 ml dropper vials
	Ointment 3 mg/g	3 g and 5 g tubes
Sisomicin	Solution 0.3%	In 3 and 5 ml dropper vials
	Ointment 3 mg/g	3 g and 5 g tubes
Neomycin	Solution 0.17%	In 5 and 10 ml dropper vials
	Ointment 5 mg/gm	3 g and 5 g tubes
Framycetin	Solution 0.5 %	In 5 and 10 ml dropper vials
	Ointment 0.5% and 1%	3 and 5 gm tubes
Amikacin	Solution 1%	In 5 ml dropper vial
Tetracyclines		
	Solution 1%	In 5 ml dropper vial
	Ointment 1%	3 and 5 gm tubes
Oxytetracycline	Ointment 1%	3 and 5 gm tubes
Sulphacetamide		
	Solution 10%,20%, 30%	In 5 and 10 ml dropper vial
	Ointment 10% and 30%	3 and 5 gm tubes
Sulfasoxazole Diolamine	Solution 4%	In 10 and 15 ml dropper vial
Chloramphenicol		
	Solution 0.4-1%	3,5 and 10 ml dropper vial
	Ointment 5 mg/g and 10 mg/g	3 and 5 gm tubes
	Powder for solution/	Preservative free
	Injection 25 mg/vial	15 ml pack with diluent
Microlides		
Erythromycin	Ointment 0.5%(5 mg/g)	In 3 and 5 gm tubes
Roxithromycin	Ointment 0.5%	In 3 and 5 gm tubes
Polypeptides		
Polymixin B	Solution 0.5-1%	5 and 10 ml dropper vial
	Ointment 1-1.5 mg/gm	3 and 5 gm tubes
	Powder for solution 500,000 units	In 20 ml vial
Bacitracin	Ointment 500 units/g and 10000 units/gm	Preservative free in 3 and 5 gm tubes

Drug name (Generic)	Dosage form/strength	Commercial packing
Fluoroquinolones		
Norfloxacin	Solution 0.3%	In 5 and 10 ml dropper vials
	Ointment 3 mg/g (0.3%)	3 and 5 gm tubes
Ciprofloxacin	Solution 0.3%	In 5 and 10 ml dropper vials
	Ointment 3 mg/g	3 and 5 gm tubes
Ofloxacin	Solution 0.3%	In 5 and 10 ml dropper vials
	Ointment 3mg/g	3 and 5 gm tubes
Pefloxacin	Solution 0.3%	In 5 ml dropper vials
Lomefloxacin	Solution 0.3%	In 5 ml dropper vials
	Ointment 3 mg/g	3 and 5 gm tubes
Sparfloxacin	Solution 0.3%	In 5 ml dropper vials
	Ointment 3 mg/g	3 gm tubes
Levofloxacin	Solution 0.5% and 1.5%	In 5 ml dropper vials
Gatifloxacin	Solution 0.3%	In 5 ml dropper vials
Moxifloxacin	Solution 0.5%	In 5 ml dropper vials
Under clinical trials (Phase-III)		
Grepafloxacin	Solution 0.3%	
Gemifloxacin	Solution 0.3%	
Trovafloxacin	Solution 0.3%	
Clinafloxacin	Solution 0.3%	
COMBINATION ANTIBIOTICS		
Bacitracin, neomycin and Polymixin B	Combination solution/ Ointment containing	
	Polymixin B sulfate 10000 units/g	In 5 and 10 dropper vials
	Neomycin sulfate 3.5 mg/g	In 5 mg tube
	Bacitracin 400 units/g	
Neomycin sulfate, Polymixin B sulfate Gramicidin	Combination solution/ointment containing Polymixin B sulfate 10000 units/g,	In 5 and 10 ml dropper vials
	Neomycin sulfate 1.75 mg/g	In 3 and 5 gm tubes
	Gramicidin 0.025 mg/ml	
Bacitracin zinc and Polymixin B sulfate	Combi solution/ointment Polymixin B sulfate 10000 units/g	In 5 and 10 ml dropper vials
	Bacitracin zinc 500 units/g	In 5 gm tube
Polymixin B sulfate and Oxytetracycline	Ointment containing Polymixin B sulfate 10000 units/g and oxytetracycline HCl 5 mg/g	In 3 and 5 gm tubes

Drug name (Generic)	Dosage form/strength	Commercial packing
Trimethoprim sulfate and Polymixin B	Combination solution containing Polymixin B sulfate 10000 units/g Trimethoprim: 1 mg/ml	In 5 and 10 ml dropper vials
Sodium sulphacetamide and Phenylephirine	Combination solution containing Sulphacetamide 15% Phenylephrine HCl 0.125%	In 5 and 15 ml dropper vials
Gentamicin and Vancomycin	Combination solution containing Gentamicin 8 μg/ml Vancomycin 20 μg/ml	In 5 ml dropper vials

ANTI-INFLAMMATORY DRUGS

Topical Steroidal Agents

	as	
Hydrocortisone	Acetate solution 2%	3 and 5 ml dropper vials
	Acetate suspension 0.5-2.5%	3 and 5 ml dropper vials
	Acetate ointment 1.5%	3 and 5 gm tubes
Prednisolone	as	
	Acetate suspension 0.12%, 0.25% and 1%	5 ml dropper vials
	Sodium phosphate solution 0.12%, 0.5% and 1.0%	5 ml dropper vials
	Phosphate ointment—0.25%	3 and 5 gm tubes
Dexamethasone	as	
	Sodium phosphate Solution—0.1%, 0.05% and 0.01%	5 ml dropper vial
	Suspension 0.1%, Sodium Phosphate	5 ml dropper vial
	Ointment 0.05%	3 and 5 g tubes
Betamethasone	Sodium phosphate Solution 0.1%	In 5 and 10 ml dropper vial
	Sodium phosphate Ointment 0.1%	3 and 5 g tubes
Triamcinolone acetonide	Suspension 0.1%	5 ml dropper vials
	Ointment 0.1%	3 and 5 g tubes
Medrysone	Suspension 1%	In 5 and 10 ml dropper vials
Fluorometholone	Suspension 0.1%,0.25%	In 5,10 and 15 ml dropper vials
	Ointment 0.1%	3 and 5 gm tubes
Rimexolone	Suspension 0.1%	5 ml and 10 ml dropper vials
Loteprednol etabonate	Solution 0.2% and 0.5%	In 2.5,5 and 10 ml dropper vials

Drug name (Generic)	Dosage form/strength	Commercial packing
Non Steroidal Anti-inflammatory Agents (NSAIDs)		
Flurbiprofen	Solution 0.03%	in 2.5,5 and 10 ml dropper vials
Ketorolac tromethamine	Solution 0.5% and 0.4%	In 5 ml dropper vial and single Use 0.4 ml unims
Suprofen	Solution 1%	In 2.5 and 5 ml dropper vials
Diclofenac sodium	Solution 0.1%	In 2.5 and 5 ml dropper vials
Indomethacin	Suspension 1% Solution 0.1%	In 3 and 5 ml dropper vials
Aspirin	Solution 1%	In 5 ml dropper vial
Fenoprofen	Solution 0.3%	In 5 ml dropper vial
Ibuprofen	Solution 0.5%	In 5 ml dropper vial
Ketoprofen	Solution 1.0%	In 5 ml dropper vial
Naproxen	Solution 0.5%	In 5 ml dropper vial
Piroxicam	Solution 1%	In 5 ml dropper vial
Diflunisol	Solution 0.03%	In 5 ml dropper vial
Phenyl butazone	Ointment 10%	3 and 5 gm tubes
Oxyphenbutazone	Ointment 10%	3 and 5 gm tubes

TOPICAL STEROID – ANTIBIOTIC COMBINATIONS

	Steroid per g/ml	Antibiotic per g/ml	
Dexamethasone Sodium phosphate and	Soln. 0.1%	0.5%	In 5 ml dropper vial
Neomycin sulfate	Oint. 0.1%	0.5%	3 and 5 gm tubes
Dexamethasone Sodium phosphate Neomycin sulfate and Polymixin B	Susp.0.1%	0.35 (Neomycin) 10000 units/ml Polymixin B	In 5 ml dropper vial
	Oint. 0.1%	0.35 (Neomycin) 10000 units/ml Polymixin B	3 and 5 gm tubes
Dexamethasone Sodium phosphate and Chloramphenicol	Soln. 0.1%	0.5-1%	In 5 ml dropper vial
Dexamethasone sodium phosphate and Framycetin	Susp.0.1%	0.3%	In 5 ml dropper vial
Dexamethasone sodium	Susp.0.1%	0.3%	In 5 ml dropper vial
phosphate and Tobramycin	Oint. 0.1%	0.3%	3 and 5 gm tubes
Dexamethasone sodium	Soln 0.1%	1%	In 5 ml dropper vial

Drug name (Generic)	*Dosage form/strength*		*Commercial packing*
phosphate, Chloramphenicol		Chloramphenicol	
and Polymixin B sulfate	5000 IU	Polymixin-B	
	Ointment 0.1 5000 IU	1% Chloram-phenicol	In 3 and 5 gm tubes
		Polymixin-B	
Dexamethasone sodium	Soln. 0.1%	0.3%	In 5 ml dropper vial
Phosphate and Gentamycin			
Dexamethasone sodium	Soln. 0.1%	0.3%	In 5 ml dropper vial
Phosphate and Ciprofloxacilin	Oint. 0.1%	0.3%	In 3 and 5 gm tubes
Dexamethasone sodium	Soln. 0.1%	0.3%	In 5 ml dropper vial
Phosphate and Ofloxacilin			
Dexamethasone sodium	Soln. 0.1%	0.3%	In 5 ml dropper vial
Phosphate and Lomefloxacilin			
Dexamethasone sodium	Soln. 0.1%	0.3%	In 5 ml dropper vial
Phosphate and Sparfloxacilin			
Betamethasone with Neomycin	Soln. 0.1%	0.5%	In 5 ml dropper vial
Betamethasone with Chloram-	Soln. 0.1%	0.5%	In 5 ml dropper vial
phenicol	Oint. 0.1%	0.5%	In 3 and 5 gm tubes
Betamethasone and	Soln. 0.1%	0.3%	In 5 ml droper vial
Gentamicin			
Hydrocortisone and	Soln. 0.5%	0.5%	In 5 ml dropper vial
Neomycin	1.5%	0.5%	
	Oint. 0.5-1.5%	0.5%	3 and 5 gm tubes
Hydrocortisone, Polymixin	Soln. 10mg/g	0.5 mg/g	In 5 ml dropper vial
B, Bacitracin and Neomycin		Polymixin	
	400 units/g	Bacitracin	
	5 mg/g	Neomycin	
	Oint.10 mg/g	0.5 mg/g	In 5 gm tube
		Polymixin	
	400 units/g	Bacitracin	
	5 mg/g	Neomycin	
Hydrocortisone and	Susp. 1%	0.3%	In 5 ml dropper vial
Gentamicin			
Hydrocortisone and	Soln. 0.5%	1%	In 5 ml dropper vial
Chloramphenicol	Oint. 0.5%	1%	In 5 g tube
Hydrocortisone and	Susp. 1.5%	0.5%	In 5 ml dropper vial
Oxytetracycline	Oint. 1.5%	0.5%	In 3 and 5 gm tube
Prednisolone and Gentamicin	Susp.1%	0.3%	In 5 ml dropper vial

Drug name (Generic)	Dosage form/strength		Commercial packing
Prednisolone and sulphacetamide	Soln.0.2% to 0.5%	10%(Sulpha)	In 5 ml dropper vial
	Oint. 0.5%	10%(Sulpha)	In 3 and 5 g tubes
Prednisolone, Neomycin and Polymixin B	Susp. 0.5%	0.35% (Neomycin) 10000 units (Polymixin)	In 5 and 10 ml dropper vials
Fluorometholone and Neomycin	Soln.0.1%	0.35%	In 5 ml dropper vial
Fluorometholone and Gentamicin	Soln.0.1%	0.9%	In 5 ml dropper vial
Fluorometholone and Tobramycin	Soln.0.1%	0.3%	In 5 ml dropper vial
Fluorometholone and Sodium sulfacetamide	Susp. 0.1%	1%	In 5 and 10 ml dropper vials
Loteprednol etabonate and Tobramycin	Soln 0.5%	0.3%	In 5 ml dropper vials

ANTIVIRAL THERAPY

First Generation Drugs

Drug name (Generic)	Dosage form/strength	Commercial packing
Indoxuridine (IDU)	Solution 0.1%	In 5 ml dropper vial
	Ointment 0.5%	3 and 5 g tubes
Vidarabine (Are-A)	Ointment 0.3%	In 5 g tubes
	Intravenous infusion 200 mg/ml	In 250 ml bottle
Trifluridine (TFT)	Solution 1%	In 5 ml and 10 ml dropper vials
Cytarabine	Ointment 1%	In 5 g tube
	Injection form -100 mg, 500 mg and 1000 mg/ml	1 ml and 2 ml ampoules and vials

Second Generation Drugs

Drug name (Generic)	Dosage form/strength	Commercial packing
Acyclovir	Ointment 3%	In 5 g tube
	Oral tablet 200 mg, 400 mg and 800 mg	Tablets in a pack of 50/100
	Powder 250 mg	In pack of 100 g/200 g/500 g
Bromo-vinyl deoxyuridine (BVDU)	Solution 0.1%	In 5 ml dropper vial
Interferons	Parenteral 30-400 million/ml	In 2 ml and 5 ml vials
Zidovudine (AZT)	100 mg capsule	Pack of 50/100 cap.
Famciclovir	100 and 200 mg tab.	In a pack of 50/100 tab.
Ganciclovir (DHPG)	Oral 250 mg capsule	in 100 cap pack
	Powder for injection	in 10 ml vial

Drug name (Generic)	*Dosage form/strength*	*Commercial packing*
	Lyophilized 500 mg/vial	
	Ganciclovir sodium	
	Intravitreal implant	In individual unit boxes in a
	Minimum 4.5 mg	Sterile types package
Foscarnet sodium	Injection 24 mg/ml	in 250 and 500 ml bottles
Fomivirsen	Injection 6.6 mg/ml	in 0.25 ml single use vial
Cidofovir (HPMPC)	Injection 75 mg/ml	5 ml ampoule
Lobucavir	Oral 100 and 200 mg tab.	Box of 100 tablets
Indinavir	Oral 100 and 200 mg tab.	Box of 100 tablets
Ritonavir	Oral 100 and 200 mg tab.	Box of 100 tablets
Saquinavir	Oral 100 and 200 mg tab.	Box of 100 tablets
Nelfinavir	Oral 100 and 200 mg tab.	Box of 100 tablets
Valaciclovir	Oral 100 and 200 mg tab.	Box of 100 tablets

ANTIFUNGAL THERAPY

Polyenes

Nystatin	Ointment containing	3 and 5 gm tubes
	100000 IU of Nystatin	
Amphotericin B	Soln. 0.75-3%	In 5 and 10 ml vials
Natamycin	Suspension 5%	In 5, 10 and 15 ml dropper vial

Imidazole Derivatives

Clotrimazole	Solution 1%	In 5 ml dropper vial
Miconazole	Solution 1%	In 5 ml dropper vial
	Applicaps 1%	In a pack of 30 applicaps
Econazole	Solution 1%	In 5 ml
	Ointment 1%	In 3 and 5 gm tubes
Ketoconazole	Oral tab. 200 and 400 mg	In a pack of 100 tab.
	Fresh solution 1-5%	In 5 ml dropper vial
Fluconazole	Solution 0.3%	5 ml dropper vial
	Oral tab 100 and 200 mg tablets	Pack of 100 tablets
Itraconazole	Oral tablet 200 mg	Pack of 100 tablets

Fluorinated Pyrimidines

Flucytosine	Oral as 250 and 500 mg capsules	Pack of 100 cap.
	Solution 1%	5 ml dropper vial

Silver Sulphadiazine

	Solution 1%	5 ml dropper vial
	Applicaps 1%	A pack of 30 applicaps

Drug name (Generic)	Dosage form/strength	Commercial packing
Terbinafine		
	Oral tablet of 125 mg and 250 mg	A pack of 100 tabs

ANTI-ALLERGY THERAPY

Mast cell Inhibitors

Drug name (Generic)	Dosage form/strength	Commercial packing
Cromolyn sodium	Solution 2% and 4%	2,5 and 10 ml dropper vials
Disodium cromoglycate (DSCG)	Solution 2%	5 and 10 ml dropper vials
Lodoxamide tromethamine	Solution 01.% Suspension	5 and 10 ml dropper vials
Nedocromil	Solution 1%	5 ml dropper vial
Olopatadine HCl	Solution 0.05% and 1%	5 ml dropper vial
Azelastine HCl	Solution 0.05%	5 ml dropper vial
Ketotifen fumarate	Solution 0.025% (0.25 mg/ml)	5 ml and 7 ml dropper vials
Pemirolast potassium	Solution 0.1%	In 10 ml controlled dropper tip vials

Antihistamines

Drug name (Generic)	Dosage form/strength	Commercial packing
Levocarbastine HCl	Suspension 0.05%	In 2.5, 5 and 10 ml dropper vials
Emedastine difumarate	Suspension 0.05%	5 ml opaque plastic vial
Pheniramine maleate	Solution 0.3%	5 ml and 10 ml dropper vials
Epinastine HCl	Solution 0.05%	in 5 ml dropper vials

Decongestants

Drug name (Generic)	Dosage form/strength	Commercial packing
I. Phenylephrine HCl	Solution 0.125-0.12%	In 5, 10 and 15 ml dropper vials
II. Imidazole derivatives		
Naphazoline HCl	Solution 0.012-0.1%	In 5, 10 and 15 ml dropper vials
Tetrahydrozoline	Solution 0.05%	In 5,10 ,15 and 20 ml dropper vials
Oxymetazoline HCl	Solution 0.025%	In 10,15 and 30 ml dropper vials
Ephedrine	Solution 0.05%	5 and 10 ml dropper vials
Rose petal aqueous infusion	Solution (Aqueous infusion in 7.5 ml with 0.1% thimerosal)	In 5 and 10 ml dropper vials

Decongestants and Anti-histamines Combination

	Anti-histamine	Decongestant	
Pheniramine maleate and Naphazoline HCl	0.3% (Pheni)	0.025% (Napha)	In 5,10 and 15 ml dropper vials
Pheniramine maleate and Phenylephrine	0.5%	0.125%	In 5,10 and 15 ml dropper vials
Pyrilamine maleate, Phenylephrine HCl and Antipyrine	Pyrilamine 0.1% and Antipyrine (0.1%)	Phenylephrine 0.12%	In 5,10 and 15 ml dropper vials

Drug name (Generic)	Dosage form/strength		Commercial packing
Antazoline phosphate and naphazoline HCl	0.5% (Anta)	0.05%(Napha)	In 10 and 15 ml dropper vials
Tetrahydrozoline and Zinc sulphate	0.25% (Zinc)	0.05% (Tetrahydrozoline)	In 10 and 15 ml dropper vials

Topical NSAIDs and Topical Steroids – See Anti-inflammatory Tables

Topical Immunosuppressors

Drug name (Generic)	Dosage form/strength	Commercial packing
Cyclosporine	Solution 2%	In 5 ml dropper vials

ANTIGLAUCOMA THERAPY

Miotics

Cholinergic Agents

Drug name (Generic)	Dosage form/strength	Commercial packing
Acetyl choline chloride	Fresh solution (1:100) Acetyl choline when reconstitued	In 2 ml dual chamber univial alongwith diluent and sterile water
Pilocarpine HCl	Solution 0.25%, 0.50%, 1%, 2%, 3%, 4%, 6%, 8% and 10%	In 2, 5, 10 and 15 ml dropper vials
Pilocarpine nitrate	Solution 1%, 2% and 4%	In 5,10 and 15 ml dropper vials
Pilocarpine HCl	Gel 4%	In 3 and 5 g tubes
Pilocarpine ocular therapeutic system (Ocusert)	Ocusert Pilo-20 releases 20 mcg pilocarpine per hour for one week	In a pack of 8 individual sterile system
	Ocusert Pilo-40 releases 40 mcg pilocarpine per hour for one week	In a pack of 8 individual sterile system
Pilocarpine Combinations		
Pilocarpine HCl and Epinephrine	Solution containing Pilocarpine 1-6% and Epinephrine (1%) (Epilo1 – Epilo6)	In 5 and 10 ml dropper vials
Pilocarpine HCl and Physostigmine	Solution having Pilocarpine(2%) and Physostigmine 0.25%	In 5 ml dropper vials
Pilocarpine nitrate and Clonidine	Solution having Pilocarpine nitrate (1%) and Clonidine(0.125%)	In 5 ml dropper vials
Carbachol	Solution 0.75%, 1.5%, 2.25% and 3%	In 5,10 and 15 ml drop containers
	Intraocular solution 0.01%	In 1.5 ml ampoules/vials

Anticholinesterase Agents

Drug name (Generic)	Dosage form/strength	Commercial packing
Physostigmine sulfate	Solution 0.25% and 0.5%	5 ml dropper vial
	Ointment 0.25%	3.5 g tube
Demecarium bromide	Solution 0.125% and 0.25%	5 ml dropper vial
Echothiophate	as Powder for Reconstitution 1.5 mg to make solution 0.03% other strengths are 0.06%, 0.125% and 0.25%	Powder pack with 5 ml diluent
Isofluorophate	Ointment 0.025% in poly-ethylene mineral oil gel.	3 and 5 g tubes

Drug name (Generic)	Dosage form/strength	Commercial packing
Alpha Adrenergic Agonists		
Apraclonidine	Solution 0.5% and 1%	In 5 and 10 ml dropper vials
Clonidine	Solution 0.125%, 0.25% and 0.5%	In 5 ml dropper vial
Brimonidine tartrate (Alphagan)	Solution 0.2%	In 5 and 10 ml dropper vials
Brimonidine tartrate and Timolol maleate	Solution having 0.2% Brimonidine and 0.5% Timolol maleate	In 5 ml dropper vial
Dapiprazole HCl	Powder lyophilized 25 mg (0.5%) solution when reconstituted	In vial with 5 ml diluent and dropper
Sympathomimetics		
Epinephrine	Solution 0.5-2% available as Epinephrine hydrochloride, Borate and bitartate	In 2, 7.5 and 10 ml dropper vials
Dipivefrin HCl	Solution 0.1%	In 2, 5, 10 and 15 ml dropper vials
Beta Blockers		
Betaxolol HCl	Solution 0.25% and 0.50%	In 2.5, 5, 10 and 15 ml dropper vials
Carteolol HCl	Solution 1%	In 5 and 10 ml dropper vials
Levobunolol	Solution 0.25% and 0.50%	In 5, 10 and 15 ml dropper vials
Metipranolol HCl	Solution 0.1%, 0.3% and 0.6%	In 5 ml and 10 ml dropper vials
Timolol maleate	Solution 0.25% and 0.5% Gel 0.25% and 0.5% (GFS)	In 5,10 and 15 ml dropper vials 5 g tube
Timolol hemihydrate	Solution 0.25% and 0.50%	In 2.5, 5, 10 and 15 ml polyvials
Carbonic Anhydrase Inhibitors		
Acetazolamide	Solution 5%	In 5 ml dropper vial
	Tablet 125 mg, 250 mg and sustained release (500 mg) capsule Powder for injection Lyophilized 500 mg	In a pack of 100 tab. In 30 and 100 cap. packing in vials
Dichlorphenamide	Tablet 50 mg	Pack of 100 tab.
Methazolamide	Tablet as 25 mg and 50 mg	Pack of 100 tab.
Dorzolamide	Solution 2%	In 5 and 10 ml dropper vials
Dorzolamide and Timolol	Solution having 2% Dorzolamide and 0.5% Timolol	In 5 and 10 ml dropper vials
Brinzolamide	Suspension 1%	In 2.5, 5 and 10 and 15 ml dropper vials
Ethoxazolamide	Oral 125 mg tab.	In a pack of 100 tab.
Prostaglandins		
Latanoprost	Solution 0.005%	In 2.5 ml plastic bottle with dropper tip
Latanoprost and Timolol	Solution having 0.005% Latanoprost and 0.5% Timolol	In 3 ml plastic bottle with dropper vials

Drug name (Generic)	Dosage form/strength	Commercial packing
Unoprostone	Solution 0.15%	In 3 ml polypack with dropper tip
Bimatoprost	Solution 0.03%	In 3 ml polypack with dropper tip
Travoprost	Solution 0.004%	In 3 ml polypack with dropper tip

Hyperosmotic Agents

Drug name (Generic)	Dosage form/strength	Commercial packing
Glycerine	Oral solution as 50% and 70%	In 7.5 and 15 ml pack
	Ointment 40%	In 3.5 g tube
Isosorbide	Oral solution as 45% (10 g per 220 ml)	In 220 ml pack
Mannitol	As injection solution 5-25%	In 50, 250, 500 and 1000 ml bottles
Urea powder	as 30% solution	In 100 ml bottle

Ocular Hypotensive Lipid (OHL)

Drug name (Generic)	Dosage form/strength	Commercial packing
	Solution 0.01%	In 5 ml and 10 ml dropper vials

Antimetabolites

Drug name (Generic)	Dosage form/strength	Commercial packing
5-Fluorouracil(5FU)	As powder and reconstituted soln (0.5 c.c. of solution contain 5 mgm of 5 FU)	Available as 50-10 mg/ml in physiological saline
Mitomycin C	3 x 2 mm cellular Sponge moistened with 0.02-0.04 mg/ml of Mitomycin C	As powder with diluent
Daunorubicin	4 x 4 mm cellulose sponge soaked in Daunorubicin (0.2 mg/ml)	Powder with diluent

LOCAL ANESTHETIC AGENTS

Injectable Agents

Esters

Drug name (Generic)	Dosage form/strength	Commercial packing
Procaine	Solution 1%	In 2 ml ampoules
Chloroprocaine	Solution 0.5-2%	2 ml ampoule
Tetracaine	Solution 0.25-2%	30 ml vial

Amides

Drug name (Generic)	Dosage form/strength	Commercial packing
Lidocaine HCl	Injection 0.5-4%	In 5 ml prefilled syringe and 30 ml pack
	Ointment 5%	In 35 g tube
	Ampoule 1%(Preservative free) for intracameral use.	2 ml ampoule
Lidocaine with Epinephrine	Combination soln. having 0.5-2% Lidocaine and 1:100000/ vials 200000 epinephrine	In 10 ml ampoule and 20, 30 and 50 ml vials
Lidocaine with Dextrose	Combination soln. containing 1.5-5% Lidocaine and 7.5% Dextrose	In 2 ml ampoule

Drug name (Generic)	Dosage form/strength	Commercial packing
Prilocaine	Solution 0.5-3%	In 2 ml ampoule and 30 ml vial
Mepivacaine	Injectable soln 1-2%	In 30 and 50 ml vials
Bupivacaine	Injectable solution 0.25-0.75%	In 30 ml vials
Bupivacaine and Epinephrine	Solution having 0.75% (Bupi) and	In 2 ml ampoules and
	1:200000 Epinephrine solution	In 30 ml vials
Etidocaine	As 0.5-1%	In 30 ml vials
Etidocaine and	Solution having 1.0-1.5%	
Epinephrine	Etidocaine and 1:200000 Epinephrine	In 30 ml vials
Centbucridine	Injectable solution 0.5%	In 30 ml vials

Topical Anesthetic Agents

Benoxinate HCl	Topical solution 0.4%	In 5 and 15 ml dropper vials
Proparacaine HCl	Solution 0.5% and 0.75%	In 10 and 15 ml dropper vials
Tetracaine HCl	Solution 0.5% and 1%	In 10 and 15 ml dropper vials
Lidocaine HCl	Solution 4%	In 10 and 30 ml dropper vials
Centbucridine HCl	Solution 1%	In 10 ml and 15 ml dropper vials
Coccaine	Solution 2%	In 10 and 15 ml dropper vials
Phenocaine	Solution 1%	In 10 and 15 ml dropper vials
Dimethocaine	Solution 2.5%	In 10 ml dropper vials
Piperocaine	Solution 2%	In 10 ml dropper vials
Dibucaine	Solution 0.1%	In 5 and 10 ml dropper vials
Naepaine	Solution 2-4%	In 10 ml dropper vials
Butacaine	Solution 2%	In 10 ml dropper vials
Local anesthetic combination		
Proparacaine and Fluorescein sodium	Combination solutioin having 0.5% Proparacaine and 0.25% Flourescein sodium	In 5 ml dropper vial
Benoxinate and Fluorescein sodium	Combination solution having 0.4% benoxinate and 0.25% Fluorescein sodium	In 5 ml dropper vial

MYDRIATICS AND CYCLOPLEGICS

Mydriatic Adrenergic Agents

Adrenaline (Epinephrine)	Solution 1:1000	2 ml ampoule and 5 ml vials
Coccaine HCl	Solution 2% and 4%	5 ml and 10 ml dropper vials
Phenylephrine	Solution 2.5% and 10%	2, 5 and 15 ml dropper vials
Hydroxy amphetamine	Solution 1%	5 ml vial

Drug name (Generic)	Dosage form/strength	Commercial packing

Cholinergic Antagonist as Cycloplegic Mydriatics

Drug name (Generic)	Dosage form/strength	Commercial packing
Atropine sulphate	Solution 0.5%, 1%, 2% and 3%	In 2,5 and 10 ml vials
	Ointment 0.5% and 1%	3.5 and 5 g tubes
Homatropine	Solution 2% and 5%	2, 5,10 and 15 ml dropper vials
Scopolamine	Solution 0.25%	In 5 and 15 ml dropper vials
Cyclopentolate HCl	Solution 0.05%, 1% and 2%	2,5,10 and 15 ml dropper vials
Tropicamide	Solution 0.5%, 1%	3, 5 and 10 ml dropper vials

Mydriatic Combinations

Drug name (Generic)	Dosage form/strength	Commercial packing
Phenylephrine HCl and Cyclopentolate HCl	Combination solution having 0.2-1% Cyclopentolate 1-5% phenylephrine	In 2 and 5 ml dropper vials In 2 and 5 ml dropper vials
Scopolamine HBr and Phenylephrine HCl	Combination solution having 0.3% scopolamine and 10% Phenylephrine	5 ml dropper vial
Tropicamide and Hydroxyamphetamine HBr	Combination solution containing 1% hydroxyamphetamine and 0.25% tropicamide	In 5 and 15 ml dropper vial
Phenylephrine HCl and Tropicamide	Combination solution having Phenylephrine 5% and Tropicamide 0.8%	In 5 and 10 ml dropper vial
Cyclopentolate HCl and Dexamethasone sodium phosphate	Combination solution having 1% cyclopentolate and 0.1%Dexamethasone	In 5 ml and 10 ml dropper vials

OPHTHALMIC VISCOSURGICAL DEVICES (OVD) AND SURGICAL ADJUNCTS

Viscoelastic Substances (OVD)

Drug name (Generic)	Dosage form/strength	Commercial packing
Sodium hyaluronate	Injection 10 mg/ml, 12 mg/ml, 14 mg/ml, 16 mg/ml and 30 mg/ml	In 0.4,0.55,0.85 and 2 ml preloaded disp. syringes with 27G or 30 G cannula
	Highly viscous 1% solution of sodium Hyaluronate of lower molecular weight	2 ml preloaded disposable syringe
Sodium hyaluronate and Chondrtion sulfate	Injection Solution Containing (3.1 mixture) Of 3% Sodium hyaluronate, 4% Chondrotin sulfate with 0.45 mg Sodium dihydrogen phosphate hydrate and 4.3 mg NaCl per ml	0.5 ml in preloaded disposable syringe
Sodium hyaluronate and Fluorescein sodium	Solution containing 10 mg Sodium hyaluronate, 0.005 mg Fluorescein sodium per ml.	In 0.55 or 0.85 ml preloaded disposable syringe cannula
Chondrotin sulfate	Injection solution 20%	In 2 ml vial with 30 G cannula.
Polyacrylamide (oscolon)	Injection solution 4.5 mg/ml	2 ml vial with 27 G cannula
Hydroxypropyl methyl Cellulose (HPMC)	Injection solution 2% and 2.5%	In 2 ml or 15 ml vial or 2 ml prefilled sterile disposable syringe with 27G cannula

Drug name (Generic)	Dosage form/strength	Commercial packing
Poly TEGMA (Triethyleneglycol monomethacrylate)	Injection solution as 40%	In 2 ml prefilled disposable syringe with cannula
Collagan	Injection solution 1.4% collagen type IV	In 2 ml disposable syringe with cannula

Irrigating Solutions

Intraocular Irrigating Solutions

Drug name (Generic)	Dosage form/strength	Commercial packing
BSS (Balanced salt solution)	Solution containing 0.64 NaCl, 0.75% KCl, 0.3% magnesium chloride, 0.43% calcium chloride, 0.39% Sodium acetate 0.17% Sodium citrate and Sodium hydroxide	In 15,30, 300 and 500 ml sterile packs
BSS plus (Mix aseptically just before use)	Solution having **Part-I** (480 ml) containing 7.44 mg NaCl, 0.395 mg KCl, 0.433 mg sodiumphosphate, 2.19 mg sodium bicarbonate Hydrochloric acid or sodium bicarbonate Hydrochloric acid or sodium hydroxide/ml **Part II** (20 ml) containing 3.85 mg Calcium Chloride dehydrate, 5 mg magnesium chloride hexahydrate, 23 mg dextrose and 4.6 mg glutathione disulfide/ml	Preservative free in 10 ml, 30, 50 and 500 ml packs

Extraocular Irrigating Solutions (EIS)

Drug name (Generic)	Dosage form/strength	Commercial packing
EIS Type I	Solution containing 0.49% NaCl, 0.075% KCl 0.048%CaCl,0.03% mgcl 0.39% Sodium acetate, 0.17% Sodium citrate and 0.013% Benzalkonium chloride	In 15, 30 and 120 ml packs
EIS Type II	Solution containing Boric acid, Sodium borate with 0.004% Phenyl Mercuric nitrate or 0.002% Thimerosal	In 15, 30,120 and 180 ml packs
EIS Type III	Solution containing 1.2%, Boric acid, 0.38% KCl, 0.014% Sodium carbonate anhydrous, 0.05% EDTA and 0.01% Benzalkonium chloride	In 30 ml and 120 ml packs
EIS Type IV	Solution containing 0.05% Tetrahydrozoline HCl with NaCl, Sodium borate, Boric acid, 0.01% Benzalkonium chloride and 0.1% EDTA	In 15 ml pack
EIS Type V	Solution containing NaCl, Sodium proprionate, Sodium borate,	In 60 and 180 ml packs

Drug name (Generic)	Dosage form/strength	Commercial packing
	Boric acid, Glycerin, Rose water, Camphor, Extract of witch hazel, Berbrine bisulfate and Benzalkonium chloride	
EIS Type VI	Solution having 0.49 NaCl, 0.4% Sodium biphosphate, 0.45% Sodium phosphate with 0.005% Benzalkonium chloride	In 180 ml pack
Eye wash	Solution containing NaCl, mono or dibasic Sodium phosphate, Benzalkonium chloride and EDTA.	In 120 ml pack with eye cup
Surgical Enzymes		
Alpha chymotrypsin	Available as powder containing 150 units or 300 units of alpha chymotrypsin with 2 ml sodium chloride diluent per dual chamber univial	As powder pack of 750 units per vial with 9 ml BSS diluent
Urokinase	As powder 5000 units of Urokinase are dissolved in 2 ml normal saline	Powder pack with 9 ml BSS diluent
Hyaluronidase	Fluffy powder containing 300 units of activity/mg	Ampoule containing 1500 IU
Chelating Agents and Mycolytics		
Sodium EDTA	Solution containing 0.01% sodium EDTA	In 5 ml and 10 ml dropper vials
Calcium EDTA	Solution containing 0.2% calcium EDTA	In 5 ml and 10 ml dropper vials
Acetylcysteine	As solution in conc. of 5%, 10% and 20% can be diluted in artificial tears or physiological saline	In 10 and 15 ml dropper vials
Laevocysteine	Solution in conc. of 0.1-0.2 molar of Laevocysteine	In 10 and 15 ml vials
Caustic Preparations		
Pure alcohol	Solution as 100% alcohol	In 60 and 120 ml pack
Hydrogen peroxide	Solution as 2%	In 30 and 60 ml pack
Cyanoacrylate Tissue Adhesive		
	As liquid tissue adhesive	In 15 and 30 g tubes
Surgical Adjuncts		
Fractionated purified Silicone oil	Injection silicone oil	10 ml vial with special flip off seal In a sterile pouch (single use)
Polydimethyl siloxane (Silicone oil)	Injection (poly dimethyl Siloxane oil)	In sterile single use 10 and 15 ml vials

Drug name (Generic)	Dosage form/strength	Commercial packing
Botulinum toxin Type A	Powder for injection (Lyophilized) 100 units of lyophilized Clostridium Botulinum Toxin Type A	Preservative free powder in vial along with 0.05 mg albumin and 0.9 mg sodium chloride in vials
Ovine hyaluronidase (Vitrase)	Injection form containing 55 IU or 75 IU OH	For vitreous hemorrhage
Anecortane acetate (Angiostatic cortisine)	3 mg and 15 mg tablets	For ARMD
Povidone iodine	Solution containing 5% povidone iodine.	In 15 and 50 ml packs
Absorbable gelatin film sterile	Sterile film in sizes of 100 mm x 125 mm and 25 mm x 50 mm	Single sterile pack and pack of 6 sterile films

OPHTHALMIC DYES

Drug name (Generic)	Dosage form/strength	Commercial packing
Fluorescein sodium	(i) Topical solution 2% contains	In 5 ml pack
	0.25% Fluorescein sodium	
	0.1% Proparacaine HCl or 0.4% Benoxinate HCl	
	0.01% Thimerosal preservative	
	(ii) Topical solution 2% Fluorescein sodium plain packs	In 1, 2 and 15 ml
	(iii) Topical solution containing	
	0.25% Flourescein sodium	
	0.05% Proparacaine HCl	In 5 ml pack
	0.01% Thimerosal with povidone, boric acid and polysorbate 80	
	(iv) Injection 10% and 25% Fluorescein sodium	In 1, 2, 5, 10 and 15 ml packs
	(v) Fluorescein strips as 0.6 mg, 1 mg and 9 mg strips (with Boric acid, polysorbate 80 and 0.5% Chlorbutanol) and high molecular Fluorescein (Higlo) Strips for soft Contact lenses	In a pack containing 100 or 300 strips Pack of 100 strips
Fluorexon	Solution as 0.35%	In 0.5 ml pipette (12 N)
Rose Bengal	Topical solution 1% containing 1% Rose Bengal with povidone, Sodium borate PEG10 and 0.01% thimerosal as 1.3 mg strip.	5 ml dropper vial Pack of 100 strips
Lissamine Green	Solution 0.1%, 0.5% and 1% Sterile strips containing 15 mg of Lissamine green	5 ml dropper vial Pack of 100 strips
Indocyanine Green	Powder for injection As 25 mg and 50 mg	Powder pack with 10 ml ampoule of aqueous solvent
Trypan Blue	Solution containing 0.6 mg Trypan Blue, 1.9 mg of sodium mono hydrogen	1 ml ampoule (Pack of 10 ampoules)

Drug name (Generic)	Dosage form/strength	Commercial packing
	orthophosphate, 0.3 mg of sodium dihydrogen orthophosphate, 8.2 mg sodium chloride and sodium hydroxide	
Verteporfin (Visudyne)	As sterile lipid based freeze dried powder Requires reconstitution with sterile water and dilution with 5% dextrose before infusion.	As single use 15 mg vial with sterile water and ampoules

LUBRICANTS AND ARTIFICIAL TEAR SOLUTIONS

Methylcellulose and Ethylcellulose Base

Drug name (Generic)	Dosage form/strength	Commercial packing
Hydroxy propyl methyl cellulose (HPMC)	i) Solution containing 0.5 or 1% HPMC and 0.01% Benzalkonium chloride.	In 10,15 ml dropper vials
	ii) Solution containing 0.5%, HPMC, Gelatin A, Chlorbutanol 0.5%, NaCl and polysorbate 80	In 10,15 and 30 ml vials
	iii) Solution containing 0.5% HPMC, boric acid, NaCl, KCl, Phosphoric acid and Sodium perborate	In 15 ml vials
	iv) Solution containing 0.5% HPMC, Dextran 40 (0.1%). 0.01% Benzalkonium Cl EDTA, NaCl and Boric acid solution	In 10 and 15 ml vials
	v) 0.5% HPMC,Dextran 70 (0.1%) Benzalkonium Chloride (0.01%) and EDTA	In 15 ml vials
	vi) Solution: HPMC 1%, Propylene-glycol, NaCl, Boric acid and paraben	In 10 and 15 ml vials
	(vii) Solution 0.8% HPMC, 0.1% Dextran 70, Sodium phosphate, KCl, NaCl, Dextrose	Preservative free in 0.5 ml single dose containers (28s)
	viii) Solution: 0.3% HPMC 2910, 0.1% Dextran 70, NaCl, KCl Sodium bicarbonate	Preservative free in single use 0.45 ml packs (28s)
	ix) Solution: 0.4% HPMC 2910, Diabasic phosphate, Potassium chloride, NaCl and 0.01% Benzalkonium Cl.	In 15 ml dropper vial
	x) Solution: 0.3% HPMC 2910, 0.1% Dextran, 0.01% polyquarterrnium-1 NaCl, KCl, Sodium borate	In 15 and 30 ml dropper vials
Hydroxy ethyl cellulose (HEC)	i) Solution containing 0.5% hydroxy ethyl cellulose (HEC), 1.67% povidone with water soluble polymers, Thimerosal 0.004% and EDTA(1%).	In 10 and 15 ml vials
	ii) Solution :0.5% HEC, Polyvinyl alcohol 1% and 0.01% Benzalkonium chloride, EDTA and NaCl	In 15 ml vials

Drug name (Generic)	Dosage form/strength	Commercial packing
	iii) Solution : 0.5% HEC in a hypertonic base, 0.25% sorbic acid 0.01% EDTA.	In 10 and 15 ml vials
	iv) Solution : 0.5% HEC 0.44% Nacl.	In 10 and 15 ml vials
Carboxy methylcellulose (CMC)	i) Solution containing 1% CMC, NaCl, KCl and sodium lactate	Preservative free in 0.3 ml unims (30 single dose pack)
	ii) Soluiton: 0.25% sodium carboxy-methylcellulose, NaCl, KCl and sodium phosphate	Preservative free in 0.6 ml single dose containers
	iii) Solution: 0.5% CMC, KCl, NaCl	Preservative free in 0.3 ml single use containers
	iv) Solution : 0.5% CMC, Boric acid, CaCl, KCl, NaCl and Magnesium chloride	In 15 ml vial
Polyvinyl Alcohol Base Solutions		
	i) Solution containing 1.4% Polyvinylalcohol (PVA) and 0.6% Povidine, 0.5% chlorbutanol and NaCl.	In 15 ml vials
	ii) Solution: 1.4%, 0.6% Povidone, Retinyl palmitate, Boric acid, 0.09% EDTA, 0.001% WSCP, NaCl, KCl.	In 15 ml dropper vials
	iii) Solution : 1% PVA, PEG-400, 1% Dextrose, 0.01% Benzalkonium, EDTA	In 15 and 30 ml vials
	iv) Solution: 1.4% PVA, 0.5% Chlorbutanol, NaCl	In 15 x 30 ml vials
	v) Solution: 0.5% PVA, 0.6% Povidone, Benzalkonium Cl, Dextrose, EDTA, NaCl, Sodium bicarbonate and Sodium phosphate	In 15 and 30 ml vials
	vi) Solution: 1.4% PVA, 0.6% Povidone and NaCl	Preservative free in 0.3 ml single dose containers (30 and 50 UD)
	vii) Solution: 3% PVA, 0.002% Thimerosal, NaCl and EDTA.	In 15 ml vial
Miscellaneous Artificial Tear Solutions		
	i) Solution: Polysorbate 80, Sodium Chloride, EDTA, Retinyl Palmitate, Mannitol, Sodium citrate and pyruvate.	Preservative free in 10 and 15 ml packs
	ii) Solution: 0.3% Glycerin, Nacl, KCl, Sodium citrate and Sodium phosphate	Preservative free in 0.3 ml (UD 32s)
	iii) Solution: 0.25% Glycerin, EDTA, Sodium chloride and Benzalkonium Cl.	In 15 ml vial
	iv) Adsorbonac NaCl 2% or 5% solution	In 5 and 10 ml vials

Drug name (Generic)	Dosage form/strength	Commercial packing
Ointments		
	i) Ointment containing petrolatum (55.5%) Lanolin (2%) and mineral oil (42.5%)	Preservative free in 3.5 and 5 g tubes
	ii) Ointment: 2% HPMC, NaCl, KCl, CaCl, MgCl, Sodium acetate and Sodium citrate	Preservative free in 3.5 and 5 g tubes
	iii) Lubricant gel carbopal 980 (Poly Acryclic acid) which transforms from gel to liquid in contact with ocular tissue.	In 5 g tube
	iv) Gel: 0.3% HPMC	In 10 ml pack
	v) Ointment: 56.8% white petrolatum, 42.5% mineral oil, Chlorobutanol, Lanolin alcohols.	In 3.5 and 7g tubes
	vi) Ointment: White)etrolatum	Preservative free in 0.5 gm pack
	vii) Ointment: 55% white petrolatum, 32% mineral oil, Boric acid, Stearic acid and wheat germ oil	In 3.5 g tube
Ocular Inserts		
Lacriset	Polymeric insert having 5 mg of HPMC	Preservative free in 60s with applicator
Punctal Plugs		
Collagen implant	Intra canalicular Collagen implant Consists of 0.2, 0.3, 0.4, 0.5 and 0.6 mm diameter inserts packed at the edge of a foam strip.	In a pack of 10 or 72 plugs with inserter tool.
Silicone plugs	Punctum silicone Plug in 1.6, 2 and 2.8 mm Sizes	In a pack of 2 or 10 plugs with inserter tool
Lubricant for Artificial Eyes		
	Solution containing 0.25% Tyloxapol and 0.02% Benzalkonium Chloride	In 15 ml dropper vials
	Solution containing 2.5% HPMC with 0.004 Thimerosal and 0.1% EDTA	In 15 ml dropper vials for gonioscopic exam.
Cyclosporine	Emulsion 0.05% (Preservative free)	5 ml poly vials
Diquafosol	Phase-III Clinical Trials	Lubricant
TOPICAL IMMUNE THERAPY		
Aspac(Topical)	Ophthalmic solution Containing 0.1% each of IgA, IgG and IgM in fixed concentrations	Preservative free In 5 and 10 ml dropper vial with controlled tip

Drug name (Generic)	Dosage form/strength	Commercial packing
TOPICAL HYPEROSMOTIC AGENTS		
Sodium chloride (Hypertonic)	i) Solution as 2% or 5% NaCl with 0.004% water soluble polymer Thimerosal and 0.1% EDTA.	In 10 and 15 ml dropper vials
	ii) Topical NaCl solution 2% or 5% with HPMC and parabens.	In 10 and 15 ml dropper vials
	iii) Topical 5% NaCl Solution with propylene Glycol, Sodium borate and boric acid	In 10 ml dropper vials
	iv) Ointment containing 6% NaCl gel with petrolatum and Lanolin.	In 3.5 and 5 g tubes
Glycerine	i) Topical solution as 50% (0.6 g glycerine/ml) with 0.55% chlorobutanol	In 7.5 ml vial
	ii) Ointment as 40% with petrolatum and lanolin parabens	
CONTACT LENS CARE PRODUCTS		
Hard Lenses		
Cleaning/Soaking/Wetting Solutions for Hard Lenses (Complete)		
Total solution	Containing buffered Isotonic Polyvinyl Alcohol, Benzalkonium chloride, EDTA	In 60 and 120 ml packs
Wetting Solutions (Hard Lenses)		
	i) Solution containing 0.004% Benzalkonium Cl, EDTA, HPMC, NaCl, KCl and Polyvinyl alcohol	In 60 ml pack
	ii) Solution: Buffered 0.1% EDTA, 0.01% Benzalkonium Cl	In 60 and 120 ml packs
Wetting/Soaking Solutions (Hard Lenses)		
	i) Solution containing buffered isotonic 0.1% EDTA and 0.05% Benzalkonium Cl	In 120 ml pack
	ii) Solution: Buffered isotonic 0.003% Benzalkonium chloride, Polyvinyl alcohol and EDTA	In 120 and 180 ml pack
Rewetting Solutions (Hard Lenses)		
	i) Solution containing Povidone, water soluble polymers, sorbic acid and EDTA (Isotonic).	In 15 ml pack

Drug name (Generic)	Dosage form/strength	Commercial packing
	ii) Solution (Isotonic) Hydroxyethyl cellulose sorbic acid, poloxamer 407, 0.1% EDTA, NaCl, KCl, Sodium borate, boric acid	In 5, 15 and 30 ml packs
	iii) Solution: Isotonic 0.04%, thimerosal,0.1%, EDTA, povidone and polyoxyethylene	In 15 ml packs
	iv) Solution: Isotonic 0.1% EDTA, 0.001% polyquaterniuml-1, Dextran, NaCl, KCl, and HPMC	Thimerosal free in 15 ml pack
	v) Solution: Buffered, isotonic NaCl, Carbamide, poloxamer 407, 0.2% EDTA, 0.15% Sorbic acid.	In 15 ml pack
	vi) Buffered Solution with polyoxyl 40 stearate PEG 300 and 0.5% Chlorobutanol	In 15 ml pack
Cleaning Solutions (Hard Lenses)		
	i) Solution with anionic sulfate surfactant, friction enhancing Agents and NaCl	In 15 and 60 ml pack
	ii) Solution: 15.7% isopropyl alcohol, poloxamer 407 and amphoteric 10	Preservative free in 12 ml
	iii) Solution: Buffered isotonic Tween 21, Polymeric cleaners, 0.1% EDTA and 0.001% poly quaternium-1.	Thimerosal free in 12 and 20 ml packs
	iv) Buffered solution Cocoampho carboxy Glycinate, sodium lauryl Sulfate, hexylene glycol, Alkyl ether sulfate, Fatty acid amide surfactants	Preservative free in 30 ml pack
	v) Solution: Cocoampho diacetate, glycol, 0.1% EDTA and 0.01% benzal-konium Cl.	In 60 ml pack
	vi) Solution with Poloxamer 188, 0.01% Benzalkonium chloride and 0.2% EDTA	In 15 and 30 ml
	vii) Solution with Hydrophilic polyelectrolyte, Polyvinyl alcohol, Hydroxyethyl cellulose, Chlorhexidine gluconate and EDTA.	In 15 and 30 ml packs
Cleaning and Soaking Solution (Hard Lenses)		
	i) Solution: Buffered surfactant cleaning agent with 0.004% Phenylmercuric nitrate	In 120 ml pack

Drug name (Generic)	Dosage form/strength	Commercial packing
Rigid Gas Permeable Lenses (RGP)		
Wetting/Soaking solutions (RGP Lenses)		
	i) Buffered solution containing 0.0015% polyaminopropyl biguanide 0.05% EDTA, Cationic cellular derivative polymer	In 120 ml pack
	ii) Buffered solution low viscosity, 0.5% EDTA, 0.006% Chlorhexidine gluconate, Cationic cellulose derivative polymer as wetting agent	In 120 ml pack
	iii) Solution having EDTA and Chlorhexidine	In 120 ml pack
	iv) Solution: Isotonic Hydroxyethyl cellulose, 0.006% polixetonium chloride	Thimerosal free in 120 ml pack
	v) Buffered solution: 0.005% Chlorhexidine gluconate, 0.02% EDTA Octylphenoxy, Ethanol, Povidone, Polyvinyl alcohol, Propylene glycol and HEC, NaCl.	In 120 and 240 ml packs
	vi) Buffered solution: Sodium and potassium chloride, PVA, PVP, HEC, Sodium bisulfite, 0.02%, Benzyl alcohol 0.1%, Sorbic acid 0.05% and Disodium edetate 0.1%	In 120 ml pack
	vii) Buffered isotonic, 0.003% Benzalkonium chloride, Polyvinyl alcohol, EDTA	In 120 and 180 ml packs
Disinfecting/Cleaning Solutions (RGP Lenses)		
	i) Buffered isotonic sterile saline solution having sodium edetate with biguanide copolymer 0.0031%	In 350 ml pack
	ii) Solution: Lauryl sulfate salt of imidazoline octylphenoxy, 0.3% benzyl alcohol and 0.5% trisodium EDTA	Thimerosal free in 120 ml pack
	iii) Solution: Lauryl sulfate salt, benzyl alcohol 0.1% and disodium edetate 0.5%	In 120 ml pack
	iv) Buffered solution; sorbitan monolaurate, betaine surfactant, silicone glycol, polyethylene glycol, 0.003% chlorhexidine gluconate, 0.005% polyamino propyl biguanide and 0.05% edetate disodium	In 120 ml pack

Drug name (Generic)	Dosage form/strength	Commercial packing
Surfactant Cleaning Solutions (RGP Lenses)		
	i) Solution: Concentrated homogenous surfactant, alkyl ether sulfate, ethoxylated alkylphenol, cocoa based phospholipid silica gel	In 30 ml pack
	ii) Surfactant solution with alkyl ether sulfate silica gel	In 30 ml pack
	iii) Buffered isotonic solution 0.004% thimerosal 0.1% EDTA, Tween 21, Hydroxyethyl cellulose and Polymeric cleaners.	In 12 and 20 ml pack
	iv) Solution: Edetate disodium 0.1%, Polyquad packs 0.001%, Tween 21, Polymeric cleaning agents	In 12 and 118 ml pack
	v) Buffered isotonic solution 0.1%, EDTA, 0.001% polyquaternium-1, Polymeric cleaners, Tween-21.	Thimerosal free in 12 and 20 ml packs
Enzymatic Cleaners (RGP Lenses)		
	i) Liquid containing subtilism and glycerol	Preservative free in 1 ml pack
	ii) Tablets: Highly Purified post-pancreatin	Pack of 24 and 36 tablets
	iii) Tablet: Papain, NaCl, Sodium carbonate, Sodium borate and EDTA	Pack of 16 and 24 tablets
	iv) Liquid: Preservative free containing propylene glycol sodium borate and pancreatin	
Rewetting Solutions (RGP Lenses)		
	i) Solution: Containing Polyquad 0.1%, Edetate disodium, Citrate buffer Dextran NaCl, KCl.	In 15 ml pack
	ii) Solution: Sorbic acid 0.1%, Edetate disodium 0.2%, HEC, Sodium borate, Boric acid and NaCl.	In 15 ml pack
	iii) Solution: Buffered, Hypertonic 0.006%, Chlorhexidine gluconate, 0.05% EDTA, Cationic cellulose derivative polymer as—wetting agent	In 10 ml pack
Soft Lenses (Hydrogel)		
Disinfection Non-hydrogen Peroxide Soft Lenses		
	i) Buffered solution containing NaCl, 0.0001% polyhexamethylene biguanide, tromethamine, tyloxapol and EDTA	Thimerosal free 120 and 360 ml packs

Drug name (Generic)	Dosage form/strength	Commercial packing
	ii) Buffered isotonic solution 0.005% Chlorhexidine 0.1% EDTA, 0.001% Thimerosal, NaCl, Sodium borate and boric acid.	In 360 ml pack
	iii) Buffered isotonic solution 0.05% EDTA, 0.001% polyquaternium-1 sodium citrate and NaCl	In 120 ml pack
	iv) Solution: Isotonic 0.00005% Polyamino propyl biguanide, 0.01% EDTA, NaCl sodium borate, Boric acid and Poloxamine	In 120 and 355 ml pack
Disinfection Hydrogen Peroxide Soft Lenses		
	i) **Disinfectant/Soaking** Solution: 3% Hydrogen peroxide, 0.85% Stablized with phosphonic acid, Phosphate buffer and	In 120, 240 and 360 ml pack
	Cleaner/Rinser isotonic Boric acid, Sodium borate, Sodium perborate, 0.006% hydrogen peroxide.	In 12 ml pack
Saline Solutions (Preserved) Soft Lenses		
	i) Solution: Buffered isotonic, 0.01% EDTA, 0.001% thimerosal, Nacl, Sodium hexameta phosphate, boric acid and sodium borate	In 240 and 360 ml packs
	ii) Solution: Isotonic 0.1% EDTA, 0.001% poly quaternium-1, Nacl, borate	Thimerosal free in 360 ml pack
	iii) Solution: Buffered isotonic 0.1% sorbic acid, 0.025% EDTA, Nacl, boric acid, Sodium borate.	Thimerosal free in 120, 240 and 360 ml packs
	iv) Buffer solution: 0.1% Sorbic acid, Boric buffer, EDTA, NaCl.	In 60 and 360 ml packs
	v) Isotonic solution: NaCl, Boric acid, Sodium borate, Sodium perborate, Hydrogen peroxide, Phosphoric acid	In 120, 240 and 360 ml packs
Preservative Free Saline Solutions (Soft Lenses)		
	i) Buffer solution containing NaCl, Boric acid and Sodium borate	In 120, 240 and 360 ml packs
	ii) Buffered isotonic solution: NaCl, Catalytic neutralizing agent, EDTA, Mono and Dibasic sodium phosphates	In 15 ml single use containers
Rinsing/Storage Solutions(Soft Lenses)		
	i) Solution containing NaCl, Sodium hexameta phosphate, Sodium hydroxide,	120 and 240 ml packs

Drug name (Generic)	Dosage form/strength	Commercial packing
	boric acid, sodium borate 0.001% EDTA and 0.001% thimerosal	
	ii) Isotonic buffered solution of NaCl, Boric acid, 0.0003% Polyaminopropyl biguanide and EDTA	In 120 and 340 ml pack
	iii) Isotonic solution with 0.9% NaCl	Preservative free 120 and 240 ml packs
	iv) Buffered isotonic with NaCl and EDTA or NaCl with boric acid and sodium borate	Preservative free 120 and 240 ml packs
Surfactant Cleaning Solutions (Soft Lenses)		
	i) Solution containing 0.001% thimerosal, EDTA.	In 15 and 60 ml pack
	ii) Buffered isotonic solution NaCl, Sodium phosphate, Tyloxapol, Hydroxyl ethyl cellulose, Polyvinyl alcohol, EDTA, Sorbic acid	In 30 ml pack
	iii) Solution with Cocoamphor carboxy glycinate, Sodium lauryl sulfate, Hexylene glycol,0.1% Sorbic acid, 0.2% EDTA	In 15 ml pack
	iv) Solution: 15.7% Isopropyl alcohol, Poloxamer 407, Amphoteric 10.	Thimerosal free in 15 and 30 ml packs
	v) Solution: Buffered Isotonic: 0.15% Sorbic acid, 0.1% EDTA, Boric acid, Poloxamine, Sodium borate, NaCl	In 240 ml pack
	vi) Solution: Propylene glycol, Sodium borate, Highly purified porcine Pancreatin enzymes	Preservative free in 5 ml and 10 ml packs
	vii) Solution: 0.25% Sorbic acid, 0.5% EDTA NaCl, KCl, Poloxamer 407	In 25 ml pack
Enzymatic Cleaners (Soft Lenses)		
	i) Tablet containing papain, NaCl, Sodium carbonate, Sodium borate, EDTA	In pack of 12, 24, 36 and 48 tablets
	ii) Tablet containing subtilisin A, Polyethylene glycol, Sodium carbonate, Nacl and Tartaric acid	In pack of 8 tablets
	iii) Tablets: Effervescing buffering and tableting agents subtilisin A. To make solution for soaking dilute in 3% hydrogen peroxide solution	In pack of 5, 10, 15 and 20 tablets
Disinfecting/Wetting/Soaking solution (Soft Lenses)		
ReNu Multiplus	i) Solution containing Hydranate, boric acid, Edetate sodium, Sodium borate, NaCl, Dymed (polyamino-	In 120, 240 and 360 ml packs

Drug name (Generic)	*Dosage form/strength*	*Commercial packing*
	Propyl biguanide) 0.001% and 1% poloxamine	
	ii) Solution: 0.001% Polyhexa-methylene biguanide (PHMB), 0.025% Tyloxapol, 1.2% Tromethamine and 0.05% edetate disodium	In 120, 240 and 360 ml packs
Rewetting Solutions (Soft Lenses)		
	i) Isotonic solution containing 0.25% sorbic acid, 0.1% EDTA, borate buffer, NaCl, HPMC and glycerin	Thimerosal free in 15 ml pack
	ii) Isotonic solution NaCl, KCl, Hydroxyethyl cellulose, poloxamer 407, Sodium borate, Boric acid, Sorbic acid and EDTA	Thimerosal free in 5,15 and 30 ml packs
	iii) Buffered isotonic solution NaCl, 0.0001% Polyhexamethylene biguanide, Tromethamine, Tyloxapol, EDTA	In 15 ml pack
	iv) Solution: Sorbic acid, 0.15% and Edetate disodium 0.2%	In 15 ml pack
	v) Buffered isotonic NaCl, Boric acid	Preservative free in 0.035 ml pack
	vi) Isotonic solution: Citrate buffer, NaCl, 0.05% EDTA, 0.001% Poly quaternium-1	In 10 and 20 ml packs
	vii) Solution: Sorbic acid 0.1% and Edetate disodium	In 15 ml pack
	viii) Isotonic solution with NaCl, 0.13% Potassium sorbate and 0.025% EDTA	Thimerosal free in 15 ml pack
NON SURGICAL ADJUNCTS		
Lid Scrubs		
	i) Solution containing PET-200 glyceryl Tallowate, Disodium Laureth sulfosuccinate cocoamido propyl amine oxide, PEG-78 glyceryl cocoate, Benzyl alcohol and EDTA	In a pack of 30/60 pads and solution (120 ml)
	ii) Solution: PEG 80 sorbitan laurate, Sodium trideceth sulfate, PEG-150 distearate, cocoamido propyl hydroxy sutlaine, Lauroamphacarboxy-Glycinate, sodium Laureth 13 carboxylate PEG-15 tallow polyamine, Quaternium-15	Alcohol free. In 30,120 and 240 ml pack compliance kit (120 ml and 100 pads)
Tear Test Strips		
Schirmer test strip	Sterile test strips	Pack of 250 strips
Snostrips	Sterile tear flow test strips	In a pack of 100 strips
Zone quick	Phenol red threads (PRT)	In 50 aluminium packing sets (100 threads)

Drug name (Generic)	Dosage form/strength	Commercial packing
Hamameli's water	Solution containing aqueous and glycerin solution of senecio Compositae, hamameli's water and boric acid	In 7 ml vial
Boric acid	As powder	In a pack of 15 g powder
Astringent Ophthalmic Solution		
	i) Zinc sulphate 0.12% Boric acid 1.25% Naphazoline HCl 0.056% and Chlorpheniramine maleate 0.01%	In 5 and 10 ml dropper vials
	ii) Zinc sulphate 0.25% Tetrahydrozoline 0.05% EDTA and Benzalkonium Cl. (0.004%)	In 10 and 15 ml dropper vials
	iii) Zinc sulphate 0.1% Bolax 0.05%, Boric acid 1.9%, Sodium chloride bottle 0.45%, KCl 0.45, HPMC 0.7%	In 10 ml dropper vial and 120 ml
Vitamin and Antioxidants		
i) Vitamin A palmitate	Tablets/Cap. Containing 5000 IU/10000 IU/15000 IU/ 25000 IU vitamin-A	In pack of 100/250 Tab./Cap.
Antioxidants	i) Capsule containing vitamin A 6000 IU, Zinc 30 mg, Copper 1.5 mg, Selenium 60 mcg, Manganese 5 mg, Vitamin B_{12} 20 mg Vitamin C 200 mg and Vitamin E 60 IU	In a pack of 100 capsules.
	ii) Mixcarotin cap. Containing 15.44 mg Of mixed carotenoids in oily suspension (Alpha carotene, beta carotene, lutein, cryptoxanthin and zeaxanthine) equivalent to 25000 IU of vitamin A.	Soft gel capsules (in a pack of 100 capsules)
	iii) Tablets containing 5000 IU beta-carotene, 150 IU E, 20 mg B_1, B_2, B_6 each, 10 mcg B_{12},15 mg elemental Zn, 50 mcg, Selenium, 20 mg calcium pantothenate, 40 mg glutathion 40 mg B_3 100 mg C, 75 mg L-cysteine	In a pack of 100/250 tablets
	iv) Capsule: 5000 IU Vitamin A, 400 mg C, 200 IU E, 40 mg Zn, 5 mg L-glutathione, 3 mg sodium pyruvate, 2 mg copper and 40 mcg selenium.	In a pack of 60 cap.
	v) Capsules soft gel: Vitamin A 5000 IU, 200 IU, vitamin E, 200 mg vitamin C, 7.5 mg zinc, 1 mg copper, 15 mcg selenium and 1.5 mg Mn.	In a pack of 50 cap.

Drug name (Generic)	Dosage form/strength	Commercial packing
	vi)Tablets: 5000 vitamin A 30 IU vitamin E, 60 mg vitamin C, 40 mg Zinc, 2 mg copper and 40 mcg selenium	Film coated tab. in a pack of 60.

Topical Anticataract Therapy

Drug name (Generic)	Dosage form/strength	Commercial packing
(i) Catalin	Solution containing pyridophenoxazine (catalin) in concentrationof 0.75 mg/15 ml solvent	Pack of tablet alongwith 15 ml solvent
(ii) Cineraria	Solution containing large quantity of organic potassium	In 15 ml dropper vial
(iii) Anti-cataract solution	Solution containing 3.3% potassium iodide, 0.83% NaCl and 1.0% Calcium chloride	In 10 ml dropper vial
(iv) Aspirin	Topical solution as 1%	In 15 ml dropper vial
(v) Vitamin E therapy	Capsule containing 100/200 mg of vitamin E (alpha tocopherol)	In a pack of 100 capsules

Medical Therapy for Diabetic Retinopathy

Drug name (Generic)	Dosage form/strength	Commercial packing
i. D400	Tablet : Herbomineral preparation	In a pack of 100 tablets
ii. Calcium debesilate	Capsule (500 mg)	In a pack of 50 capsules
iii. Aspirin	Tablet (325 mg)	In a pack of 100 tab.
iv. Dipyridamol	Tablet (225 mg)	In a pack of 60 tablets
v. Ticlopidine	Tablet (500 mg)	In a pack of 100 tablets
vi. Cyclandelate	Capsule (400 mg)	In a pack of 100 capsules
vii. Ponalrestat	Tablet (600 mg)	In a pack of 50 tablets
viii. Sulindac	Tablet (250 mg)	In a pack of 100 tablets

DISINFECTIVE AND ANTISEPTIC AGENTS IN OPHTHALMOLOGY

Drug name (Generic)	Dosage form/strength	Commercial packing
a) Formaldehyde (Formalin)	i) as 10% aqueous soln	In 60 ml, 400 ml 1 liter and 5 liter packings.
	ii) as 10% tablets	In a pack of 60/100 tablets
b) Ethylene oxide	As 3% colorless liquid	In 400 ml and 1 liter packing
c) Glutaraldehyde	2% solution	As 60 ml, 400 ml and 1 liter packings
d) Sodium hypochlorite	As 1% solution	In 60 ml and 400 ml and 1 liter packings
e) Isopropyl alcohol	As 70% isopropyl alcohol	Pre sterilized individual swabs (A pack of 100 swabs)
f) Biguanides		
i) Polyhexanide (PHMB)	As stock 20% solution For ocular conditions diluted solution (1:1000) as 0.02% is prepared	In 60 ml, 100 ml and 400 ml packings
ii) Chlorhexidine	As 5% stock solution 0.2% diluted solution is prepared in isotonic saline for ophthalmic use	In 100 ml, 400 ml and 1 liter packings

Drug name (Generic)	Dosage form/strength	Commercial packing
g) Povidone Iodine (Halogens)	5% sterile prep. solution	In 5 ml, 15 ml dropper vials
h) Acetone	As 58.8% solution	In 60 ml,100 ml,400 ml and 1 liter packings
i) Cetrimide	10% solution	In 400 ml and 1 liter packings
j) Beta propiolactone (BPL)	0.2% solution/condensed product of ketone and formaldehyde	On 100 ml, 400 ml and 1 liter packings
k) Alcoholic rub-in-hand Disinfectant (Sterillium)	As solution containing 100 ml 2-propanol 45.0 g 1-propanol 30.0g Ethyl hexadecyl 2 g Dimethyl ammonium, Ethyl sulfate	In 100 ml pack
l) Cutasept (Antiseptic)	As solution containing 2-propanaol 63 g, Benzalkonium Cl-0.025 g] 10 g	100 ml and 500 ml pack
m) Korsolex disinfectant	As solution containing (Each 100 gm contains) Glutaraldehyde 7.0 g Formaldehyde 8.2 g Polymethylol urea derivative 17.6 g	As 500 ml pack
n) Bacillol disinfectant	As solution (Each 100 gm contains) Ethanol—10 gms 2-Propanol—9 gms 1-Propanol—6 gms	As 200 ml pack with spray
o) Baktolin (Antiseptic)	As solution (Each 100 gm contains) Propylene glycol 0.52% Sodium salicylate 0.46% Sodium lauryl sulphate 4.08% Sodium benzoate 5.9% with Coco Glucoside, PEG 120, Glycerine, Glycol stearate and sodium citrate	As 500 ml pack with dispenser
p) HIV disinfectant	Solution containing 45 g 2-propanol, 30 g 1-propanol, 0.2 g mecetronium ethyl sulfate (INN)	In 500 ml and 1 liter packs
q) Hydrogen peroxide	As stock solution (6%) for ophthalmic use can be diluted to 3%.	In 100 ml, 500 ml packs

37

Recent Advances in the Surgical Management of Age-related Macular Degeneration

- MACULAR TRANSLOCATION
- SUBMACULAR HEMORRHAGE IN ARMD-CNVM
- SURGICAL REMOVAL OF CHOROIDAL NEOVASCULAR MEMBRANE
- ENDOSCOPIC PEELS
- MACULAR BUCKLE IN EXUDATIVE AGE-RELATED MACULAR DEGENERATION
- IMPLANT RADIOTHERAPY FOR EXUDATIVE MACULAR DEGENERATION
- RETINAL PROSTHESIS
- RPE TRANSPLANTATION
- IRIS PIGMENT EPITHELIAL CELL TRANSPLANTATION
- RETINAL CELL TRANSPLANTATION
- STEM CELL RESEARCH
- GENE THERAPY
- ANTIANGIOGENIC THERAPY
- IMPLANTABLE MINIATURED TELESCOPE (IMT)
- TENSMAC (TRANSCUTANEOUS ELECTRICAL NERVE STIMULATION OF THE MACULA)
- RHEOPHERESIS

S Natarajan, Nishant Patel, Hitendra Mehta, Suhas Dongargaonkar (India)

INTRODUCTION

Age-related macular degeneration is the one of the leading cause of blindness in old age population throughout the world, especially more in developed countries. Now with better quality of life and increased life expectancy in developing countries like India it is soon becoming one of the most common pathology encountered by ophthalmologist in geriatric population. It is a well known fact that though wet AMD accounts for much less number of cases as compared to dry AMD it accounts for most of the cases of severe visual loss due to AMD. Different surgical options have been tried to manage the pathology and in this chapter we will discuss about some of them.

MACULAR TRANSLOCATION

Macular translocation involves moving the neurosensory retina of the macular region in an eye with recent onset subfoveal pathology to a new location with presumable healthier RPE and choriocapillaris. The most common indication of macular translocation is recent onset subfoveal CNV other being RPE defects created after removal of subfoveal CNV and cases having central geographic atrophy.

The basic pathology of AMD is usually limited to macular area. The inner aspect of Bruch's membrane is diffuse thickened, impending adequate passage of nutrients from the choroids to the pigments epithelium and metabolic products form the RPE to choroid. Multiple modalities of treatment like laser photocoagulation, photodynamic therapy or transpupillary thermotherapy (TTT) have shown to be helpful to stabilize the vision in about 70 percent of cases but one limitation in all these treatments is the inability to correct for the absence of RPE- Bruch's membrane choriocapillaris support of the photoreceptors that occurs with macular degeneration.

The mechanisms responsible for visual loss in eye with AMD may be either reversible or irreversible. In early stage of neovascular AMD, the visual loss may be due to subretinal fluid or hemorrhage in the macular region. In later stages of the disease fibrovascular proliferation causes permanent damage of the photoreceptors. Therefore by moving the neurosensory retina in an eye with recent onset subfoveal lesion to a new location with presumably healthier RPE and choriocapillaris away from the area of pathology, the fovea may be able to recover or maintain its visual function. In addition by moving the fovea away, removal or destruction of CNVs may be possible.[1]

Macular translocation has been defined[2] as any surgery that has a primary goal of relocation the central neurosensory retinal or fovea intraoperatively or postoperatively specifically for the management of macular disease.

Effective macular translocation is defined as successful intraoperative or postoperative relocation of the fovea overlying subfoveal lesion to an area outside the border of the lesion.

Classification of Macular Translocation Surgery[3]

- MT with large curvilinear incision of the retina
- MT with 360° retinotomy.
- MT with large retinotomy.
- MT with punctate or not retinotomy.
- MT with chorioscleral shortening.
- MT with infolding (imbrication or inpouching)
- MT with chorioscleral outfolding (outpouching)
- MT without chorioscleral shortening.

Basic Principles of Surgery

As a general principle vitrectomy is followed by creation of retinal detachment by infusion of fluid under the retina either through sclera or from inside through the retina. Once detachment is created either complete or incomplete the retinal is rotated around the optic nerve head to a desired degree and reattached. Many modification have been made by leading vitreoretinal surgeon do get optimum visual results by minimize manipulation and thereby surgical complications.

- ***Machemer*** advocated total RD with 360° peripheral retinotomy with created around 4500 μm of macular translocation.[4]
- ***Toth*** and ***Machemer***, alongwith ***Eckardt*** and ***Conrad*** have used transretinal infusion to create detachment, using wide field chandelier illumination

or illuminated cannula, wide field viewing systems[5] or performing oblique or rectus muscle transposition.[6]

- ***Ninomiya*** and ***Tano*** described detachment of temporal retina only and created 180° peripheral retinotomy with a superior or inferior radial incision to move the fovea superiorly or inferiorly.[7]
- A retinal detachment may be created on the temporal side without a retinotomy after which sclera is shortened by scleral resection resulting in shift of choroid and sclera in relation to the fovea.[8,9]
- ***De Juan*** has described method of limited translocation in which only temporal retina is detached and limbal parallel arcuate shortening of choroid and sclera is done thereby achieving about 1500 μm of translocation and later CNV was photocoagulated.[9]

Complications

Complication of the macular translocation surgery include retinal detachment, PVR, cataract, neovascularization of iris, corneal decompensation, recurrence of membrane, CME, diplopia. The rate of retinal detachment after MT surgery has decreased in past few years largely due to refinement in surgical techniques, use of PFCL, wide angle viewing system, wide field illumination and technique of inducing retinal detachment using fine gauge needles for fluid injection.[5]

SUBMACULAR HEMORRHAGE IN ARMD-CNVM

Submacular hemorrhage results in a large scotoma and poor vision[10-14] if left alone. Submacular hemorrhage associated with certain clinical features like submacular hemorrhage extending beyond the vascular arcades, associated subfoveal hemorrhagic pigment epithelial detachment or with associated breakthrough vitreous hemorrhage usually has poor visual prognosis.

Surgical Management

Different techniques are applied for the surgical management of submacular hemorrhage. Here we will discuss in brief about them.

a. Pneumatic displacement with prone position– intravitreal injection of 0.4-0.5 ml of perfluoropropane gas followed by prone position has been tried to temporarily displace the blood.[15]
b. Pneumatic displacement with intravitreal Tissue Plasminogen Activator (t-PA), followed by prone positioning—A simple technique to treat above condition is to inject t-PA intravitreally (25-100 μg) followed by a separated injection of either SF6 or C3F8.[16-18] The patient is reviewed after clearance of the blood from the macular area.
c. Intravitreal t-PA, vitrectomy with perfluorocarbon liquid injection followed by subretinal t-PA – in this technique[19,20] preoperative intravitreal Tpa is injected followed by vitrectomy and intravitreal injection of PFCL to displace liquified subretinal blood through a retinotomy. Again subretinal space is irrigated with Tpa to remove remaining solid clots.
d. Vitrectomy with subretinal irrigation/aspiration of Tpa– here initial vitrectomy is followed by subretinal irrigation of Tpa. A time interval of about 20 to 45 minutes is allowed for the Tpa to cause clot lysis after which it is aspirated along with the blood from the subretinal space.[21-23]
e. Direct surgical removal of submacular clots with subretinal dissection through large retinal incision. Due to high incidence of complications this technique is almost out of use now.

SURGICAL REMOVAL OF CHOROIDAL NEOVASCULAR MEMBRANE

Choroidal neovascular membrane usually causes a decline in visual function either due to exudative fluid, hemorrhage or the neovascular tissue itself especially if it extends beneath the central macula and interferes with normal metabolic interaction between photoreceptors and RPE.[24, 25] The goal of the surgery is to remove the CNVM while preserving as much normal RPE, choriocapillaris and neurosensory retina as possible, which may result in resolution of exudative fluid and/or hemorrhage and return of normal interaction between photoreceptors and RPE thereby restoring the visual function.

Eyes with CNVM due to AMD are not considered good candidates for surgical treatment as the widespread nature of the disease involving the RPE/Bruch's membrane/Photoreceptor complex and extensive fibrovascular growth posterior to RPE.[1-4]

Table 37.1: Morphological features of CNVM

Membranes anterior to RPE	*Membranes posterior to RPE*
Clinical features • A discernible, well defined edge of membrane • The membrane may be seen to lie anterior to the plane of underlying RPE • A thin rim of blood/ pigmented border varying between dark brown and tan indicating the presence of a plane between the membrane and the RPE	*Clinical features* • Edge of the membrane indistinguishable from the surrounding tissue • RPE itself appears elevated-RPE surrounding the membrane gradually slopes back to the plane of the normal RPE • Subretinal blood if present does not outline the edge of the membrane and the blood may appear darker suggesting a sub- RPE location
Angiographic features • A well defined boundary/a rim of blocked fluorescence between the hyperfluorescence of the membrane and the background choroidal fluorescence • Angiographically compact membrane with regular distinct borders is seen • Relative homogenous pattern of fluorescence in the membrane • Late staining of tissue outside membrane is absent	*Angiography features* • A ill defined edge or irregular border between membrane fluorescence and background choroidal fluorescence • Uneven filling of fluorescein dye suggest sub-RPE • Late hyperfluprescence in adjacent tissue implies occult or sub- RPE membrane • Angiographic evidence of RPE detachment is highly suggestive of sub-RPE membrane

Location of the membrane whether anterior or posterior to the RPE plays an important role in the prognosis and results of surgery. Table 37.1 highlights few morphological features depending on the location of the membrane.

In this technique a small retinotomy is created after complete vitrectomy and removal of posterior hyaloid. BSS if gently infused through the retinotomy to create a localized RD after which the CNVM is removed with a subretinal pick forceps taking care to minimize RPE loss (Table 37.2). During the above maneuver the IOP can be elevated to avoid bleeding. Fluid gas exchange is done and patient is given a prone position. Special instruments (33 to 36 gauge with about 130 degree bend and 3 mm long blades) are used to remove the CNVM with minimal trauma to the RPE and photoreceptors.[26,27] Complications of the surgery mainly include recurrence the others being cataract formation, macular pucker, retinal detachment, retinal holes, hemorrhage, endophthalmitis and light toxicity.

ENDOSCOPIC PEELS

Pigment epithelial endoscopic laser surgery is a surgical modality of treatment where precise laser photocoagulation of the CNVM complex and choroidal feeder vessels is possible using endoscopic laser. Surgical technique

Table 37.2: Results of surgical removal of CNVM[28-29]

Better surgical results	*Poor surgical results*
Type I (Pre-RPE membrane) Presumed ocular histoplasmosis idiopathic multifocal choroiditis	***Type II (Post-RPE membrane)*** Age-related macular degeneration High myopia Angioid streaks.
Subretinal pigment halo around CNVM Sharply defined borders and plaque-like elevation of CNV Normal fellow eye	Associated PED CNV adherent to the retina or the adjacent scar Age > 50 years

includes standard three-port pars plana vitrectomy with proper and complete separation and removal of posterior hyaloid with induction of localized retinal detachment through a retinotomy. Endoscope is introduced through the retinotomy and laser is applied to the CNVM (Figures 37.1 to 37.5).

MACULAR BUCKLE IN EXUDATIVE AGE-RELATED MACULAR DEGENERATION

Morphometric analysis of the retina and choroid at and around the macula in patients with age-related macular degeneration has demonstrated a relative choriocapillary congestion and vasodilation under the macula.[30] Moreover, color Doppler analysis of eyes with AMD has also demonstrated decreased velocity.

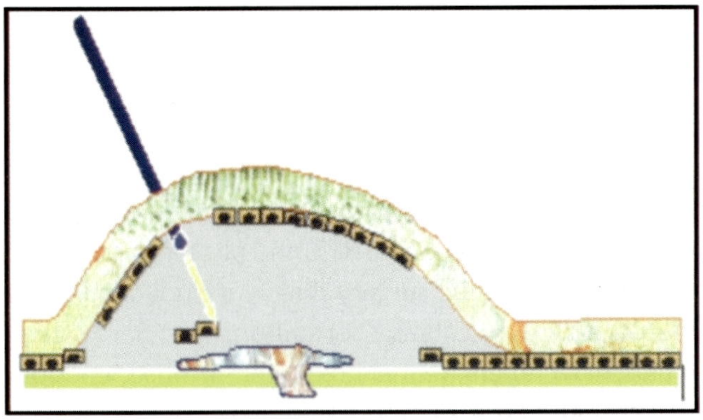

Figure 37.1: Schematic diagram of PEELS

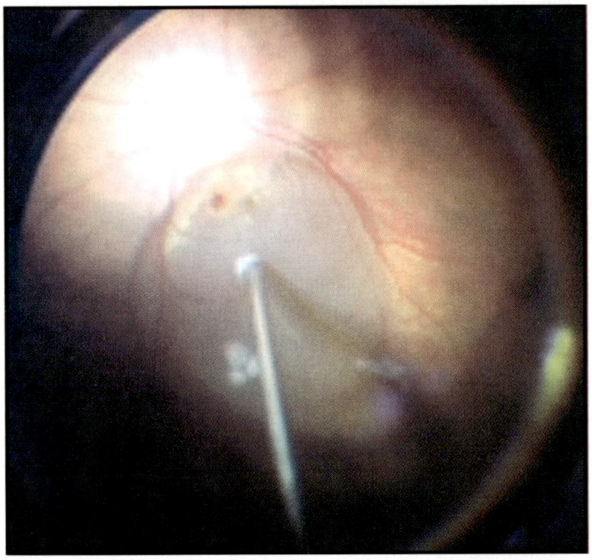

Figure 37.2: Induction of retinal detachment

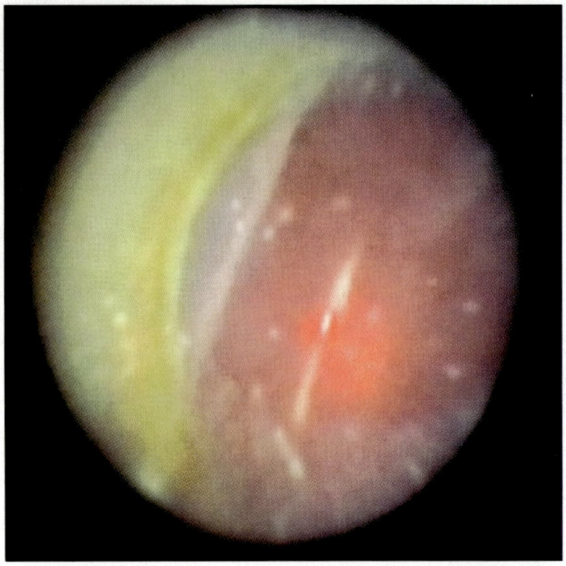

Figure 37.3: Laser delivery to the choroidal neovascular membrane

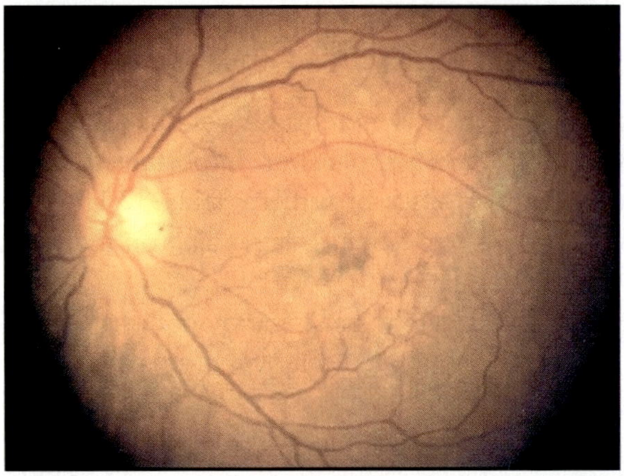

Figure 37.4: Preoperative subfoveal CNV with RCA (VA : 6/60)

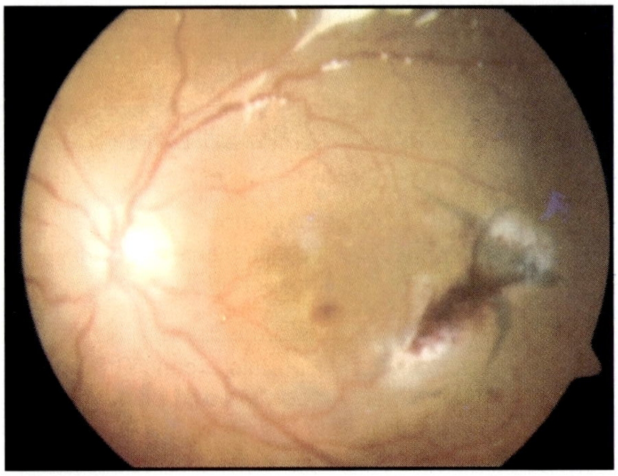

Figure 37.5: Immediate postoperative

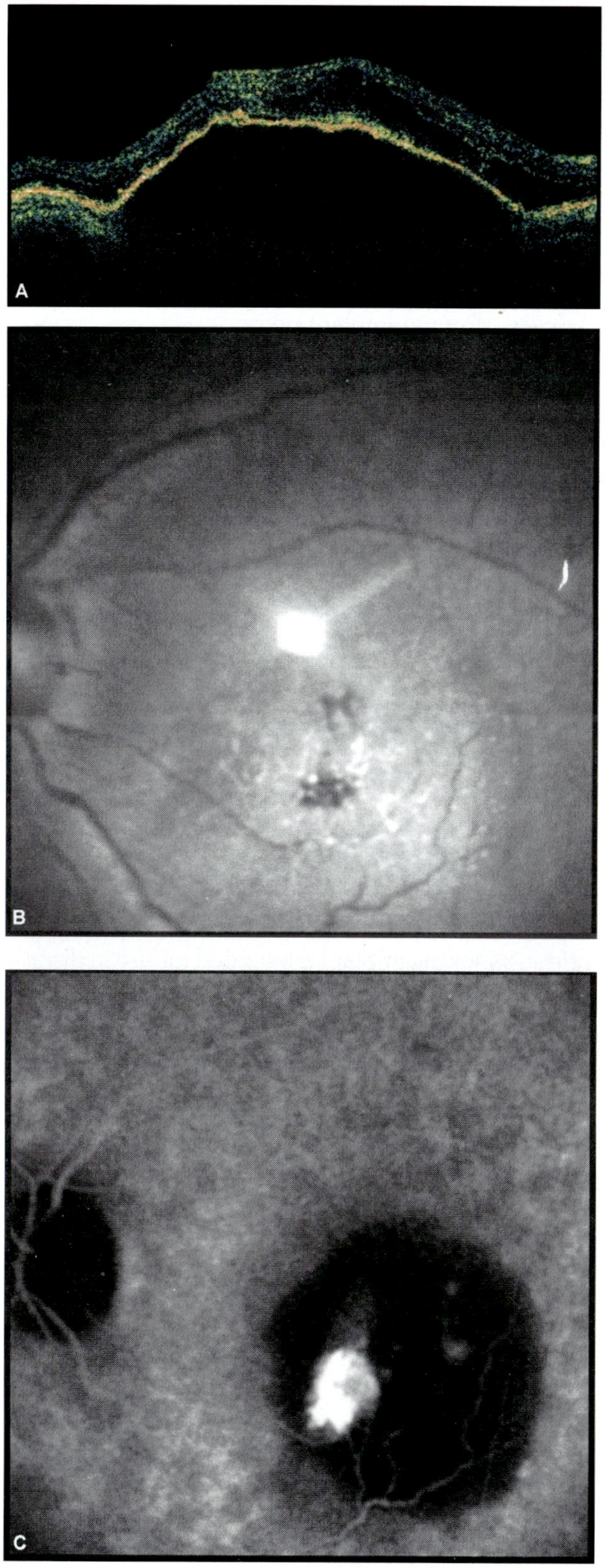

Figures 37.6A to C: Immediate postoperative

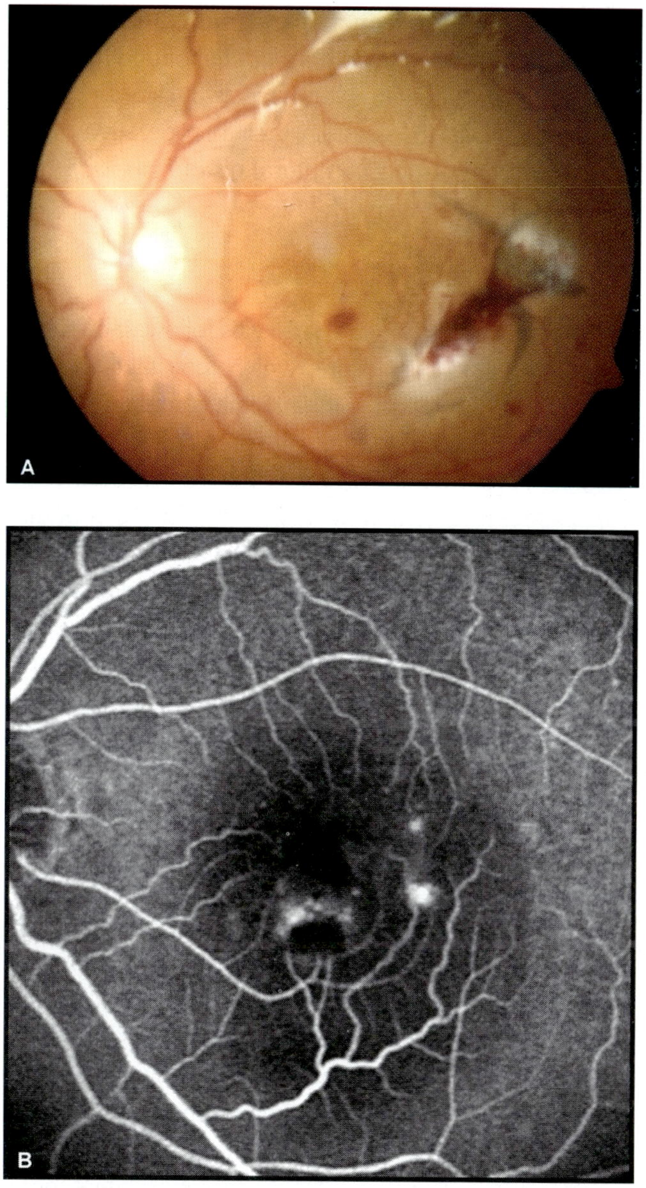

Figures 37.7A and B: 3months postoperative (VA: 6/24)

And increased pulsatility of ocular arterial blood flow.[31] The resulting vascular congestion may increase exudation, bleeding and growth from the CNVM.

In the attempt to reduce the choroidal engorgement, vascular leakage and bleeding in AMD patients, an external posterior macular buckle has been used. The macular buckle consists of a strip of Gore-Tex material with an additional 8.5 to 9 mm piece of silicone sponge buckling material. This produces a scleral indentation at the level of the fovea centered underneath the CNVM, thereby helping to reduce the choroidal congestion. Limited studies done with this modality of treatment has shown that eyes treated with macular buckle placement were more likely to maintain their preoperative vision compared to retrospective natural history studies.[32]

IMPLANT RADIOTHERAPY FOR EXUDATIVE MACULAR DEGENERATION

Radiation can induce acute vasculitis followed by slowly progressive vascular closure, which may take years to develop.[33-35] Radiation to the macula containing CNVM can affect the angiogenesis. Moreover, it has been suggested that radiotherapy may inhibit the scar formation associated with end-stage exudative macular degeneration.[36]

External beam radiotherapy has been tried for the treatment of CNVM as it is widely available, nonsurgical and comparatively less expensive. However, it not only irradiates both the eyes but also sinuses and /or the brain. Proton beam therapy also has been used with the advantage of being nonsurgical and unilateral. However the disadvantage of this technique is that it can be affected by ocular movements and it is not widely available.

Implant radiotherapy or brachytherapy involves placement of radiation source directly near the macula. Here, the macula receives larger dose than with EBRT but the normal ocular structures receive less radiation. Moreover, it allows high dose of irradiation over a relatively short duration and moreover almost no radiation to the other eye and the surrounding parts of the body.

Pallidium –103[37] or strontium –90[38] have been employed for implant radiotherapy. Studies with above modality of treatment have shown resolution of hemorrhages, exudates and subretinal fluid.

RETINAL PROSTHESIS

Currently two different kinds of retinal prosthesis are being investigated, epiretinal or subretinal. The epiretinal one does not disturb the relationship between the RPE and retina, however its position should remain same after implantation and should be able to remain steady despite ocular movements.

The subretinal one disturbs the relationship between the RPE and choroid but can access the visual signal integration system at the earliest possible and thereby allowing the signals to be processed by the maximal amount. Described below are some of the investigators who are currently involved with retinal prosthesis.

Epiretinal

Eckmiller—Retinal implant news.

Bonn Rizzo—The retinal implant group, MIT, Harvad; the chip is positioned near ganglion cells. A camera is mounted on the eyeglasses to capture image and a digital signal processor transmits a light image to the chip. Two computer chips are used along with a tiny solar panel and a long circuit.

Humayun – Intraocular retinal prosthesis group, North Carolina state prosthesis project.

Johns Hopkins – Small external camera is used to capture image and a chip is implanted near ganglion cell layer resulting in a 10x10 pixel capability.

Subretinal

Zrenner – Retinal implant,

Tubingen Yagi – Hybrid retinal implant

Chow – Optobionics; composed of micro-photodiode subunits the implant is intended for use in disorders where photoreceptors are lose, while the remaining retinal layers are spared, e.g. Retinitis pigmentosa, ARMD. It is stimulated by light, which is converted to electric impulses inducing biological visual signals in the remaining functional retinal cells. Several initial studies have been carried out in animals with success. The device has been implanted in 6 human eyes with RP and 1year follow-up has shown no major complications. Patients have reported improved vision and appreciation of black and white images in well-lit room. US FDA approval is awaited for larger human trials.

As these early stages of research, predicting the time of availability and ultimate efficacy of retinal prosthesis is difficult. However, progress has been made in the last decade, and human subjects have been able to identify crude shapes and phophenes, and animal testing has been encouraging.

RPE TRANSPLANTATION

RPE dysfunction is believed to be the main cause of many debilitating diseases of which ARMD and retinitis pigmentosa are the most common problems. In these diseases, photoreceptors ultimately are affected, causing severe vision loss because of the loss or dysfunction of RPE cells rather than any abnormality of the photoreceptor themselves. In last few years tremendous amount of research has been made in the area of RPD transplantation. Two techniques have been used, the external (anterior transvitreal) approach and the internal (posterior transcleral) approach. In both the cases RPE cells are introduced into the subretinal space as cell suspension or sheets of RPE cells.

The types of cells currently being used for transplanting are: human fetal RPE immortalized RPE, porcine fetal RPE and autologous (obtained from the same eye that is being transplanted, from a remote location. RPE cells can be harvested from cadever eyes within 24 hours of death and can be preserved at 4° for upto 48 hours. Cryoprecipitate obtained from human blood donors can be used for adhesion cultivation and transfer of RPE cells.

Survival of the grafted transplanted RPE cells can be monitored by labeling them with carbon particles, fluorescent dye, radioactive level (3-H thymidine) and lad –2. Studies have shown that fetal RPE cells do not survive and repopulate because of the unavailability of extracellular matrix receptors required for attachment and spreading. However, cleaning and resurfacing the inner collagenous layer increased the RPE attachment, decreased apoptosis, and allowed cells to repopulate.

As a part of FDA controlled phase 1 clinical trail, intact sheets of RPE cells are transplanted, at least till 3 months, no rejection has been reported. Rejection has been shown to occur early in patients with wet AMD than in patients with dry AMD, most likely because of compromised blood retinal barrier in wet AMD.

Rejection seems to be worse in patients with both major histocompatibility complex incompatibilities.

Predinisone has been shown to play role in delaying rejection by suppressing humoral response.

Cyclosporine, given intravitreally prolongs the survival of transplanted RPE cells by inhibiting the first phase of T cell activation while azathioprine delays rejection by inhibiting delayed hypersensitivity reaction and cellular cytotoxic activity.

Some of the issues which still need to be addressed before RPE cell transplantation becomes a clinically viable surgical procedure are collection and preservation techniques, prolongation of survival of grafted cells, control of long-term immune responses, and techniques that would allow a monolayer formation of the grafted cells.

IRIS PIGMENT EPITHELIAL CELL TRANSPLANTATION

This method was introduced by Gelance et al.[39,40] There are two different methods by which the procedure can be performed.

One Step Surgery

Here IPE cells are harvested from one or two basal iridectomies and reinjected into the subretinal space in 20 percent serum. An injection of 20,000-50,000 cells has shown a viability of 70-80 percent.

Two Step Surgery[41]

IPE cells are harvested through iridectomy and cultured until a desired number is reached after which they are injected in the subretinal space near macula after removal of any subretinal membranes. Here approximately about 20,000 to 2,00,000 cells are injected.

RETINAL CELL TRANSPLANTATION

The main aim of transplanting retinal photoreceptors is to re-establish appropriate cellular connections and thereby some functional capacity. During surgical experiments on animals, transplanted fetal tissue do survive and differentiate, but do not show normal retinal orientation.[42] While enzymatically separated adult photoreceptor cells transplanted into subretinal space survive and tend to develop synaptic terminals but outer segments tend to degenerate.[43,44] However, the functional capacity of these transplanted cells has not been tested since the visually directed behavior of these animals was not assessed. Despite the paucity of evidence that this technique is useful, mechanically dissociated fetal retinal of 14 to 18 weeks gestation have been grafted in patients with advanced RP. No rejection or complications have been reported and some patients have reported improvement of vision.[45]

STEM CELL RESEARCH

Scientists have discovered stem cells (immature precursor cells) in the eye of adult rodents, and studies are now under way to see if these cells can be transplanted into humans to replace diseased photoreceptors.

Experiments are also underway to use stem cells for drug delivery devices to deliver vascular endothelial growth factor inhibitors, lutein and zeaxanthin as well as other drugs.

GENE THERAPY

A replication deficient adenovirus gene trangene vector, Ad, (GV) PEDF 11D, having the tansgene cDNA for human pigment epithelium-derived factor (PEDF) is under research. PEDF is a potent antiangiogenic factor in normal human eye and the intravitreal delivery of Ad (GV) PEDF 11D will administer PEDF to the target cells in the human eye.[46] VEGF is a potent factor in many of the disease, which result in neovascularization, and CNV is no exception. VEGF soluble receptor gene transfection can inhibit CNV.[47]

ANTIANGIOGENIC THERAPY

Examination of CNVMs removed postoperatively and after postmortem has shown it to be immunoreactive to growth factors (e.g. VEGF, TGF – B, PDGF, b- FGF), which are thought to be angiogenic.

A new rationale for an attack on vascular endothelial growth factor (VEGF), a mediator for angiogenesis in many experimental and clinical situations is on the horizon. VEGF is also a vascular permeability factor and is actually 50,000 times more potent than histamine in inducing leakage of the blood vessels and upregulation of VEGF has been shown with both increased permeability of ocular blood vessels and development of neovascularization in the eye. Drugs under research as anti-VEGF therapy include pagaptanib (Macugen) an aptamer that block the VEGF receptor when given intravitreally, an antibody fragment called rhuFab V2 that is also given intravitreally.

An antiangiogenic steroid, anecortave acetate, which is angiostatic but having less glucocorticoid activity, is under investigation as a monotherapy as well as an adjunct. Role of steroids is treating increased vascular permeability is being explored. Intravitreal injection of a steroid (triamcinolone), a biodegradable implant (Oculex, which delivers dexamethasone and a reservoir implant (releasing fluocinolone) are under investigation as adjunct to the above mentioned treatment modalities.

IMPLANTABLE MINIATURED TELESCOPE (IMT)

IMT is a new approach to aid vision in patients with age-related macular degeneration. The telescope consists of 3X telescope that is contained in carrying device made of PMMA that can be implanted in the capsular bad. It provides improvement of the central visual acuity in the implanted eye for reading, while the other eye can be used for peripheral navigational vision. The implant has a universal power; fine adjustment of vision can be achieved by wearing low power plus or minus spectacles. The advantage of the implant is that it provides magnification of vision without the need to hold the device patient may notice transient difficulty in orientation.

TENSMAC (TRANSCUTANEOUS ELECTRICAL NERVE STIMULATION OF THE MACULA)

This form of treatment is under research currently. It involves rejuvenation of the diseased cells before they degenerate by using electrostimulation given by small electrodes placed in the troubled area, which pass micro-electric current.

RHEOPHERESIS

Here blood filtration is performed to remove toxic protein and waste material that hinder blood flow, thus increasing capillary blood flow to the macula, is done by using a membrane differential filtration system. (The RheoFilter and Plamsflo MDF system). This modality of treatment is under considerable debate.

Most of the surgical treatment is only directed to treat the pathological conditions arising due to AMD rather than the cause. We hope that in the near future more effective treatment options to manage the cause of AMD come into vogue so that this disease, which is climbing in prevalence, can be taken care of in very early stage and/or prevented from becoming so severe that it causes visual loss.

REFERENCES

1. Machmer R. Macular translocation. Editorial Am J Ophthalmol 1998;125:698-700.
2. Kah – Guan Au Enong, Dante J, Peiramici, et al. Macular translocation: Unifying concepts, terminology and classification. Am J Ophthalmol 2001;131:244-53.
3. Adapted from Au Eong KG, Piermici Dj, Fuji GY, De Juan E, jr. Limited macular translocation in age related macular degeneration. In: Alberti WE, RichardG, Sagerman RH (Eds.) Age related macular degeneration: Current treatment concepts Berlin Heidelberg: Springer – Verlag 2001;37-54.
4. Machemer R. retinal separation, retinotromy and macular translocation, 2: a surgical approach to age related macular degeneration? Graefes Arch Clin Exp Ophthalmol 1993; 231:635-41.
5. Cynthia Toth, Sharon Freedman. Macular translocation with 360° peripheral retinectomy- Impact of technique and surgical experience on visual outcomes. Retina 2001; 21: 293-303.
6. Eckardt C. macular rotation with and without outer rotation of the globe in patients with age related macular degeneration; Graefed Archive for clinical and experimental. Ophthalmology 1999; 237; 313-25.
7. Ninomiya Y et al. retinotomy and foveal translocation for surgical management of subfoveal choroidal neovascular membrane. Am J Ophthalmol 1996; 122: 613-21.
8. Imai K, Anat Loewenstein, De Juan E, Jr. Translocation of the retinal for management of subfoveal choroidal neovascularisation 1: A preliminary report in humans. Am J Ophthalmol 1998; 125: 635-46.
9. Eugene De Juan Jr, Anat Loewenstein et al. Translocation of the retina for management of subfoveal choroidal neovascularization 2: A preliminary report in humans. Am J Ophthalmol 1998; 125: 635-46.
10. A very RL, Fekart S, Hawkins BS, Bressler NM. Natural history of subfoveal hemorrhages in age related macular degeneration. Retina 1996; 16: 183-89.
11. Scupola A, Coscas G, Soubrane G, Balestrazzi E. Natural history of macular subretina haemorrahage in age related macular degeneration. Ophthalmologica 1999; 213:97-102.
12. Berrocal MH, Lewis ML, Flynn HW Jr. Variations in the clinical course of submacular haemorrhage. Am J Ophthalmol 1996; 122:486-93.
13. Chen WL, Liu JH, Lee FL Natural course of submacular haemorrhage. Chung Hua I Hsueh Tsa Chih (Taipei) 1999; 62: 268-77.
14. Bennett Sr, Folk JC, Boldi FC, Klugman M. Factors Prognostic of visual outcome in patients with subretinal haemorrhage. Am J Ophthalmol 1990; 109: 33-37.
15. Ohji M,Saito Y,Hayashi A, et al. Pneumatic displacement of subretinal haemorrhage without tissue plasminogen activation. Arch Ophthamol 1998;116:1326-32
16. Lim JI. Subretinal haemorrhage. In Sternberg P, Lin JI (Eds): Macular disease. Int Ophthalmol Clin 1995; 35: 95-104.
17. Peyman GA, Nelson et al. tissue Plasminogen activating factor assisted removal of subretinal haemorrhage. Ophthalmic Surg 1991; 22:57-82.
18. Heriot WJ, Further experience in management of submacular hemorrhage with intravitreal tpa. In: Proceedings of the 1997 Update on macular surgery. San Francisco: American Academy of Ophthalmology 1997;82-84.
19. Kimura M, Tano Y, Maeno T, et al. Removal of subretinal haemorrhage facilitated by prooperative intravitreal tissue plaminogen activator, Retina 1994;14:83-84.
20. Kamei M, Tano Y, Maeno T, et al. Surgical removal of submacular hemorrhage using tissue plasminogen atcivator and perfluorocarbon liquid. Am J Opthalmol 1996; 121:267-75.
21. Peyman GA, Nelson NC Jr, Altruki W, et al. Tissue plasminogen activating factor assisted removal of subretinal haemorrhage, Ophthalmic Surg 1991;22: 575-82.
22. Millsap MC, Peyman GA, Greve MDJ. Subretinal hemorrhage removal with multiple retinotomy sites in age-related macular degeneration, Opthalmic Surg 1994;25:723-25.
23. Lewis H. Intraoperative fibrolysis of submacular hemorrhage wit tissue plasminogen activator and surgical drainage, Am J Ophthamol 1994;118:559-68.
24. Sabates NR, Crane WG, Sabates FN, Schuchard RA, Fletcher DC. Scanning laser ophthalmoscope macular perimetry in the evaluation of submacular surgery. Retina 16:296-304.
25. Tezel TH, Del LV, Flowers PF, Lambert HM, Sternberg P, L'Hernault N. Ultrastructural features of surgically excised subretinal neovascular membranes in the ocular histoplasmosis syndrome. Arch Ophthalmol 1993;111:88-95.
26. Thomas MA, Grand MG, Williams DG, Lee cm, Pesin SR, Lowe MA. Surgical management of subfoveal choroidal neovascularization. Ophthalmology 1992;99:952-68.
27. Thomas MA, Lee CM, Pesin SR, Lowe MA. New instruments for submacular surgery. Am J Ophthalmol 1991;112:733-24 (letter).
28. Gass JD. Biomicroscopic and Histopathologic consideration regarding the feasibility of surgical excision of subfoveal neovascular membranes. Am J Ophthalmol 1994;118:285-98.

29. Thomas MA. Vitrectomy surgery for choroidal neovascularisation, Macula Society Rosenthal Lecture, Boca Raton, FL, 1995.
30. Spraul CW, Lang GE, Grossniklaus HE. Morphometric analysis of the choroid, Bruch's membrane, and retinal pigment epithelium in eyes with age-related macular degeneration. Invest Ophthalmol Vis Sci 1996;37:2724-35.
31. Friedman E, Krumpsky S, Lane AM, et al. Ocular blood flow velocity in age-related macular degeneration. Ophthalmology 1995;102:640-46.
32. Peyman GA, Conway MD, Recansens MA, et al. Use of a macular buckle for exudative age-related macular degeneration. Ophthalmic Surg Lasers 1999;30:619-30.
33. Chakravarthy U, Biggart JH, Gardiner TA, et al. Focal irradiation of perforating eye injuries. Curr Eye Res 1989; 8:1241-50.
34. Charkarvarthy U, Gardiner TA, Archer DB, Maguire CJ. A light microscopic and autoradiographic study of non irradiated and irradiated ocular wounds. Curr Eye Res 1989; 8:337-48.
35. Flickinger JC, Pollock BE, Kondziolka D, Lunsford LD. A dose-response analysis fo arteriovenous malformation obliteration after radiosurgery. Int J Radiat Oncol Biol Phys 1996;36:873-79.
36. Hart PM, Archer DP, Chakarvarthy V. Asymmetry of disciform scarring in bilateral disease when one eye is treated with radiotherapy. Br J Ophthalmol 1995;79:562-68.
37. Finger PT, Lu D, Buffa A, et al. Palladium – 103 versus iodine – 125 for ophthalmic plaque radiotherapy. Int J Radiat Oncol Biol Phys 1993;27:849-54.
38. Brady LW, Freire JE, Longton WA, et al. Radiation therapy for macular degeneration: technical considerations and preliminary results. Int Radiat Oncol Biol Phys 1997;39:945-48.
39. Gelanee M, Breipohl W, Weidmann P, Baib-Majani W, Heinmann K. First experimental iris pigment epithelial transplantation in subretinal space of RCS rat. Invest Ophthalmol Vis Sci 1997;38:334-39.
40. Gelance M, Meneses P, Rosenfeld MR, Duvoisin RM, Coleman D. Long term results of autologous transplantation of iris pigment epithelial cells into the subretinal space. Invest Ophthalmol Vis Sci 1997;38:334-39.
41. Tamai M, Abe T, Tomita H. Yoshida M. Kano T, Sato M. Autologous iris pigment transplantation in age related macular degeneration. In: Das T (Ed): Retina. Current Practice and Future Trends. Hyderabad Paras Publishing 1999;151-61.
42. Aramant RB, Seiler MJ, Turner JE. Donor age influences on the success of retinal transplants to adult retina. Invest Ophthalmol Vis Sci 1988;29:498-503.
43. Gouras P, Du J, Gelanze M, et al. Survival and synapse formation of transplanted rat rods. J Neural Transplant Plast 1991;2:91-100.
44. Gouras P, Du J, Gelanze M, et al. Transplantation of photoreceptors labelled with tritiated thymidine into RCS rats. Invest Ophthalmol Vis Sci 1991;32:1704-07.
45. Del Cerro M, Das TP, Lazar ES, et al. Neural retinal transplantaton into twelve RP patients. Invest Ophthalmol Vis Sci (Suppl) 1997;38;1204.
46. Rasmussen H, Chu KW, Campochiaro P, Gehlbach PL, Haller JA, Handa JT, et al. Clinical Research and Regulatory Affairs, USA.
47. Honda M, Sakamoto T, Ishibashi T, Inomata H, Uneo H. Adenovirus–mediate soluble VEGF/flt-1 receptor gene transfection: a role of VEGF and possible treatment for SRN in age related macular degeneration. Department of Ophthalmology, Faculty of Medicine, Kyushu University, Fukuoka, Japan.

38

Recent Advances in Lid, Orbital and Lacrimal Surgery

- LID SURGERY
- ORBITAL SURGERY
- LACRIMAL SURGERY
- MISCELLANEOUS MODES OF TREATMENT

AK Grover, Sarmi Malik, Zia Chaudhuri (India)

INTRODUCTION

The recent years have seen a number of advances in the armamentarium of the oculoplastic surgeon. Grafts and tissue substitutes have become an area with an ever expanding choice of tissue, natural or synthetic. Many of these products were initially used in non-ophthalmic fields and later found their way into oculoplasty surgery. Some of these new products are high quality *banked fascia* on a widespread manufactured basis, manufactured *sclera, Alloderm* (Lifecall Corp, Woodlands, Tex)- an acellular dermal product that can be used as a good *eyelid spacer, pericardial grafts, hydroxyapatite granules, Medpor and Alloderm sheets*—all of which can be used to replace orbital volume in enophthalmos. The use of integrated implants after enucleation has necessitated the need to cover these, especially when hydroxyapatite implants are used. These have included *fascia, vicryl mesh, sclera, pericardium*, etc. The use of other replacement tissues would continue as man's quest for perfection continues.[1]

This chapter deals with some of these aspects, which have seen substantial changes, and puts the current status in these subjects in a proper perspective.

LID SURGERY

Materials used in Frontalis Sling Surgery

A number of materials have been used for sling surgery in ptosis. Some alternatives to fresh autologous fascia lata have been used. These include both naturally occurring materials like *banked fascia lata* and *palmaris longus tendon*, and synthetic materials like *silicon rod, ePTFE* (Figures 38.1A and B) suture (Gore-Tex), 1-0 *Prolene, Mersilene* and *polyester* sutures.

Autologous/Homologous Materials

It is interesting to note that fresh fascia lata (Figures 38.2A and B) has shown better results than stored fascia lata. It has been found to have less chances of tissue reaction in the form of granulomas, as compared to the stored fascia. In addition, the failure rate after using stored fascia lata has been reported to be 40-50 percent after a ten-year follow-up.[2]

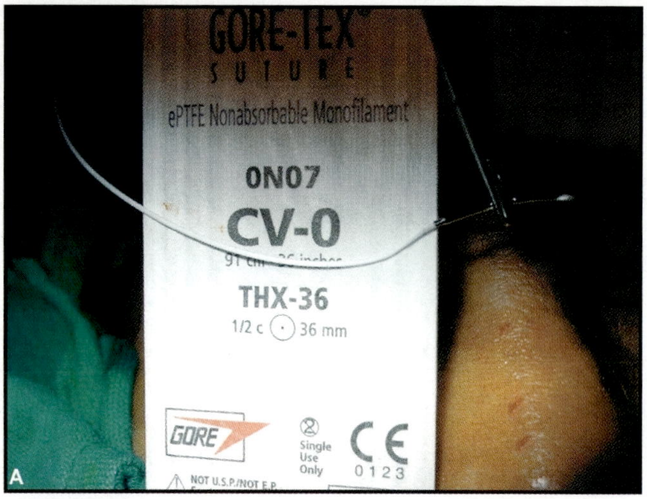

Figure 38.1A: ePTFE suture, which is frequently used to perform a frontalis sling surgery

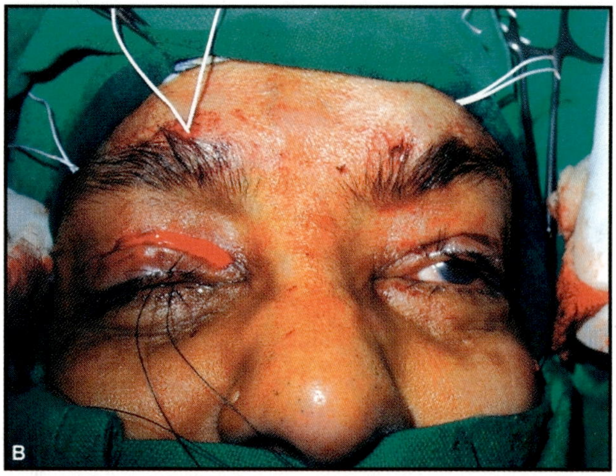

Figure 38.1B: A double triangle frontalis sling surgery being performed with ePTFE sutures

In a histopathological study of frontalis suspension materials in rabbit, autogenous fascia lata, 1-0 Prolene and silicon bands were compared. It was found that fascia lata showed better incorporation into surrounding tissues and least inflammatory reaction as compared to synthetic materials.[3]

Thus, autogenous fascia lata has been proven to be the material of choice in sling surgery for ptosis, provided there are no contraindications (Figures 38.2C to G).

Some known complications of using fascia lata include an unsightly scar in the thigh region, hematoma formation, keloid formation and herniation of the muscle belly. These complications have been reported in the

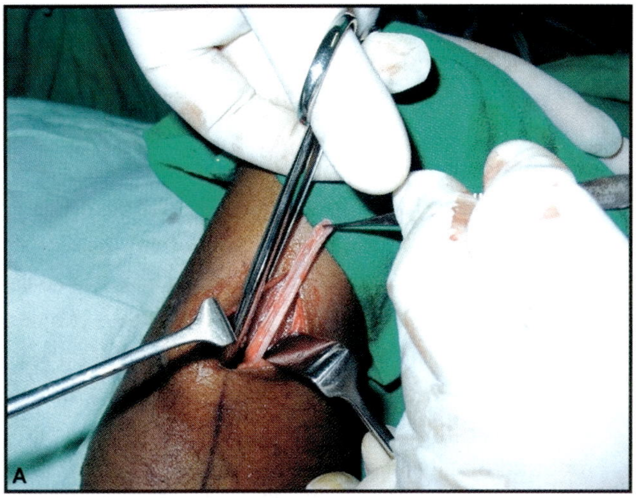

Figure 38.2A: Fresh autogenous fascia lata being dissected out from the thigh for use as slinging material in frontalis sling surgery

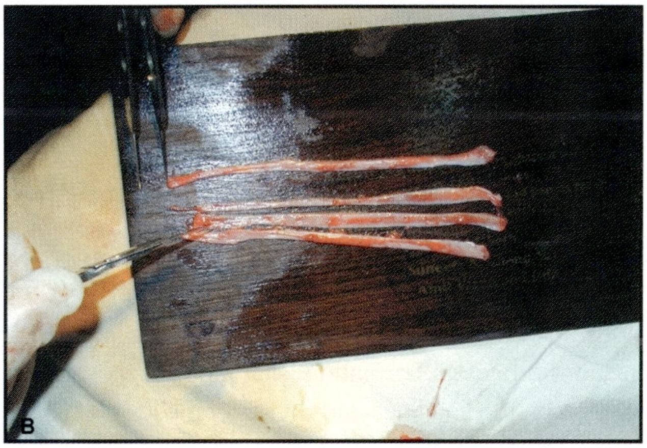

Figure 38.2B: Dissected fascia lata cut into 4 pieces of equal width

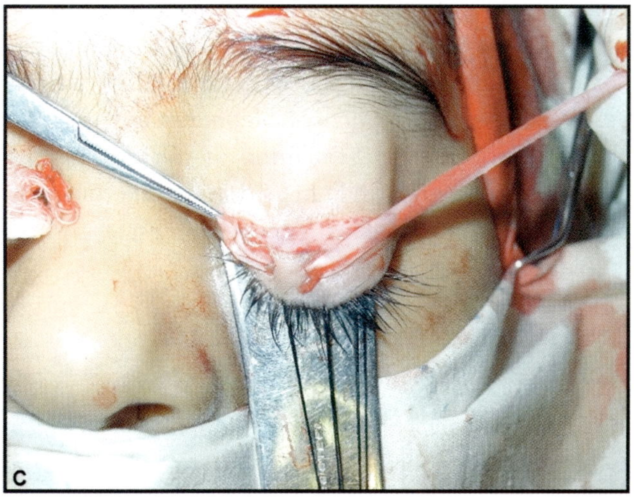

Figure 38.2C: Fascia lata inserted through the lid incision

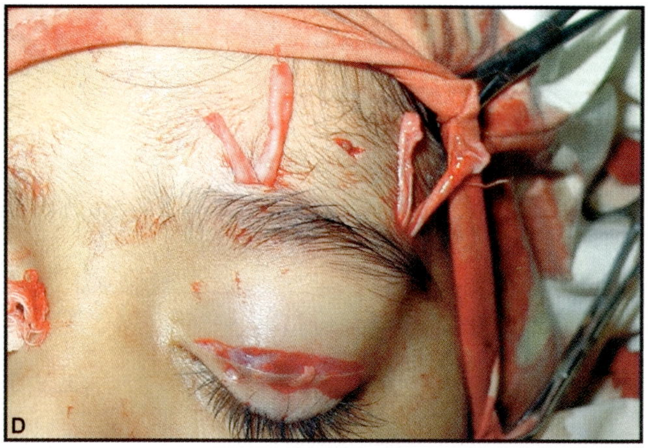

Figure 38.2D: The sling taken out through the forehead incision

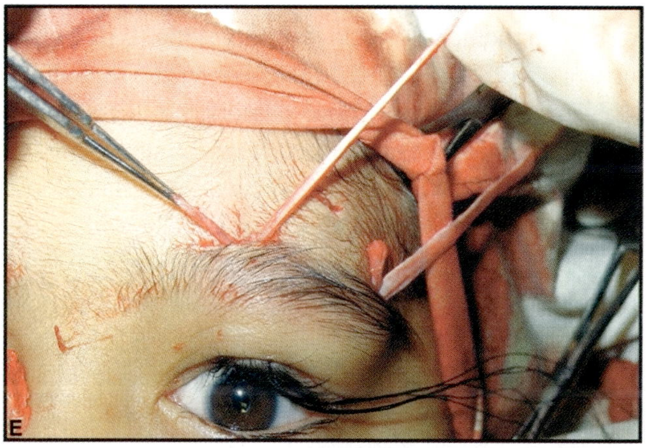

Figure 38.2E: Knots tied through the forehead incision

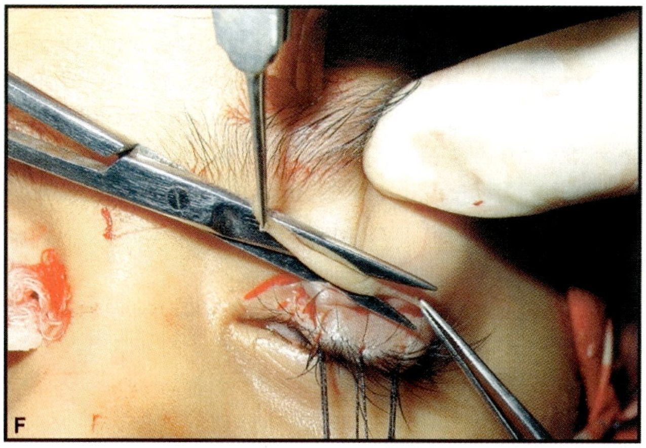

Figure 38.2F: Blepharoplasty of lid performed to remove redundant skin

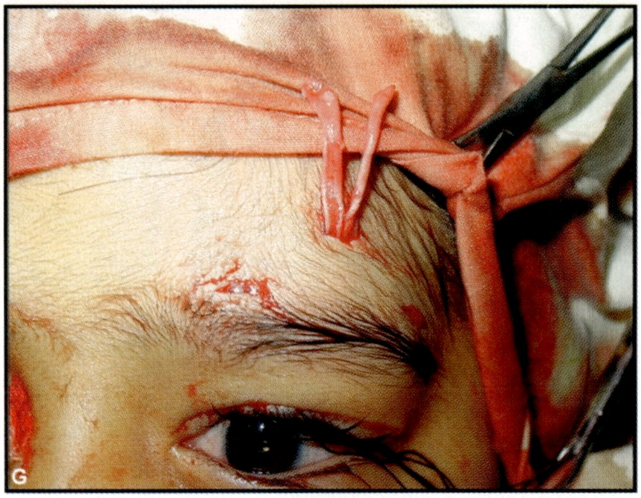

Figure 38.2G: Knots tied on the central forehead incision

traditional method of fascia lata harvesting as described by Callahan and Beard.[4] In order to prevent these problems, Naugle et al[5] have described a technique in which fascia lata was harvested from the upper part of the thigh. They have reported lower rates of hematoma formation, herniation of the muscle belly and a less conspicuous scar. This scar, being on the upper part of the thigh, can be easily concealed by short pants or swimming costumes.

A naturally occurring alternative to fascia lata is autogenous palmaris longus tendon. It has been shown to have comparable results to fascia lata, when used in sling surgery.[6]

Synthetic Materials

The use of synthetic materials in sling suspension surgery for ptosis has three-fold advantages. It cuts down valuable operating time and occasionally obviates the need for general anesthesia There is no unsightly scar on the thigh region and no chances of complications like hematoma, keloid formation, and herniation of the muscle belly.

Synthetic materials have been traditionally used in certain selected conditions.

1. *Very young children:* Fascia lata is not usually harvested before the age of 3 years.
2. *Poor Bell's phenomenon or unpredictable results:* In post-traumatic ptosis, chronic progressive external ophthalmoplegia, myasthenia gravis and third nerve palsy, there is a chance that postoperative suture adjustment may be required. Thus, it is preferable to use a synthetic material.
3. *Mechanical ptosis:* Among artificial materials, *silicon* has been used in the form of 1 mm silicon rod[7] and No. 40 silicon bands.[8] It has the advantage of its greater elasticity as compared to fascia lata. It is easily available and relatively cheaper priced, thus making it one of the more economical options for the patient. *Polyester fiber mesh* has also been used as a synthetic alternative to fascia lata. However, it has been reported that it is difficult to pass this material through submuscular planes.[9] The major problems encountered with synthetic material are extrusion, granuloma formation, infection, slipping of sutures and delayed recurrence of ptosis. The complications of granuloma formation and infection, which may necessitate suture removal, have been specially reported in regard to *Mersilene* suture and *ePTFE* (Gore-Tex) sutures.

Transconjunctival Blepharoplasty with Lower Eyelid CO_2 Laser Rejuvenation

With age, changes occur in the lower eyelid, which includes orbital fat herniation, skin redundancy, and an increase in the fine lines and rhytids of the lower lid skin. The conventional method to correct the same has included the *lower incisional blepharoplasty.* Lower lid retraction with lateral canthal rounding is common complications seen with lower incisional blepharoplasty. Resurfacing the lower eyelid *CO_2 laser* at the time of performing *transconjunctival blepharoplasty* or after about 2 months from the time of performing the procedure has significantly helped in the improvement of the lower lid wrinkles, skin redundancy and fat herniation in such patients.[10]

Isobutyl Cyanoacrylate Tissue Adhesive to Stabilize External Weights in Facial Palsies

Implanted gold weights have been found to be effective in the treatment of ocular exposure in patients with facial nerve palsies. *External weights* may be used for the same purpose. However, these require to be secured with an adhesive tape to the eyelid. These tapes lose their adhesiveness quickly and may not be effective after a while. Besides, they may not be tolerated for extended periods. *Isobutyl Cyanoacrylate tissue adhesive* is a simple, quick, and inexpensive method of securing temporary external weights to the eyes of patients with facial nerve palsy with ocular exposure. Additionally, it is better tolerated and lasts longer.[11]

Management of Facial Nerve Palsy

Management of facial nerve palsies can be a tricky affair. A lot depends on the stage of the palsy and the particular problem requiring correction. Some of the problems require emergency management while other problems can be dealt with electively. A staged approach has been developed for the management of facial nerve palsy.[12-18]

Stage 1: Supportive Care

During this stage a special note is made of presence or absence of Bell's phenomenon and corneal sensation. Papilloedema is ruled out. Initial therapy includes liberal use of lubricant ointments and drops. Taping of the eyelids may be carried out. Tarsorrhaphy as a management option is not favored much. A temporary tarsorrhaphy may be considered, only if it is absolutely imperative.

Stage 2: General Facial Re-animation

The procedures available include anastomosis of the 12th cranial to 7th cranial nerve, 7th nerve grafts and temporalis muscle transfer. These procedures help in providing facial tone.

Stage 3: Lower Lid and Canthal Support

In order to protect the globe and minimize paralytic ectropion lateral canthal suspension and medial canthoplasty may be done to provide lower lid and canthal support. Sub-orbicularis oculi fat lift is a relatively newer procedure, which may be used in the management of paralytic lower lid retraction.[30,31] In this procedure, the midfacial structures are repositioned and supported. However, overtime, the unopposed gravitational force on the paralyzed lid causes it to assume an unstable position.

Stage 4: Passive Upper Lid Animation

For this purpose, upper eyelid weights are easy to insert (and if necessary, to remove) and provide passive lid closure, thus minimizing the chances of corneal exposure. The size of the weight to be used must be titrated against the amount of lid closure and corneal coverage. It is recommended by Seiff et al[17] that the superior edge of the weight must be placed at the top of the tarsus through an eyelid crease incision, in order to provide maximum effectivity, while minimizing the chance of migration (see Figure 38.1).

Stage 5: Dynamic Eyelid Animation

A palpebral sling or Arion silicone sling may be used for this purpose. Palpebral spring provides dynamic lid closure with mechanical upper lid lowering, while the Arion sling has the advantage of re-animation of both the upper and the lower lid.

Stage 6: Soft Tissue Repositioning

This includes repositioning of the eyebrow. A conservative blepharoplasty may also be considered, provided the cornea is not decompensated.

Botulinum toxin A injections have been useful in the management of facial nerve palsy, during the stage of aberrant regeneration. This helps in restoring facial symmetry. However, its long-term use remains controversial.

Small Incision External Levator Repair[19]

Taking into consideration the recent trends towards "minimally invasive surgery" in all surgical fields, including ophthalmology, methods have been described to perform levator surgery through a small incision. Though smaller incisions allow quicker healing, there are some inherent disadvantages in performing any procedure without proper visualization like inadequate visualization in cases of excessive bleeding, having to extend the incision in case more exposure is required.

In a study conducted by Lucarelli et al,[19] a new surgical technique of small incision levator repair through an 8mm incision on patients with aponeurogenic blepharoptosis was described. The results were satisfactory with no significant intraoperative complications and appropriate surgical correction in 25 out of 28 cases undergoing the procedure. No patients required resurgery. The procedure was considered to be safe and effective in selected cases. However, the long-term results of the procedure need to be evaluated vis-à-vis the conventional method.

ORBITAL SURGERY

Materials used in Orbital Floor Fracture

The goal of management in orbital floor fractures is to restore the normal anatomy of the orbit, to minimize edema, bony instability and tissue shrinkage, which may result in enophthalmos, hypophthalmos, soft tissue incarceration and facial asymmetry.[20]

Open reduction of orbital floor fractures along with freeing of the incarcerated tissues is done by various approaches, e.g. transantral, transorbital or a combination of both. After freeing the incarcerated tissues from the fracture site, the size and nature of the defect in the orbital floor is evaluated. Implants are inserted subperiosteally and the periosteum is positioned back above the implant. Implants may be autogenous, homogenous, heterogeneous or synthetic. Endoscopic endonasal repair of fractures has also been described.

Several materials have been used in the repair of orbital floor fractures. Controversy persists regarding the decision to use *autologous* versus *alloplastic* materials in orbital repair and reconstruction. Advantages of any alloplastic material are cutting down of the operating time, as no time is required for harvesting bone or cartilage. In addition there is no scarring or morbidity from a donor site. Some complications of alloplastic materials are fistula formation, cyst formation, migration, motility restriction, infection, globe elevation, proptosis and optic nerve trauma.[21-23] Wolfe[24] believes that a blanket condemnation or endorsement of alloplastic materials is wrong and more effort should be directed to teaching proper harvesting of the bone grafts and to defining the indications for alloplastic materials.

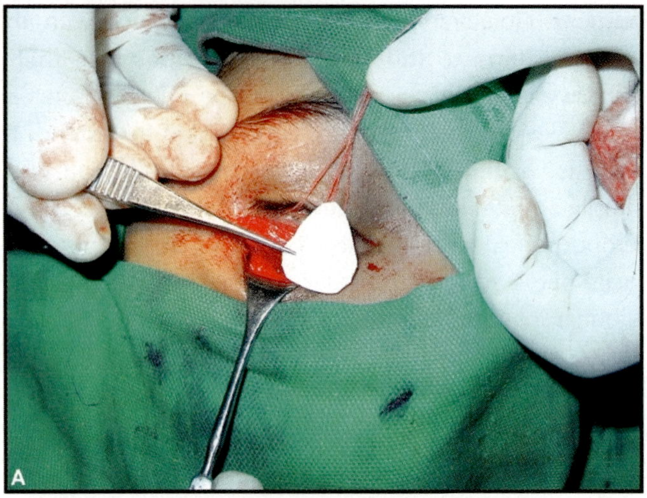

Figure 38.3A: Medpor implant being implanted over the floor defect

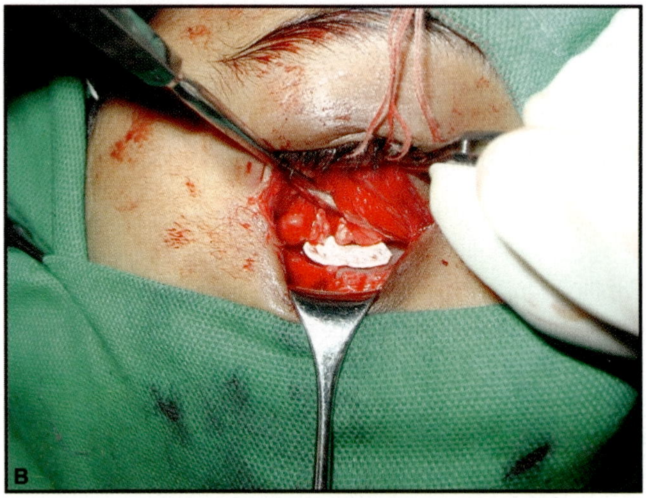

Figure 38.3B: The Medpor implant is inserted in its appropriate position

Autogenous implants used in orbital floor repair include *bone* and *fascia lata. Calvarium split grafts* have been found to be particularly suitable.

Synthetic materials include *methyl methacrylate, ePTFE (Goretex), polyvinyl sponge, Teflon, silicones* and *porous polyethylene channel (Medpor)*—(Figures 38.3A and B).

Teflon has been used in the repair of orbital floor fractures for the past several years. It has been shown to be well tolerated in the orbit even in long-term studies. It has also been shown to effectively improve the deviation of the eyeball. It has a very low incidence of infection and rejection.[25] However, late extrusion of these implants have been seen ten years after implantation.[26] Complications of Teflon, like migration and implant pocket infection are reduced by measures such as proper fixation of the implant and by avoiding packing of the maxillary antrum at the time of implantation.[27]

Silicone is well tolerated and has satisfactory results in the treatment of orbital floor fractures. It has been reported to have no incidence of infection, tissue reaction or extrusion.[28] However, as in the case of Teflon, late extrusion has been reported.[26]

ePTFE is suitable for use in orbital floor repair as it is biocompatible, easy to handle, chemically stable, low in cost, with properties of elasticity and ductility. In addition, in a study by Cozollino et al, no case of post-operative inflammation occurred in a group of patients after a two-year follow-up.[29]

Porous polyethylene channels (Medpor) are especially useful for compound orbital fractures. They have internal channels that accept microplates from conventional plating systems facilitating fixation of bones.

Some absorbable materials that have been used include *polydioxanone plate,*[30] *poltglycolic* and *polylactic acid*[31] and *vicryl mesh.*[32] The advantage of using absorbable materials is decreased chance of postoperative infection, while retaining the advantages of alloplastic over autogenous materials. Layered poly glactin (vicryl) mesh has also been used in orbital floor fracture repair.[32] It has also been used in a variety of complicated orbital fractures. It is available in the form of 26.5 by 24 mm sheets, packaged in 24 layers. A varying thickness of mesh may be used according to the thickness required, after measuring the defect in the orbital floor. It does not require fixation to orbital tissues.

Anophthalmic Implants

Coralline Hydroxyapatite Orbital Implant

Coralline hydroxyapatite orbital implant was introduced in 1985. Arthur C Perry of California, USA, designed it. This implant, comprising a natural component of coral reefs, known as porous hydroxyapatite, was different in that it becomes integrated as a living part of the recipient's orbital tissue.[33] At the time, this implant appeared to offer advantages over all previously used materials. By its biocompatibility and its providing a scaffolding for fibrovascular ingrowth, it was regarded as the ideal orbital implant for several years. It provided improved ocular motility as well as decreased incidence of migration and extrusion. However, time and experience have disclosed certain disadvantages, risks and complications of this material. Besides the disadvantage of its prohibitive cost, a major concern has been the rate of implant exposure. The rate of exposure of hydroxyapatite implants has been reported from 2.5 percent to as high as 21.6 percent.[34-36] In order to overcome these problems, newer materials are being investigated.

Porous Polyethylene (Medpor)

Porous polyethylene (Medpor) is a synthetic plastic material (Figures 38.4A and B), which has been used as a viable alternative to hydroxyapatite. Like hydroxyapatite, it has the properties of biocompatibility, fibrovascular ingrowth and high tensile strength. Compared to hydroxyapatite, it has a smooth external surface, thus eliminating the need for a wrapping material. In addition, it is far more economical to the patient. (The cost of a Medpor implant is roughly half that of a hydroxyapatite one). The implant may be used after a primary enucleation or evisceration or as a secondary implant, if the implant needs to be removed for some reason. After a routine enucleation, the Medpor implant is inserted and the extraocular muscles are directly sutured onto the surface of the implant with the help of 5-0 vicryl suture (Figures 38.4C and D). This differs from a hydroxyapatite, in which the muscles are sutured onto a wrapping material. Significantly, Medpor implants have been reported to have a lower rate of implant exposure.[37] However, it does not provide as complete a scaffolding for fibrovascular ingrowth as hydroxyapatite. The long-term risks and consequences of using this material are yet to be seen.

Newer wrapping materials for hydroxyapatite implants have also been investigated. The usual materials used are naturally occurring substances obtained from the patient or donors, e.g. *sclera, fascia lata,* etc. A newer material being investigated for this purpose is *polyglactin mesh.* The advantages of using polyglactin mesh as a wrapping material include the ease of use, longer shelf

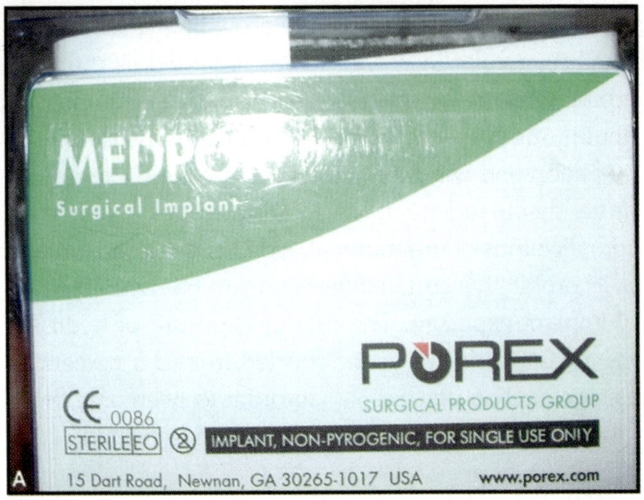

Figure 38.4A: The Medpor implant for use as an orbital implant in an anophthalmic socket

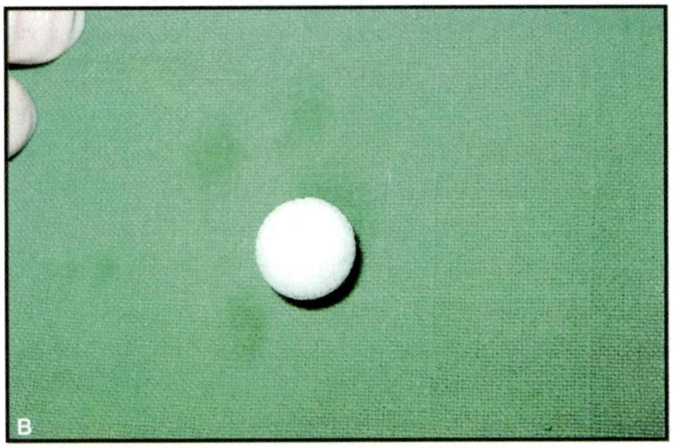

Figure 38.4B: The medpor implant

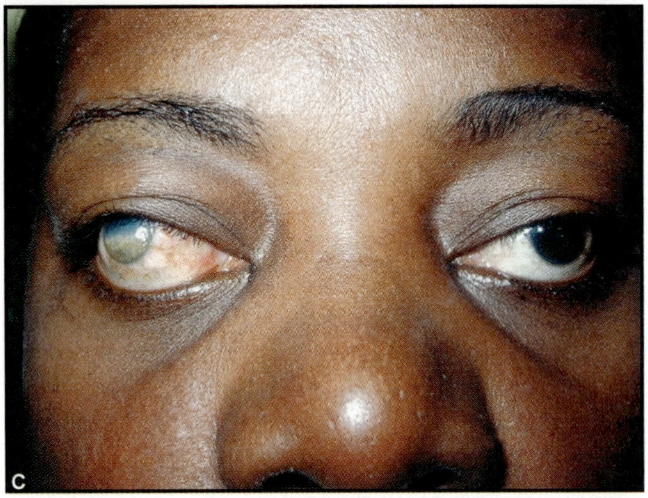

Figure 38.4C: Patient with right sided badly disfigured eye who underwent evisceration with primary implantation with Medpor

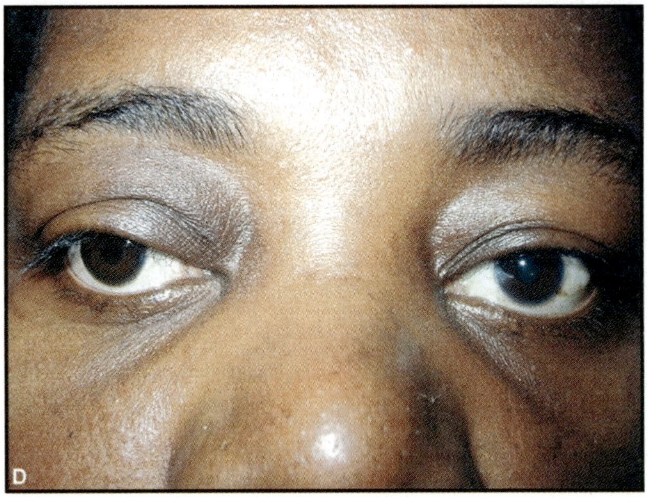

Figure 38.4D: Postoperative appearance of the same patient

life, and no need for donor tissue and less tissue reaction. In case of donor materials, the risk of transmission of infectious diseases is also abolished. The mesh is characterized by 360° entry of fibro vascular tissue, as compared to selective entry in sclera wrapped implants. It has also been found to have a lower rate of exposure as compared to sclera wrapped implants. Again, as in the case of Medpor, further study is warranted on the subject.

Orbital Epidural Catheter for Pain Control after Orbital Implant Surgery[38]

The surgical placement of orbital implants for patients undergoing eviscerations and enucleations is associated with significant post-surgical pain. Retrobulbar injections of local anesthetics have been described to counteract this pain. The effect is rapid but short lasting in these cases. Besides, the inherent problems of retrobulbar anesthesia cannot be ignored. An ingenious method to control this severe postoperative pain, seen especially in patients having undergone surgeries with hydroxyapatite implant is the use of an orbital epidural catheter connected to a patient controlled analgesia Bupivacaine Hydrochloride pump. Fezza et al[38] have reported good results with the use of this pump after orbital implant surgery. Keeping the cost factor in mind, this can be tried in some patients as a secondary procedure.

LACRIMAL SURGERY

Endoscopic Lacrimal Surgery[39]

Endoscopic DCR surgery can be done as a primary procedure or in the revision of failed DCR. Advantages of the procedure include the excellent hemostasis, decreased postoperative pain and absence of external scarring, swelling and bruising. There are definite disadvantages of the procedure, which includes the high cost of instruments and a steep learning curve. Contraindications to the procedure include lacrimal sac tumors, lacrimal abscesses and dacryoliths. Appropriate evaluation of potential benefits should be performed in every patient taken up for this surgery. As with every new procedure, the benefits of the new procedure should be evaluated completely prior to abandoning the old procedure.

Balloon Catheter Dilatation[40,41]

Balloon catheter dilatation, used as a primary procedure, has been generally found to be effective in cases of congenital as well acquired NLD obstruction. The advantages of the procedure include its simplicity, short time taken and easy repeatability. A lacrimal probe is advanced through the lacrimal passages into the nose. A balloon catheter over a guide wire is then inserted into the lacrimal sac and inflated repeatedly for about 10 times. Success rates in cases of congenital NLD obstructions have been reported to be as high as 95 percent. It is of excellent use is adult patients with partial obstructions of the NLD.

Anti-metabolites in Lacrimal Surgery

Mitomycin C has been used in a dose of 0.2 mg/ml in patients with re-surgery after failed DCR. It has been shown that the use of Mitomycin C results in a larger osteotomy size.[42] This is attributed to its anti-scarring and anti-fibrotic effects. Its judicious use in appropriate conditions may be performed.

Partial Lacrimal Carunculectomy in the Management of Epiphora[43]

Treatment of patients with epiphora without anatomic obstruction of the lacrimal drainage system is difficult. The lacrimal caruncle is thought to have an important role in tear drainage. A large caruncle may create the problems of eyelid malposition, a lacrimal pump problem, redundant conjunctival tissue over the puncta, or may mechanically push the eyelid out creating a localized ectropion. A partial carunculectomy may be effective in treating such patients.

MISCELLANEOUS MODES OF TREATMENT

Benign Essential Blepharospasm

Essential blepharospasm is an idiopathic, involuntary spasm of the eyelids, which is chronic and progressive in nature and may become visually disabling. Essential blepharospasm must be differentiated from similar conditions like Meige's syndrome and hemifacial spasm. Some patients have psychological problems, which lead to frequent blinking. In order to identify true essential blepharospasm, Gladstone and Putterman have developed a "blepharospasm test".[18] The patient is asked to repeatedly open and close his eyes and then to keep his eyes open. In essential blepharospasm, this triggers an involuntary spasm and the patient's eyelids close at the time he is instructed to open them. Treatment of essential blepharospasm may be non-surgical or surgical. Non-surgical management options include psychotherapy, drug treatment and botulinum toxin injection.

Psychotherapy

Although the psychiatric implications of the disease were dismissed in earlier literature, it has been seen that emotional crises occasionally trigger the onset of essential blepharospasm. The Benign Essential Blepharospasm Research Foundation (BEBRF) provides patient education and support to help them understand and cope with the disease. It was found in a survey, that helps from the BEBRF benefited 90 percent patients with essential blepharospasm with a patient acceptance rate of 96 percent.[44] These figures go in favor of the psychological implications of the disease. It is evident that education and patient support must be a primary part of successful treatment of this condition.

Drug Therapy

A variety of drugs have been tried in the treatment of essential blepharospasm. Amantidine is one such drug that has been found to be effective in about 10 percent of cases. It is prescribed in the dose of 100 mg twice a day.[45] However, side effects of this drug include depression, orthostatic hypotension, psychosis, urinary retention, congestive heart failure, headaches and fatigue.

Botulinum Toxin Injection

Botulinum toxin injection leads to a selective paralysis of the muscles into which it is injected. The main disadvantage of the drug is its temporary action and the eventual need for further injections. This drug has been found to effectively relieve blepharospasm for an average of 25 weeks after the initial injection. Its advantage lies in its simplicity and efficacy. However, side effects can occur, such as upper lid ptosis, lower lid ectropion and diplopia. In a study of 17 patients with essential blepharospasm and hemifacial spasm, botulinum toxin was found to consistently give relief to patients.[46] It is used in a dose of 12.5 to 25 units (0.005-0.010 micrograms) injected into the orbicularis oculi muscle of each effected eye at multiple points, with a 27-gauge needle.

Surgical Management

Surgical options available in the management of essential blepharospasm include selective avulsion of branches of the facial nerve and orbicularis myectomy.

In selective neurectomy, the upper branches of the facial nerve are selectively avulsed. Selective avulsion along with upper face lift (rhytidectomy) was found to have a 94 percent successful resolution of handicapping blepharospasm over a period of 8-162 months.[47] Complications of the procedure include upper facial paralysis, lagophthalmos, secondary exposure keratopathy, brow ptosis, paralytic lower lid ectropion and secondary epiphora.

Gillum and Anderson described an orbicularis myectomy including excision of the entire orbicularis, procerus and corrugator muscles and reported a success rate of approximately 85 percent.[48] The procedure involved a direct brow lift, excision of upper lid skin and levator advancement along with the excision of muscles. Side effects of the procedure include marked lid edema, ptosis, ecchymosis, and brow ptosis and exposure keratopathy.

Lasers in Oculoplastic Surgery[10, 49]

As in the field of medicine in general and oculoplastic surgery in particular, lasers have increasingly made their presence felt in the last few years.

The three lasers used in oculoplasty are argon laser, carbon dioxide laser and YAG contact laser. In laser corrective surgery, as in any oculoplasty procedure, the expectations of the patient must be realistic. The doctor must explain to the patient in detail what to expect and the possible complications of the procedure.

Argon Laser

Argon laser has its energy output between 488 to 514 nm, which falls in the blue green range of the visible spectrum. It is selectively absorbed by hemoglobin of red blood cells, and it creates a thermal effect leading to vessel obliteration. Thus, it is highly effective in the treatment of vascular malformations and tumors including port wine hemangiomas, superficial varicose veins, capillary and cavernous hemangiomas, and superficial telangiectasias. Because of the selective absorption by hemoglobin, the energy required in these conditions is relatively less and there is minimal damage to surrounding structures.

Argon laser is also selectively absorbed by melanin, which renders it less effective in dark skinned individuals. Greater power is required in the case of pigmented lesions, like tattoos and naevi, leading to more tissue destruction and scarring.

As the argon laser energy is fully absorbed to a depth of 1-2 mm in skin and mucous membrane, it is not useful where blood vessels are larger or located in the deeper portions of the skin. Needless to say, all safety precautions for protection of the eyes of the patient as well as the operation theater personnel are essential.

Nd-YAG Laser

Nd-YAG laser is a near infrared laser of 1064 nm. This is maximally absorbed by protein. The energy is focused and concentrated at the tip of a synthetic sapphire probe. The probe is used as a surgical scalpel to cut, vaporize and coagulate tissues. A precise incision can be made with minimum blood loss with the help of this laser. This is particularly useful while performing procedures that are usually associated with significant blood loss e.g. Dacryocystorhinostomy, excision of vascular tissues and debulking of orbital tumors. As the YAG laser can affect tissues to a depth of 3-5 mm, it is effective for hemostasis even when active bleeding is encountered. A disadvantage of this laser is the documented delay in wound healing, so the sutures have to be removed a little later than in conventional surgery.

Carbon Dioxide Laser

Carbon dioxide laser, with energy of 10,600 nm, operates in the infrared range. It may be used in pulsed or continuous mode. When focused it can be used to incise tissues and when defocused it can be used to vaporize tissues. Carbon dioxide laser is absorbed by water, in contrast to Nd-YAG, which is absorbed by protein and argon laser, which is absorbed by chromophores. Carbon dioxide laser absorption occurs up to a depth of 0.1mm of soft tissue. The advantage of this laser is that it precisely destroys target tissue while sparing the surrounding structures. It also offers an advantage in deep surgical cavities like orbit and nasal cavity. It is useful as an alternative to a surgical scalpel blade in excision of hemangiomatous lesions, adenoma sebaceum, naevi and port wine stains. It is also used in blepharoplasty procedures, excision of xanthelasma, lymphangioma, exenteration, etc. A relatively newer use of the carbon dioxide laser is "skin resurfacing" for the treatment of superficial wrinkles of the skin of the face. The advantage of the carbon dioxide laser is the easy control of depth of resurfacing it affords. It thus gives the skin a more youthful appearance. However, the long-term effectiveness of this technology will only be proved with time.

The main contraindication to any laser procedure is unrealistic expectations of the patient. Other contraindications are active infection of the skin, history of keloid formation or hypertrophic scarring. Some complications of laser procedures are infection, hypopigmentation and scarring. There is also evidence that laser incisions do not attain the same tensile strength as scalpel incisions until at least 3 weeks postoperatively.

Oculoplastic Applications of Acellular Dermal Allografts[50]

Autologous and alloplastic implants are extensively used to treat clinical conditions like contracted conjunctival fornices, superior sulcus defects, and soft tissue contour defects in the periorbital region. The efficacy of an acellular dermal graft (Alloderm, Lifecell Corp, Woodlands, Tex) was assessed in different oculoplastic procedures categorized as either barrier/scaffolding group (primary and secondary implant coverage and lid spacer graft) or the volume augmentation group (superior sulcus and other periorbital soft tissue contour defects). Conclusions derived were that acellular human dermis is an excellent barrier and reconstructive grafting material, which can be a good alternative to autologous and alloplastic grafts. It has excellent handling properties, avoids harvesting autologous tissue and produces minimal inflammation. It is, however, important to realize that Alloderm does not provide an epithelial surface and may not be of use in patients with ocular surface disorders like Stevens Johnson's syndrome or chemical burns. Its long-term use thus warrants further study.

REFERENCES

1. Penne RB. Oculoplastic Surgery. In: Wilson RP (Ed): Year Book of Ophthalmology; Wills Eye Hospital; CV Mosby; St Louis; 2000 Edition: 2000;157-86.
2. Wilson ME, Johnson RW. Congenital ptosis: Long-term results of treatment using lyophilized fascia lata for frontalis suspensions. Ophthalmology 1991;98:1234-37.
3. Jeong S, Ma YR, Park YG. Histopathological study of frontalis suspension materials. Jap J Ophth 2000;44(2):171-74.
4. Callahan MA, Beard C. Beard's ptosis 4th Edition. Birmingham: Aesculapius Publishing Co, 1990;151.
5. Naugle TC Jr, Fry CL, Sabatier RE, Elliot LF. High leg incision fascia lata harvesting. Ophthal 1997;104(9):1480-88.
6. Lam DS, Ng JS, Cheng GP, et al. Autogenous palmaris longus tendon as frontalis suspension material for ptosis correction in children. Am J Ophth 1998;126(1):109-15.

7. Leone CR Jr, Shore JW, Van Gemert JV. Silicone rod frontalis sling for the correction of blepharoptosis. Ophth Surg 1981;12(12):881-87.
8. Leone CR Jr, Rylander G. A modified silicone frontalis sling for the correction of blepharoptosis. Am J Ophth 1978; 85(6):802-05.
9. Lim BA, Choo CT. The use of sodium hyaluronate as a lubricant in brow suspension ptosis surgery using polyester fibre mesh. Ophth Surg and Laser 1998;29(7):606-07.
10. Carter SR, Seiff SR, Choo PH et al. Lower Eyelid CO_2 Laser Rejuvenation: A randomized, prospective, clinical study. Ophthalmology 2001;108:437–41.
11. Shepler TR, Seiff SR. Use of Cyanoacrylate tissue adhesive to stabilize external eyelid weights in the temporary treatment of facial palsies. Oph Plast and Reconstr Surg 2001;17:169-73.
12. Seiff SR, Chang J. The staged management of ophthalmic complications of facial nerve palsy. Ophthal Plast Reconstr Surg 1993;9:241-59.
13. Seiff SR, Carter SR. Re-animation of the paretic eyelid complex. Facial Plast Surg Clin North Am 1998;6:21-30.
14. Boerner M, Seiff S. Etiology and management of facial nerve palsy. Curr Opin Ophthalmol 1994;5:61-66.
15. Hoenig JA, Shorr N, Shorr J. The sub-orbicularis oculi fat lift in aesthetic and reconstructive surgery. Int Ophthalmol Clin 1997;3:179-91.
16. Seiff Sr, Choo PH, Carter SR. Facial nerve paralysis. In: Mauriello JA, (Ed). Unfavourable results in eyelid and lacrimal surgery. Boston: Butterworth-Heinemann 2000;227-34.
17. Seiff SR, Carter SR. Facial nerve paralysis. Int Ophthal Clin 2002;42(2):103-12.
18. Gladstone G, Putterman AM. A repetitive forced closure test. Arch Ophthalmol 1985;103:477-80.
19. Lucarelli MJ, Lemke BN. Small Incision Levator repair: Techniques and Early results. Am J Oph 1999;127:637-44.
20. Antonyshyn O, Gruss JS. Complex orbital trauma: the role of rigid fixation and primary bone grafting. Adv Ophthalmic Plast Reconstr Surg 1985;75(1):17-24.
21. Browning CW. Alloplastic materials in orbital repair. Am J Ophthal 1967;63(5):955-62.
22. Jordan DR, St. Onge P, Anderson RL, et al. Complications associated with alloplastic implants used in orbital fracture repair. Ophthalmology 1992;99(10):1600-08.
23. Mauriello JA, Hargrave S,Yee S, et al. Infection after insertion of alloplastic orbital floor Implants. Am J Ophthal 1994;117:246-52.
24. Wolfe SA. Autogenous bone grafts versus alloplastic materials in maxillofacial surgery. Clin Plast Surg 1982;9(4): 539-40.
25. Otto AJ, Borghouts JM. Orbital correction with the use of alloplastic material. Mod Probl Ophthalmol 1975;14:641-44.
26. Brown AE, Banks P. Late extrusion of alloplastic orbital floor implants. Br J Oral Maxillofac Surg 1993;31(3):154-57.
27. Aronowitz JA, Freeman BS, Spira M. Long term stability of Teflon orbital implants. Plast Reconstr Surg 1986;78(2):166-73.
28. Mwanza JC, Ngoy DK, Kayembe DL. Reconstruction of orbital floor blow out fracture with silicone implant. Bull Soc Belge Ophthalmol 2001;280:57-61.
29. Cozzolino A, Piane R, Pasalli GC, Ruggiero G. Use of PTFE membranes in the orbital floor fractures. Minerva Stomatol 2001;50(11-12):373-79.
30. Iizuka T, Mikkonen P, Paukku P, Lindquist C. Reconstruction of orbital floor with polydioxanone plate. Int J Oral Maxillofac Surg 1991;20(2):83-87.
31. Hollier LH, Rogers N, Berzin E, Stal S. Reabsorbable mesh in the treatment of orbital floor fractures. J Craniofac Surg 2001;12(3):242-46.
32. Mauriella JA Jr, Wasserman B, Kraut R. Use of vicryl mesh implant for repair of orbital floor fractures causing diplopia: a study of 28 patients over 5 years. Ophthal Plastic and Reconstructive Surgery 1993;9(3):191-95.
33. Flanagan JC. A new orbital implant to increase enucleation prosthesis motility. In Laibson PR, Adams RE, Arentson JJ et al, Eds. Year Book of Ophthalmology 1990. St Louis: Mosby, 1990;95-96.
34. Buettner H, Bartley GB. Tissue breakdown and exposure associated with orbital hydroxyapatite implants. Am J Ophth 1992;113:669-73.
35. Jordan DR, Klapper S. Wrapping hydroxyapatite implants. Ophth Surg Lasers 1989;30(5):403-07.
36. Oestreicher JH, Liu E, Berkowitz M. Comparison of hydroxyapatite orbital implants: A review of 100 consecutive cases and comparison of Dexon mesh and scleral wrapping. Ophthalmology 1995;102:586-93.
37. Jordan DR. Anophthalmic orbital implants. Ophthal Clin of North America 2000;13(4):587-608.
38. Fezza JP, Klippenstein KA, Wesley RE. Use of Orbital catheter to control pain after Orbital Implant Surgery. Arch Ophthalmol 1999;117:784-88.
39. Hartikainen J, Grenman R, Puukke R, et al. Prospective randomized comparison of external DCR and endonasal DCR. Ophthalmology 1998;105:1106-13.
40. Becker BB, Berry FD, Koller H. Balloon catheter dilatation for treatment of congenital NLD obstruction. Am J Oph 1996;121:304-09.
41. Janssen AG, Mansour K, Bos JJ. Obstructed NLD Duct in Epiphora: Long Term Results of dacryocystoplasty by means of balloon dilatation. Radiology 1997;205:791-96.
42. Kao SCS, Liao CL, Tseng JHS et al. DCR with intra-operative MMC. Ophthalmology 1997;104:86-91.
43. Mombaerts I, Colla B. Partial Lacrimal Carunclectomy: A simple procedure for epiphora. Ophthalmology 2001; 108:793-97.
44. Anderson RL, Patel BCK, Holds JB et al. Blepharospasm: Past, Present and Future. Ophthal Plast Reconstr Surg 1998; 14:305-17.

45. Putterman AM. Symmetrel in the treatment of essential blepharospasm. In Bosniak (Ed): Advances in Ophthalmic Plastic Reconstructive Surgery, Elmsford, N.Y., Pergamon Press, 1985;4:227-28.
46. Shorr N, Stuart R, Seiff, Kopelman J. The use of Botulinum toxin in Blepharospasm. Am J Ophthal 1985;99:542-46.
47. Felt DR, Putterman AM, Weingarten CZ. Facial Nerve Avulsion and primary rhytidectomy in the treatment of essential blepharospasm. In: Bosniak (Ed): Advances in Ophthalmic Plastic Reconstructive Surgery, Elmsford, N.Y., Pergamon Press, 1985;4:349-60.
48. Gillium W, Anderson R. Blepharospasm surgery. Arch Oph 1981;99:1058-62.
49. Biesman BS. Cutaneous facial resurfacing with CO2 laser. Oph Surg Lasers 1996;27:685-98.
50. Rubin PAD, Fay AM, Remulla HD, et al. Ophthalmic Plastic Applications of Acellular Dermal Allografts. Ophthalmology 1999;106:2091-97.

39

Endoscopic Conjunctivo-dacryocystorhinostomy

- ENDOSCOPIC SURGERY
- INDICATIONS AND CONTRAINDICATIONS FOR CDRC AND THE ALTERNATIVES AVAILABLE
- PREOPERATIVE WORK-UP
- POSTOPERATIVE WORK-UP
- COMPLICATIONS
- UNBREAKABLE TUBE AND INJECTOR
- WHY USE ENDOSCOPIC CDRC?

Stefano Cavazza (Italy)

INTRODUCTION

Jones pioneered the conjunctivodacyocystorhinostomy (CDRC) and used a glass tube to by-pass the lacrimal canaliculi and sac forming, in symptomatic ephiphora, a direct conduit for tears from the conjunctival lake to the nasal cavity.[1]

CDRC is indicated as the treatment for obstruction of the upper, lower, or common canaliculi or any combination of these. Additional indications are severe lacrimal pump dysfunction in facial nerve palsy and failed dacryocystorhinostomy (DCR).[1-3]

There are several causes of canalicular obstruction: idiopathic, congenital anomalies, trauma, inflammation, herpetic infection, tumors, Stevens-Jonson syndrome, systemic chemotherapy, radiation therapy.[2-4]

In terms of etiology, trauma (dog bites, motor vehicle accidents, assault, and spike injury) and infection were the most usual of lacrimal canalicular obstruction.[2-4]

When possible, the classic surgical technique of CDRC, was performed under general anesthesia and after suturing the posterior flaps of lacrimal and nasal mucosa, a standard step of the external DCR technique, a portion of caruncle was excised with scissors, and a tract between this site and the nose was created using a 18-gauge needle or a 15-degree blade: this tract was then widened using a Beaver knife or a lacrimal probe. Liu[5] proposed a conjunctival approach to avoiding skin scarring.

The Jones or the Putterman-Gladstone[6] tube (a modified Jones tube with an extra flange that anchors the tube in the medial canthal soft tissues) was inserted into the fistula with the aid of a lacrimal probe and then sutured in place with 6-0 silk or polyglycolate absorbable suture. The anterior nasal and lacrimal mucosal flaps were sutured together, and the overlying tissue closed.

ENDOSCOPIC SURGERY

Nasal and transcanalicular endoscopy are now well-established procedures in the diagnosis and treatment of lacrimal pathways stenosis or obstructions. They follow the trend towards minimally invasive microsurgery procedures, which characterizes all branches of ophthalmology from bimanual phaco to vitreoretinal surgery. If, on the one hand it requires more expensive equipment, such as the endoscopes, light sources, monitors and lasers, on the other hand, trauma, pain and scarring are minimally and recovery is more rapid. Also surgical time is reduced: according to Hartikainen[7] the surgical duration of endonasal DCR was three times shorter the time required for external DCR, the average duration being 23 minutes and 78 minutes respectively ($P<0.0001$).

Endoscopic CDRC can be performed under local or general anesthesia: for both techniques we used preoperative nasal packing with 5 percent xylocaine-naphazoline soaked cotton pledgelets. Under local anethesia, the area of the medial canthus was infiltrated with 2 percent lidocaine/1:100,000 epinephrine, and by means of direct endoscopic vision, the lateral wall of the nose and the middle meatus area were infiltrated with the same combination of anesthetics using a tuberculin syringe and 27-gauge needle.

After a minimal excision of the caruncle with Westcott scissors, a 14-gauge needle was passed from the medial fornix at the medial canthal angle and angled down 45° through the thin lacrimal bone, we feel the maxillary-lacrimal suture, into the middle meatus.

Using the nasal endoscope we looked for the tip of the needle, paying special attention to avoid damaging the nasal septum, an area highly prone to bleeding from accidental trauma: this may also increase postoperative synechiae and the failure of the surgical procedure.

Under direct endoscopic vision, the track was widened first with the needle and then with a lacrimal probe or blunt scissors. A Bowman probe (Figure 39.1) was used as a guide to position the tube: ideally the tube should protrude into the nose for approximately 2 mm, with the slanted end pointed downwards and it must clear the nasal septum by at least 3 mm (Figure 39.2). The length of the tube(18-20-22 mm) can be changed if these criteria are not respected.

Anterior turbinate resection can also be performed if the anterior turbinate obstructs the tube.

Then in order to confirm patency of the tube, it was irrigated with a 5 percent Iodopovidone solution and the proximal end of the tube (Figure 39.3) was secured at the medial canthus with a 5-0 polyester suture.

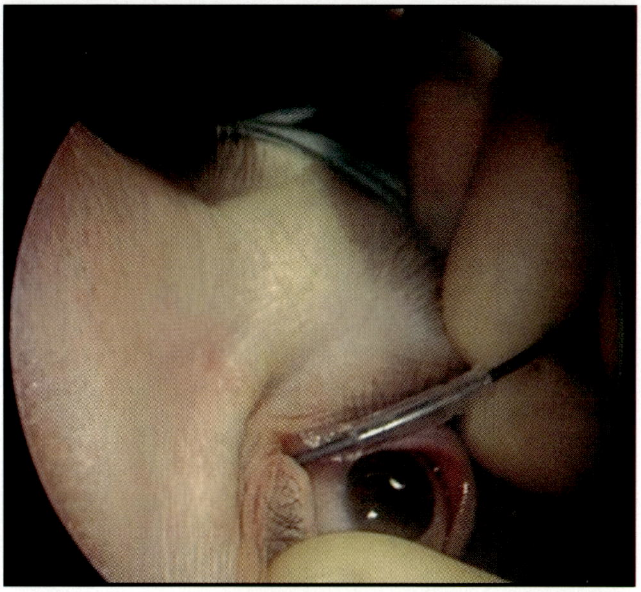

Figure 39.1: (Tube 1) The Bowmann probe was used as a guide to position the tube

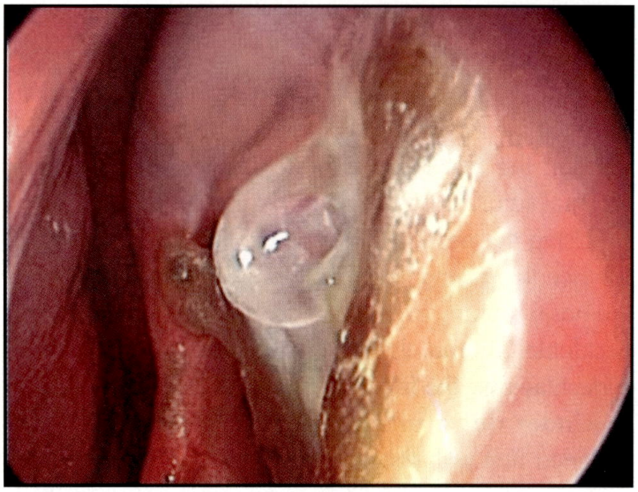

Figure 39.2: (Tube 2) Good position of the tube in the lacrimal region of the nose,10 days after surgery

INDICATIONS AND CONTRAINDICATIONS FOR CDRC AND THE ALTERNATIVES AVAILABLE

CDRC is indicated for some, but not all, cases of canalicular obstruction. Despite the presence of obstruction, the technique should be avoided in patients affected by keratoconjunctivitis sicca, in very young patients, patients affected by occasional ephipora and in generally in patients who cannot adequately manage long-term tube maintenance.

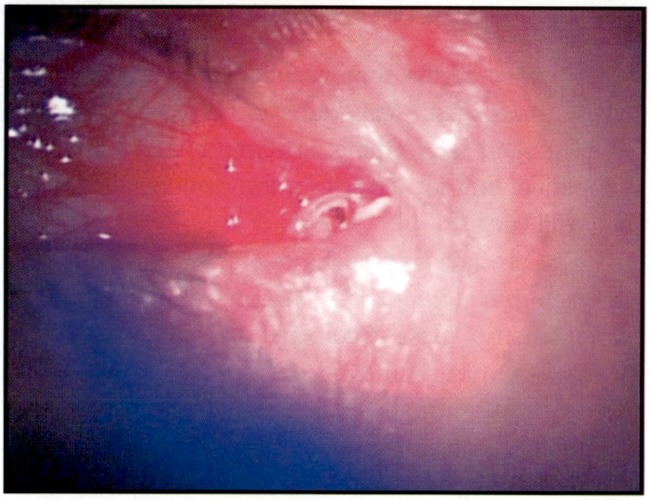

Figure 39.3: (Tube 3) Lateral end of the tube in the medial fornix 4 after surgery

In the event of previous DCR, prior to CDRC surgery, we normally perform an endoscopic or external revision that includes granuloma and scar resection, middle turbinectomy or widening the bony ostium if it is too small. Is very important to request a consultation with an otolaryngology colleague if there is extensive involvement of the nasal septum in the scar tissue mass.[8]

If patency is observed in at least 8 mm of the upper or lower canaliculi (or both) it is possible to perform a canaliculodacryocystorhinostomy as an alternative to CDRC.[9] This is a procedure in which the upper, lower, or common canaliculi, (or a combination of these), is sutured to the lacrimal sac, which is then sutured to the nasal mucosa. When successful, (50-60% when it is performed for more lateral obstructions), it has the advantage of highlighting the need for a permanent tube.[9]

New technology: transcanalicular endoscopy, diffused primarily throughout Europe, using very small flexible fiberoptic scopes, under direct observation, we can treat the canalicular obstruction that can be by-passed using a trephine or a variety of lasers. Although this new technology has potential for minimally invasive canalicular surgery, greater success rates are need before it becomes more widely accepted.[10]

PREOPERATIVE WORK-UP

It is important to carefully review the patient's medical history preoperatively. Any medication that increases bleeding, such as aspirin (acetylsalicylic acid, ASA), non-steroid anti-inflammatory agents (NSAIDS), Coumadin or other anticoagulants should be noted. ASA should be suspended at least one week before surgery and Coumadin four days prior the operation.[8]

A CT should be performed to rule out the presence of any underlying sinus disease or bone destruction which would point to lacrimal sac tumor. A CT scan provides the best information on post-traumatic bony anatomy.[8]

Anterior rhinoscopy, or better still nasal endoscopy, must be performed on all patients.

These permit the identification of nasal disease and tumors and also gives the surgeon an idea of the anatomical nasal space. The patient can then be informed about the need for a resection of the middle turbinate and/or septoplasty.

CDRC can produced good results but only following a careful preoperative selection of well-informed patients.

POSTOPERATIVE WORK-UP

In the postoperative, an association of antibiotic-cortisone drops and cortisone nasal spray were prescribed for 10 days. Patients were instructed how to care for the tube, including regular sniffing to clear it and placing a finger over the medial canthus when sneezing or blowing the nose. Follow-up visits were weekly during the first month and monthly over the first year. Patients were then told to return to their doctor immediately if any problems arose.

Like all DCRs, we used nasal endoscopy for the follow-up especially during in the first month.

Using endoscopy, we initially control the intranasal position of the tube and subsequently any early post-operative problems such as synechiae and granulomas can be treated successfully.

COMPLICATIONS

Several types of complications have been reported following the insertion of the Jones tubes. They include extrusion, malposition, obstruction, infection, discomfort, diplopia, reflux of nasal secretion onto the eye, systemic toxicity from topical eyedrops and tube breakage.[2-11]

In a recent retrospective analysis on 49 eyes operated with CDRC by Lim and colleagues,[3] the most common complication was extrusion and the second most frequent was obstruction of the tube.

Extrusion is the complete displacement of the tube from its intended position. Lateral obstruction is caused by conjunctival overgrowth or by granulation tissue, medial obstruction is caused by overgrowth of the nasal mucosal or granulation tissue or granuloma.[3-4]

In the early postoperative period, two of the six patients in the our endoscopic CDCR group, required the excision of conjunctival overgrowth which was performed as office procedure with topical anesthesia.

UNBREAKABLE TUBE AND INJECTOR

We have modified the design of the original Jones tube and most importantly we have changed the material. We feel that unbreakable tubes are safer and can be easily injected in the soft tissue of the lacrimal region by means of specific injector that will soon be produced by Janach (Italy).

Our tubes are made from PMMA or Teflon: these materials are biocompatible, hydrophobic, non-porous, rigid and inert, and are already being used in all sorts of ocular implants.

We have a slight preference for PMMA tubes because they are more transparent and therefore less visible than the Teflon tubes, but a greater amount of time is required for observations.

WHY USE ENDOSCOPIC CDRC?

With the advent of new technology, older procedures will inevitably be challenged. This has already happened with external and endonasal DCR.

Endoscopic CDRC avoids the formation of cutaneous scars, it is more rapid procedure and there is less blood loss.[2-12]

The smaller, 3 mm diameter track, the less traumatic approach, and the new materials used should cause a weaker scarring reaction in the surrounding tissue, and this should produce longer stability, reducing the occurrence of extrusion which is the most common complication observed with this type of surgery.

REFERENCES

1. Jones LT. Conjunctivodacryocystorhinostomy. Am J Ophthalmol 1965;59:773-83.
2. Trotter WL, Meyer DR. Endoscopic conjunctivo dacryocystorhinostomy with Jones tube placement. Ophthalmology 2000;107:1206-9.
3. Lim C, Martin P, Benger R, Kourt G, Ghabrial R. Lacrimal canalicular bypass surgery with the Lester Jones tube. Am J Ophthalmol 2004;137:101-08.
4. Steinsapir KD, Glatt HJ, Putterman AL. A 16-year study of conjunctival dacryocystorhinostomy. Am J Ophthalmol 1990;109:387-93.
5. Liu D. Conjunctival incision for primary conjunctivodacryocystorhinostomy with Jones tube. Am J Ophthalmol 2000;129:244-5.
6. Gladstone GJ, Putterman AM. A modified glass tube for conjunctivodacryocystorhinostomy. Arch Ophthalmol 1985;103:1229-30.
7. Hartikainen J, Grenman R, Pukka P, Seppa H. Prospective randomized comparison of external dacryocystorhinostomy and endonasal laser dacryocystorhinostomy. Ophthalmology 1998;105:1106-12.
8. Jordan DR. Standard external dacryocystorhinostomy. In: Mauriello JA (Ed): Unfavorable result of eyelid and lacrimal surgery. Woburn, Butterworth-Heinemann, 2000;519-49.
9. Glatt HJ, Putterman AM. Conjunctivo dacryocystorhinostomy. In: Mauriello JA (Ed): Unfavorable Result of Eyelid and Lacrimal Surgery. Woburn, Butterworth-Heinemann, 2000;575-89.
10. Mandeville JTH, Woog JJ. Obstruction of the lacrimal drainage system. Current Opinion in Ophthalmology 2002;13: 303-9
11. Bartley GB, Gustafson RO. Complications of malpositioned Jones tubes. Am J Ophthalmol 1990;109:66-69.
12. Watkins LM, Janfaza P, Rubin P. The evolution of endonasal dacryocystorhinostomy. Survey of Ophthalmol 2003;48:73-84.

40

Surgical Procedure in Stem Cell Transplantation

- LIMBAL STEM CELL DEFICIENCY
- LIMBAL STEM CELL TRANSPLANTATION
- PREOPERATIVE PREPARATION
- SURGICAL TECHNIQUE FOR LIMBAL ALLOGRAFT
- RECIPIENT EYE
- AMNIOGRAFT
- SURGICAL TECHNIQUE FOR LIMBAL AUTOGRAFT
- LIMBAL STEM CELL TRANSPLANTATION WITH KERATOPLASTY
- LIMBAL STEM CELL TRANSPLANTATION WITH AMNIOTIC MEMBRANE GRAFT
- POSTOPERATIVE COURSE
- POSTOPERATIVE DRUG THERAPY
- SUCCESS RATES
- RECENT ADVANCES

Sunita Agarwal, Soosan Jacob (India)

INTRODUCTION

The corneal epithelium continuously sheds its surface epithelium, and is replaced by stem cells originating from beneath and peripheral to the central desquamating epithelium.[1,2] Stem cells are the ultimate source of the rapidly self-renewing corneal epithelium and are located in the basal layer of the limbal epithelium.[3-5] They are present in the crypts of Vogt or the palisades of Vogt, which are principally located at the sclerocorneal limbus.[6] These cells, like all stem cells are poorly differentiated[7,8-10] and have a low mitotic rate and asymmetrical DNA segregation. They have the potential for clonogenic cell division and are essential for the maintenance of a healthy corneal surface. Limbal stem cells evolve into the transiently amplifying cells (TAC). Both of these undergo cell division and remain in the poorly differentiated stage. They are both located in the limbal region, with the stem cells in the basal epithelium[7,11,12] and TAC occurring in the basal and suprabasal levels, extending up to the superficial layers. These cells divide into the non-dividing post-mitotic cells (PMCs), which then undergo terminal differentiation and migrate onto the central cornea as terminally differentiated cells (TDCs) to form the new corneal epithelium.

LIMBAL STEM CELL DEFICIENCY

Loss of limbal stem cells, or corneal stem cell deficiency, can be partial or total, unilateral or bilateral. The absence or malfunction of corneal stem cells, either primary (aniridia, congenital erythrokeratoderma etc.) or secondary [(chemical burns, Stevens-Johnson syndrome, ocular cicatricial pemphigoid (Figure 40.1) etc.)],[8,12,13] results in loss of the regenerative capacity of the corneal epithelium. This results in "transdifferentiated" conjunctivally-derived epithelium surfacing the cornea or, sometimes, failure to resurface at all leading to a persistent epithelial defect, with corneal neovascularization (Figure 40.2) and scarring, melting, ulceration and perforation of the cornea, corneal calcification, and band keratopathy.[14-19] The patient may complain of decreased vision, photophobia, tearing, blepharospasm, and recurrent episodes of pain, as well as a history of chronic inflammation with redness.

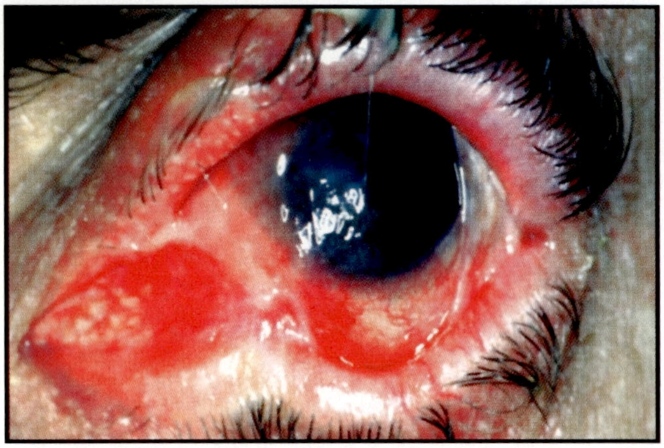

Figure 40.1: Pemphigoid (Courtesy-Guillermo Simon-Castellvi, Spain)

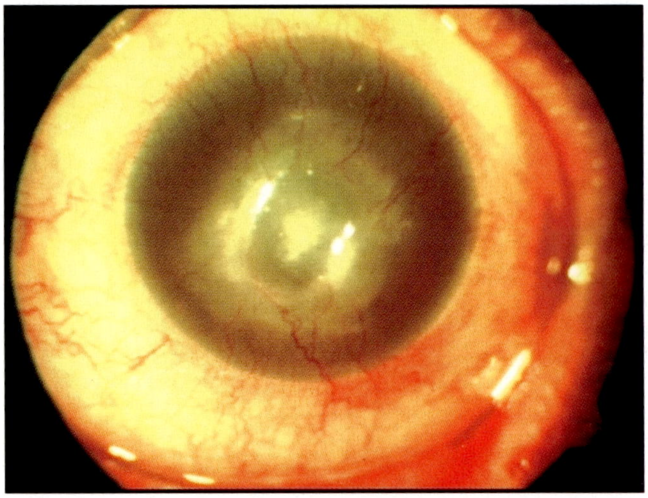

Figure 40.2: Patient with dry eye, corneal vascularization and epithelial defect

A keratoplasty in these patients, whether lamellar or penetrating, is generally not successful as the host's corneal epithelium is only temporarily replaced and the limbal function continues to remain poor.[20-21] Limbal stem cell transplantation is a surgical modality, described by Kenyon and Tseng, to replenish or repopulate the ocular surface epithelium in an eye with limbal stem cell deficiency. Limbal transplantation for these patients restores the corneal limbal stem cells and long-term corneal epithelial healing may be achieved.[22-29] A keratoplasty may be combined with this or done at a later sitting. Any underlying primary problem should also be corrected.

LIMBAL STEM CELL TRANSPLANTATION

A variety of techniques of limbal transplantation have been reported.[30-41] All these procedures remove the host's altered corneal epithelium and pannus and provide a new source of epithelium for a diseased ocular surface. From the donor tissue, transient amplifying cells are generated which migrate onto the denuded corneal surface of the host. A successful transplantation leads to the host's cornea (or grafted cornea) being permanently covered by epithelium from the donor. The donor tissue can be obtained from the other eye (**limbal autograft**) in cases of unilateral disease. In case of bilateral disease, cadaveric whole globe or corneoscleral rim of a living relative (**limbal allograft**) can be used. Limbal transplantation procedures may also be classified depending on the carrier tissue used for the transfer of the limbal stem cells. Either conjunctiva (**conjunctival limbal graft**) or corneal/limbal stroma (**keratolimbal graft**) have been used as carrier tissue for limbal stem cells.[36]

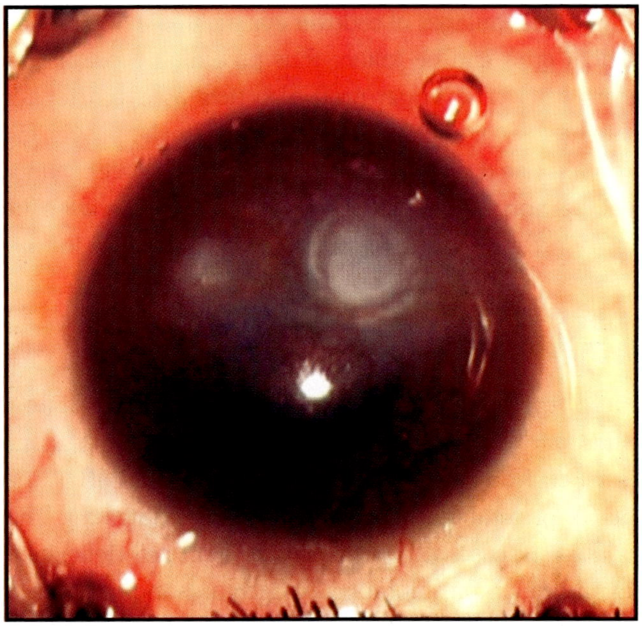

Figure 40.3: Patient to undergo limbal stem cell transplantation. Note the corneal vascularization and corneal opacity

PREOPERATIVE PREPARATION

Any preexisting problem such as dry eye, corneal anesthesia, conjunctival scarring, corneal epithelial keratinisation, mucous depletion, meibomitis, entropion, ectropion, trichiasis, etc. should be taken care of. Procedures-like punctal occlusion, autologous serum eye drops, lid margin eversion, scleral contact lens and topical retinoid acid ointment may be used preoperatively to augment ocular surface defense. The patient (Figure 40.3) can be put on preoperative steroids and immunosuppressives to decrease coexisting inflammation. In case of allograft, HLA typing and matching can be done.

SURGICAL TECHNIQUE FOR LIMBAL ALLOGRAFT

From Cadaver Eye

As success depends on transplantation of healthy limbal stem cells, fresh donor eyes are preferred. In case of cadaver eye, whole globe is preferred as it provides better stability while dissecting the donor tissue. Several variations of limbal autografts[30-37]and allografts[32-41] have been reported. Dua HS, Azuara-Blanco et al have described a modified procedure for limbal allograft.[42] The eye is first made tense by injecting air into the vitreous cavity through the optic nerve using a 26 gauge needle and the nerve is clamped. The eye is held in a Tudor Thomas stand. A trephine 3 mm smaller than the corneal diameter is used to make a well centered, superficial, partial thickness cut in the donor tissue (approximately 150 μm depth). The cornea peripheral to the cut is then dissected using a bevel up dissector. The dissection is carried all the way through the limbus into a small peripheral rim of sclera, approximately 1mm, any conjunctiva, if present being retained. This corneoscleral rim is then cut free from the cadaver globe. The recipient bed is prepared by doing a 360 degree peritomy, and removing the conjunctivalized epithelium and underlying scar tissue off the cornea by blunt dissection. The donor graft is then placed at the host limbus and sutured in place using 10-0 nylon. Any gap is filled with a "spacer" made from donor corneal stroma or a piece of donor limbal tissue from the other eye of the same donor. The host conjunctiva is reapproximated to the limbus using interrupted sutures. If required, a tarsorrhaphy can be done.

The advantages of cadaver eye are that a 360 degree limbal graft can be taken, thus providing more limbal stem cells. The larger graft also acts as a barrier for migration of conjunctivally derived epithelium over the cornea. The disadvantage is that there is a greater chance of rejection of the graft and the patient may even be required to be put on immunosuppressives for his lifetime.

From Live Related Donor

Here, the procedure followed is the same as limbal autograft (explained next) except that the donor tissue is taken from a live, related donor (Figures 40.4 and 40.5), preferably after HLA typing and matching. This is done in case of bilateral limbal stem cell deficiency. Even though this theoretically decreases the chances of rejection as compared to cadaver graft, yet postoperative systemic immunosuppressive therapy may be required for the patient's lifetime.

RECIPIENT EYE

The recipient bed is then prepared by doing a peritomy in the involved area and removing the conjunctivalized epithelium and underlying scar tissue off the cornea by blunt dissection. A bed is prepared for the graft by excising a rim of corneolimbal tissue corresponding in size to the donor. A thin rim of conjunctiva is also excised.

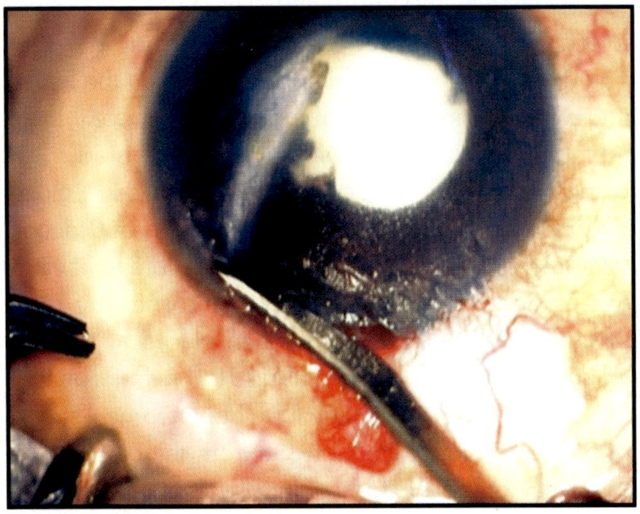

Figure 40.4: Dissection done in the live related donors eye to get a limbal graft

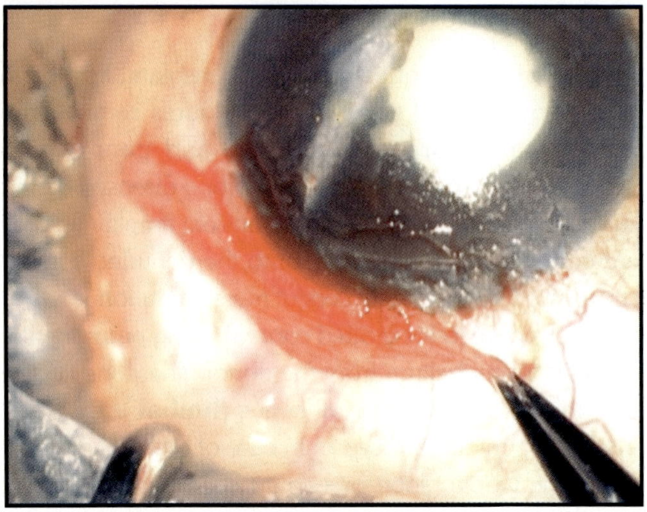

Figure 40.5: Limbal graft dissection complete

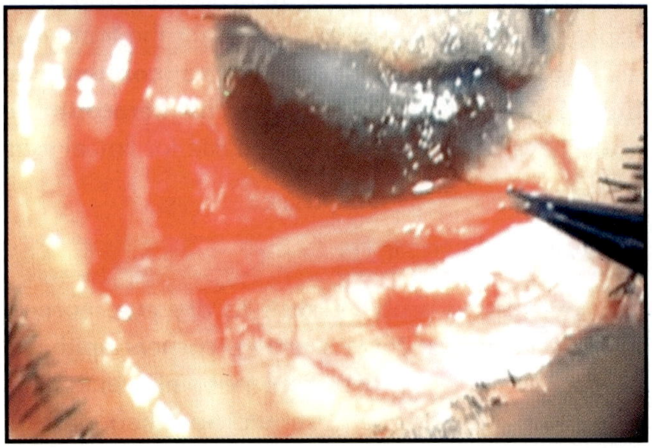

Figure 40.6: Dissection done in the recipient eye and graft kept over the area for suturing to start

The donor graft is then kept in place (Figure 40.6) and sutured in place using 10-0 nylon (Figure 40.7). The host conjunctiva is approximated to the donor conjunctiva using interrupted sutures. If required, a tarsorrhaphy can be done. At the end if necessary an amniotic membrane transplantation can also be done (Figure 40.8).

AMNIOGRAFT

Amniotic membrane can be got from a maternity ward. This way one can use fresh amniotic membrane. One can also use Amniograft (Bio-tissue Inc, Miami, USA). Amniograft is the brand name from Bio-tissue. This has been recovered aseptically from a donated placental tissue through elective caesarian section delivery and

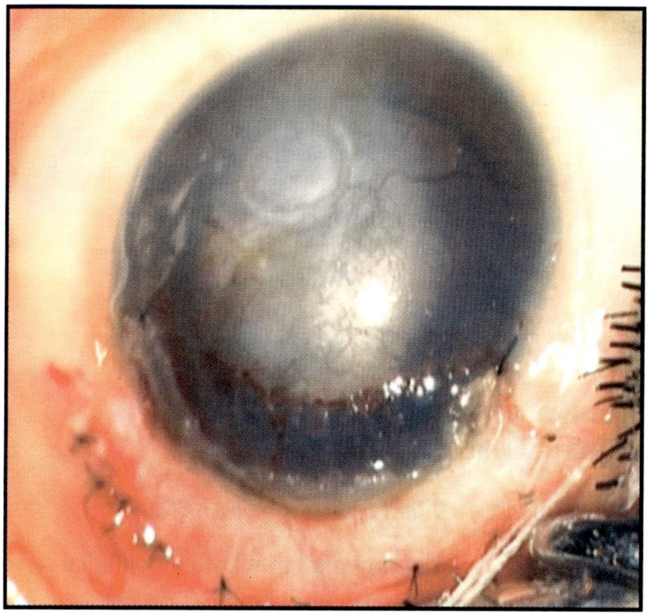

Figure 40.7: Suturing done of the limbal graft

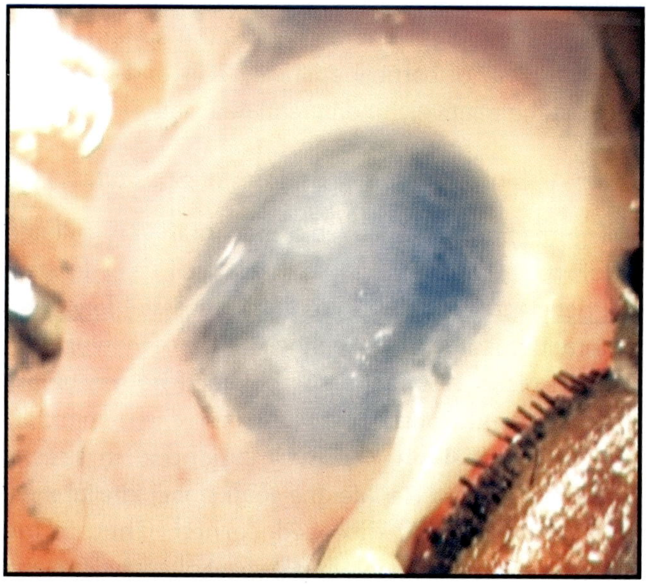

Figure 40.8: Amniotic membrane transplantation done

processed under class 100 condition. The donor is screened for H1V, HBsAg etc. Amniograft is preserved in a validated and patented storage medium made of Dulbecco's modified eagle medium and glycerol (1:1) with antiobiotics. No preservatives or additives are added. The tissue is stored at 80°C prior to distribution.

Amniograft is attached to a white nitrocellulose paper with the stromal (sticky) side adherent to the filter paper, and the basement membrane side away from the paper. If orientation is questionable after detaching the membrane from the paper, one can use a dry Weckcel or cotton tip to check. Weckcell will only adhere to the (sticky) stromal side.

Bio-tissue have also brought out Prokera which is a clinically proven amniograft which is mounted on a corneal shaped ring so that you can use a sutureless graft for ocular surface reconstruction. This way there is quicker healing, no scars and it takes less time.

SURGICAL TECHNIQUE FOR LIMBAL AUTOGRAFT

Here, the donor tissue is taken from the same or the opposite eye.[43,44] Hence, it can be performed only in conditions with limited or unilateral limbal stem cell deficiency.[22] The advantage is that the risk of graft rejection is very low.

Dua HS, Azuara-Blanco et al have described a modified procedure for limbal allograft.[22] The donor tissue is taken from the contralateral eye and transplanted onto the diseased eye. It may also be taken from a different site on the same eye in case of localized disease. Approximately 2 clock hours of the donor tissue consisting of 2 mm of superficial (about 150 μm) peripheral cornea, limbus and 3 mm of conjunctiva is dissected from the donor eye.

The number of grafts taken depends on the severity and extent of involvement of the diseased eye. A maximum of upto 180 degrees of limbal tissue may be excised from the donor eye without inducing iatrogenic limbal stem cell deficiency.

LIMBAL STEM CELL TRANSPLANTATION WITH KERATOPLASTY

In case of both allografts and autografts, if a penetrating keratoplasty is also planned for the same sitting, it is done after the limbal grafts are sutured in place. The corneal graft has generally to be kept to within 7 mm in size to avoid encroaching onto the limbal graft.

LIMBAL STEM CELL TRANSPLANTATION WITH AMNIOTIC MEMBRANE GRAFT

Limbal stem cell transplantation can be combined with an amniotic membrane graft in severe cases (see Figure 40.8). Amniotic membrane graft may be sufficient by itself in cases with partial limbal stem cell deficiency but in cases with total stem cell deficiency, it is combined with limbal stem cell transplantation.

Amniotic membrane serves as a "transplanted basement membrane." It facilitates migration of epithelial cells and reinforces epithelial cell adhesion. It provides a potential substrate and is a source of various growth factors that promote epithelialization and enhance wound healing.[13, 23,24]

POSTOPERATIVE COURSE

The patients should be on frequent follow up until epithelialization is complete. Generally, the epithelium starts growing from the graft within two to three days and becomes complete within two weeks.[42] If at any stage, conjunctival epithelium is seen to grow over the limbus or cornea again, it is scraped off to allow the epithelialization to occur from the graft. The signs which are indicative of graft rejection include graft edema, graft neovascularization, vascularization over the graft onto the cornea, focal conjunctival injection, or focal corneal epithelial defect in the sector of rejection.

POSTOPERATIVE DRUG THERAPY

Postoperatively, the patient is maintained on topical antibiotic steroid drops and preservative-free artificial tears. Autologous serum eyedrops are also seen to be useful. In case of allografts, steroids may be continued for a longer period at a low dosage (one drop per day). Immunosuppressive therapy is also given postoperatively for allografts.

SUCCESS RATES

Tsubota and coauthors[45] in 1999, published a large case series in *the New England Journal of Medicine,* where they used a cadaver source for the donor LSC, and all patients underwent concomitant amniotic membrane grafting. Success rates as denoted by successful epithelialization with phenotypic corneal epithelium, presence of a clear cornea, and visual acuity were 71 percent, 50 percent, and 0.04 (count fingers) respectively in burn patients and were lower: 50 percent, 28 percent, and 0.02 (hand motion) respectively in ocular cicatricial pemphigoid/Stevens-Johnson syndrome group. Their conclusion was that limbal stem cell transplantation with amniotic membrane grafting was successful in certain patients. These results, though not as satisfactory from the point of final visual acuity are acceptable as the only other alternative for these patients would be a keratoprosthesis.

RECENT ADVANCES

Transplantation of ex vivo Expanded Limbal Epithelial Stem Cells

Using Collagen Shield as Transfer Substrate

He and Macully[46]documented that limbal epithelial stem cells can be grown in vitro and stratified on collagen gel substrate. They transferred these collagen shields with epithelial cells to denuded ex vivo human corneal stroma in organic cultures. The 3T3 coculture system allows clonal growth of corneal epithelial cells and maintains them in the relatively undifferentiated state.[47]

Using Amniotic Membrane as Transfer Substrate

Pellegrini et al[25] transplanted a sheet of in vitro cultured autologous limbal corneal epithelial cell layer to stem cell deficient cornea and reported successful long-term restoration of the corneal epithelial surface in two cases. A small piece of limbal tissue obtained from a biopsy from the contralateral eye was digested enzymatically and the epithelium was then expanded in special medium. Three weeks later the confluent epithelial sheet was grafted to the diseased cornea. They found difficulties in handling this fragile sheet of epithelium and hence the search for a suitable carrier was begun, the role being fulfilled by amniotic membrane. When the expanded cell population reached 40-50 percent confluence, they were passed on to human amniotic membrane and allowed to attach to the AM for 10-14 days. This was then used for limbal stem cell transplantation. The biopsy can be taken from the same patient in case of unilateral or limited disease and from a living related donor or a cadaver eye[28, 48] in case of bilateral total involvement. Culturing the cells takes three to four weeks. It may then be cryo-preserved for any length of time in liquid nitrogen. In case of allografts, the patient may need to be placed on immunosuppressive therapy postoperatively.

Using Fibrin as Transfer Substrate

Limbal stem cells can be cultured using fibrin as a medium and can be transferred to the eye.[49]

Gene Therapy

Genes expressing anti-inflammatory proteins or growth factors can be used to prevent inflammation and to supply components for healthy epithelial turn over.[50]

KEY POINTS

1. The corneal epithelium continuously sheds its surface layers, and is replaced by epithelial cells beneath and peripheral to the central desquamating epithelium. The origin of these cells is thought to be from the crypts of Vogt or the palisades of Vogt located at the sclerocorneal limbus, where the stem cells reside.
2. These cells have the potential for clonogenic cell division and are essential for the maintenance of a healthy corneal surface.
3. In patients with limbal stem cell deficiency, limbal autotransplantation or allotransplantation should be considered for corneal surface reconstruction. This may be combined with or followed by keratoplasty.
4. The donor tissue can be obtained from the fellow eye (**limbal autograft**) in cases of unilateral disease. Cadaveric whole globe or corneoscleral rim of a living relative (**limbal allograft**) can be used when both eyes are affected.
5. Limbal transplantation procedures vary depending on the carrier tissue used for the transfer of the limbal stem cells. Carrier tissue is needed in limbal transplantation because it is not possible to transfer limbal stem cells alone. Either conjunctiva (**conjunctival limbal graft**) or corneal/limbal stroma (**keratolimbal graft**) have been used as carrier tissue for limbal stem cells.
6. The future lies in transplanting **ex vivo expanded limbal epithelial stem cells** using a suitable transfer substrate. **Gene therapy** can be implemented by incorporating suitable genes into these cells to decrease inflammation or to express growth factors.
7. Amniotic membrane can be got from a maternity ward. This way one can use fresh amniotic membrane. One can also use Amniograft (Bio-tissue Inc, Miami, USA).

REFERENCES

1. Maumenee A, Scholz R. Histopathology of the ocular lesions produced by the sulphur and nitrogen mustards. Johns Hopkins Hospital Bull 1948;82:121-47.
2. Buschke W. Morphologic changes in cells of corneal epithelium in wound healing. Arch Ophthalmol 1949;41:306(16):703.
3. Kinoshita S, Friend J, Thoft RA. Biphasic cell proliferation in transdifferentiation of conjunctival to corneal epithelium in rabbits. Invest Ophthalmol Vis Sci 1983;24:1008-14.
4. Lajtha LG. Stem cell concepts. Differentiation 1979;14:23-34.
5. Potten CS, Morris RJ. Epithelial stem cells in vivo. J Cell Sci 1988;10(Suppl):45-62.
6. Davanger M, Evensen A. Role of the pericorneal papillary structure in renewal of corneal epithelium. Nature 1971;229:560-61.
7. Cotsarelis G, Cheng SZ, Dong G, Sun TT, Lavker RM. Existence of slow-cycling limbal epithelial basal cells that can be preferentially stimulated to proliferate: implications on epithelial stem cells. Cell 1989;57:201-09.
8. Tseng SC. Regulation and clinical implications of corneal epithelial stem cells. Mol Biol Rep 1996;23:47-58.
9. Ebato B, Friend J, Thoft RA. Comparison of central and peripheral human corneal epithelium in tissue culture. Invest Ophthalmol Vis Sci 1987;28:1450-6.
10. Pellegrini G, Golisano O, Paterna P, et al. Location and clonal analysis of stem cells and their differentiated progeny in the human ocular surface. J Cell Biol 1999;145:769-82.
11. Kruse FE, Volcker HE. Stem cells, wound healing, growth factors, and angiogenesis in the cornea. Curr Opin Ophthalmol 1997;8:46-54.
12. Kruse FE. Stem cells and corneal epithelial regeneration. Eye 1994;8:170-83.
13. Dua HS, Azuara-Blanco A. Limbal stem cells of the corneal epithelium. Surv Ophthalmol 2000;44:415-25.
14. Chen JJY, Tseng SCG. Corneal epithelial wound healing in partial limbal deficiency. Invest Ophthalmol Vis Sci 1990;31:1301-14.
15. Huang AJW, Tseng SCG. Corneal epithelial wound healing in the absence of limbal epithelium. Invest Ophthalmol Vis Sci 1991;32:96-105.
16. Kenyon KR, Bulusoglu G, Ziske JD. Clinical pathologic correlations of limbal autograft transplantation. Am J Ophthalmol 1990;31:1.
17. Kinoshita S, Kiorpes T, Friend J, et al. Limbal epithelium in ocular surface wound healing. Invest Ophthalmol Vis Sci 1982;23:73-80.
18. Nishida K, F S, Ohashi Y, et al. Ocular surface abnormalities in aniridia. Am J Ophthalmol 1995;120:368-75.
19. Tseng SCG. Concept and application of limbal stem cells. Eye 1989;57:201-09.
20. Brown SI, Bloomfield SE, Pearce DB. Follow-up report on transplantation of the alkali burned cornea. Am J Ophthalmol 1974;77:538-42.

21. Abel R Jr, Binder PS, Pilack FM, et al. The results of penetrating keratoplasty after chemical burns. Trans Am Acad Ophthalmol Otolaryngol 1975;79:584-95.
22. Dua HS, Azuara-Blanco A. Autologous limbal transplantation in patients with unilateral corneal stem cell deficiency. Br J Ophthalmol 2000; 84: 273-8.
23. Azuara-Blanco A, Pillai CT, Dua HS. Amniotic membrane transplantation for ocular surface reconstruction. Br J Ophthalmol 1999;83:399-402.
24. Dua HS, Azuara-Blanco A. Amniotic membrane transplantation. Br J Ophthalmol 1999;83:748-52.
25. Pellegrini G, Traverso CE, Franzi AT, Zingirian M. Long term restoration of damaged corneal surface with autologous cultivated corneal epithelium. Lancet 1997;349:990-93.
26. Schwab IR. Cultured corneal epithelia for ocular surface disease. Trans Am Ophthalmol Soc 1999;97:891-986.
27. Schwab IR, Isseroff RR. Bioengineered corneas–the promise and the challenge. N Engl J Med 2000;343:136-8.
28. Schwab IR, Reyes M, Isseroff RR. Successful transplantation of bioengineered tissue replacements in patients with ocular surface disease. Cornea 2000;19:421-26.
29. Tsai RJ, Li LM, Chen JK. Reconstruction of damaged corneas by transplantation of autologous limbal epithelial cells. N Engl J Med 2000;343:86-93.
30. Copeland RA, Char DH. Limbal autograft reconstruction after conjunctival squamous cell carcinoma. Am J Ophthalmol 1990;110:412-15.
31. Jenkins C, Tuft S, Liu C, et al. Limbal transplantation in the management of chronic contact-lens associated epitheliopathy. Eye 1993;7:629-33.
32. Pfister R. Corneal stem cell disease: concepts, categorization, and treatment by auto- and homotransplantation of limbal stem cells. CLAO J 1994;20:64-72
33. Kwitko S, Marinho D, Barcaro S, et al. Allograft conjunctival transplantation for bilateral ocular surface disorders. Ophthalmology 1995;102:1020-25.
34. Kenyon KR, Rapoza PA. Limbal allograft transplantation for ocular surface disorders. Ophthalmology 1995;102 (suppl):101-02.
35. Holland EJ. Epithelial transplantation for the management of severe ocular surface disease. Trans Am Ophthalmol Soc 1996;94:677-743.
36. Holland EJ, Schwartz GS. The evolution of epithelial transplantation for severe ocular surface disease and a proposed classification system. Cornea 1996;15:549-56.
37. Tan DTH, Ficker LA, Buckley RJ. Limbal transplantation. Ophthalmology 1996;103:29-36.
38. Tsai RJF, Tseng SCG. Human allograft limbal transplantation for corneal surface reconstruction. Cornea 1994;13:389-400.
39. Tsubota K, Toda I, Saito H, et al. Reconstruction of the corneal epithelium by limbal allograft transplantation for severe ocular surface disorders. Ophthalmology 1995;102:1486-96.
40. Sundmacher R, Reinhard T. Central corneolimbal transplantation under systemic ciclosporin A cover for severe limbal stem cell insuficiency. Graefes Arch Clin Exp Ophthalmol 1996;234(suppl):s122-s125.
41. Tseng S, Prabhasawat P, Barton K, et al. Amniotic membrane transplantation with or wihout limbal allografts for corneal surface reconstruction in patients with limbal stem cell deficiency. Arch Ophthalmol 1998;116:431-41.
42. Harminder S Dua, Augusto Azuara-Blanco. Allo-limbal transplantation in patients with limbal stem cell deficiency Br J Ophthalmol 1999;83:414-19.
43. Kenyon KR, Tseng SC. Limbal autograft transplantation for ocular surface disorders. Ophthalmology 1989;96:709-22; Discussion 722-23.
44. Kenyon KR. Limbal autograft transplantation for chemical and thermal burns. Dev Ophthalmol 1989;18:53-58.
45. Tsubota K, Satake Y, Kaido M, et al. Treatment of severe ocular-surface disorders with corneal epithelial stem-cell transplantation. N Engl J Med 1999;340:1697-703.
46. He YG, McCulley JP. Growing human corneal epitheli-um on collagen shield and subsequent transfer to de-nuded cornea in vitro. Curr Eye Res 1991;10:851-63.
47. Rheinwald JG, Green H. Serial cultivation of strains of human epidermal keratinocytes: the formation of keratinizing colonies from single cells. Cell 1975;6:331-43.
48. Koizumi N, Inatomi T, Suzuki T, Sotozono C, Kinoshita S. Cultivated corneal epithelial transplantation for ocular surface reconstruction in acute phase of Stevens-Johnson syndrome. Arch Ophthalmol 2001;119:298-300.
49. Rama P, Bonini S, Lambiase A, et al. Autologous fibrin-cultured limbal stem cells permanently restore the corneal surface of patients with total limbal stem cell deficiency. Transplantation 2001;72:1478-85.
50. Hauswirth WW, Beaufrere L. Ocular gene therapy: quo vadis? Invest Ophthalmol Vis Sci 2000;41:2821-26.

41

Artificial Vision

- RELEVANCE OF PROBLEM
- VISUAL PATHWAYS
- BACKGROUND AND HISTORY OF ARTIFICIAL VISION
- INTRAOCULAR RETINAL PROSTHESIS (HUMAYUN ET AL)

Mark S Humayun, Rohit R Lakhanpal (USA)

RELEVANCE OF PROBLEM

More than 1 million Americans are legally blind and 10 percent have no light perception from various causes.[1] Certain experimental approaches, such as gene and drug therapy may be a preventative or therapeutic option.[2,3] However, once photoreceptors are nearly completely lost, such as in end-stage retinitis pigmentosa (RP) or age-related macular degeneration (AMD), very few approaches[4] can restore useful vision to blind patients. Retinitis pigmentosa (RP) is the leading inherited cause of blindness with 1.5 million people worldwide affected and an incidence of 1/3,500 live births.[5] Also, AMD is the leading cause of visual loss among adults older than 65, with 700,000 newly diagnosed patients annually in the United States, 10 percent of whom become legally blind each year.[6]

With increased average lifespan, the number of Americans with age-related eye disease and resulting visual impairment is expected to double during the next three decades.[7] Photodynamic or conventional laser therapy are two effective methods in slowing the progression of AMD, while gene therapy and new surgical interventions,[8-10] including localized ocular drugs,[11-15] are examples of approaches currently being researched to help reverse the development of blindness caused by retinal disease.

In addition to the retinopathies described above, cortical tumors and trauma involving the visual pathways or occipital cortex have traditionally represented treatment hurdles to affected patients. Thus far, physicians have been in a limited position of offering low-vision devices to enhance remaining vision rather than therapeutically targeting and reversing the underlying disease process. Using artificial means to treat extreme vision impairment has come closer to reality during the past few decades. The goal of this research has been to create an implantable medical device to provide useful vision for those patients who are left with no alternatives. This chapter will briefly summarize the history and evolution of visual prostheses, including retinal implants, and present the current state of the field with remaining challenges that lie ahead.

VISUAL PATHWAYS

Normal physiologic vision is initiated when light passes through the cornea and lens of the eye to the rods and cones of the photoreceptor layer on the outer surface of the retina initiating photochemical Artificial Vision 3 MSH, RRL transduction (Figure 41.1A). The cell bodies of these receptors synapse with horizontal and bipolar cells. Bipolar cells synapse either directly with ganglion cells or indirectly by first synapsing with amacrine cells. The axons of the ganglion cells converge to form the optic nerve, acquire mylenation upon exiting the orbit, and travel posteriorly, joining the contralateral optic nerve to form the optic chiasm. The visual pathway continues around the cerebral peduncle, via optic tracts to the lateral geniculate nucleus, and posteriorly via optic radiations to the primary visual cortex in the occipital lobe (Figure 41.1B). Visual information is then relayed from V1 to higher cortical association and processing areas.

BACKGROUND AND HISTORY OF ARTIFICIAL VISION

Improvement and restoration of vision has long been a goal of science and medicine. As far back as 1665, English natural philosopher Robert Hooke wrote:

> The next care to be taken, in respect to the Senses, is a supplying of their infirmities with instruments, and as it were, the adding of artificial organs to the natural . . . and as glasses have highly promoted our seeing, so it is not improbable, but that there may be found many mechanical inventions to improve our other senses of hearing, smelling, tasting, and touching.[16]

Hooke's statement demonstrates both a keen insight that all the senses could be improved by artificial means and a lack of understanding that living things use electricity as a signaling mechanism. As scientists began to understand electricity and apply it to living things, this knowledge improved understanding of human body systems and eased human suffering. For example, in the 19th century, Galvani and Volterra performed experiments demonstrating that both muscles and the auditory system responded to electrical stimuli.

Later, C. H. Wilkinson, an English surgeon, published a brochure in 1799 touting that at a cost of "one guinea

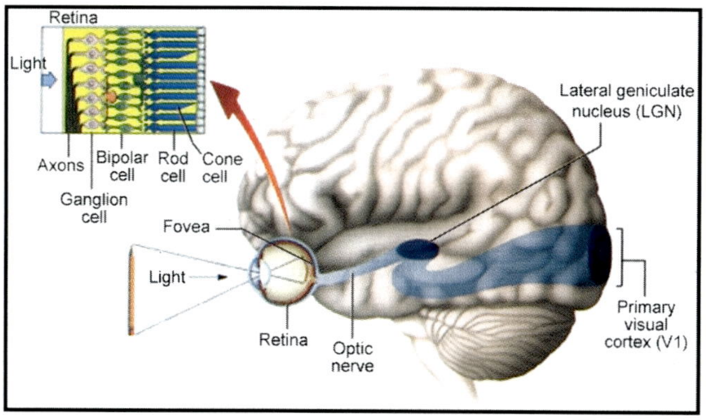

(A) Light travels through the tear film, cornea, aqueous, lens and vitreous to activate the light-sensitive, multilayered neural network of cells and transsynaptic connections of the retina at the photoreceptor layer

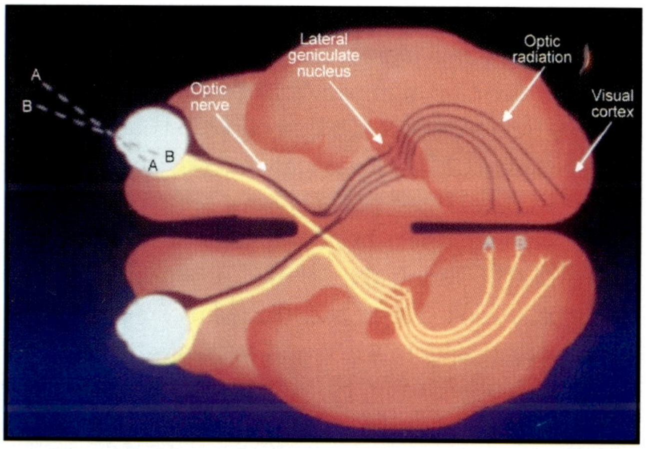

(B) The image is processed and transmitted through retinal ganglion cells which merge to form the optic nerve, myelinate posterior to the orbit and merge with contralateral fibers to form the optic chiasm. The pathway terminates at the primary visual cortex in the occipital lobe

Figures 41.1A and B: Human visual system

per week" he would treat patients with a variety of ailments (including blindness) in his "Medico-Electric" rooms. Although highly anecdotal, these reports do demonstrate mankind's emerging understanding that the human body is an electrical system and that electricity may have therapeutic uses. Today, electrical stimulation continues to find valid therapeutic applications in the human body. However, Artificial Vision 4 MSH, RRL therapeutic electrical stimulation to treat disease is not the same as electrical stimulation to replace lost function, and the two should not be confused.[16]

Historically, several methods of supplementing remaining functional vision have been pursued via interventions at several points along the visual pathway, including the retina, optic nerve, and occipital cortex. Visual prostheses are based on neuronal electrical stimulation at different locations along the visual pathway (i.e. cortical, optic nerve, epiretinal, subretinal). Each of the different approaches will be discussed. In terms of retinal prostheses, advances in microtechnology have allowed for the development of sophisticated, high-density integrated circuit devices that may be implanted either in the subretinal or epiretinal space. Analogous to the cochlear implants for some forms of deafness, these devices propose to restore useful vision by converting visual information into patterns of electrical stimulation that would excite the remaining spared inner retinal neurons in diseases such as retinitis pigmentosa and age-related macular degeneration. However, the approach in the visual system is more complex than in the auditory system. In the eye, information processing occurs simultaneously and in parallel within millions of neurons that transform the incoming light stimuli into electrical impulses, processing these impulses within the retina before sending the results through axons via the lateral geniculate nucleus to the visual cortex. Thus, the relative complexity of the visual system presents challenges to researchers attempting visual prostheses. In this chapter, we will focus upon the epiretinal implant as developed by Humayun et al.

Epiretinal implants rely on imaging devices such as a camera and then transform this visual information to patterns of electrical stimulation to excite remaining retinal neurons. Designs tend to vary in terms of how much required electronic circuitry is contained in an intraocular device versus extraocular elements. Power sources and signal transmission may be accomplished by induction coils, penetrating wires, or lasers.

INTRAOCULAR RETINAL PROSTHESIS (HUMAYUN ET AL.)

Our group, Humayun et al, has pioneered research in the development of a device called the intraocular retinal prosthesis (IRP). This IRP includes both an external, wearable component and an implantable, intraocular component (Figure 41.2A). The external portion is comprised of a lightweight Artificial Vision 5 MSH, RRL camera built into spectacles, pocket batteries, and a small pager-sized visual processing unit. Power and data are sent wirelessly from this external unit to the internal portion of the prosthesis. The implanted portion of the device consists of a receiver/stimulating microelectronic chip and a micro-electrode array, currently including 16 platinum electrodes of approximately 500 μm diameter (Figure 41.2B). The electrode array is affixed to the epiretinal surface by a retinal tack. This Model 1 allows for digital video capture and translation to a pixilated image to occur externally, with only the final processed data and power transferred to the implanted portion of the prosthesis. The implanted part of the device then converts the transferred visual data into controlled patterns of electrical pulses to stimulate the remaining retinal neurons.

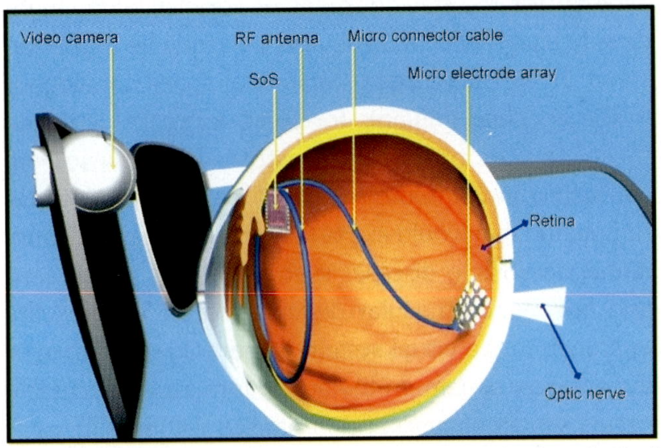

(A) Illustrated view of the intraocular retinal prosthesis epiretinal prosthesis apparatus including the camera, connector cable, and microelectrode array is noted. Visual percepts are formed and transmitted through the optic nerve to the visual cortex

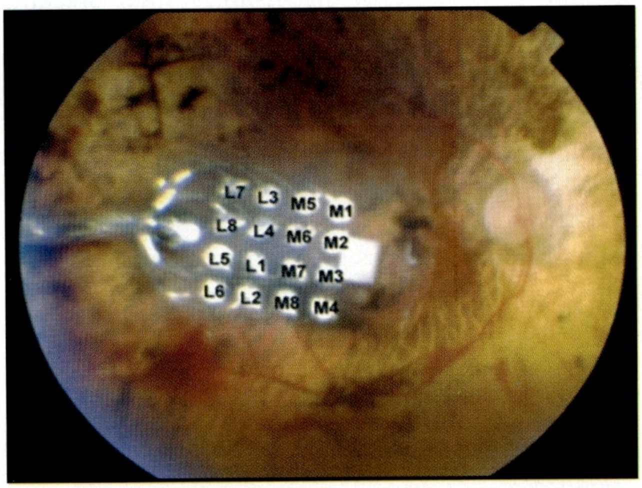

(B) Fundus photograph of implanted epiretinal prosthesis in a patient with retinitis pigmentosa. Note that each platinum electrode is labeled with a unique designation for localization of percepts. This implant is located in the macula

Figures 41.2A and B: Epiretinal macular apparatus and implant

Preliminary tests of epiretinal electronic stimulation were performed in humans using temporary devices without tack fixation in the operating room.[17-19] During these short periods of electrical stimulation, patients were able to identify crude forms such as letters or a box shape. Further, they reported no persistence of the image pursuant to stimulation.[18] Based on these encouraging results, a permanent implant trial began in 2002 at the Doheny Retina Institute (DRI) as part of a Food and Drug Administration (FDA) Investigational Device Exemption study. To date, three patients have received implants, each including 16-electrode, model 1 devices [Second Sight, LLC]. During the follow-up period, objective (electrically evoked responses [EERs] recorded from the visual cortex) (Figure 41.3) and subjective evidence of visual perceptions using psychophysical tests have been obtained. Patients reported visual percepts in locations consistent with the implanted electrodes, the ability to discriminate between percepts created by different

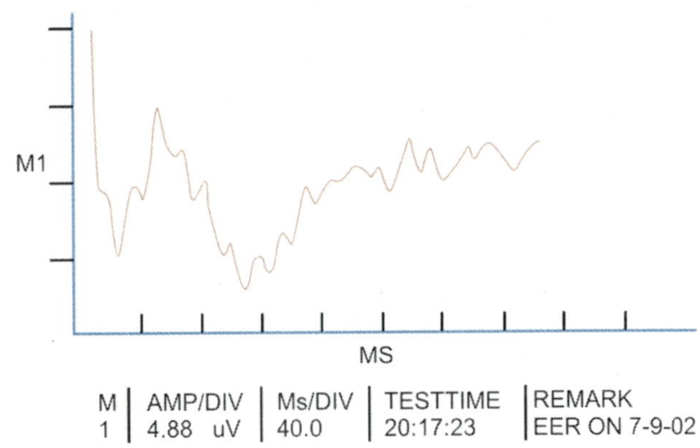

Figure 41.3: Electrical-evoked Response after epiretinal implantation. Electrical-evoked response (EER) elicited from a patient with retinitis pigmentosa implanted with the intraocular retinal prosthesis epiretinal prosthesis during electrical stimulation

electrodes based on the locations of the percepts, the ability to discern brighter or dimmer percepts with varying levels of current, and the ability to distinguish the direction of motion of objects.[19]

These preliminary patient tests are most encouraging because they provide further evidence of plasticity/ learning curve of the visual pathway and demonstrate that epiretinal stimulation can be conducted in a retinotopic manner. While RGC are located in closest proximity to the microelectrode array and require less current, stimulation of these cells would require more image processing, complex stimulation patterns to account for lost retinal processing, and sub-optimal, larger, and ill-defined Artificial Vision 6 MSH, RRL percepts.[20, 21] It is more desirable to stimulate the deeper bipolar cells, thereby utilizing the intact processing capability of inner retina cell layers.

Experiments done in the past by Greenberg et al have found that although the epiretinal stimulating electrodes are physically in closer proximity to the retinal ganglion cell axons and retinal ganglion cell bodies, that by varying the pulse width of the stimulating current that the electrodes can be 'tuned' to selectively stimulate retinal bipolar cells rather than retinal ganglion cells.[22] RGC responded to shorter pulse durations (<0.5 msec) while deeper retinal neural layers responded to longer pulse durations (>0.5 msec).[22]

This experimental result, if consistently produced in the patient, would enable an epiretinal prosthesis to employ the processing from the entire retina as it would initiate the electrical signal propagation at the level of the retinal bipolar cell. The histological retinal changes associated with the mechanical effects of epiretinal implantation are also less severe than with subretinal implantation. Since the epiretinal implant does not intervene between the RPE/choroid and the retina, there is less of an inflammatory reaction and fewer retinal architecture changes noted. For example, in both normal and retinal rod-cone degenerate (rcd1) dogs, chronic stimulation over a period of months followed by histological examination revealed that there is minimal effect on the retinal layers.[23] Thus, chronic implantation and stimulation appear to be safe.

Our group has also incorporated the use of optical coherence tomography (OCT) as a non-invasive method to acquire qualitative and quantitative information about the retina-implant interface.[24] This approach and the ability to resolve any lift-off of the array from the retina are critical as tens of microns separation of the electrode from the retina markedly increases the current requirements. Thus, using OCT will improve our ability to anatomically follow the epiretinal implants in both animal models and patients while also monitoring local changes around the implant site.[24]

Screening in the clinic before surgery has also markedly improved our ability to judge the implant requirements in blind patients. From correlating preoperative electrically evoked responses (EERs) and certain psychophysical tests in the clinic with electrical thresholds obtained with direct retinal stimulation from both our short-term and long-term implant tests, we have learned that these preoperative EERs and Artificial Vision 7 MSH, RRL psychophysical tests were highly predictive of the current level needed to elicit visual perception by direct electrical stimulation.[25]

Finally, the next model for the IRP is undergoing development. The Model 2 device may incorporate MEMS component so that the retina-implant interface may be a more flexible frame for attachment. This new prosthesis will also possess more than the 16 electrodes currently provided. Such a device will require improved technology that simultaneously reduces the size and increases the capability to 60-100 electrode contacts on the retina. While the ever increasing capability of microelectronics will partially solve this problem, specific technology in the areas of microelectrode fabrication and hermetic packaging will need to be developed to enable implementation of an even higher resolution (1,000 electrodes) epiretinal prosthesis.

CONCLUSIONS

The advantages of the epiretinal approach include the following: (1) the epiretinal placement allows for the vitreous to act as a sink for heat-dissipation from the microelectronic device; (2) a minimal number of microelectronics are incorporated into the implantable portion of the device; the wearable portion of electronics allows for easy upgrades without requiring subsequent surgery; and (3) the electronics allow the user and the doctor full control over every electrode parameter and digital signal processing involved in imaging objects allowing the implant to be customized for each patient. The disadvantages to this approach include: (1) requirement of techniques that will provide prolonged adhesion of the device to the inner retina; and (2) further distance of the epiretinal device to the target bipolar cells than the subretinal device requires increased current.

Future research for all parties involved in the epiretinal prostheses need to address not only microfabricated electrode arrays that will last over long-term but also microelectronics that are efficient and dissipate minimal heat and packaging for microelectronics that will allow for the microelectronics to survive in the warm saline environment of the eye. In addition, significant attention needs to be given to the manner in which visual images will be encoded and delivered in patterns of electrical stimulation to the retina. Artificial Vision 8 MSH, RRL.

REFERENCES

1. Ross RD. Is perception of light useful to the blind patient? (Editorial and Comments). Arch Ophthalmol 1998;116:236-8.
2. Berson EL, Rosner B, Sandberg MA, et al. A randomized trial of Vitamin A and Vitamin E supplementation for retinitis. (Comments) Arch Ophthalmol 1993;111:761-72.
3. Sharma RK, Ehinger B. Management of hereditary retinal degenerations: present status and future directions. Surv Ophthalmol 1999;43:427-44.
4. del Cerro M, Gash DM, Rao GN, et al. Retinal transplants into the anterior chamber of the rat eye. Neuroscience 1987; 21:707-23.
5. Bunker CH, et al. Prevalence of retinitis pigmentosa in Maine. American Journal of Ophthalmology. 1984;97(3): 357-65.
6. Curcio CA, Medeiros NE, Millican CL. Photoreceptor loss in age-related macular degeneration. Investigative Ophthalmology and Visual Science. 1996.;7(7):1236-49.
7. Humayun MS, de Juan E Jr. Artificial vision. Eye 1998;12 (Pt 3b):605-07.
8. Fujii GY, et al. Initial experience of inferior limited macular translocation for subfoveal choroidal neovascularization resulting from causes other than age-related macular degeneration. American Journal of Ophthalmology 2001; 131(1):90-100.
9. Fujii GY, et al. Patient selection for macular translocation surgery using the scanning laser ophthalmoscope. Ophthalmology 2002;109(9):1737-44.
10. Ng EW, et al. Iatrogenic choroidal neovascularization occurring in patients undergoing macular surgery. Retina., 2002;22(6):711-18.
11. Krzystolik MG, Afshari MA, Adamis AP, et al. Prevention of experimental choroidal neovascularization with intravitreal anti-vascular endothelial growth factor antibody fragment. Arch Ophthalmol 2002;120(3):338-46.
12. D'Amico DJ, Goldberg MF, Hudson H, et al. Anecortave acetate as monotherapy for the treatment of subfoveal lesions in patients with exudative age-related macular degeneration (AMD): interim (month 6) analysis of clinical safety and efficacy. Retina 2003;23(1):14-23.
13. Slakter JS. Anecortave Acetate Clinical Study Group. Anecortave acetate as monotherapy for treatment of subfoveal neovascularization in age-related macular degeneration: twelve-month clinical outcomes. Ophthalmology. 2003;110(12):2372-83; discussion 2384-5.
14. Gragoudas ES. VEGF Inhibition Study in Ocular Neovascularization-1 (VISION-1): Efficacy Results From Phase II/III MacugenTM (Pegaptanib Sodium) Clinical Trials. [ARVO abstract] Invest Ophthalmol Vis Sci. 2004. Abstract nr 2364.
15. D'Amico DJ, Bird AC. VEGF Inhibition Study in Ocular Neovascularization-1 (VISION-1): Safety Evaluation From the Pivotal MacugenTM (Pegaptanib Sodium) Clinical Trials. [ARVO abstract] Invest Ophthalmol Vis Sci. 2004. Abstract nr 2363.
16. Weiland JD, Humayun MS. Past, present, and future of artificial vision. Artif Organs 2003;27(11):961-2.
17. Humayun MS, de Juan E Jr, Dagnelie G, et al. Visual perception elicited by electrical stimulation of retina in blind humans. Archives of Ophthalmology 1996;114(1):40-46.
18. Humayun MS, de Juan E Jr, Weiland JD, et al. Pattern electrical stimulation of the human retina. Vision Research 1999;39(15):2569-76.
19. Humayun MSW, Fujii J, Greenberg GY, et al. Visual Perception in a Blind Subject with a Chronic Microelectronic Retinal Prosthesis. In Press 2003.
20. Greenberg RJ, Velte TJ, Humayun MS, et al. A computational model of electrical stimulation of the retinal ganglion cell. IEEE Transactions on Biomedical Engineering., 1999;46(5):505-14.
21. Lakhanpal R, Yanai D, Weiland JD, et al. Advances in the development of visual prostheses. Current Opinion in Ophthalmology 2003;(14):122-27.
22. Greenberg R. Analysis of electrical stimulation of the vertebrate retina- work towards a retinal prosthesis. in PhD Dissertation. 1998, The Johns Hopkins University: Baltimore, MD.
23. Piyathaisere DV, Margalit E, Chen SJ, et al. Heat effects on the retina. Ophthalmic Surg Lasers Imaging 2003;34:114-20.
24. Panzan CQ, Guven D, Weiland JD, et al. Retinal Thickness in Normal and RCD1 Dogs Using Optical Coherence Tomography (In Press).
25. Yanai D, Lakhanpal RR, Weiland JD, et al. The Value of Preoperative Tests in the Selection of Blind Patients for a Permanent Microelectronic Implant. Trans Am Ophthalmol Soc 2003;101.

42

Nanotechnology in Ophthalmology

- MEDICINE AND NOTECHNOLOGY
- NANOTECHNOLOGY IN OPHTHALMOLOGY
- ETHICS
- POTENTIAL PROBLEMS
- THE CHALLENGE AHEAD

NR Biswas, Alok K Ravi, Madhurjya Gogoi (India)

INTRODUCTION

Nanotechnology is a field of science comprising the body of theories and techniques that allow the production and manipulation of minute objects that measure a little as one billionth of a meter (the nanometer). Although research in this field dates back to Richard P Feynman's work 1959, the term nanotechnology was first coined by K Eric Drexler in 1986 in the book *Engines of Creation.*

Nanotechnology involves research and technology development at the atomic, molecular, or macro-molecular levels in the critical dimension range of approximately 1-100 nanometers. Nanotechnology research and development includes control at the nanoscale and integration of nanoscale structures into larger material components and systems. Within these larger scale assemblies, the control and construction of their structures and components remains at the nanometer scale.

Nanobiotechnology is an emerging area that applies the tools and processes of nano / microfabrication to build devices for studying biosystems. Vice-versa, researchers also learn from biology how to create better micro-nanoscale devices. The field is highly interdisciplinary and features a close collaboration between life scientists, physical scientists, and engineers.

Of relevance to medicine is **Nanomedicine**, which may be defined as the monitoring, repair, construction and control of human biological systems at the molecular level, using engineered nanodevices and nanostructures. The goal is to deliver the potential benefit of discoveries in the laboratory to society.

The power of nanotechnology can be encapsulated in an apparently simple and minute device. Packed with miniature chemical processors, computing, and robotics, it will produce a wide-range of items quickly, cleanly, and inexpensively, building products directly from blueprints. The enabling technologies include optics, nanolithography, mechanochemistry and 3D prototyping.

Although nanotechnology is in the research stage as of now, it is likely to arrive in 20 to 30 years from now. It is being extensively pursued for research on ageing, cancer, and drug development and delivery.

MEDICINE AND NANOTECHNOLOGY

Medicine attempts to make the best use of the body's natural healing powers and homeostatic mechanisms. The underlying principle is that, all else being equal, those interventions are best that intervene least. The promise of nanotechnology in medicine lies in the potential to achieve this by target specific and controlled delivery of intervention measures at the cellular level. Nanosystems have significantly different biological properties from large-sized systems (e.g. implants or microparticles) that could be used effectively to overcome problems in drug and gene therapy using programmable and controllable microscale robots. This will hopefully unlock the indefinite extension of human health and the expansion of human abilities. The possibility of applying nanotechnology in even traditional Chinese medicine has been explored.[1]

THE MEDICAL NANODEVICE

Composition

The typical medical nanodevice will probably be a micron-scale robot assembled from nanoscale parts ranging from 1-100 nm (1 nm = 10^{-9} meter), and might be fitted together to make a working machine measuring perhaps 0.5-3 microns (1 micron = 10^{-6} meter) in diameter. Three microns is about the maximum size for blood borne medical nanorobots, the limiting factor being capillary passage.

Carbon will likely be the principal element comprising the bulk of a medical nanorobot, probably in the form of diamond or diamondoid/fullerene nanocomposites—largerly because of the tremendous strength and chemical inertness of diamond. Other elements such as hydrogen, sulfur, oxygen, nitrogen, fluorine, silicon, etc. will be used for special purposes.

Properties

The medical nanodevice should be visualized as two spaces: Its interior and its exterior. The exterior will be exposed to the diverse chemical brew that makes up our human biochemistry. But the interior of the nanorobot may be a highly controlled environment into which external liquids would not normally intrude, except in specific instance.

The ideal model of the medical nanodevice will consist of an injection of a few cubic centimeters of micron-sized nanorobots. The circulating nanorobots will be designed to accomplish a specific task, and would remain absolutely inactive outside of the target volume. Even once inside the target treatment volume, nanorobots would still remain inactive until the physician tells them to begin the active treatment, or the precise antigenic signature of the target tissue is detected. Knowledge of these antigens will become extensive, soon after the completion of the *Human Genome Project* early in the 21st century.

Nanorobots will communicate their positions, operational status, and the outcome of treatment using encoded acoustic messaging for internal communications as well as for communication with the physician, who will retain complete control. It may not be necessary to image the nanodevices directly, and procedures such as biopsy should be rarely needed. They will have a high level of redundancy to ensure effectiveness and safety. *In vivo* medical nanodevices could metabolize local glucose and oxygen for energy, or use externally supplied acoustic power. Their exfusion from the body will occur via the usual excretory channels or other scavenger systems. The only physical change to be seen in the patient will hopefully be his recovery.

The Question of Immune Response

Many medical nanorobots will have only temporary residence in the body, and the issue of nanodevice biocompatibility is in principle similar to the biocompatibility of medical implants generally. It is not expected to be a major problem. The design of the exteriors will be critical to minimize bioactivity and opsonization. Passive diamond is one such design.

Replication

Replication is a crucial basic capability for molecular manufacturing, but medical nanorobots need not ever replicate *in vivo* except in the most unusual of circumstances. Replicators will almost certainly be very tightly regulated by governments everywhere.Many medical nanorobots will have very simple computers on board each device. The risk of human like artificial intelligence is unfounded.

Genetics

Of great importance is the use of nanotechnology in genetics. DNA is a unique material for nanotechnology since it is possible to use base sequences to encode instructions for assembly in a predetermined fashion at the nanometer scale. This emerging field of DNA-nanotechnology is now exploring DNA-programed processes for the assembly of organic compounds, biomolecules, and inorganic materials.[2] Bioconjugated nanoparticles are being evaluated for biosensing and bioimaging, such as cell staining, DNA detection and separation, rapid single bacterium detection, and biotechnological application in DNA protection.[3]

Drug Development

Nanosystems comprising nanoparticles and nanodevices such as nanobiosensors and nanobiochips, are being developed for targeted drug therapy. Among these nanomaterials, carbon nanotubes (CNT) have emerged as an efficient and safe tool for transporting and translocating therapeutic molecules such as bioactive peptides, proteins, nucleic acids and drugs.[4-6]

Many polymerizable surfactants have been synthesized with all possible combination of the various types (anionic, cationic, zwitterionic or non-ionic group) and of classical polymerizable groups (acrylate, methacrylate, acrylamide, vinyl, allyle, diallyle, etc.). The polymerizable group can be located at different parts of the surfactant molecule most often near the polar head or at the end of hydrophobic tail, or even in the counterion (Figure 42.1).

Another importan parameter, which synergies the release kinetics in different pH, solutions, is the swelling behavior of the polymer. One of the most important characteristics of the present copoly(NIPAAM-VP-AA) micelles is their ability to ionize/deionize at different pH-senstive polymer. The key to the controlling of the pores of the particles include both overall -COOH content and the ionization of –COOH groups. At acidic pH, the carboxylic groups exhibit inter-chain hydrogen bonding creating a tighter overall network and hence the pore

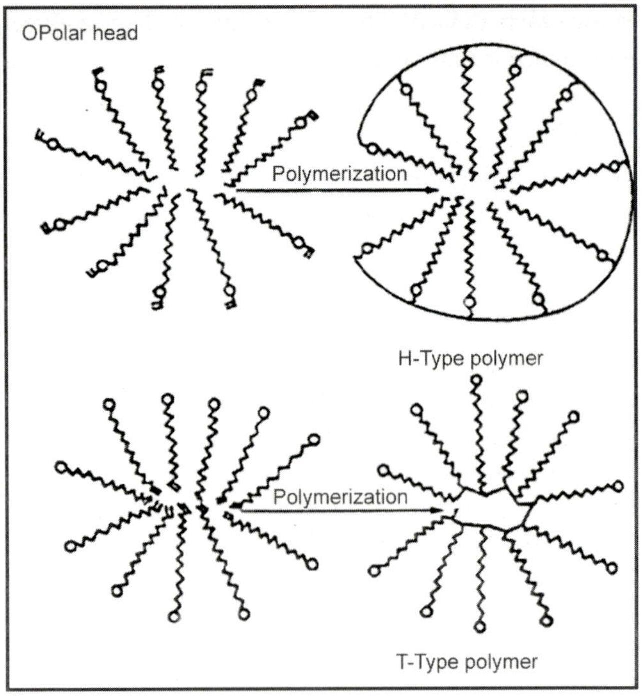

Figure 42.1: Schematic ideal representation of head and tail monomeric and polymeric

size becomes smaller. Consequently due to small pore size, the release of drug from the micelles is quite slow. At alkaline pH, -COOH groups become ionized and due to repulsion among the ionized –COO groups swelling take place. As a result of swelling, pore size of the polymer increases and the drug release becomes faster (Figure 42.2).

NANOTECHNOLOGY IN OPHTHALMOLOGY

The application of nanotechnology in ophthalmology has so far mainly been on the development of drug delivery systems. A few such examples are:

1. Experimental studies have been reported on ocular hypotensive formulation containing biodegradable calcium phosphate nanoparticles (CAP) and 7-hydroxy-2-dipropyl-aminotetralin (7-OH-DPAT) for achieving controlled and targeted drug delivery for treatment of ocular diseases.[7]
2. Gelatin nanoparticles encapsulating pilocarpine HCl or hydrocortisone as model drugs have been produced using a desolvation method.[8]
3. The successful topical application of non-steroidal anti-inflammatory drugs sodium ibuprofen as well as flurbiprofen loaded polymeric nanoparticle suspensions made from inert polymer resins on the eye to counteract the miosis induced by surgical traumas, such as cataract extraction.[9,10]
4. The use of albumin nanoparticles to enhance the antiviral activity of ganciclovir while decreasing its intrinsic toxicity have been evaluated in human fibroblasts.[11]
5. Intravitreal injection of ganciclovir-loaded bovine serum albumin nanoparticles in rats has been studied for treatment of cytomegalovirus infection.[12]

Nanoparticles for Ocular Drug Delivery

Studies that have investigated the potential of nanoparticles for ocular drug delivery have been limited and have yet to demonstrate conclusively if they are superior to the conventional eye drop; however, there have been some promising results. Using a radiotracer technique, the ocular disposition of nanoparticles following topical instillation to the rabbit eye was investigated by Wood et al.[14] It was found that although nanoparticles composed of poly-hexyl-2-cyanoacrylate

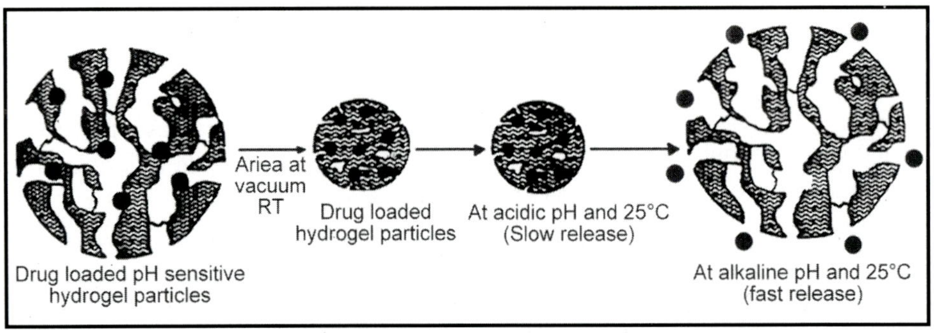

Figure 42.2:

were rapidly cleared from the precorneal site, approximately 1 percent of the instilled dose was able to adhere to corneal and conjunctival surfaces.

The elimination of ^{111}In-labeled nanoparticles from tear fluid was compared to liposomes and control solutions by gamma-ray scintigraphy.[15] All three preparations were cleared from the cornea much faster than from the inner canthus. Clearance half-life of the solution from the cornea and inner canthus were 1.3 and 5 min, respectively. Positively charged liposomes displayed the longest corneal half-life at 3.7 min, while nanoparticles had the longest inner canthal half-life at 17.3 min and an intermediate value of 2.2 min in the cornea. In comparison, radiotracer technique indicated that polyalkylcyanoacrylate nanoparticles had a half-life in tears of about 20 min.[14] The residence time of these same nanoparticles in inflamed eye tissues was about 4 times higher than that observed in healthy tissues.[16]

The main objective of employing nanoparticles as a carrier for ophthalmic drug delivery is to provide sustained drug release and prolonged therapeutic activity. Using pilocarpine as a model drug, Harmia et al[17] were able to demonstrate prolonged miosis in rabbits following topical administration of drug adsorbed to polybutylcyanoacrylate nanoparticles. A commercial pilocarpine solution was used as a control. Interestingly, when pilocarpine was incorporated into nanoparticle matrix, no significant prolongation of the miotic was observed. It was suggested that an insufficient amount of drug was released from the nanoparticles prior to their removal from the precorneal site; thus, there was also a limited quantity of drug available for absorption. Conversely, when drug was adsorbed to the surface of the nanoparticles, drug release did not restrict the amount of drug available for absorption and may have facilitated a direct interaction with epithelial surfaces of tissues in the precorneal site. In another study, the use of polyalkylcyanoacrylate nanoparticles prolonged the intraocular pressure-reducing effect of pilocarpine for more than 9 h in a rabbit model.[18]

Ocular Distribution of Nanoparticles

The fate of nanoparticles in the body depends on the physicochemical properties of the nanoparticles.[19] Properties such as pH, surfactant, and stabilizers influence the mucoadhesion properties to the ocular membrane and thereby modify the precorneal retention of the nanoparticles. It has been shown that the molecular weight of the polymer influences the residence time of nanoparticles in the precorneal area.[20] As the molecular weight increases, the polymer becomes poorly retained, whereas low molecular weight polymers are retained for a longer time. Experimental data on the disposition of polyhexylcyanoacrylate nanoparticles in tears, the aqueous humor, cornea, and conjunctiva of albino rabbits clearly showed adhesion of nanoparticles to absorbing tissue.[21]

Drug Used in Particulate Ocular Delivery

A polybutylcyanoacrylate nanoparticle delivery system for pilocarpine nitrate has been evaluated in comparison to the solution of the drug for pharmacokinetic and pharmacodynamic aspects.[22] Emulsion polymerization technique was employed in preparing nanoparticles, and *in vivo* experiments were performed by application of the formulations to the eyes of New Zealand white rabbits pretreated with betamethasone to create an elevated intraocular pressure mimicking glaucoma conditions. The results indicated an increase of 23 percent in pilocarpine levels in aqueous humor and prolonged t½ for the polybutylcyanoacrylate nanoparticle preparation compared to the aqueous control solution. It was possible to prolong the miosis with nanoparticles with lower drug content compared to the control solution. Betaxolol[23] and amikacin sulfate[24] loaded polyalkylcyanoacrylate nanoparticles have shown similar effects. The superficial charge and binding type of the drug onto the nanoparticles are important factors playing a role in the improvement of the therapeutic response. In another study, adsorption of pilocarpine onto polybutylcyanoacrylate nanoparticles enhanced the miotic response by about 22 percent compared to the control aqueous drug solution.[25]

In a clinical study with Piloplex® (latex emulsion of pilocarpine hydrochloride) a lower level of the drug with less fluctuation compared to the corresponding control solution was observed on the third day of treatment. This study involving nine subjects showed a reduction by

5.25 mm Hg of the average diurnal intraocular pressure value compared to the control. Only one out of 30 patients complained of a local sensitivity reaction with Piloplex in the yearlong.[26] Similar results were obtained in yet another study involving 50 patients, where 67.6 percent of the eyes treated with the formulation were under control, while only 45.2 percent were under control with the pilocrpine solution.[27]

Nanoparticles appear to offer several advantages in the area of ophthalmic drug delivery. Particularly attractive are their bioadhesive properties which, if optimized, may overcome a major shortcoming of most ophthalmic products, i.e. inadequate retention time in the prcorneal site. Another important feature is the versatility of nanoparticles as a drug carrier. Many different types of compounds can be incorporated or adsorbed to nanoparticles, and depending on the composition, nanoparticles with different release characteristic can be designed. Furthermore, nanoparticles are easy to manufacture and form a stable, yet biodegradable product. Biodegradability suggests that nanoparticles will have low toxicity.

Although most of the investigations provided results that promised an advantage of the nanoparticle ophthalmic drug delivery, there is a need for further studies to elucidate the pharmacodynamic and pharmacokinetic fate of nanoparticle ophthalmic products, the safety of long-term use of this new type of ophthalmic dosage form, and also the aspects of the industrial product development.

ETHICS

The ethical debate has seen extreme and opposite positions being adopted. Optimists visualize the best case scenarios, possibly utopian, whereas others present all manner of apocalyptic visions. Many of these are based on incomplete, simplified and outdated visions of a nanotechnology. Therefore, updated information must be made available for an informed debate on ethics. A framework for such a debate has been suggested.[28]

POTENTIAL PROBLEMS

Problems could relate to biocompatibility, design constraints, and onboard computers malfunctions, and the human factor, a bit small. However, the most serious problems may devolve from the inherent complexity of a multitude of nanodevices independently trying to cooperatively work on a very complex biological task in a short timeframe. Moreover, there is always the possibility of the unexpected.

THE CHALLENGE AHEAD

No actual working nanorobot has yet been built. Development in these disciplines has proved to be more difficult than expected. The field of nanomedicine is rapidly evolving, and it is necessary to verify realistically how such high technologies may support medicine. The biggest benefit to be gained for human society from nanomedicine is the elimination of all common diseases, medical pain and suffering, and allow for the extension of human capabilities, most especially our mental faculties. Issues of ownership, regulation, ethics, and others will have to be continually addressed as new information becomes available.

REFERENCES

1. Gao YT, Shi SQ, Pan HW. [Possibility of applying nanotechnology to research on the basic theory of traditional Chinese medicine.] Zhong Xi Yi Jie He Xue Bao 2005;3(6):426-28. [Article in Chinese]
2. Gothelf KV, Labean TH. DNA-programmed assembly of nanostructures. Org Biomol Chem 2005;21;3(22):4023-37.
3. Tan W, Wang K, He X, Zhao XJ, Drake T, Wang L, Bagwe RP.Bionanotechnology based on silica nanoparticles. Med Res Rev 2004;24(5):621-38.
4. Bianco A, Kostarelos K, Prato M. Applications of carbon nanotubes in drug delivery. Curr Opin Chem Biol 2005.
5. Jain KK.The role of nanobiotechnology in drug discovery. Drug Discov Today 2005;10(21):1435-42.
6. Labhasetwar V. Nanotechnology for drug and gene therapy: the importance of understanding molecular mechanisms of delivery. Curr Opin Biotechnol 2005;28.
7. Chu TC, He Q, Potter DE. Biodegradable calcium phosphate nanoparticles as a new vehicle for delivery of a potential ocular hypotensive agent. J Ocul Pharmacol Ther 2002; 18(6):507-14.
8. Vandervoort J, Ludwig A. Preparation and evaluation of drug-loaded gelatin nanoparticles for topical ophthalmic use. Eur J Pharm Biopharm 2004 ;57(2):251-61.
9. Pignatello R, Bucolo C, Ferrara P, Maltese A, Puleo A, Puglisi G. Eudragit RS100 nanosuspensions for the ophthalmic controlled delivery of ibuprofen. Eur J Pharm Sci 2002; 16(1-2):53-61.

10. Pignatello R, Bucolo C, Spedalieri G, Maltese A, Puglisi G. Flurbiprofen-loaded acrylate polymer nanosuspensions for ophthalmic application. Biomaterials 2002;23(15):3148-55.
11. Pignatello R, Bucolo C, Spedalieri G, Maltese A, Puglisi G. Flurbiprofen-loaded acrylate polymer nanosuspensions for ophthalmic application. Biomaterials 2002;23(15):3247-55.
12. Merodio M, Espuelas MS, Mirshahi M, Arnedo A, Irache JM. Efficacy of ganciclovir-loaded nanoparticles in human cytomegalovirus (HCMV)-infected cells. J Drug Target 2002; 10(3):231-38.
13. Merodio M, Irache JM, Valamanesh F, Mirshahi M. Ocular disposition and tolerance of ganciclovir-loaded albumin nanoparticles after intravitreal injection in rats. Biomaterials 2002;23(7):1587-94.
14. Wood RW, Li VHK, Kreuter J, Robinson JR. Ocular disposition of polyhexyl-2-cyano[3-^{14}C] acrylate nanoparticles in the albino rabbit. Int J Pharm 1985;23:175.
15. Kreuter J. Nanoparticles and liposomes in ophthalmic drug delivery, in Ophthalmic Drug Delivery. Biopharmaceutical, Technological and Clinical Aspects, Saettone MS, Bucci G, Speiser P (Eds): Liviana Press, Padua, Italy, 1987;101.
16. Diepold R, Kreuter J, Guggenbuhl P, Robinson JR. Distribution of polyhexyl-2-cyano-[3-^{14}C] acrylate nanoparticles in healthy and chronically inflamed rabbits eyes. Int J Pharm 1989;54:149.
17. Harmia T, Kreuter J, Speiser P, Boye T, Gurny R, Kubis A. Enhancement of myotic response of rabbits with pilocarpine-loaded polybutylcyanoacrylate nanoparticles. Int J Pharm 1986;33:187.
18. Diepold R, Kreuter J, Himber J, Gurny R, Lee VHL, Robinson JR, et al. Comparison of different models for the testing of pilocarpine eyedrops using conventional eye drops and a novel depot formulation (nanoparticles), Albercht von Graefes Arch Klin Exp Ophthalmol 1989;227:188.
19. Davis SS, Illum L. The targeting of drugs using polymeric microspheres. Br Polym J 1983;15:160.
20. Das SK, Tucker IG, Davies NM. A gamma scintigraphic evaluation of the effect of molecular weight of poly(isobutyl cyanoacrylate) Nanoparticles on the precorneal residence in rabbit. Proc Int Symp Control Rel Matter Controlled Release Society, Inc 1992;19:395.
21. Vezin W, Florence A. *In vitro* degradation rates of biodegradable poly-N-alkylcyanoacrylates. J Pharm Pharmacol 1978;30:5P.
22. Zimmer A, Mutschler E, Lambrecht G, Mayer D, Kreuter J. Pharmacokinetic and pharmacodynamic aspects of an ophthalmic pilocarpine nanoparticle-delivery system. Pharm Res 1994;11:1435.
23. Marchal-Heussler L, Maincent P, Hoffman H, Spittler J, Couvreur P. Antiglaucomatous activity of betaxolol chlorhydrate sorbed onto different isobutyl cyanoacrylate nanoparticles preparations. Int J Pharm 1990;58:115.
24. Losa C, Valvo P, Castro E, Vila-Jato JL, Alonso MJ. Improvement of ocular penetration of amikacin sulphate by association to poly(butyl cyanoacrylate) nanoparticles. J Pharm Pharmacol 1991;43:548.
25. Harima T, Kreuter J, Speiser P, Boye T, Gurny R, Kubis A. Enhancement of miotic response of rabbits with pilocarpine-loaded polybutylcyanoacrylate nanoparticles. Int J Pharm 1986;33:187.
26. Ticho U, Blumenthal M, Zonis S, Gal A, Blank I, Mazor ZW. Piloplex, a new long-acting pilocarpine polymer salt. A long-term study. Br J Ophthalmol 1979;63:48.
27. Ticho U, Blumenthal M, Zonis S, Gal A, Blank I, Mazor ZW. A clinical trial with Piloplex-a new long-acting pilocarpine compound: Preliminary report. Ann Ophthalmol 1979;11:555.
28. Gordijn B. Nanoethics: From Utopian Dreams and Apocalyptic Nightmares towards a more Balanced View. Sci Eng Ethics 2005;11(4):521-33.

43

Glaucoma Surgery Techniques with the Fugo Blade®

- FUGO BLADE®
- THE IMPORTANCE OF CONJUNCTIVAL LYMPHATICS IN GLAUCOMA SURGERY
- GLAUCOMA SURGERY TECHNIQUES WITH THE FUGO BLADE®

Daljit Singh (India), Richard J Fugo (USA)

INTRODUCTION

The glaucoma filtration surgery technique has remained nearly static during the past century, mainly for the reason that the surgical tools have remained more or less the same.[1] The instruments have become smaller and finer, as well as the operating microscope has become a standard aid for improved magnification. Nonetheless, the only palpable 'revolution' has been the making of a scleral flap. The introduction of mitomycin has improved certain case results, but it has also added many new serious complications. In spite of the availability of antibiotics, steroids, and non-steroidal anti-inflammatory medication, there has been no real breakthrough. Results remain unpredictable and there are too many serious side effects, often related to immediate collapse of the anterior chamber. For these reasons, most anterior segment surgeons avoid glaucoma filtration surgery.[2] In this scenario, the arrival of a new ablative surgical tool in the form of the Fugo Plasma Blade has brought about a fundamental change in the approach to filtration surgery. This new approach could only happen thanks to the unique ability of Fugo Plasma Blade to ablate the surface of the sclera with a hair thin plasma cloud. The Fugo Blade can ablate permanent tracks through tissues such as cornea, sclera and ciliary body in a resistance free fashion. And, the plasma ablation of tissue occurs without any clinically significant collateral damage or postoperative reaction to the incision wall.

FUGO BLADE®

The Fugo Blade® is a unique cutting instrument, which employs plasma, the 4th state of matter, for ablating incision paths in tissue in a manner similar to the eximer laser and is the only electrosurgical device approved for intraocular use by the food and drug administration (FDA) in the USA.[3]

The Fugo Blade is also known as the Plasma Blade in many other parts of the world, since it ablates with plasma energy.[4] It consists of a console, a handpiece with a disposable tip and an activation footswitch (Figure 43.1). Four rechargeable "C" cell flashlight size batteries provide the energy. The power generated is about 1watt for little energy is needed to energize the cutting tip, thereby, one charge of the batteries lasts for about an hour of cutting time. The plasma is visible under high magnification, looking like bees on a honey cone or a miniature fluorescent light bulb. This plasma ablates in such a fashion that it creates a smooth wall along the ablation/incision path. The secret is that the electromagnetic waves are brought to a sharp focus by the electronics in the console and in the handle, onto the tip of the blunt incising filament which has the thickness of a human hair[5] The electromagnetic oscillations knock electrons from their orbits in the atoms of the tissue. Thus plasma, the fourth state of matter, consisting of charged atoms and electrons is produced. This plasma cloud at the activated tip-tissue junction becomes visible to the naked eye. Surgeons such as Prof. Randal Olson (Utah, USA), Prof. Ike Ahmed (Toronto, Canada) and Dr I Howard Fine (Washington State, USA) have all emphatically stated that this device has nothing to do with classic electrosurgery or diathermy.

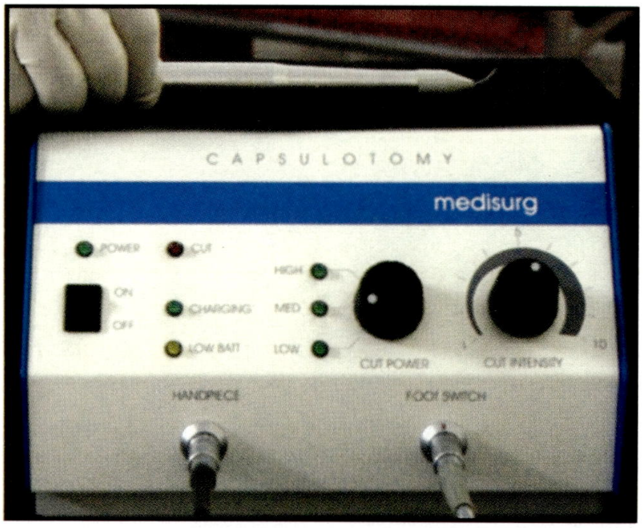

Figure 43.1: The Fugo Blade® console and the handpiece with attached disposable tip. There is an outlet for the handpiece and one for the foot-switch. There are controls to regulate the cutting power of the tip

Under a high power microscope, the plasma cloud is visible as a 25-50 microns wide pulsating yellow cloud on the hair thin, blunt activated tip (Figure 43.2).[6] Around the plasma cloud, there is reddish much wider photon cloud. The cutting power resides in the inner thin

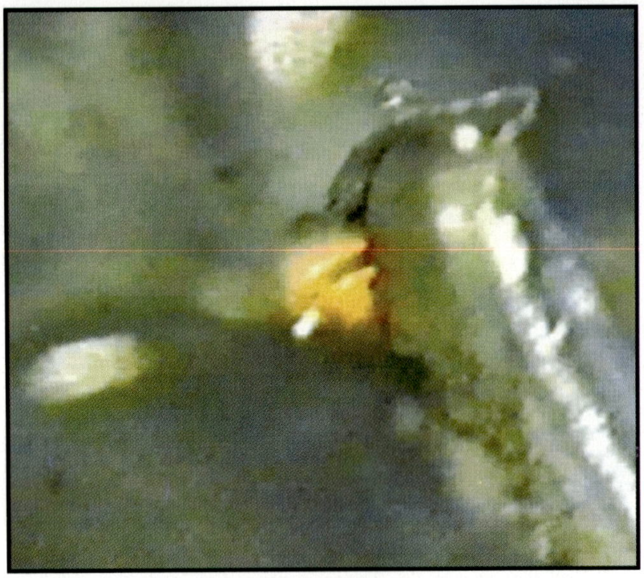

Figure 43.2: The cutting power resides in the thin, inner yellow looking plasma cloud surrounding the activated filament of Fugo Blade® tip. The much wider, outer non-cutting photon cloud looks orange

plasma cloud. The plasma sustains itself as long as the electromagnetic oscillations from the activated tip keep interacting with the tissue, which is ablated in the truest sense.[7] The plasma cloud oscillations instantly shatter the macromolecules of the tissue into small fragments. The micro-molecular fragments thus produced mix with water vapor and are discharged at great speed as a plume; just as is seen with the eximer laser.[8] During extraocular procedures such as touching a bleeding area, the molecular oscillation throws the particles millimeters away. This produces a process called "Autostasis" wherein these small particles plug the top of small vessels thereby producing a non-cauterizing hemostasis. Histologic sections show that cautery produces charred, blistered wound margins whereas the Fugo Blade wound margins have been shown to be pristine clean, thereby reducing swelling, redness, pain and scarring.[9] The plasma energy at the tip is at a very high energy density, while possessing very low total energy since the plasma cloud has a very small volume. However, the energy field does not extend beyond 25 microns from the plasma, meaning that little or no heat is generated in tissue outside of the incision. Therefore, the Fugo Blade does not burn or cauterize. This has been demonstrated by ablating through visible conjunctival or muscle vessels, as well as the creation of bloodless pupiloplasties in seconds.[10] The Fugo Blade® possesses this important function of non-cauterizing during incision of cut tissue. It does this in two ways-firstly by the ablation of the vessels in the cutting path and secondly by the particle oscillation, which tends to plug the small bleeding vessels. Finally, it should be made clear that the Fugo Blade® is completely different from a diathermy unit. The Fugo Blade® uses minute amounts of energy yet cuts sharper than a diamond blade whereas diathermy uses large amounts of energy but cuts poorly and damages the wall of the incision path, as seen on histologic sections.[11]

THE IMPORTANCE OF CONJUNCTIVAL LYMPHATICS IN GLAUCOMA SURGERY

Conjunctival lymphatics are generally ignored in discussions of ocular fluid dynamics.[12] However, if we visualize the extremely well knit lymphatic network under the conjunctiva, we soon realize that it has a role in fluid drainage in normal and operated eyes. Normally, over 30 percent of the aqueous humor filters out of the eye through uveoscleral outflow. There is an additional leakage from the anterior chamber through the aqueous veins. All this interstitial fluid has a substantial chance of being trapped by the lymphatics and then drained away from the eye. Post-surgical drainage is nothing short of managing a flood of aqueous – the lymphatics act as flood drains.[13]

The lymphatics and the Pallisades of Vogt are frequently visible under slit-lamp microscope as transparent channels and columns running parallel to the limbus (Figure 43.3).[14] However, the most spectacular view is seen in some patients who have pigmentation around the limbus. The pigment outlines the finest lymphatic channels at the limbus as well as the Pallisades of Vogt., (Figure 43.4).[15]

Once it is realized that the lymphatics have a role in the drainage of the aqueous, the surgeons will then begin to understand the importance of doing minimal dissection, minimal cautery and minimal use of mitomycin C. The greater the trauma and destruction to the lymphatics, the greater the chance of scar and tenon cyst formation

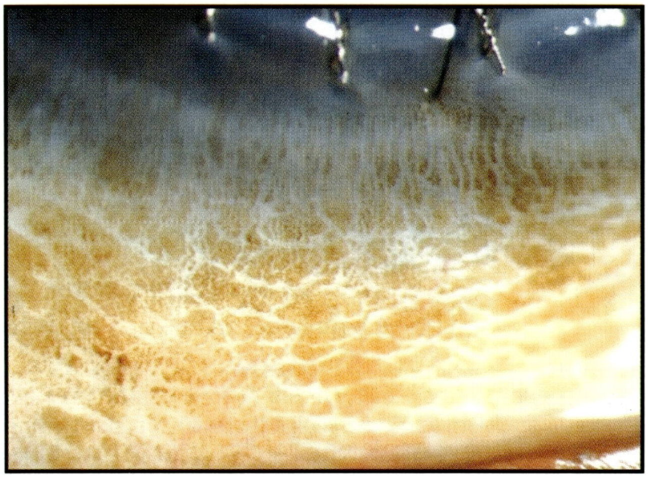

Figure 43.3: It shows beautifully outlined small and large lymphatic vessels as well as the Pallisades of Vogt. The channels on the limbus are vertically placed. Beyond the limbus they form a dense network with the larger vessels having a general direction parallel to the limbus

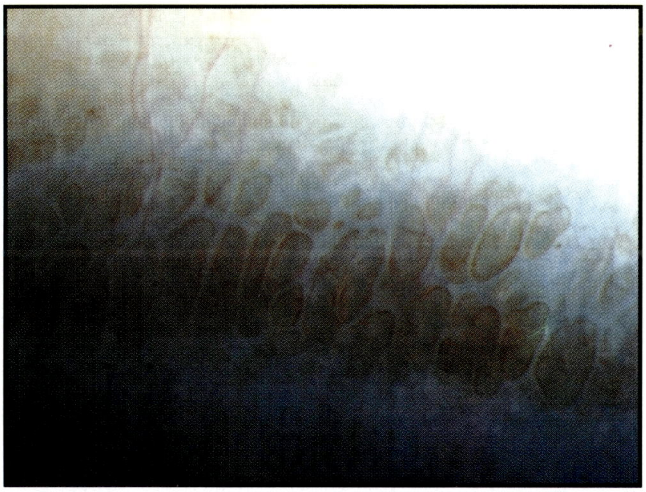

Figure 43.4: This shows beautifully outlined lymphatics at the limbus. There is pigment around the lymphatics and the Pallisades of Vogt

with subsequent decrease of aqueous flow from the subconjunctival space and back into the vascular tree.[16]

GLAUCOMA SURGERY TECHNIQUES WITH THE FUGO BLADE®

Four different techniques of glaucoma surgery have been developed and practiced. They are:

1. Transciliary filtration (TCF).
2. Transconjunctival transciliary filtration (TC-TCF).
3. Microtrack filtration (MTF).
4. Non-perforating filtration (NPF).

Transciliary Filtration (Singh Filtration)[17]

The technique of surgery is as follows:

1. The conjunctiva is detached from the limbus for about 6-7 mm and it is retracted away from the limbus.
2. The Tenon capsule from the exposed sclera is excised with scissors.
3. The bleeding spots on the sclera are closed with the lowest energy of the Fugo Blade. A 600 microns tip is used for this purpose.
4. A scleral ablation point behind the surgical limbus is chosen for TCF. There is a variation dependent upon ocular type from high myopia to high hyperopia. The experienced TCF surgeon can easily identify the correct spot for scleral ablation, whereas the novice TCF surgeon can quickly and easily identify the location of the iris root employing anterior chamber transillumination. Instructional tapes on this are available from Medisurg, Ltd, USA (Tel 610-277-3937).[18]
5. The 600 microns tip is chosen to ablate the sclera at the chosen point. A scleral pit is formed (Figure 43.5).The energy at medium settings is applied in

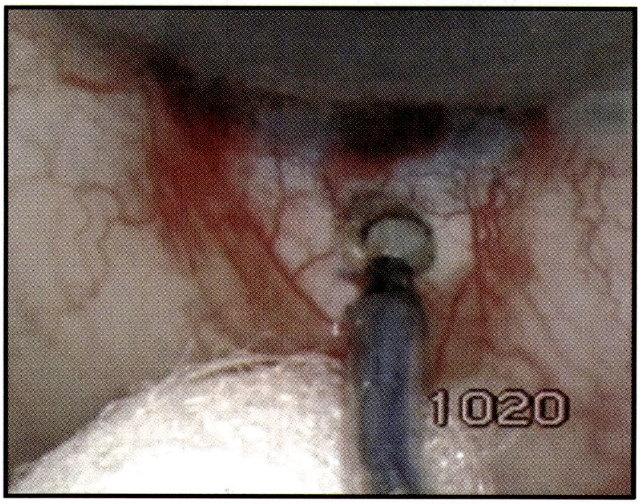

Figure 43.5: The conjunctiva has been detached from the limbus.A pit is getting formed on the sclera, about 1 mm behind the surgical limbus, with the help of activated 600 microns tip of Fugo Blade

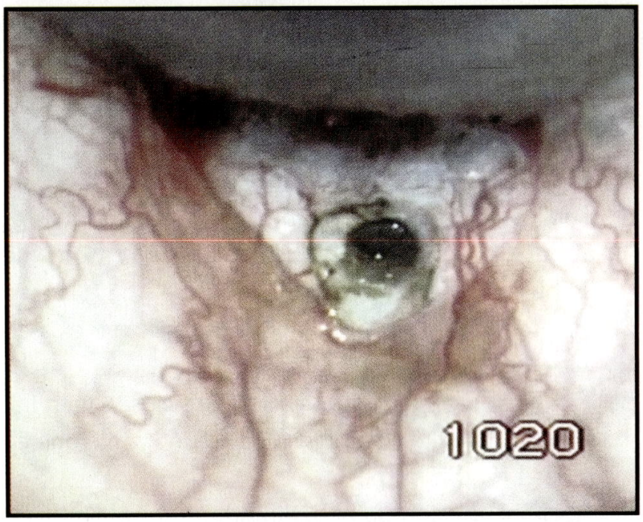

Figure 43.6: The scleral pit has reached to the depth of the anterior part of the ciliary body.The edge of the scleral pit has been beveled with Fugo Blade. Any part of the sclera that is merely touched by activated Fugo Blade, it just disappears

small steps, until the ciliary body is visible. The edges of the pit are beveled especially at the proximal edge (Figure 43.6).

6. There is a choice of a 100 microns or a 300 microns tip for the next step, which is the next step of the creation of a track through the ciliary body into the posterior chamber (Figure 43.7). The tip is directed behind the iris root, through the anterior part of the pars plicata. The tissue is touched a couple of times

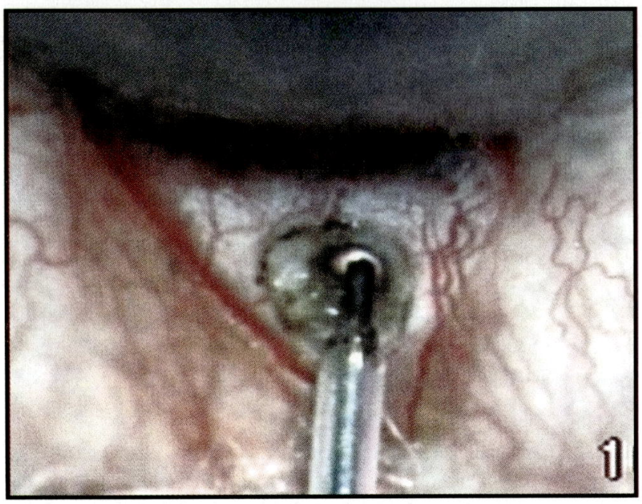

Figure 43.7: A 300 microns activated Fugo Blade tip is in the process of going through the most anterior part of the ciliary body.The plasma energy is visible to the naked eye

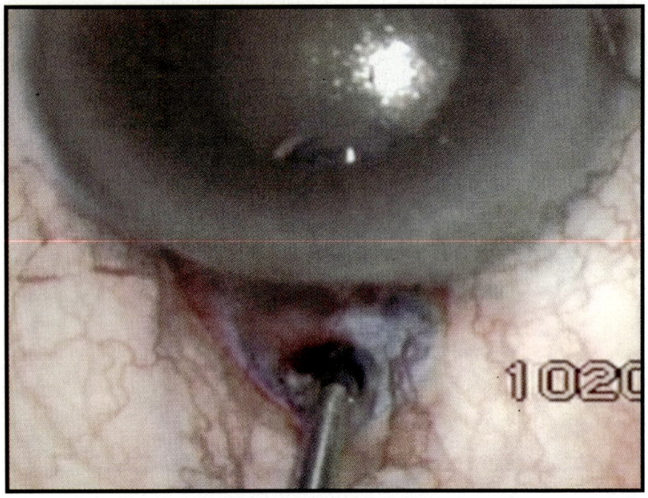

Figure 43.8: Injection of air in the filtering track shows the air bubble is appearing in the papillary area, from under the iris, confirming that the track is through the ciliary body

with the activated Fugo Blade tip until suddenly there is a rush of posterior chamber fluid along with small particles of ciliary body epithelium. The track formation is over in several seconds.

7. For demonstration purpose, air may be injected through the track with a 22-gauge cannula. The air appears in the anterior chamber from under the iris (Figure 43.8). The posterior chamber may be irrigated in a similar fashion to wash out any pigment or blood. A drop of trypan blue placed on the track is washed away by outflow of aqueous.
8. Finally, the conjunctiva is lifted back to the limbus and sutured with one or more sutures (Figure 43.9).[19]

TCF is done without a scleral flap or under a scleral flap. Atwal has modified the technique such that he makes two tracks- one transciliary and another one is made into the anterior chamber from under the base of the scleral flap. He terms the procedure the "Atwal Balanced Approach" or "ABA".[20] As of this writing, Dr Atwal has performed over 100 ABA procedures with a maximum follow-up time of slightly more than 4 months and with only 3 failed filters but with not a single collaped anterior chamber. Mitomycin is normally not used in the TCF operation. However, it can be judiciously used in high risk cases before making the scleral pit, or inside the pit before making the track through the ciliary body. Recall that this must only be performed with minimal exposure of the tissue to the mitomycin.

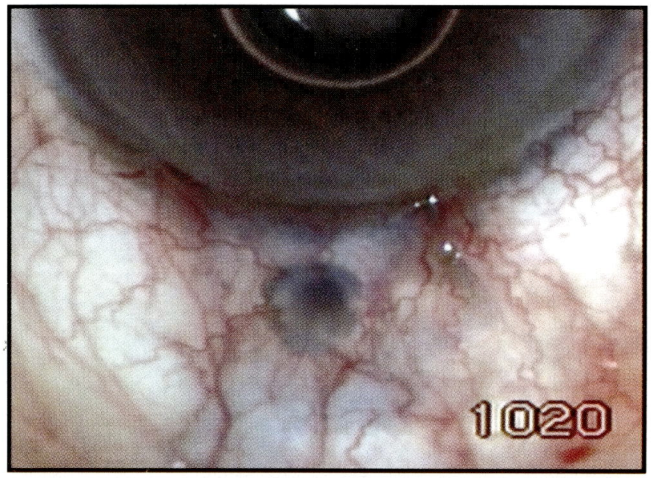

Figure 43.9: The conjunctiva has been sutured back to the limbus with 30 microns stainless steel suture

TCF is suitable for phakic eyes and pseudophakic eyes with an intact posterior capsule. Surgical errors are possible and manageable. A posteriorly directed perforating tip can disturb vitreous, which then may plug the TCF pore and therefore does not allow the aqueous to flow out. Repeating the ablation in an in and out movement of the activated Fugo Blade ablation probe into the area of vitreous causes plasma ablation of vitreous strands and thereby may open up ablation pits clogged with errant vitreous strands. If the surgeon wishes to reverse the TCF, the sclera may be closed at the site of the error with a suture. Then another site may be selected for a TCF track. The scleral pit may bleed excessively if the patient has a coagulation deficiency. This can occur with standard anticoagulation medication or with natural herbs or food such as high intake of fish, flax seed, ginsing balboa, vitamin E, etc. Make sure that there is no bleeding before proceeding to the next step of making a track through the ciliary body. In case there is any doubt, this site is abandoned and another close by site is chosen for restarting the procedure. Recall that the scleral pit takes seconds to create. Sometimes misdirection of the operating tip opens the track into the anterior chamber. Agitation of aqueous in the anterior chamber or formation of air bubbles in the anterior chamber is a diagnostic sign. In such a case, the anterior chamber is filled with air and another track is made somewhat posteriorly through the ciliary body into the posterior chamber—it becomes the Atwal procedure in reverse. It is imperative to make the posterior chamber ablation pit since this decompression of the posterior chamber all but eliminates flat anterior chambers postoperative, even with an eye pressure of 2-3 mm Hg.[21]

Postoperative management of the Fugo Blade procedures is much easier and more pleasant for both patient and physician than it is with trabeculectomy. There is practically never a flattening of the anterior chamber. Any bleeding into the anterior chamber is either from the angle or from the posterior chamber. It is uncommon. The blood is absorbed very slowly, since the greater fluid flow is through the posterior chamber. Choroidal detachment is comparable to that of trabeculectomy and is usually self absorbing.

Failure of the procedure is possible. In the first few days, the filtration track or the scleral pit may be closed by a blood clot. Another cause could be 'posterior iris bombe' which closes the internal opening. The track may be reopened after waiting for 2-3 days. The conjunctiva is detached from the limbus and then sutured back after the corrective procedure. Late failure can occur due to the formation of scar tissue or the formation of Tenon cyst. These are relatively easy to diagnose. The condition is treated by reopening the operation site and removing the scar tissue. The filtration track is usually found functional underneath the scar or the cyst. Mitomycin may be used with discretion and pinpoint application.

A primary success rate of over 80 percent is expected in cases of primary glaucoma. Furthermore, TCF is a filtering procedure that most anterior surgeons can perform rapidly and with a small amount of tissue manipulation. Importantly, postoperative chair time is minimized because flat anterior chambers are rarely seen, even with eye pressures of 2-3 mm Hg.[22] Cases of angle closure glaucoma achieve chamber deepening with the procedure. The use of mitomycin increases the success rate in these cases, but it also seems to increase the rate of avascular bleb formation.

The procedure of TCF reduces surgery time, decreases tissue trauma and decreases the number and severity of early and late postoperative complications. Reoperation at the old site or an adjoining site is easy and without excessive trauma to tissues.[23]

The learning curve is low but there are techniques which must be mastered.[24] There is significant surgeon variation in preference to surgical approach, e.g. ABA versus pure TCF. For example, Dr Myron Wilson (Georgia, USA) and his associate Dr Johnny Gayton have performed over 30 pure TCF procedures (personal correspondence). They no longer employ anterior chamber transillumination and are now performing 3 TCF patients in a 15 minutes surgical block. They have had 2 failures in their group but note that re-ops are simple to perform. Most notably, they have stated that a large percentage of their TCF patients have the "most horrible pathology in our practice with no good option to treat" their glaucoma. Dr Herbert Kaufmann, Director of the LSU Eye Center, (USA) relayed a similar sentiment regarding his "worse eyes" glaucoma patients to one of the authors (RJF).

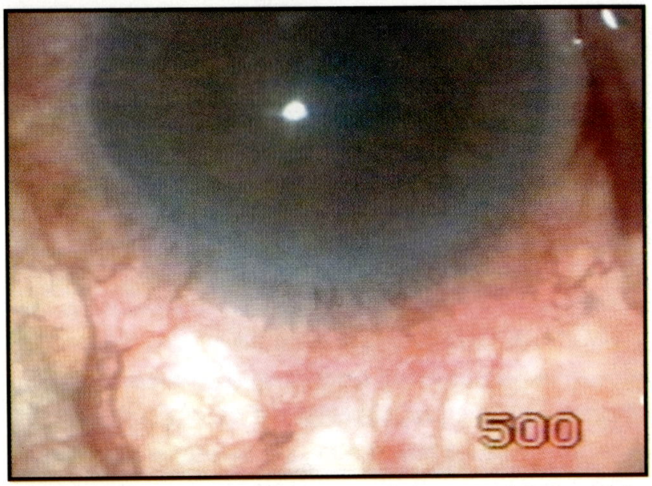

Figure 43.10: A case of malignant glaucoma, of three weeks duration, causing very severe constant pain and loss of eyesight. Notice the posterior edge of the surgical limbus visible under the conjunctiva.This edge is about 1 mm from the attachment of the conjunctiva to the cornea

Transconjunctival Transciliary Filtration (Singh TC-TCF)[25]

In this technique, the posterior chamber is connected to the subconjunctival space without any dissection. This technique comes in handy in a number of situations like malignant glaucoma, painful neovascular glaucoma, pseudophakic glaucoma with iris bombe, and phakomorphic glaucoma preliminary to cataract surgery with or without IOL implantation. It is also helpful in such glaucomatous eyes that have extensive scarring, so that it is difficult to dissect close to the limbus. The operation is done under full local or a short general anesthesia. The steps are as follows:

1. The most important landmark is the point of reflection of the conjunctiva from the cornea. The second landmark is the posterior edge of the bluish looking surgical limbus (Figure 43.10). The relationship between the first and the second landmarks should be clearly visualized. The scleral entry has to be about a mm posterior to the surgical limbus. Keep that point in sight. It should be away from any big vessel on the sclera. Nonetheless, anterior chamber transillumination is simple to perform and gives the new TCF surgeon a definite location for a scleral ablation pit.

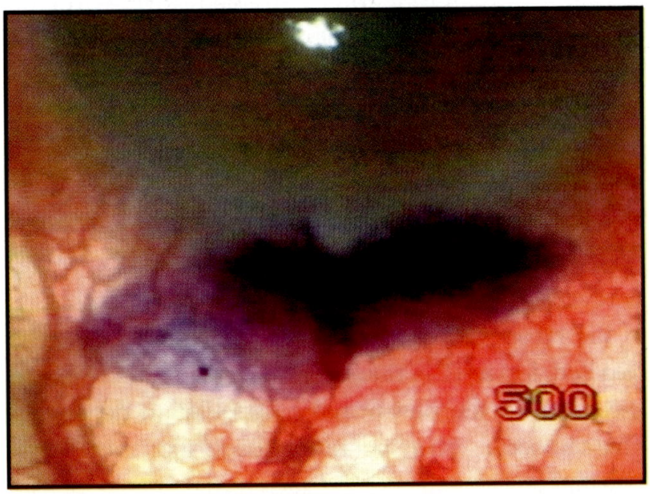

Figure 43.11: The conjunctiva in the region of the limbus is stained with gentian violet

2. Gentian violet is applied on the conjunctiva over the limbus (Figure 43.11). The conjunctiva is gripped with a forceps about 7-8 mm away from and parallel to the limbus. The conjunctiva is pulled down over the cornea. The attachment of the conjunctiva to the cornea becomes sharply visible as a blue line (Figure 43.12). At this point, we press down on the conjunctiva with the dull edge of a razor blade fragment, held in a blade holder, so that the conjunctiva shall not slide back.

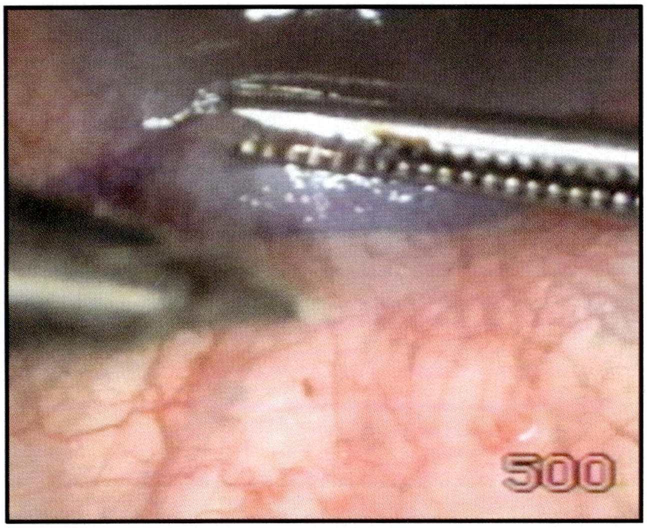

Figure 43.12: A conjunctival fold is pulled down with forceps, revealing the sharp edge of the conjunctival limbus.A blade holder with a blade fragment is ready to be placed at the sharp line

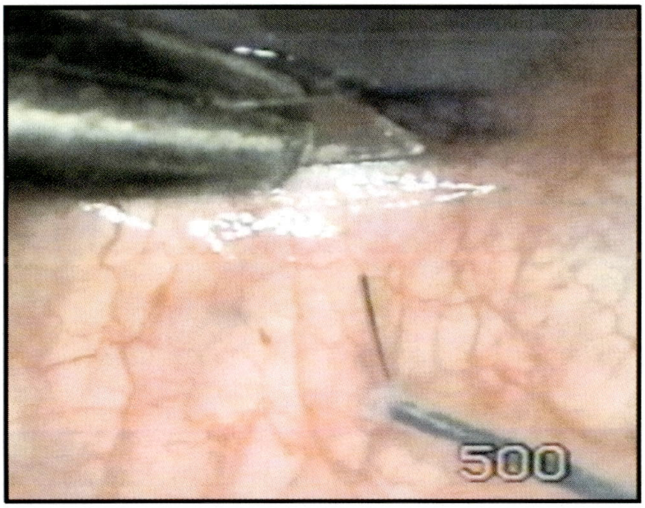

Figure 43.13: The conjunctiva is being restrained with the dull side of the razor fragment.The Fugo Blade tip 100 microns size is brought close to the conjunctiva, about 2 mm behind and aimed behind the iris towards the posterior chamber

3. A Fugo Blade tip of 100 microns or 300 microns is chosen according to the surgeon's choice. The tip is placed at the chosen pre-selected point and directed towards the plane just posterior to and parallel with the iris (Figure 43.13).[26]

   The tip is activated and made to ablate a track between the posterior chamber and the subconjunctival space (Figure 43.14). The system energy is turned off and the tip is withdrawn.

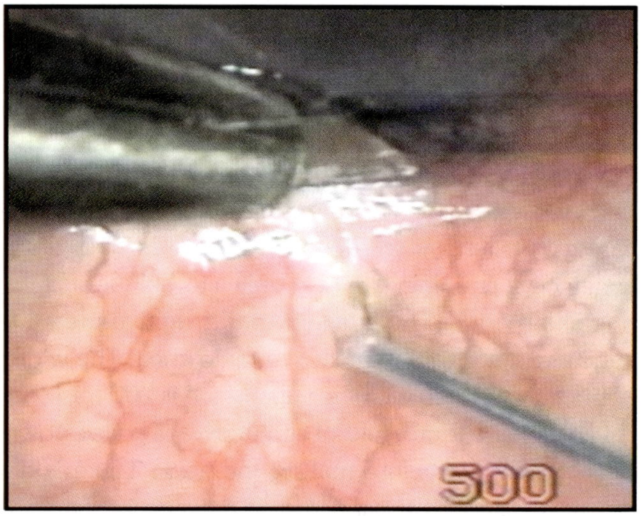

Figure 43.14: The activated 100 micron filament passes through the conjunctiva, sclera and ciliary body in a fraction of a second. The escaping fluid inactivates the filament.The filament is withdrawn immediately

   The completion of the track is signaled by the flow of fluid and sometimes uveal pigment.

4. The conjunctiva is allowed to fall back (Figures 43.15). The filtering fluid begins elevating the conjunctiva. The hole in the conjunctiva may be closed with a suture.

Microtrack Filtration (Singh MTF)[27]

This technique employs a transconjunctival approach using a 100 microns Fugo Blade filament to create a filtering track between the anterior chamber and the

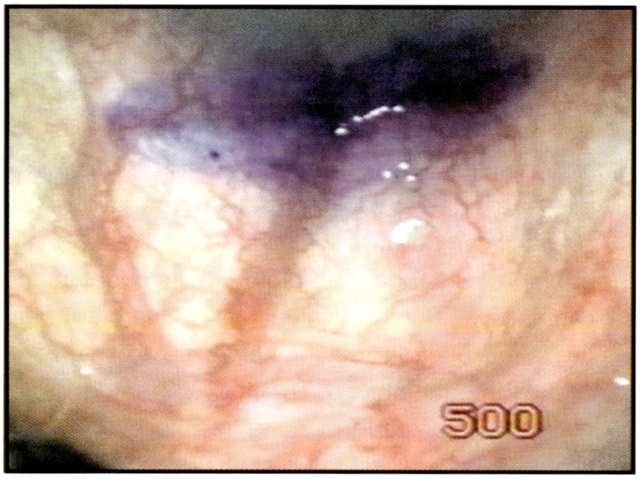

Figure 43.15: A filtering bleb starts getting raised, as the conjunctiva is allowed to fall back to its normal place

subconjunctival space. The objective is to have a minimally invasive procedure for a variety of glaucoma cases having normal or deep anterior chambers. It can deal with emergency situations such as traumatic and inflammatory glaucomas if the intraocular pressure is uncontrolled by medical means. Sometimes there is a case with extensive scarring with a small area of virgin conjunctiva remaining, therein only a technique such as this shall work. The track is made right under the attachment of the conjunctiva to the cornea. The width of the track created with the Fugo Blade is 200 microns. A very small 1-2 mm fold of conjunctiva is pulled down over the cornea before making the track. There is no involvement of the uveal tissues in the surgery. There is minimal disturbance of the reactive Tenon tissue. The fine microtrack is created with the hope that the iris shall not block the internal pore opening and scarring shall not occur over the external pore opening. The procedure is as follows:

The pupil is constricted prior to the operation.

The operation may be performed under topical anaesthesia, subconjunctival anesthesia or general anaesthesia. The important point is that the eye should not move during the fraction of a second that it takes to perform the actual operation.

1. Make a note of the attachment of the conjunctiva to the cornea. The track has to be made right under it without creating a buttonhole.
2. The conjunctiva has to be brought down not with a forceps but with a dull sapphire or ruby knife (Figure 43.16).The dull knife should be able to hold the conjunctiva down but not cut it. One can use a diamond knife with 0.6 mm or 1 mm tip. Even a sharp knife shall not cut the conjunctiva if it is not moved side to side and is not pressed to firmly. Why use such a sharp tool for bringing down the conjunctiva? Because we need a moderately sharp but poor electrical conductor to hold down the conjunctiva. The inactivated Fugo Blade Plasma tip has to touch this instrument before it is activated and pushed into the anterior chamber (Figure 43.17). A plastic tool may perform the same function but is not yet available. A metallic tool possesses a high electrical conductivity.

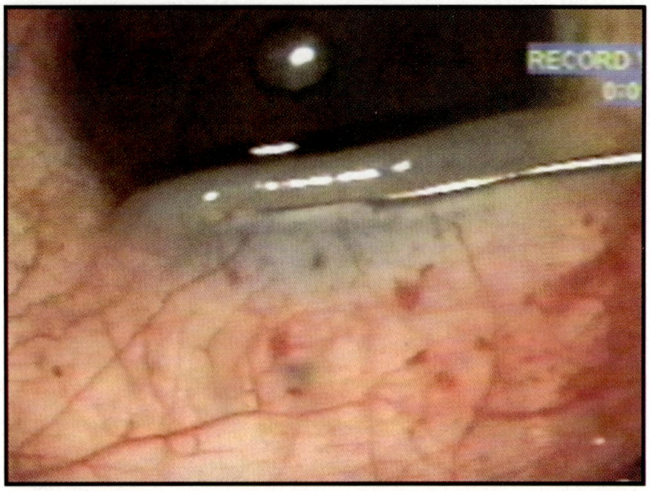

Figure 43.16: The conjunctiva is being pushed down to show the 'root' of the conjunctiva, where it is attached to the cornea.The microtrack in to the anterior chamber has to be made close the 'root'

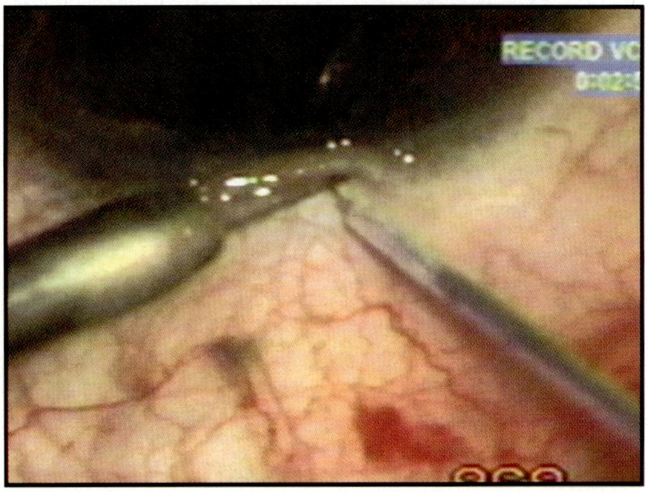

Figure 43.17: The conjunctival fold is held at the 'root' with the edge of a diamond knife, while the Fugo Blade is touch it in an inactivated state, poised and ready to move. The tip should be kept at the desired angle, before it is activated

The knife edge is placed lightly about 1 to 1.5 mm from the conjunctival limbus. It is used to press and push the conjunctival towards the cornea, until its further progress is stopped by the root of the conjunctiva. In other words, the conjunctival flap cannot be pulled further because of traction from its attachment at the lumbus.

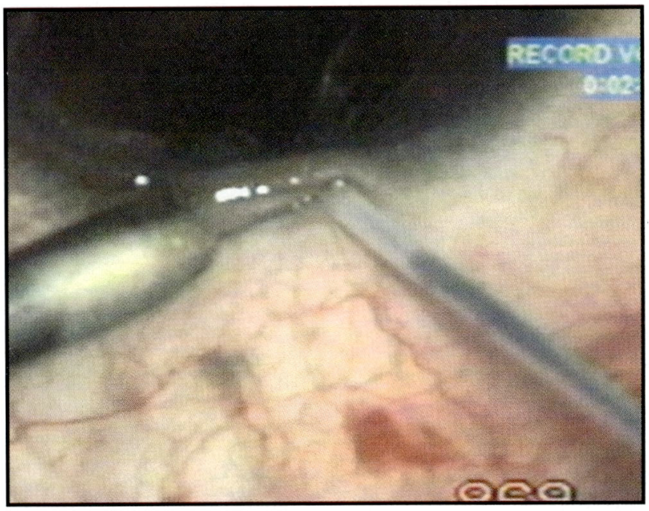

Figure 43.18: The moment the tip is activated, it enters the anterior chamber in a minute fraction of a second.It is withdrawn immediately. It is just an 'in and out' operation

3. The inactivated Fugo Blade tip is pressed against the conjunctiva retracting knife, then it is activated with the foot switch. With a smart jab, the activated Fugo Blade tip is pushed in then out of the anterior chamber (Figure 43.18). A track is instantly created in a resistance free fashion. A small air bubble may be injected if desired.

4. The conjunctival fold steadying knife is lifted and the conjunctiva is allowed to retract back to normal. The aqueous seepage through the track starts raising a bleb (Figure 43.19).
5. A bandage contact lens is put in place, to prevent excessive leakage (Figure 43.20). It is removed after 2 weeks.

Following creation of the MTF, the lymphatics are seen to fill at the limbus (Figure 43.21). The bandage contact lens slows down the movement of aqueous in order to inhibit excessive anterior chamber decompression with subsequent collapse of the anterior chamber. Soon the lymphatics become invisible due to bleb formation.

Postoperative management requires close attention. The pupil is kept constricted for at least one month when the fluid movement through the track becomes stabile, and there is no further tendency of the iris to block the internal opening. If the track becomes blocked with iris, the intraocular pressure will rapidly rise. On gonioscopy, the blocked internal opening of the Microtransciliary Filtration track shall be seen to be plugged with a fine wick of iris (Figure 43.22). This wick can be blown away with a single shot of YAG laser and the filtration will be restored (Figure 43.23). The idea of making the track under the most distal part of the conjunctiva is to minimize the chance of iris blockage as well as to minimize Tenon scarring. In case of failure, the procedure can be easily and quickly redone in an adjoining area. The procedure is not suitable as such for angle closure cases. An additional manual iridectomy is needed.

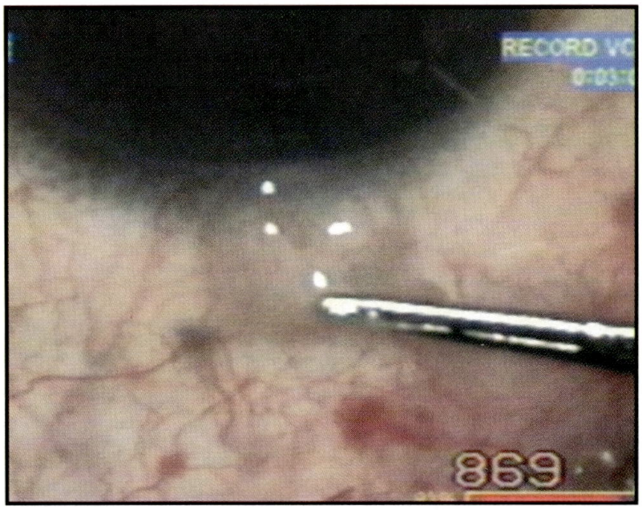

Figure 43.19: The conjunctival hole is held with a plane forceps for a few seconds

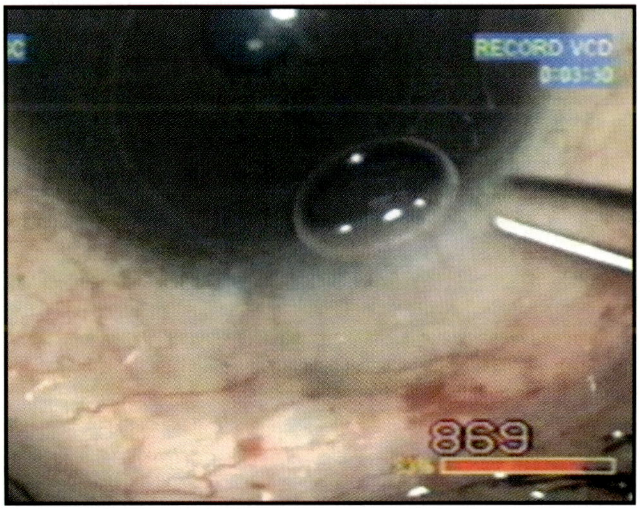

Figure 43.20: A bandage contact lens is placed to cover the filtration track

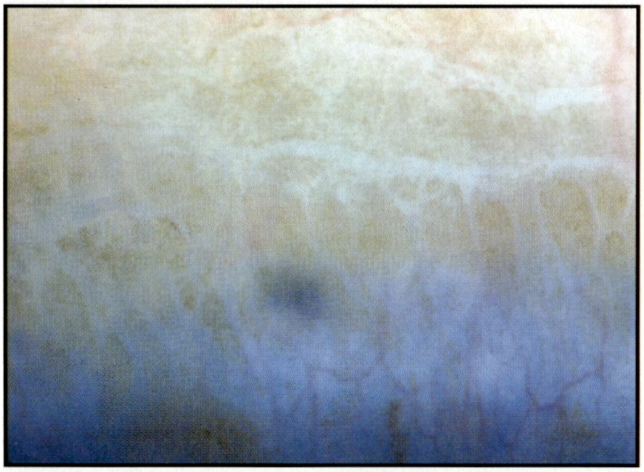

Figure 43.21: It shows MTF opening and filled up lymphatics at the limbus, 4 hours after operation.There is a bandage contact lens in place, which slows down the movement of aqueous and sometimes fills up the lymphatics. The presence of pigmentation at the limbus helps in the visualization of the lyphatics

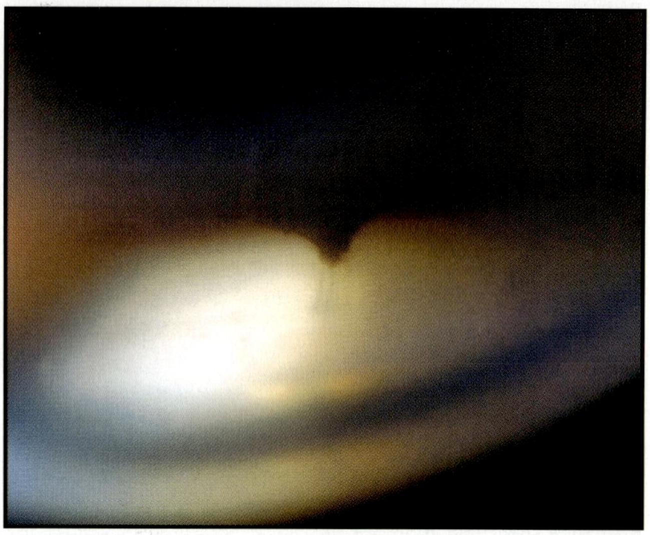

Figure 43.22: It shows the blockage of the internal opening of MTF with a small nipple of iris tissue,two days after the operation

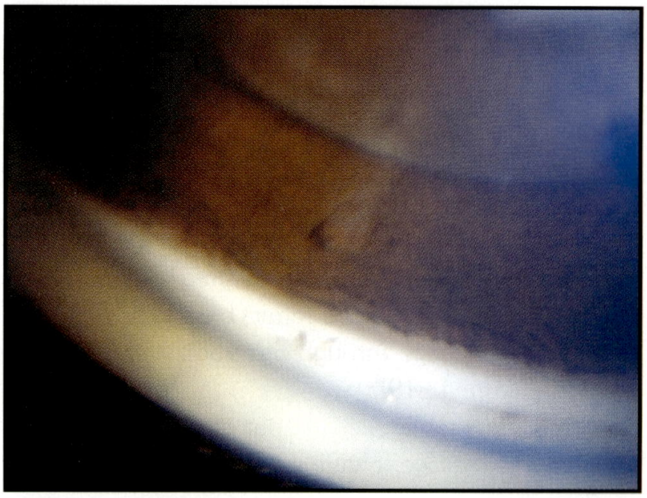

Figure 43.23: Same patient as above.The iris tissue blocking the internal opening has been blown away, which restored the filtration.Notice that the intrnal MTF opening is anterior to the cornea-scleral trabeculae. The more anterior the better

Since the procedure is minimally traumatic and completed in a minute or two, it has the possibility of becoming a frontline field tool to fight worldwide glaucoma. It is particularly suitable for very sick and uncooperative patients. A primary success rate of over 80 percent is achievable. MTF fills a void in the vast world, where millions go blind for lack of costly glaucoma medication and for lack of costly surgical care. Like all other filtration procedures, there is need for regular follow-up. Since we are decompressing the anterior chamber of the eye, the possibility of postoperative collapsed anterior chamber is a consideration.

Non-perforating Filtration (NPF)

Non-perforating filtration has been around for some years in the form of visco-canalostomy and deep sclerectomy with or without a collagen implant. The objective is to tap Schlemm's canal and not to open the anterior chamber. Both of these techniques require meticulous dissection under high magnification of the microscope. The techniques have not attracted many converts, mainly because they are considered more difficult to perform and the reported results have shown uneven success, compared to the "gold standard" trabeculectomy. The basic problem has been that surgeons must first perform a standard trabeculectomy type scleral flap, then proceed to perform a second scleral flap under the first flap. This second flap requires the surgeon to use a blade to bisect the thin scleral layer under the first scleral flap – truly a daunting surgical feat. This maneuver cannot be repeatedly performed by most surgeons. Dr

Ike Ahmed is performing a series of non-perforating glaucoma filtration procedures at the University of Toronto with the Fugo Blade. Dr Ahmed and his fellows now use the Fugo Blade to perform what they have coined "erasing tissue" from the scleral flap bed. They erase the scleral tissue until aqueous percolates through the thinned scleral window. This procedure requires less than a minute to perform and according to Dr Ahmed eliminates the last remaining hurdle for all ophthalmologists to perform the non-perforating glaucoma procedure (personal communication).

There are many ways to perform NPF with the Fugo Blade. They are:

a. Open non-perforating filtration.
b. NPF under a limbus based sclerocorneal flap.
c. NPF under a fornix based corneoscleral flap.

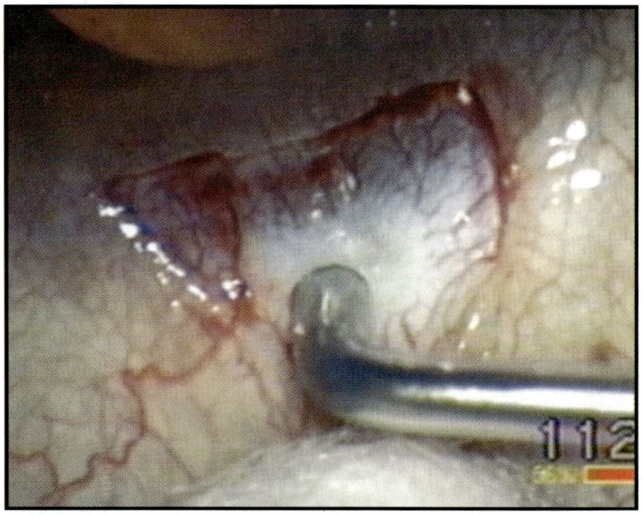

Figure 43.24: The conjunctiva has been detached from the limbus. The blood vessels in the area of surgery are being ablated with 600 microns tip of Fugo Blade

Open Non-perforating Filtration (Singh NPF)

The surgery is done under local anesthesia as described previously.

1. The conjunctiva is detached from the limbus for about 5 mm.
2. Any blood ooze is hemostased with a minimum energy setting of the Fugo Blade 600 micron tip (Figure 43. 24).
3. Any Tenon capsule in the exposed area is cut with forceps and scissors.
4. Fugo Blade Ablation of the limbal area to expose the canal of Schlemm. A 600 microns Fugo Blade tip is used to ablate the limbal area by moving the tip from the corneal to the scleral side. With every passage, the limbal pit becomes deeper (Figure 43.25). The pit is also widened in a sloping fashion to facilitate deeper ablation in the center. The ablation involves the tissues on either side of the surgical limbus. The surgical limbus overlies the anterior corneoscleral trabeculae. Thus, we would expect to find the canal of Schlemm just posterior to it. Thinning of the cornea anterior to the surgical limbus may help later on in producing a filtration pore with the YAG laser, in cases where enhancement of filtration is needed. The thinning of the limbal tissues by Fugo Blade ablation is continued at the lowest energy settings, until an aqueous ooze is observed. Once the ooze starts (Figure 43.26) ,the Fugo Blade tip becomes less effective at erasing tissue because the fluid causes a decrease in resonance of the ablation energy at the Fugo Blade tip and thereby damps the energy transfer into the scleral tissue.[28] Observe the oozing area for a minimum of one minute. The ooze may be highlighted by putting a drop of trypan blue (Figure 43.27), which is then washed away.
5. The conjunctiva is sutured back to the limbus (Figure 43.28). We use 30 microns steel suture or other minimally reactive suture.

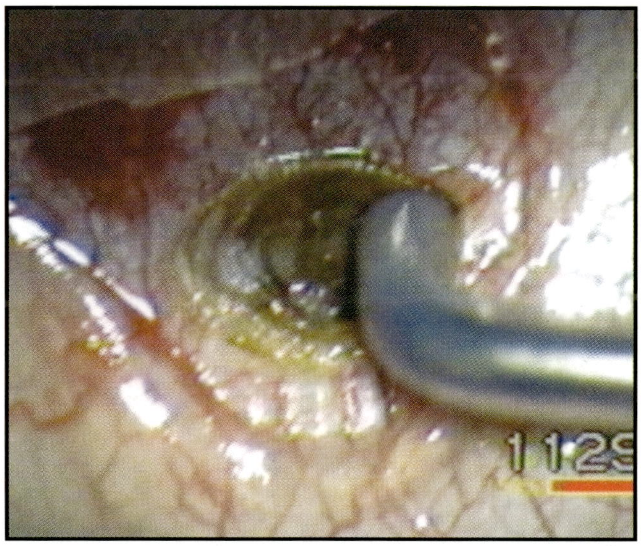

Figure 43.25: The scleral pit over the Schlemm canal is being deepened and widened with 600 microns tip of Fugo Blade

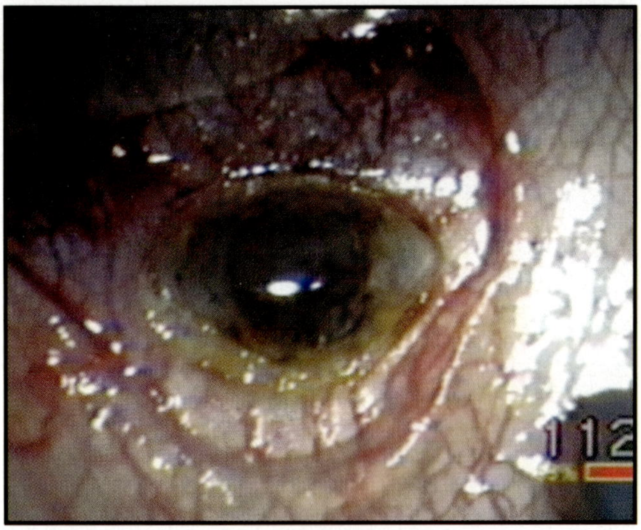

Figure 43.26: The ooze is evident in the scleral pit over Schlemm's canal

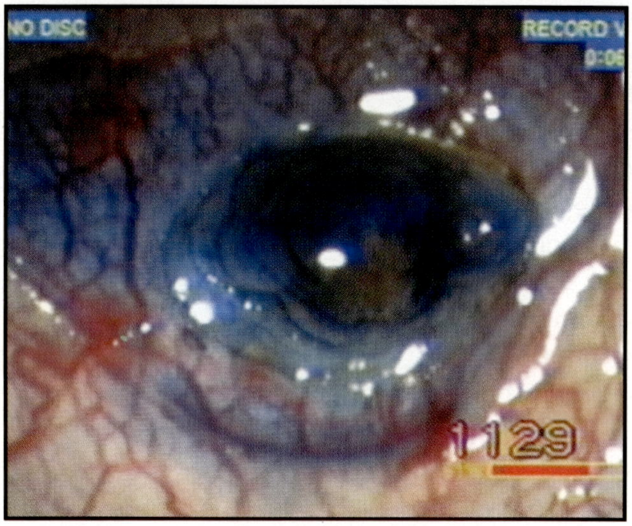

Figure 43.27: The oozing aqueous is washing away the trypan blue that was dropped on the scleral pit

There is scope for innovation in this technique. The filtration can be done with a 200 microns tip and without a wider limbal pit.

NPF Under a Limbus based Sclero-corneal Flap

The steps of operation are as follows.

1. The limbus is detached as usual and the scleral surface is cleared of Tenon capsule and bleeding points.
2. A triangular scleral flap about 1/3 mm thick and 2 mm wide is made with its base towards the limbus.
3. The flap is held with a forceps, while ablation of the limbal tissues is performed as before until aqueous begins to percolate though the thinned window.
4. The conjunctiva is sutured back to the limbus.

Note that the scleral flap is not sutured, since it is not required. Mitomycin may be applied under the flap before the exteriorization of the Schlemm's canal, in selected cases. In case a collagen implant is desired, a rectangular scleral flap is fashioned, which is sutured back at the end of surgery. Collagen implants create a space under the flap and are absorbed in about 6 months.

NPF Under a Fornix Based Corneoscleral Flap (Singh)

The steps of operation are as follows:

1. The conjunctiva is detached for 6-7 mm.

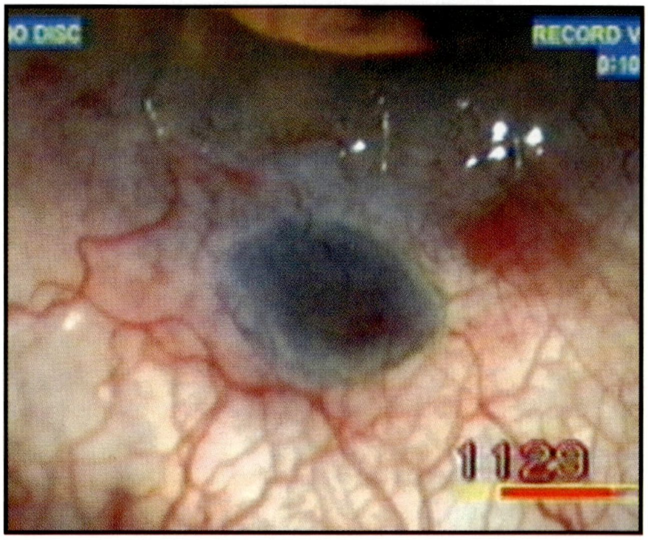

Figure 43.28:The conjunctiva has been sutured back to the limbus with multiple sutures

2. A 0.3 mm thick and 2.5 mm wide flap of corneo-sclera is raised anterio-posteriorly.
3. The exposed base is ablation-thinned. The edges of the base are also ablated.
4. The tissue ablation is done as before to start seepage of fluid from the area of Schlemm's canal.
5. The corneoscleral flap is sutured back with two 30 microns sutures.
6. The conjunctiva is sutured back at the limbus.

The point to note is that there is no trauma to the Tenon capsule and the episcleral blood vessels. The filtering aqueous escapes from the ablated edges of the base under the corneo-scleral flap.

A careful follow-up of non-perforating filtration cases is required. In the first few days, the filtration may become blocked by a blood clot. A pressure bandage may relieve the block. Sluggish aqueous flow may raise the intraocular pressure beyond normal. In such a case, the fluid flow can be augmented by making a YAG laser pore in the thinned limbal area.

The surgery of non-perforating filtration has a learning curve. The filtration area may not be found as desired. It may open into the anterior chamber, in which case a peripheral iridectomy is done with the Fugo Blade and the case finished like any anterior chamber filtration. In this case, placement of a TCF pore may serve to protect against anterior chamber collapse. On the other hand, the ciliary body area may be exposed without finding Schlemm's canal. In this case, the operation is finished with a transciliary filtration (TCF) procedure. A case may be finished as double filtration track—one in the anterior chamber and the other transciliary (Atwal procedure). With a little experience, Fugo Blade filtration procedures may be performed with 6 X or 8 X head worn loop magnification, which underscores the value for Third World glaucoma, especially since the procedures require minutes to perform.

Besides the techniques described above, the Fugo Blade is helpful in the placement of valves and setons.[29] It can make a gutter on the sclera that accommodates and holds the silicone tubing of the valve. It can be used to remove Tenon cyst formation around the valve and tubing to restart the function of the valve. The Fugo Blade is an excellent tool to cut and destroy Tenon cysts without extensive dissection. The conjunctiva is ballooned around the cyst. A special 300 or 600 micron Fugo Blade tip is introduced from one side to ablate the walls of the tenon cyst from edge to edge, at the same time removing much of the scar tissue. A suture is applied to the entry point of the tip.

The Fugo Blade is an important surgical tool that is fundamentally different from all the previous devices that have been employed in surgery.[30] It does not cut, but it ablates much like excimer laser, with clinically insignificant collateral damage.[31] This has been confirmed by such leaders in our field such as Dr I Howard Fine, Dr Ike Ahmed, Dr Herbert Kaufman and Dr F Hampton Roy. Rather, the Fugo Blade creates tracks even through vascular tissues such as the ciliary body. It closes the blood vessels as it makes an ablation path in the tissues by autostasis. It is not a cautery, and causes no charring. A note of extreme caution is warranted wherein no surgeon should attempt the herein presented procedures with any other electrosurgical device besides the Fugo Blade.[32] The Fugo Blade uses a small amount of energy in the form of plasma to ablate, remove, or "erase" tissue. It has the potential for application in every field of ophthalmology, general surgery, even dentistry.[33]

Glaucoma surgery shall never be the same with the introduction of Fugo Blade. Transciliary filtration and non-perforating techniques substantially remove all worries connected with anterior chamber integrity. Microtrack filtration needs further development and refinement for an application on a mass scale to fight the worldwide menace of glaucoma. The future surgical techniques shall take into account the importance of preserving a healthy lymphatic network under the conjunctiva and strive for minimally traumatic operations.

During the time of Galen Circa 150AD, Roman physicians possessed over 150 distinct operations in their surgical repertoire in areas such as abdominal surgery, brain surgery and eye surgery. The surgical trays from the era of Galen had impressive, refined surgical equipment which if examined carefully were not much different from present day equipment except for the material used in their production. Over the last century, we have added standard electrosurgery, fiberoptics and laser. Now, ophthalmology has introduced a technology which shall provide a quantum leap in surgical capability. This technology is known as the Fugo Blade wherein tissue is "erased" by thin layers of plasma. This requires minimal energy, cuts resistance free and leaves incision walls pristine clean. This work represents an intense collaboration between the two authors. With a solid background in biophysics, Dr Fugo has concentrated on the equipment while Dr Singh has focused on truly remarkable clinical applications which require a combination of imagination and the skill of a master surgeon. This work has been accomplished at much personal sacrifice. Nonetheless, it is an honor to be a part of a project that has the potential to elevate the quality of health care worldwide....for the industrialized world but also for the poorest of the poor. One of the authors (DS) refers to this new technology as "the great equalizer". This new solid state technology will allow the poorest clinic in a remote part of the world to have access to the most advanced medical technology in the world.

REFERENCES

1. Sabbagh LB. The never-ending quest: Creating a better way to remove the lens. Eyeworld 1998;3(4):50-53.
2. Kent C. Transciliary Filtration—Without Bleeding. Ophthalmology Management 2002;6(11):84-87.
3. Sabbagh LB. The leading edge: Harnessing electrons for a faster, smarter incision. Eyeworld 1998;3(4):88.
4. Kronemyer B. Fugo Blade uses low-level energy to create anterior capsulotomy. Ocular Surgery News 2000;18(21): 45-46.
5. Kellan R, Fugo RJ. Device increases safety, efficiency of cataract surgery. Ophthalmology Times 2000;25(22):7-9.
6. Fugo RJ, DelCampo DM. The Fugo Blade™: The next step after capsulorhexis. Annals of Ophthalmology 2001; 33(1):12-20.
7. Kent C. Plasma Capsulotomy. Ophthalmology Management. 2001;5(8):72-73.
8. Fine IH, Hoffman RS, Packer M. Highlights of the 2002 ASCRS Symposium, Part I. Eyeworld 2002;7(7):38.
9. Hidalgo-Simon A. Plasma Knife Provides Clean and Accurate Cut for Capsulorhexis. Eurotimes 2002;7(11):27.
10. Singh D, et al. Plasma Powered Squint Surgery with the Fugo Blade. Annals of Ophthalmology 2003;35(1):12-14.
11. Izak, Andrea M, et al. Analysis of the capsule edge after Fugo plasma blade capsulotomy, continuous curvilinear capsulorhexis, and can-opener capsulotomy. Journal of Cataract and Refractive Surgery 2004;30(12):2606-11.
12. Kent C. Revealed: The Eye's Lymphatic System. Ophthalmology Management 2002;6(5):114.
13. Singh D. Letters: Conjunctival Lymphatic System. Journal of Cataract and Refractive Surgery 2003;29(4):632-33.
14. Singh D, et al. The Conjunctival Lymphatic System. Annals of Ophthalmology 2003;35(2):99-104.
15. Singh D. Transciliary Filtration and Lymphatics of Conjunctiva: A Tale of Discovery. Tropical Ophthalmology. 2002;2(1):9-13.
16. Bethke WC. A New Clue to Lymphatic Drainage? Review of Ophthalmology 2002;9(3):12.
17. Singh D, Singh K. Transciliary Filtration Using the Fugo Blade. Annals of Ophthalmology 2002;34(3):183-87.
18. Roy FH. Course for Fugo Blade is enlightening, surgeon says. Ocular Surgery News 2001;19(17):35-38.
19. Scimeca G. Phaco with Transciliary Filtration an Alternative to Triple Procedure. Ocular Surgery News 2005;23(11):58.
20. Atwal A. 'Atwal's Balanced Approach' for Glaucoma Filtration Surgery Presented. Ocular Surgery News 9/15/ 2005.
21. Fugo R. A New Way to Perform Trabeculectomy. Ophthalmology Management 2005.
22. Fugo R. Transciliary Filtration Procedure Offers New Approach to Glaucoma. Ocular Surgery News 2005;23(5): 4-26.
23. Fugo R. Transciliary Filtration Procedure Offers New Approach to Glaucoma. Ocular Surgery News 2005;16(6): 18-19.
24. Wolf K. Surgeon Describes Learning Curve with Fugo Blade. Ocular Surgery News 2004;22(10):10.
25. Guttman C. Transciliary filtration provides improved safety and simplicity. Ophthalmology Times 2005;30(3):28.
26. Fugo R. Regarding Transciliary Filtration. Tropical Ophthalmology 2002;2(1):7-8.
27. Singh D. Singh Microfiltration for Glaucoma; A New Technique. Tropical Ophthalmology 2001;1(6):7-11.
28. Singh SK. Fugo Blade Capsulotomy: A New High Tech Cutting Technology. Tropical Ophthalmology 2001;1(1): 14-16.
29. Fugo R. The Fugo Blade Allows New Surgical Maneuvers. Ocular Surgery News 2003;21(22):5-7.
30. Singh D, Singh RSJ. Applications of the Fugo Blade. In Wilson ME, Triverdi RH, Pandey SK, (Eds): Pediatric Cataract Surgery: Techniques, Complications, and Management. 1st Edition. Lippincott Williams and Wilkins, 2005; 97-100.
31. Peponis E, Rosenberg P, Reddy SV, Herz JB, Kaufman HE. The Use of the Fugo Blade in Cornea Surgery: A Preliminary Animal Report. Cornea (In Press).
32. Video Journal of Cataract and Refractive Surgery. New Developments: New Devices- Fugo Blade. Vol. XVIII, Issue 1, 2002.
33. Kent C. Corneal Pits May Relieve Edema. Review of Ophthalmology 12,9. September 2005.

Index